Diagnosis and Treatment of Vestibular Disorders

Jacob C. Lucas • Christopher A. Schutt
Dennis I. Bojrab • Seilesh Babu
Editors

Diagnosis and Treatment of Vestibular Disorders

Second Edition

Springer

Editors
Jacob C. Lucas
Department of Otology and Neurotology
Michigan Ear Institute
Farmington Hills, MI, USA

Christopher A. Schutt
Department of Neurotology
Providence Hospital, Michigan Ear Institute
Farmington Hills, MI, USA

Dennis I. Bojrab
Department of Otology and Neurotology
Michigan Ear Institute
Farmington Hills, MI, USA

Seilesh Babu
Department of Neurotology
Providence Hospital, Michigan Ear Institute
Farmington Hills, MI, USA

ISBN 978-3-032-11739-7 ISBN 978-3-032-11740-3 (eBook)
https://doi.org/10.1007/978-3-032-11740-3

This Springer imprint is published by the registered company Springer Nature Switzerland AG
The registered company address is: Gewerbestrasse 11, 6330 Cham, Switzerland

Preface to the First Edition

Vestibular disorders can result in devastating and frightful symptoms, creating dramatic changes in immediate and long-term quality of life. Diagnosis and management of the patient afflicted with vestibular disorders is rewarding to the patient and the physician. This task is complex and begins with a thorough clinical history and neurotologic physical examination. With a judicious use of diagnostic tests, a diagnosis may be obtained in the majority of patients.

Afterwards, an effective treatment plan can be initiated.

Patients with dizziness present to the primary care physician, the emergency room physician, the neurologist, or the otolaryngologist. This textbook was developed for these physicians in order to provide a useful, practical approach to evaluate and treat patients with dizziness. Its intent is to improve the ability to accurately diagnose specific vestibular disorders, initiate appropriate therapy, reduce the unnecessary cost burden by knowing when to refer, and most importantly improve patient's quality of life.

To accomplish this task the book is separated into several parts. The anatomy and physiology of the vestibular system is discussed to provide a necessary background for the disease process. A thorough history and neurotologic examination is described to allow implementation into practice. Audiologic and vestibular testing is described in order to facilitate appropriate referrals and interpretation of test results. Finally, pathophysiology, diagnosis, and management strategies for common vestibular diseases are discussed with an evidence-based review.

Understanding the vestibular system and disorders began centuries ago and continues to evolve to this day. Some notable influences include Prosper Meniere, Ernest Ewald and Robert Barany. In 1861, Meniere, a French researcher, described a series of patients with episodic vertigo and hearing loss, placing the inner ear as the pathologic source of the vertigo. In the late 1800s, Ernest Ewald a physiologist from Germany established the labyrinthine origin of nystagmus and described eye movement correlated with vestibular involvement. Robert Barany, who won the Nobel Prize in 1914 as an Austro-Hungarian otologist, developed testing theories and methods of testing the labyrinth. Continuation of identification of new vestibular disorders has occurred as recent as 1998 with the description of superior canal dehiscence by Lloyd Minor.

The field of Neurotology became a subspecialty thanks to the foresight, research and unselfish dedication to teaching of many physicians. William House is considered the father of Neurotology with his endeavors in the care of Acoustic Neuromas, treatment of the patient with vestibular disorders and development of the Cochlear Implant. His unselfish and tireless efforts to share his knowledge with temporal bone laboratory teaching and the beginning of a fellowship program to teach this subspecialty to Otolaryngologists is unparalleled. His approaches and management matured and spread to hundreds of physicians throughout the world. Michael Glasscock and Malcolm Graham, who both trained and worked at the House Ear Institute, brought skull base surgery to the Midwest in Tennessee and Michigan respectively. Harold Schuknecht began his work with T. Manford McGee at Henry Ford Hospital prior to Schuknecht moving to Massachusetts Eye and Ear Infirmary and McGee staying in the greater Detroit area. The Michigan Ear Institute would later be formed with Drs. McGee, Graham, Bojrab, Kartush, LaRouere and Charles Stockwell, PhD and Ken Bouchard, PhD.

All of these physicians, teachers and researchers had the unrelenting desire to optimize patient care and spread knowledge through temporal bone laboratory teaching and fellowship training programs; thus, allowing them to propagate the standard of care that will continue to carry on for years to come. In addition to the above-mentioned physicians, we owe much of our understanding of clinical signs and diagnostic tests of the patient afflicted with vestibular disorders to such people as Hugh Barber, Vincente Honrubia, Robert Baloh, David Zee, Lloyd Minor, John Carey and Joel Goebel, to name a few.

We feel fortunate to have many esteemed colleagues from around the country willing to commit their tireless dedication to provide their insight and education to make this textbook better than we thought possible. To them we are grateful.

> To study the phenomenon of disease without books is to sail an uncharted sea, while to study books without patients is not to go to sea at all. Sir William Osler

Farmington Hills, MI, USA — Christopher A. Schutt
Farmington Hills, MI, USA — Seilesh Babu
Farmington Hills, MI, USA — Dennis I. Bojrab

Preface to the Second Edition

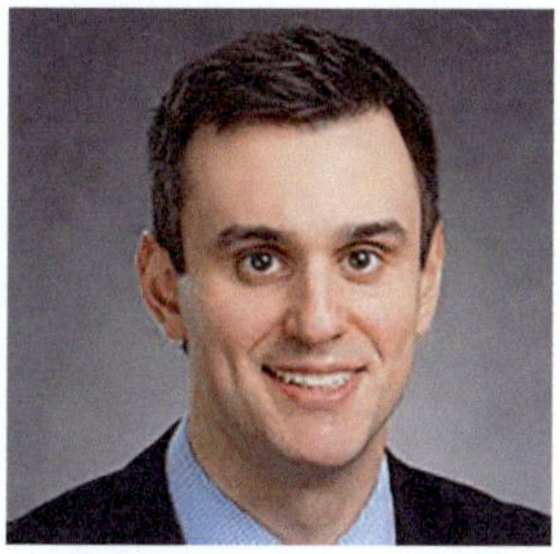

We are proud to present a thoroughly revised and expanded second edition of *Diagnosis and Treatment of Vestibular Disorders*.

Over the past several years, our understanding of vestibular disorders has continued to evolve—with advances in diagnostics, therapeutic strategies, and surgical techniques. Recognition of *third window syndromes* beyond the well-characterized superior canal dehiscence has even introduced new anatomic variants which are expanding our understanding of vestibular pathophysiology.

This new edition incorporates updated literature, expanded chapters, and contributions from both returning and new authors. As before, our goal remains: to offer a practical, evidence-based approach to the evaluation and management of vestibular disorders, for both the seasoned specialist and the primary care provider on the front lines. We remain thankful for the many collaborators who have once again shared their expertise to make this edition possible. We hope it continues to serve as a meaningful guide in the care of patients with vestibular complaints.

This edition also carries special significance. We dedicate it to the memory of our beloved colleague, Dr. Alexander Luryi. Alex's extraordinary talent and passion touched the lives of countless friends, colleagues, patients, and family members who had the privilege and honor of knowing him. He lived with purpose and pursued excellence in all he did. As a neurotologist, he cared deeply for his patients, dedicating himself to improving lives through compassionate treatment and innovative research that continues to help patients today.

At the Michigan Ear Institute, we often recall the sound of Alex playing the piano in the hospital lobby between cases—a beautiful gift that uplifted all who heard it. He was always ready with a quick joke and even quicker to lend a helping hand and a kind smile.

We honor Alex for the enduring impact of his life. Thank you, Alex, for your unwavering dedication—as a physician, a colleague, and a friend.

Farmington Hills, MI, USA Jacob C. Lucas
Farmington Hills, MI, USA Christopher A. Schutt
Farmington Hills, MI, USA Dennis I. Bojrab
Farmington Hills, MI, USA Seilesh Babu

Contents

Contributors

Oliver F. Adunka Department of Otolaryngology-Head and Neck Surgery, The Ohio State University, Wexner Medical Center, Columbus, OH, USA

Bora Agabigum Department of Otology and Neurotology, Michigan Ear Institute, Farmington Hills, MI, USA

Sumit K. Agrawal Department of Otolaryngology-Head and Neck Surgery, Schulich School of Medicine and Dentistry, Western University, London, ON, Canada

Tristan J. Allsopp Otolaryngology Department, The University of Arkansas for Medical Sciences, Little Rock, AR, USA

Emily C. Ambrose Department of Otolaryngology, University of Colorado Anschutz Medical Campus, Aurora, CO, USA

Patrick J. Antonelli Department of Otolaryngology-Head & Neck Surgery, University of Florida, Gainesville, FL, USA

Seilesh Babu Department of Otology and Neurotology, Michigan Ear Institute, Farmington Hills, MI, USA

Heather D. Balon Department of Audiology, Michigan Ear Institute, Farmington Hills, MI, USA

Marc Bennett Department of Otolaryngology Head and Neck Surgery, Vanderbilt University Medical Center, Nashville, TN, USA

Dennis Bojrab II Department of Otology and Neurotology, Michigan Ear Institute, Farmington Hills, MI, USA

Dennis I. Bojrab Department of Otology and Neurotology, Michigan Ear Institute, Farmington Hills, MI, USA

Department of Otolaryngology - Head and Neck Surgery, The University of Alabama at Birmingham, Birmingham, AL, USA

Matthew L. Bush Division of Otology, Neurotology, & Cranial Base Surgery, Department of Otolaryngology-Head and Neck Surgery, University of Kentucky, Lexington, KY, USA

Benjamin Campbell Altru Professional Center, Grand Forks, ND, USA

John P. Carey Johns Hopkins Outpatient Center, Baltimore, MD, USA

Matthew L. Carlson Department of Otolaryngology-Head and Neck Surgery, Mayo Clinic School of Medicine, Rochester, MN, USA

Stephen P. Cass Department of Otolaryngology, University of Colorado Anschutz Medical Campus, Aurora, CO, USA

Si Chen University of Florida, Gainesville, FL, USA

Robert M. Conway Department of Otology and Neurotology, Michigan Ear Institute, Farmington Hills, MI, USA

Department of Otolaryngology, Head and Neck Surgery, Ascension Macomb-Oakland Hospital, Madison Heights, MI, USA

Francis X. Creighton Johns Hopkins Outpatient Center, Baltimore, MD, USA

John L. Dornhoffer Otolaryngology Department, The University of Arkansas for Medical Sciences, Little Rock, AR, USA

Rance J. T. Fujiwara Department of Otolaryngology–Head and Neck Surgery, University of Texas Southwestern Medical Center, Dallas, TX, USA

Gerard J. Gianoli The Ear and Balance Institute, Covington, LA, USA

Department of Otolaryngology, Tulane University, New Orleans, LA, USA

A. Tucker Gleason University of Virginia, Department of Otolaryngology-Head and Neck Surgery, Charlottesville, VA, USA

Michael E. Hoffer Department of Otolaryngology, University of Miami, Miller School of Medicine, Miami, FL, USA

Department of Neurological Surgery, University of Miami, Miller School of Medicine, Miami, FL, USA

Brandon Isaacson Department of Otolaryngology–Head and Neck Surgery, University of Texas Southwestern Medical Center, Dallas, TX, USA

Neal M. Jackson Departments of Otolaryngology & Neurosurgery, Tulane University School of Medicine, New Orleans, LA, USA

Department of Otology and Neurotology, Michigan Ear Institute, Farmington Hills, MI, USA

Hyunseo D. Jung Department of Otology and Neurotology, Michigan Ear Institute, Farmington Hills, MI, USA

Brekel Kemp Department of Otolaryngology, Tulane University School of Medicine, New Orleans, LA, USA

Bradley W. Kesser University of Virginia, Department of Otolaryngology-Head and Neck Surgery, Charlottesville, VA, USA

Daniel E. Killeen Department of Otolaryngology–Head and Neck Surgery, University of Texas Southwestern Medical Center, Dallas, TX, USA

Kyle Kimura Department of Otolaryngology Head and Neck Surgery, Vanderbilt University Medical Center, Nashville, TN, USA

J. Walter Kutz Jr. Department of Otolaryngology–Head and Neck Surgery, University of Texas Southwestern Medical Center, Dallas, TX, USA

Wanda Lai Florida ENT and Allergy, Tampa, FL, USA

Department of Otology and Neurotology, Michigan Ear Institute, Farmington Hills, MI, USA

Daniel Lan Department of Otolaryngology, University of Miami, Miller School of Medicine, Miami, FL, USA

Michael J. LaRouere Department of Otology and Neurotology, Michigan Ear Institute, Farmington Hills, MI, USA

St. John Providence Hospital, Novi, MI, USA

Omolara Lawal Yale School of Medicine, Department of Neurology, New Haven, CT, USA

Jacob C. Lucas Department of Otology and Neurotology, Michigan Ear Institute, Farmington Hills, MI, USA

Alexander L. Luryi Camden, NJ, USA

Maria C. Machala Department of Otolaryngology, University of Colorado Anschutz Medical Campus, Aurora, CO, USA

Robert J. Macielak Department of Otolaryngology-Head and Neck Surgery, The Ohio State University, Wexner Medical Center, Columbus, OH, USA

Devin L. McCaslin Department of Otolaryngology-Head and Neck Surgery, Mayo Clinic School of Medicine, Rochester, MN, USA

Beth N. McNulty Division of Otology, Neurotology, & Cranial Base Surgery, Department of Otolaryngology-Head and Neck Surgery, University of Kentucky, Lexington, KY, USA

Elias Michaelides Department of Otolaryngology, Rush University College of Medicine, Chicago, IL, USA

Elliot Morse Department of Surgery, Yale University School of Medicine, New Haven, CT, USA

Lauren Mueller Department of Otolaryngology, Washington University, St. Louis, MO, USA

Dhasakumar Navaratnam Departments of Neurology (OL, DN) Neuroscience (DN) and Surgery (DN), Yale University, School of Medicine, New Haven, CT, USA

Yale School of Medicine, Department of Neurology, New Haven, CT, USA

Lorne S. Parnes Department of Otolaryngology-Head and Neck Surgery, Schulich School of Medicine and Dentistry, Western University, London, ON, Canada

Amy Schettino Department of Surgery, Yale University, School of Medicine, New Haven, CT, USA

Desi P. Schoo Department of Otolaryngology-Head and Neck Surgery, The Ohio State University, Wexner Medical Center, Columbus, OH, USA

Christopher A. Schutt Department of Otology and Neurotology, Michigan Ear Institute, Farmington Hills, MI, USA

Zachary G. Schwam Department of Otolaryngology, Icahn School of Medicine at Mount Sinai, New York, NY, USA

Saul Strieb Department of Otolaryngology-Head and Neck Surgery, The Ohio State University, Wexner Medical Center, Columbus, OH, USA

Alex D. Sweeney Baylor College of Medicine and Texas Children's Hospital, Houston, TX, USA

Varun V. Varadarajan Neurotology and Skull Base Surgery, Sacramento Ear, Nose & Throat, Sacramento, CA, USA

Erika McCarty Walsh Department of Otolaryngology, University of Alabama, Birmingham, AL, USA

George Wanna Department of Otolaryngology at New York Eye and Ear Infirmary of Mount Sinai and Mount Sinai Beth Israel, New York, NY, USA

Division of Otology-Neurotology at the Mount Sinai Health System, New York, NY, USA

Audiology, Hearing and Balance Center at the Mount Sinai Health System, New York, NY, USA

Ear Institute at the Mount Sinai Health System, New York, NY, USA

Eric Wilkinson Idaho Ear Clinic, Meridian, ID, USA

Robert Yawn College of Medicine – Memphis, Department of Otolaryngology Head-Neck Surgery, Memphis, TN, USA

Peng You Department of Otolaryngology-Head and Neck Surgery, Schulich School of Medicine and Dentistry, Western University, London, ON, Canada

Ashley C. Zaleski-King Department of Speech Language Pathology and Audiology Towson University, Towson, MD, USA

Christopher K. Zalewski Auditory and Vestibular Clinical Research Section (AVCRS), Neurotology Branch, National Institute on Deafness and Other Communication Disorders (NIDCD), National Institutes of Health (NIH), Bethesda, MD, USA

Part I
The Vestibular System

Chapter 1
Anatomy and Physiology of the Vestibular System

Ashley C. Zaleski-King, Wanda Lai, and Alex D. Sweeney

Anatomy and Physiology of the Peripheral Vestibular System

The peripheral vestibular system contains five sensory structures: three semicircular canals (the horizontal, also termed lateral; anterior, also termed superior; and posterior canals), and two otolith organs (the utricle and the saccule). Within each sensory organ, sensory hair cells are organized specifically to allow for transduction of head motion in different planes into neural impulses (Fig. 1.1).

A. C. Zaleski-King
Department of Speech Language Pathology and Audiology Towson University, Towson, MD, USA

W. Lai
Florida ENT and Allergy, Tampa, FL, USA

A. D. Sweeney (✉)
Baylor College of Medicine and Texas Children's Hospital, Houston, TX, USA
e-mail: alex.sweeney@bcm.edu

J. C. Lucas et al. (eds.), *Diagnosis and Treatment of Vestibular Disorders*, https://doi.org/10.1007/978-3-032-11740-3_1

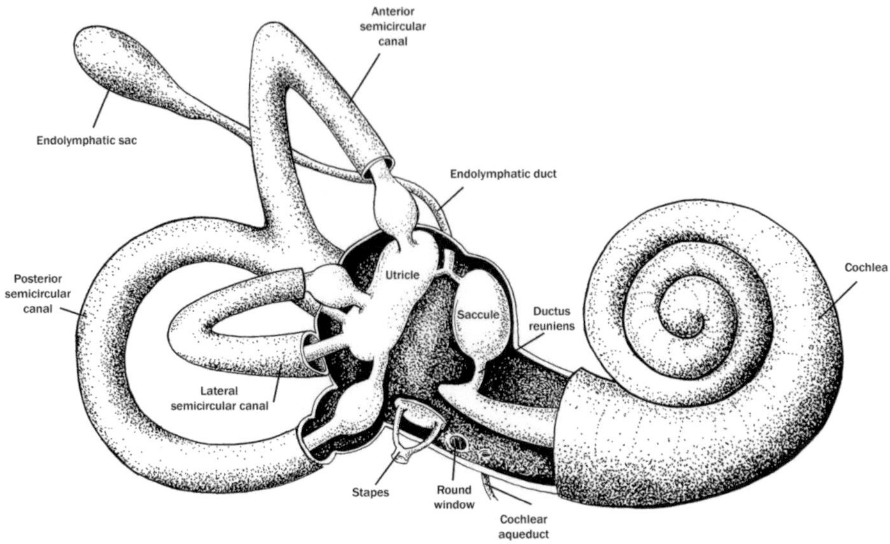

Fig. 1.1 Anatomy of the labyrinth

The Inner Ear Labyrinths

The peripheral sensory apparatus of the vestibular system lies within the inner ear, laterally adjacent to the air-filled middle ear, medially bordered by the temporal bone, posterior to the cochlea. Within the inner ear, a bony labyrinth houses a membranous labyrinth containing vestibular receptors. The two labyrinths differ in the type of fluid composition. The bony labyrinth contains perilymph, which is a substance with chemical composition similar to cerebrospinal fluid, with an increased sodium-to-potassium concentration ratio [31]. The cochlear aqueduct is thought to connect perilymph to the spinal fluid pathway. The oval window and the round window are two structures separating the middle ear and the perilymph of the inner ear.

The membranous labyrinth contains endolymph, a second type of inner ear fluid. Endolymph is composed of a higher potassium-to-sodium concentration ratio, similar to intracellular fluid [15]. Endolymph is generated in the stria vascularis in the wall of the cochlear duct [26]. The endolymphatic sac, a membranous structure within the inner ear, absorbs endolymph and connects to other endolymphatic spaces within the inner ear through the utricular duct and the ductus reuniens [8]. Separation of endolymph and perilymph fluids is maintained through a tight junctional complex surrounding the apex of each cell [16]. Partitioning of the fluids is important for mechanical reasons, to allow semicircular canals to utilize endolymph fluid dynamics to transmit semicircular canal information, and also for biophysiological reasons, to provide an electrochemical gradient necessary for hair cell transduction [16]. Though outside of the scope of this chapter, it is also noteworthy that the structural integrity of this partition is also essential to the biological basis of auditory function in the inner ear.

Inner Ear Sensory Hair Cells

Each vestibular structure contains specialized sensory hair cells. These hair cells function to transmit mechanical energy into neural activity generated as a result of head motion or as a result of gravitational changes [9]. Head motion occurs with linear and/or rotational acceleration forces that cause deflection of a specific subset of hair cell bundles in each receptor organ.

Vestibular receptor hair cells consist of cilia, the cell body, and nerve endings (afferent and efferent). The cilia are rod-shaped sensory mechanoreceptors embedded in a membrane of neuroepithelium, forming a rigid bundle on top of each cell body. The basic structure of each hair cell includes a single long hair, kinocilium, and approximately 70–100 shorter hairs, stereocilia, on the apical end [27]. These hair cells are organized in rows and positioned based on length. The tallest stereocilia are positioned in closest and the shortest in furthest proximity to the kinocilium. Tip links are filamentous structures that connect the tips of shorter sterocilia to the body of adjacent taller stereocilia [3].

The vestibular epithelium consists of two different types of cell bodies: type I and type II. Type I hair cell bodies are shaped like a flask with a rounder base, wider middle, and narrower apex and base. The calyx, a large afferent nerve ending, surrounds the type I hair cell body, and makes contact with efferent nerve ending. Type I hair cells are associated with irregular afferent activity and high variability in resting discharge rate. Type II hair cells are the most abundant and are shaped like a cylinder with several afferent and efferent direct connections. Type II hair cells mostly synapse on regular afferents with low variability of resting discharge rate. Differences in type I and type II hair cell adaptation may be related to differences in attachment of afferent and efferent nerve endings [1].

Though structurally different, Type I and type II hair cells share important functional features. Both hair cell types generate a tonic, spontaneous neural firing rate averaging around 70–90 spikes per second [12] in the absence of any stimulus (Fig. 1.2). Both types of hair cells also exhibit excitatory and inhibitory responses, though only when the hair cell bends in a plane of polarization specific to that cell body. This directional polarization functions so that during excitatory responses, deflection of stereocilia causes bending toward the kinocilium. This movement toward the kinocilium shifts the tip links, causing a mechanical opening of the transduction channels and an influx of potassium ions. Depolarization of the hair cell stimulates neurotransmitter release into the synapses, causing an increase in firing rate. This excitatory activity increases neural firing rate from the tonic level to up to 400 spikes per second. The opposite occurs during inhibition, when stereocilia are bent away from kinocilium, resulting in decreased tip link tension, mechanical closure of the channel, and a decrease in firing rate. In comparison with the change in neural firing rate during excitation, the change in neural activity during inhibition is significantly reduced from the tonic rate of around 90 spikes per second down to the disappearance of neural activity.

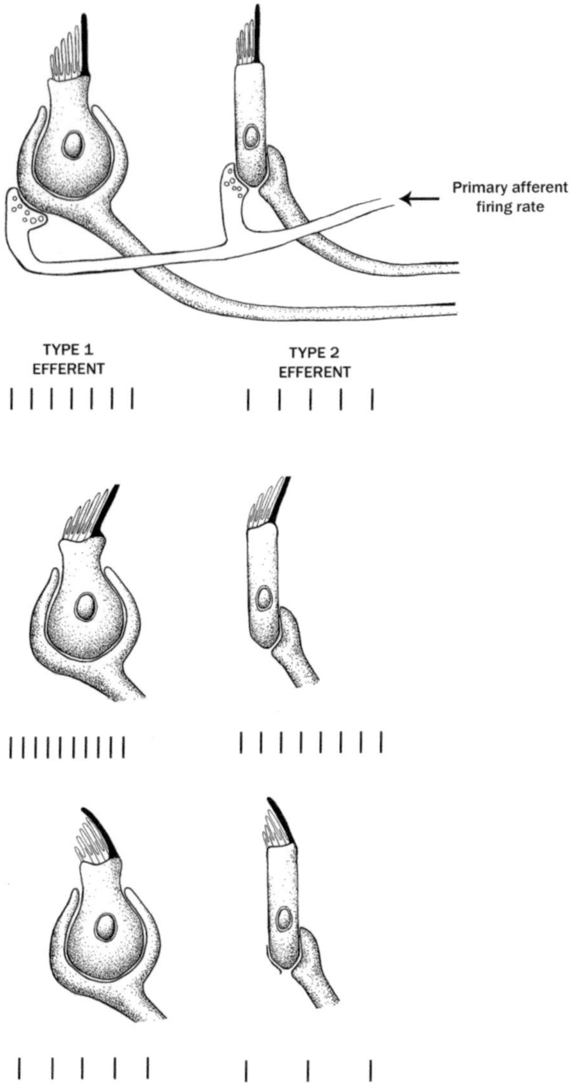

Fig. 1.2 Afferent firing rate in basal state toward kinocilium and away from kinocilium

Semicircular Canals

The three semicircular canals (SCCs) consist of the membranous labyrinth encased in bony canal structures, arranged in three mutually perpendicular planes. Together, the lateral (or horizontal), anterior (or superior), and posterior SCCs make up a unique arrangement that allow for a three-dimensional vector representation of rotational acceleration. Whereas the lateral canals are oriented in a 30 degree angle in the axial plane, the superior and posterior canals are oriented in a 45 degree angle to the sagittal plane [22]. Each SCC is sensitive to movement in a specific vector, residing in approximate parallel planes to the SCC in the opposite ear (i.e., the left ear lateral and right ear lateral, left ear anterior and right ear posterior, and left ear posterior and right ear anterior).

All SCCs open into the utricle; the other end of each SCC opens to the ampulla, a dilated sac [24]. At the base, the ampulla contains sensory neuroepithelium, the crista ampullaris, which is comprised of approximately 7000 hair cells. These hair cells are embedded into the cupula, a gelatinous surrounding attached to the epithelium at base of the crista. The cupula can be thought of as a "plug" dividing the SCCs into two compartments [2]. Within the cupula, each hair cell makes synaptic contact with nerve endings to form the primary afferent nerve fiber of each SCC.

Within each SCC, hair cells are either oriented toward or away from the utricular sac, to generate either an excitatory or inhibitory response. In the lateral canal, for example, the kinocilia are positioned pointing toward the utricular sac. An excitatory response is generated when the cupula is bent toward the utricular sac, known as ampullopetal flow, and an inhibitory response is generated when the cupula is bent away from the utricular sac, termed ampullofugal flow. The opposite is true for hair cell orientation in the anterior and posterior SCCs: ampullopetal flow (i.e., cupula bending toward the utricular sac) results in inhibition and ampulofugal (i.e., cupula bending away from utricular sac) results in excitation.

The mechanics of SCC activation are related in part to the density and viscosity characteristics of the cupula and the surrounding endolymph [2]. The cupula and the surrounding endolymph are made up comparable densities [1]. Without head motion, hair cells embedded within the cupula remain at a neutral position as the cupula floats within the endolymph.

With head motion, rotational acceleration generates endolymph movement that displaces the cupula, bending hair cells in the opposite direction of rotation. The viscous make-up of endolymph causes fluid to lag behind, producing a current in the opposite direction of rotation. The cupula and the embedded stereocilia are then deflected, and based on the direction of rotation, produce either a sudden increase or decrease in neural firing rate of the afferent neuron (Fig. 1.3) [12]. When rotational velocity of the head becomes constant, the cupula returns to an upright position, and the synaptic potential of each cell normalizes [19]. The viscosity of the endolymph and the mass of the cupula dampen the neural firing rate, limiting the amount of head velocity information generated for low-frequency head motion. Canal responses are also limited, in that they are asymmetrical at high frequencies due to the greater dynamic range of hair cells available during the excitatory response of hair cells [12].

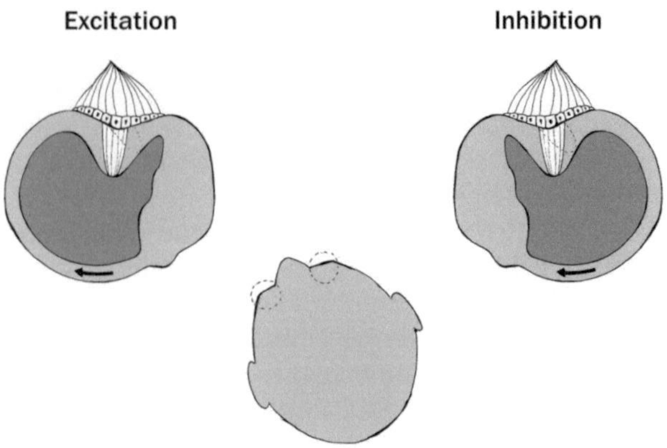

Fig. 1.3 Rotary head motion resulting in excitation and inhibition of respective paired semicircular canals

Otolith Organs

The two otolith organs, the utricle and the saccule, are housed within two cavities in the vestibule. The utricle is oval-shaped and contained within a swelling adjacent to the SCCs, the elliptical recess. The saccule is oriented perpendicular to the utricle and parallel to the sagittal plane within the spherical recess. Together, the otolith organs function to detect linear acceleration and static orientation of the head relative to gravity.

The sensory neuroepithelium is contained within the macula of each otolith organ, oriented horizontally in the utricle and vertically in the saccule. The striola is an area within the neuroepithelium dividing hair cells into two regions with different hair cell arrays. Unlike the SCCs, the stereocilia within the otolith organs are polarized in different directions: away from the kinocilium in the saccule and toward the kinocilium in the utricle. These hair cell bundles project into a gelatinous membrane, on top of which are calcium carbonate particles, or otoconia, embedded on the surface. Linear acceleration generates forces on the otoconia and gelatinous membrane, resulting in deflection of hair cell bundles. The utricle is stimulated by movement in the horizontal plane (i.e., head tilt sideways and lateral displacement) while the saccule is excited by movement in the vertical plane (i.e., sagittal plane upward, downward and forward, backward; [36]). This shearing motion between the layer of otoconia and the membrane displaces the hair cell bundles, opening mechanically gated transduction channels in the tops of the stereocilia to depolarize the hair cell and cause neurotransmitter release [36]. This neurotransmitter release generates an increase in afferent neural firing rate. For other hair cells with different orientations, the same shear force results in either a decrease in firing rate, or no change to the tonic firing rate [2]. A subset of afferent nerves fire specifically when the head is upright, before increasing or decreasing based on direction of head tilt [13].

Though conceptual and theoretical understanding of peripheral end organ innervation is fairly straightforward, activation of these pathways is more complex and sometimes restricted. The otolith organs are limited in the capacity to distinguish between tilt with respect to gravity and linear translation [36]. In some cases, this inability to distinguish between translational accelerations and changes in head orientation can be resolved using extra-otolith cues arising from either the SCCs or the visual system [38]. In most cases, human movement results in simultaneous excitation and inhibition of both SCC and otolith receptor organs in both labyrinths.

Anatomy and Physiology of the Central Vestibular System

Central vestibular connections facilitate interaction of inputs from each vestibular labyrinth, as well as other inputs from somatosensory and visual sensory systems [15]. For example, a tilt to one side of the head has opposite effects of the corresponding hair cells of the other side of the head [36]. In addition, there is a convergence of otolith and semicircular canal input at all central vestibular levels, from the vestibular nuclei (VN) to cortical centers processing vestibular information [20].

The Vestibular Nerve

After peripheral end organ excitation, labyrinthine sensory information is transmitted by the eighth cranial nerve through the internal auditory canal, entering the brainstem at the pontomedullary junction [15]. Along with the vestibular nerve, the facial nerve, cochlear nerve, and the labyrinthine artery also travel through the internal auditory canal. Starting from the periphery, the bipolar neurons of Scarpa's (vestibular) ganglion are activated by the hair cells of the crista ampullaris in the SCCs and the maculae in the otoliths [3]. The superior portion of Scarpa's ganglion arises from the cristae of the lateral and anterior SCCs, the macula of the utricle, and a branch of the saccular nerve. The inferior portion of Scarpa's ganglion connects to the cristae of the posterior SCC and the macula of the saccule. These superior and inferior bundles of Scarpa's ganglia merge with the cochlear nerve to form the eighth cranial nerve. Most vestibular nerve fibers connect centrally to the ipsilateral vestibular nuclei in the pons [5], though some innervate the cerebellum directly [5]. The central processing component begins as the eighth cranial nerve enters the brainstem, in the vestibular nucleus complex and in the cerebellum [15].

The Vestibular Nuclear Complex

The vestibular nuclei are located at the fourth ventricle and extend in two columns from the pons to the medulla. As the primary recipients of vestibular input, the VN include four major nuclei: the medial, superior, lateral, and inferior [5], which function to process vestibular input before transmission to motor centers [29]. In each ear, the vestibular nerve connects directly the ipsilateral VN, as well as to the contralateral side through several interconnecting neurons. The cerebellum, the reticular formation, the spinal cord, and the cervical junction all provide additional afferent information to the VN. Efferent information is relayed from the VN back to these same areas [2].

Motor Outputs of Vestibular System

Movement generates a complex pattern of vestibular stimulation. Information regarding head and body movement is transmitted through the central nervous system to motor centers such as the oculomotor nuclei and the spinal cord. The outputs of these systems allow individuals to walk while achieving a steady image on the retina through the vestibulo-ocular reflex (VOR) and to generate postural responses with respect to the external environments through the vestibulospinal reflex (VSR).

The Vestibulo-Ocular Reflex (VOR)

The vestibulo-ocular reflex consists of a three neuron arc. The reflex originates through peripheral organ activation, before connecting to directly to the VN through the medial longitudinal fasciculus (MLF), the tract that carries excitatory projections from the abducens nucleus to the contralateral oculomtotor nucleus. Indirect projections also arise from the reticular formation to the oculomotor nuclei. The purpose of the VOR is to preserve the image on the center of the visual field. This is accomplished through transduction of physical acceleration of the head into biological signals, directing eye movement in the equal and opposite direction of head movement (Fig. 1.4) [30].

The latency of the VOR pathway is only around 20 ms [6, 7, 18], allowing rapid and accurate stabilization of gaze without any blurring of vision during head movements. The VOR completes this reaction quickly, but imperfectly, lacking in sensitivity to slow rotations. The VOR also compensates poorly for sustained motion at constant speeds. When there is no longer vestibular input during prolonged motion in light, two overlapping visual pathways, the optokinetic and the smooth pursuit systems, supplement vestibular responses. The velocity storage system, a central phenomenon that extends the duration of rotational vestibular signals also helps. This system improves the ability of the (rotational) VOR to transduce low-frequency components of sustained head movements [21].

Six extraocular muscles are innervated to preserve the retinal image through three distinct nuclei: the oculomotor nucleus, the trochlear nucleus, and the abducens nucleus. Each muscle is balanced in such a way that the contraction of one occurs simultaneously with the relaxation of another. Each pair works

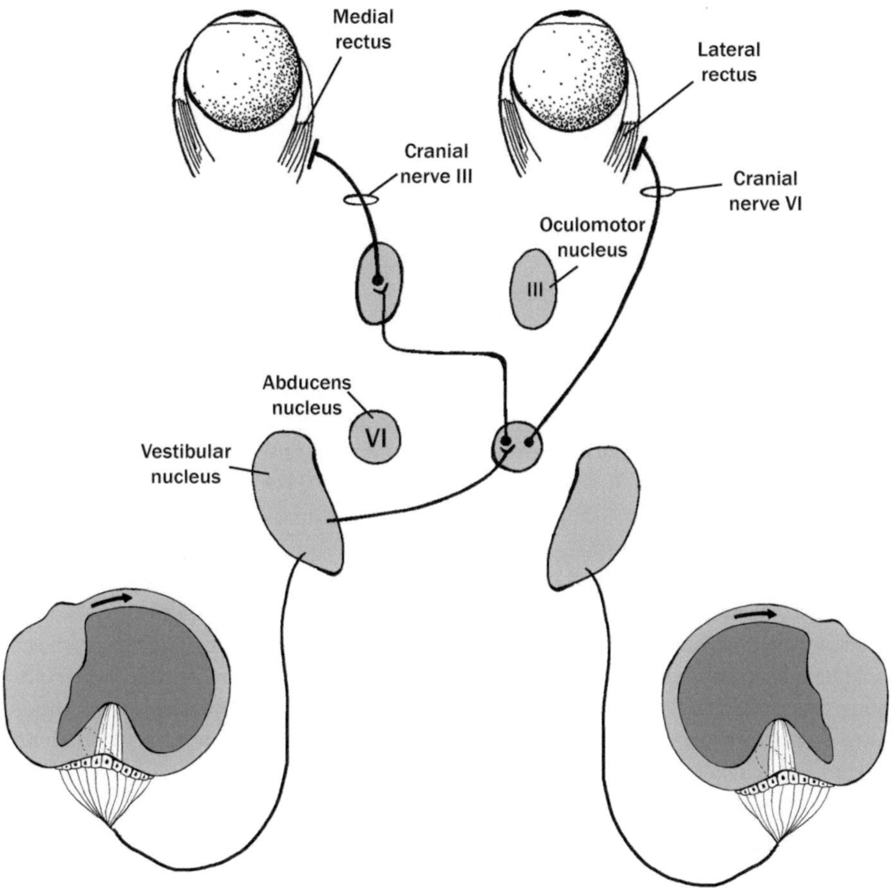

Fig. 1.4 Semicircular canal-ocular reflex

synergistically and coincides approximately with the planes of the SCCs. The VOR can be organized into three different subtypes based on planar function: the horizontal (or rotational) VOR, which compensates for head rotation, the translational VOR, which compensates for linear head movement and the ocular counter-roll, which compensates for head tilt [36].

The rotational VOR functions as the head turns, activating the SCC. During horizontal rotation, primary vestibular afferents from the horizontal SCC stimulate the ipsilateral medial and ventrolateral vestibular nuclei. These secondary vestibular neurons have axons that either decussate and ascend contralaterally to the abducens nucleus, or ascend ipsilaterally to the oculomotor nucleus. The motor neurons from the abducens nucleus synapse at the lateral rectus muscle, whereas similar motoneurons from the oculomotor nucleus synapse at the medial rectus muscles. Some neurons also connect directly from the VN to the ipsilateral medial rectus through the ascending tract of Deiters. In addition to the excitatory projections, inhibitory projections also project to the ipsilateral lateral rectus and contralateral medial rectus muscles to permit eye movement in the equal and opposite direction of head movement [36]. Vertical SCC activation functions similarly. Activation of the anterior and posterior SCCs stimulates the VN, which synapse on the oculomotor, trochlear or abducens motoneurons. These synapses innervate the inferior and superior rectus, and oblique muscles.

Relative to the rotational VOR pathway, less is understood about the translational VOR pathway and VOR the pathway resulting in the ocular counter-roll response. Stabilization of an image when the head moves sideways, forward, or is tilted is thought to be due to the otolith–ocular pathway, connecting signals from the utricle and saccule to the oculomotor neurons [36]. During linear head translation, stimulation of the lateral portion of the utricle is mediated by polysynaptic connections to the lateral and medial VN. These VN synapses project to the abducens nucleus, bilaterally through the MLF to motor neurons directing eye gaze.

During head tilt, torsional or oblique eye movements produce an ocular counter-roll [25]. The ocular counter-roll consists of eyes moving in the opposite direction of the head tilt at a much smaller amplitude of the head tilt [28]. With head tilt, the medial portions of the utricle are excited, synapsing on the lateral VN. Through the MLF, the lateral VN connect to trochlear oculomotor nuclei, which excite ipsilateral superior oblique and superior rectus and contralateral inferior oblique and inferior rectus muscles to generate ocular counter-roll. Ipsilateral projections from the VN also innervate polysynaptic inhibitory connections to the ipsilateral inferior oblique [35]. Static ocular counter-roll compensates for about 10–20% of the head roll in humans (with interindividual and intraindividual differences [37].

Vestibulospinal Reflex (VSR)

The vestibulospinal reflex (VSR) is composed of a series of motor commands, initiated from the vestibular system to help maintain postural stability. Visual and prioprioceptive sensory inputs are integrated with information from the VSR to maintain orientation of the body relative to the external environment [17]. The VSR is composed of the medial and lateral vestibulospinal tracts in addition to the reticulospinal tract.

The medial vestibulospinal tract (MVST) is primarily a contralateral pathway, originating in response to simulation from the SCCs, through the medial VN. This pathway descends through the MLF bilaterally, and terminates no lower than the mid-thoracic spinal cord [34]. The MVST is thought to mediate head position by controlling the muscles of the neck and shoulder. Another reflex controlling head position through neck muscles is the vestibulocollic reflex. The vestibulocollic reflex stabilizes the head by initiating head movement in the direction counter to the current head-in-space velocity through activation of vestibular receptors [10]. Yaw rotation of the head typically involves SCC activation through vestibulocollic innervation to the medial VN, descending through the MLF to the upper cervical levels of the spinal cord [30].

The lateral vestibulospinal tract (LVST) includes ipsilateral excitatory pathways, which originate in the lateral VN, descending through the inferior VN, to terminate on the anterior horn cells at various levels of the spinal cord, and on proximal limb extensors. Simultaneous disynaptic connections inhibit contralateral proximal extensors [27]. The LVST is thought to control postural lower limb adjustments to movement. When the head is tilted, VN in both the canals and the otoliths are activated, transmitting impulses through the LVST and MVST to the spinal cord; this action induces extensor activity on the ipsilateral head side and flexor activity on the contralateral side [15]. The third pathway originating in the reticular formation descends to the spinal cord terminating in the mediate parts of the gray matter to influence limb and trunk movement. Both VN and the reticular formation provide information to the spinal cord to maintain compensatory feedback responses to postural instability.

Vestibulocerebellum

The vestibulocerebellum is also known as the flocculonodular lobe and is composed of the nodule and the flocculus. Afferent projections from the VN connect directly to the vestibulocerebellum. Efferent projections from Purkinje cells within the vestibulocerebellum send efferent information ipsilaterally to the VN and to the fastigial nucleus. These pathways work to monitor vestibular activity and, when necessary, to support the vestibulocerebellar role as an adaptive processor. The vestibulocerebellum, for example, modifies vestibular input by adjusting the gain and duration of the VOR [19], while processing afferent activity from the macula [15]. This area also plays a role in translating vestibular and proprioceptive inputs to regulate vestibulospinal reflexes.

Vestibular Cortical Centers

In the primate brain, no isolated vestibular cortex has been identified [23]; however, the parietal insular vestibular cortex (PIVC) is one area of the cortex with a known concentration of vestibular inputs [33]. In macaques, neural activity in the PIVC has been recorded during head movement, in a position with the neck twisted and throughout motion of a visual target; similar PIVC activation is not associated with eye movement [33]. It is hypothesized that neurons in the PIVC may primarily be used as an index of movement in space to transform object movement from being self-referenced to being referenced to the environment [33].

Neurons in the PIVC also function to converge multisensory self-motion cues with external object motion information [32]. Vestibular inputs share cortical projections with other pathways processing visual and somatosensory information [11, 14]. Inhibitory vestibular–visual interaction has also been noted using large-field optokinetic visual displays inducing apparent self-motion perception, with an increase in parieto-occipital areas in the occipital cortex with a simultaneous decrease in the PIVC bilaterally [4]. In theory, this relationship allows the dominant sensorial weight to be shifted from one modality to the other, depending on which mode of stimulation predominates [4].

References

1. Baloh RW, Honrubia V. Clinical neurophysiology of the vestibular system. New York: Oxford University Press; 2001.
2. Barin K, Durrant JD. Applied physiology of the vestibular system. In: Canalis RF, Lempert PR, editors. The ear: comprehensive otology. Philadelphia: Lippincott Williams & Wilkins; 2000. p. 431–46.
3. Barrett KE, Barman SM, Boitano S, Brooks HL. Chapter 10. Hearing & equilibrium. In: Barrett KE, Barman SM, Boitano S, Brooks HL, editors. Ganong's review of medical physiology. 24th ed. New York: McGraw-Hill; 2012.
4. Brandt T, Dieterich M. The vestibular cortex: its locations, functions, and disorders. Ann N Y Acad Sci. 1999;871(1):293–312.
5. Brodal A. Anatomy of the vestibular nuclei and their connections. In: Vestibular system part 1: Basic mechanisms. Berlin, Heidelberg: Springer; 1974. p. 239–352.
6. Bronstein AM, Gresty MA. Short latency compensatory eye movement responses to transient linear head acceleration: a specific function of the otolith-ocular reflex. Exp Brain Res. 1988;71(2):406–10.
7. Collewijn H, Smeets JB. Early components of the human vestibulo-ocular response to head rotation: latency and gain. J Neurophysiol. 2000;84(1):376–89.
8. Corrales CE, Mudry A. History of the endolymphatic sac: from anatomy to surgery. Otol Neurotol. 2017;38(1):152–6.
9. Della Santina CC, Potyagaylo V, Migliaccio AA, Minor LB, Carey JP. Orientation of human semicircular canals measured by three-dimensional multiplanar CT reconstruction. J Assoc Res Otolaryngol. 2005;6(3):191–206.
10. Ezure K, Sasaki S. Frequency-response analysis of vestibular-induced neck reflex in cat. I. Characteristics of neural transmission from horizontal semicircular canal to neck motoneurons. J Neurophysiol. 1978;41(2):445–58.
11. Ferrè ER, Walther LE, Haggard P. Multisensory interactions between vestibular, visual and somatosensory signals. PLoS One. 2015;10(4):e0124573.
12. Fernandez C, Goldberg JM. Physiology of peripheral neurons innervating semicircular canals of the squirrel monkey. II. Response to sinusoidal stimulation and dynamics of peripheral vestibular system. J Neurophysiol. 1971;34(4):661–75.
13. Fernandez C, Goldberg JM. Physiology of peripheral neurons innervating otolith organs of the squirrel monkey. I. Response to static tilts and to long-duration centrifugal force. J Neurophysiol. 1976;39(5):970–84.
14. Guldin WO, Grüsser OJ. Is there a vestibular cortex? Trends Neurosci. 1998;21(6):254–9.
15. Hain TC, Helminski JO. Anatomy and physiology of the normal vestibular system. In: Herman SJ, editor. Vestibular rehabilitation. Philadelphia: F.A. Davis Company; 2007.

16. Highstein SM, Fay RR, Popper AN. The vestibular system, vol. 24. Berlin: Springer; 2004. p. 154–6.
17. Horak FB, Shupert CL. Role of the vestibular system in postural control. Vestib Rehabil. 1994;2:98–113.
18. Johnston JL, Sharpe JA. The initial vestibulo-ocular reflex and its visual enhancement and cancellation in humans. Exp Brain Res. 1994;99(2):302–8.
19. Khan S, Chang R. Anatomy of the vestibular system: a review. NeuroRehabilitation. 2013;32(3):437–43.
20. Kingma H. Function tests of the otolith or statolith system. Curr Opin Neurol. 2006;19(1):21–5.
21. Laurens J, Angelaki DE. The functional significance of velocity storage and its dependence on gravity. Exp Brain Res. 2011;210(3–4):407–22.
22. Lee SC, Abdel Razek OA, Dorfman BE. 2011. Vestibular system anatomy. Retrieved from: Emedicine. medscape.com/article/883956-overview aw2aab6c10.
23. Lopez C, Blanke O. The thalamocortical vestibular system in animals and humans. Brain Res Rev. 2011;67(1–2):119–46.
24. Lyskowski A. Anatomy of vestibular end organs and neural pathways. In: Cummings CW, et al., editors. Otolaryngology –head & neck surgery. Philadelphia: Elsevier Mosby; 2005. p. 3089–114.
25. Markham CH, Diamond SG. Ocular counterrolling in response to static and dynamic tilting: implications for human otolith function. J Vestib Res. 2003;12:127–34.
26. Mescher AL. Chapter 23. The eye and ear: special sense organis. In: Mescher AL, editor. Junqueira's basic histology: text & atlas. 12th ed. New York: McGraw-Hill Medical; 2010.
27. Oghalai JS, Brownell WE. Chapter 44. Anatomy & physiology of the ear. In: Lalwani AK, editor. Current diagnosis & treatment in otolaryngology—head & neck surgery. 3rd ed. New York: McGraw-Hill Medical; 2012.
28. Paige GD, Tomko DL. Eye movement responses to linear head motion in the squirrel monkey. I Basic characteristics. J Neurophysiol. 1991;65(5):1170–82.
29. Precht W. Vestibular mechanisms. Annu Rev Neurosci. 1979;2:265–89. https://doi.org.proxy-tu.researchport.umd.edu/10.1146/annurev.ne.02.030179.001405.
30. Purves D, Augustine GJ, Fitzpatrick D, Hall WC, LaMantia AS, McNamara JO, White LE. Neuroscience. 4th ed. Sunderland: Sinauer Associates; 2012.
31. Salt AN. The cochlear fluids: perilymph and endolymph. In: Neurobiology of hearing: the cochlea. Raven Press; 1986. p. 109–22.
32. Shinder ME, Taube JS. Differentiating ascending vestibular pathways to the cortex involved in spatial cognition. J Vestib Res. 2010;20(1, 2):3–23.
33. Shinder ME, Newlands SD. Sensory convergence in the parieto-insular vestibular cortex. J Neurophysiol. 2014;111(12):2445–64.
34. Ten Donkelaar HJ. Desending pathways from the brain stem to the spinal cord in some reptiles. I. Origin. J Comp Neurol. 1976;167(4):421–42.
35. Uchino Y, Ikegami H, Sasaki M, Endo K, Imagawa M, Isu N. Monosynaptic and disynaptic connections in the utriculo-ocular reflex arc of the cat. J Neurophysiol. 1994;71(3):950–8.
36. Wong A. Eye movement disorders. Oxford University Press; 2008.
37. Zingler VC, Kryvoshey D, Schneider E, Glasauer S, Brandt T, Strupp M. A clinical test of otolith function: static ocular counter-roll with passive head tilt. Neuroreport. 2006;17(6):611–5.
38. Zupan LH, Merfeld DM. Neural processing of gravito-inertial cues in humans. IV. Influence of visual rotational cues during roll optokinetic stimuli. J Neurophysiol. 2003;89(1):390–400.

Chapter 2
Mechanism of Compensation After Unilateral Loss

Si Chen and Eric Wilkinson

Functional Changes in Vestibular Compensation

Vestibular compensation is a neurologic phenomenon of central nervous reorganization that allows functional recovery after a peripheral vestibular input loss. Three main mechanisms are responsible for vestibular compensation: adaptation, substitution, and habituation.

Adaptation is the change in central nervous system regulation of neuronal activities that enables reduced sensitivity and clinical response to a constant environment. After unilateral peripheral vestibular weakness, both static and dynamic deficiencies are created which must be overcome. Static deficiencies are due to a constant asymmetric firing rate of the vestibular nuclei. Presenting as acute rotary vertigo symptomatically and visualized as spontaneous nystagmus, they often resolve over a short time period. Dynamic deficiencies occur with head movement and are manifested as changes in the vestibulo-ocular reflex (VOR). The normal VOR moves the eye during head movement in order to stabilize visual targets onto the fovea. Normal gain in VOR is 1, meaning the amplitude and speed of eye movement are exactly the opposite of head movement. With vestibular loss, the gain is reduced and thus patients experience retinal slip, which is interrupted as a visual disturbance. Adaptation to dynamic vestibular loss is seen when the gain of VOR increases over time to regain stable gaze and visual focus during head movement [9].

Substitution occurs with sensory, behavior, and cognitive changes. Multiple inputs contribute to one's sense of equilibrium: vestibular, visual, and

S. Chen
University of Florida, Gainesville, FL, USA
e-mail: sichen1@ufl.edu

E. Wilkinson (✉)
Idaho Ear Clinic, Meridian, ID, USA
e-mail: Eric@wilkinsonmed.com

J. C. Lucas et al. (eds.), *Diagnosis and Treatment of Vestibular Disorders*,
https://doi.org/10.1007/978-3-032-11740-3_2

proprioceptive inputs. When vestibular input is lost in a unilateral peripheral vestibular injury, the central nervous system gives more importance to sensory and proprioceptive inputs to re-establish equilibrium [18, 21]. This is known as sensory substitution. Through behavioral substitution, patients develop behaviors that improve gaze stability and dynamic visual acuity in the setting of abnormal VOR response to movement. These include saccadic eye movements and suppression of cortical visual motion processing [8, 28]. Other strategies are learned behavior such as closing eyes during head movement to the lesion side, blinking with head movement, or moving the whole body as a block [23]. Cognitive substitution describes the phenomenon when the patient moves the whole trunk and head in anticipation of head movement [9].

Some methods in vestibular rehabilitation apply the concept of habituation to ameliorate clinical symptoms. Habituation differs from adaptation, in that it is a progressive reduction in response with repetition of a stimuli. In benign paroxysmal positional vertigo (BPPV) patients who underwent Epley's maneuver, additional vestibular rehabilitation has been shown to improve gait performance [6]. Rehabilitation with rotational movements in rotatory chair is also shown to reduce VOR gain discrepancies and treat visual disturbances [30]. With habituation, patients learn to tolerate or become desensitized to dizziness and vertigo.

All three mechanisms of vestibular compensation have complex interaction in the functional recovery of a patient. Each patient goes through a unique process of vestibular compensation with differential utilization of these mechanisms.

Structural Changes in Vestibular Compensation

In addition to functional changes, structural alterations in the central nervous system have been demonstrated in a series of elegant studies in the past decade. A cascade of molecular and cellular events can be seen from the brainstem to the cortex.

At the brainstem level, acute unilateral vestibular loss creates an asymmetric resting discharge of the vestibular nucleus complexes on both sides. The ipsilateral vestibular nucleus decreases firing rate and sensitivity to inhibitory neurotransmitters. At the same time after vestibular injury, the contralateral vestibular nucleus decreases its firing rate and increases inhibitory activity. With vestibular compensation, the ipsilateral firing rate returns to normal within a week; however, the sensitivity to head velocity does not return to normal [33, 36]. In the lesioned vestibular nuclei, animal studies demonstrate increased inflammatory markers, neuroprotective and neurotrophic factors, cellular metabolism, cell proliferation, and axonal growth [10, 19, 26, 32, 37].

The acute stress response is activated in acute vestibular loss [13]. Elevated cortisol and ACTH levels are seen in Meniere's and vestibular schwannoma patients [20]. In cat models of unilateral vestibular neurectomy, increase in stress hormone (vasopressin, corticotrophin-release factor) reactive cells is see in paraventricular nucleus [38]. Stress hormones alter the milieu of neurotransmitters (glutamate, acetylcholine, GABA, and glycine) and neuromodulators (histamine, adrenaline, and noradrenaline). Clinically, patients experience anxiety with acute vestibular loss, and poorly compensated patients continue to suffer anxiety and depression [12]. Modulating neurotransmission with histaminergic ligands has been shown to improve vestibular compensation in cats. Neurochemical studies in vestibular compensation are an opportunity for pharmacological intervention to accelerate recovery.

New imaging modalities have improved our understanding of higher level cortical changes with unilateral vestibular loss and subsequent vestibular compensation. Alterations in the cortical structure, cerebral metabolism, and functional connectivity contribute to vestibular compensation.

Functional MRI of vestibular neuritis patients demonstrated gray matter volume (GMV) changes in the superior temporal gyrus, insula, inferior parietal lobe, middle temporal areas, and posterior hippocampus. In particular, the increase in GMV of the contralateral superior temporal gyrus and posterior insula (ascending vestibular pathway) correlated with the level of functional impairment [14]. The GMV increase in somatosensory and visual cortex (middle temporal areas) was also noted, which corroborates the clinical findings that patients rely on somatosensory and visual input when there is a loss of vestibular input [15]; in addition, the extent of functional recovery as measured by Dizziness Handicap Inventory also correlates with GMV increases in the visual cortex [17]. Together, these imaging evidences suggest that vestibular compensation depends on the increased use of contralateral vestibular afferents and other sensory inputs in response to defective ipsilateral vestibular input.

Cerebral glucose metabolism is altered in animal models of unilateral labyrinthectomy (UL). FDG-MicroPET studies revealed asymmetric glucose metabolism in the vestibulocerebellum, thalamus, temporoparietal cortex, hippocampus, and amygdala following UL in rats [40]. With vestibular compensation, glucose metabolism is first re-balanced in the vestibular nuclei, thalami, and temporoparietal cortices within 1–2 days. Bilateral glucose metabolism increases in the hippocampus and amygdala and later in vestibulocerebellum and hypothalamus in 7–9 days [40]. These support the neuronal plasticity and contribution of thalamo-cortical and limbic areas to vestibular compensation. Human studies of acute and chronic peripheral vestibular loss using FDG-PET demonstrate an activation pattern similar to peripheral vestibular stimulation on the contralateral side in healthy subjects. There is increase in glucose metabolism in the contralateral thalamus and vestibular cortex, which is reversed within 3 months after peripheral vestibular nerve lesion [2, 3].

Studies using fMRI revealed that functional interregional connectivity (resting-state activity) is altered with unilateral vestibular loss. Vestibular signals are conveyed to multiple cerebral regions via distinct pathways in healthy subjects. In the acute phase of vestibular neuronitis, there is decrease in functional connectivity in contralateral parietal lobe (intraparietal sulcus and supramarginal gyrus) in human subjects, which participates in spatial orientation and multisensory integration. With vestibular compensation, functional connectivity is increased over 3 months. In addition, patients with little disability demonstrate larger increase in functional connectivity on follow-up examination [16]. The changes in functional connectivity reflect the evolving changes in cortical areas responsible for spatial perception and orientation that underlie the process of vestibular compensation.

Recovery of Static Versus Dynamic Vestibular Deficits

Vestibular compensation for static versus dynamic deficits occurs through different processes. Static deficits after unilateral vestibular loss generate symptoms when the patient is stationary. Dynamic deficits result in symptoms when the patient moves.

Static symptoms are subjective vertigo or tilting of the visual vertical axis while standing in place or sitting. Patients exhibit ocular motor and postural signs, such as spontaneous nystagmus, skew deviation, eye cyclotorsion, and tilting of head and body to the lesion side. Static symptoms are compensated within a short time period in animal models and human studies. In humans, full compensation may take 3 months for the ocular motor and postural deficits, and up to 1 year for the perceptive deficits [23, 25]. Static deficits are attributed to the imbalance of spontaneously resting discharges between the two vestibular nuclei. In response, neurons of the ipsilateral vestibular nuclei demonstrate increased excitability and decreased sensitivity to inhibition by the contralateral side [7, 31, 39]. Recovery of static deficits correlates with restoration of symmetric firing rate of the vestibular nuclei [23].

Dynamic symptoms occur when the patient moves the head or body. It is demonstrated by reduced gain, phase shift, and time constant of vestibulo-ocular reflex (VOR). Recovery of dynamic function takes place slowly and some patients never fully compensate, as evidenced by little to no recovery of VOR in response to fast head movements. Catch-up saccades develop in response to lack of VOR recovery [23]. Dynamic deficits are compensated by complex neuronal processes. Increased neuronal cell proliferation and differentiation in animal models of unilateral vestibular loss indicate structural remodeling by neurogenesis, astrogenesis, and synaptogenesis within the vestibular nuclei networks [10]. Sensory substitution and behavioral substitution are two additional learning processes through which vestibular compensation takes place for dynamic deficits.

Vestibular Compensation Is Idiosyncratic

Vestibular compensation is believed to differ depending on the nature of the injury to the peripheral vestibular system [25]. Sudden complete loss of unilateral peripheral vestibular function, such as vestibular neuronitis, has been studied using animal models of unilateral vestibular neurectomy (UVN). Gradual peripheral vestibular loss, such as slow growing vestibular schwannoma or ototoxic medications, was studied using animal models of unilateral labyrinthectomy (UL). In surgical labyrinthectomy, the peripheral vestibular organs are removed while Scarpa's ganglion is preserved. This results in slow degeneration of vestibular nerve fibers, which continues for many years after UL. Afferent tonic input continues to come from the resting discharge of Scarpa's ganglion to vestibular nuclei neurons. Finally, transient vestibular weakness, such as Meniere's disease and benign paroxysmal positional vertigo, had been replicated by intratympanic tetrodotoxin (TTX). When comparing the time course of posture recovery in cat models, transient (TTX) and gradual (UL) loss of vestibular function was compensated faster than acute and sudden vestibular loss (UVN) [11]. In histopathologic studies of these cats, sudden complete loss of unilateral peripheral function (UVN model) elicited intense cell proliferation in the ipsilateral vestibular nuclei, which was not seen with transient (TTX) or gradual (UL) vestibular lesions [25]. This suggests that the mechanism of vestibular compensation in sudden unilateral vestibular loss is different from transient or gradual loss.

In addition to neuronal plasticity, behavioral plasticity in the vestibular system contributes to the time course and final outcome of vestibular compensation. For patients who suffer unilateral peripheral vestibular loss from the same pathology, individual differences in compensation are well described. Patients demonstrate interindividual variability in the utilization of behavioral strategies to compensate for vestibular loss. This is illustrated by studies of Meniere's disease patients who underwent UVN. There is a bimodal distribution of Meniere's disease patients who swayed less in eyes-open versus eyes-closed conditions after UVN. Further examination explained why. Prior to UVN, posturography studies of the patients showed two distinct subpopulations, those who are visual field dependent versus those who are not. After UVN, visual field-dependent patients exhibited more subjective vertical deviation after UVN than visual field-independent patients [21, 27]. In response to unilateral vestibular loss, some patients had an innate reliance on visual cues versus other sensory input, such as proprioception. The idiosyncratic reweighing of sensory inputs is an important concept for therapeutic interventions that aim to augment vestibular compensation [25].

Vestibular Rehabilitation

The concept of vestibular rehabilitation was developed by two British practitioners, Sir Terence Cawthorne and Harold Cooksey, during World War II. They observed that soldiers with head injury recovered their balance faster if they were mobilized early after injury instead of remaining bedbound [9]. We now understand that there is structural reorganization within the vestibular neuronal network during early vestibular compensation, which presents an opportunity window to augment recovery [23].

Animal studies have demonstrated that sensorimotor restriction following UVN significantly delays recovery of static and dynamic performance in monkeys and cats [22, 24]. Sensorimotor restriction at 1 week or 3 weeks after UVN had similar effects; however, it had no effect when applied to the animals 6 weeks after UVN. The authors argue that the period within 1 month after unilateral vestibular loss is a sensitive one, although the exact timing may differ for different etiologies of vestibular loss [22]. Early engagement in rehabilitation via active behavioral and physical training during this critical time can improve brain plasticity and functional recovery.

Vestibular rehabilitation encourages the patients to learn sensory substitution by incorporating visual and somatosensory input early in the process. Strategies to reduce stress and anxiety through behavioral and cognitive therapies can help because excessive stress impairs vestibular compensation [12, 34]. In addition to addressing the location and extent of vestibular loss, successful vestibular rehabilitation requires assessment of the global function of a patient, which includes vision, proprioception, physical health, motor strength, cerebellar function, cognitive abilities, and psychological disorders.

Specific methods in vestibular rehabilitation can augment mechanisms of vestibular compensation. Adaptation exercises are known to increase VOR and treat visual disturbances. An example is to ask the patient to keep a target in visual focus while performing head movements. Substitution exercises instruct the patients to stand with eyes closed or with moving platforms. These challenges aim to increase utilization of visual and proprioceptive cues for postural control. Habituation exercises such as Brandt and Daroff exercises are examples where repetitive vestibular stimulus can reduce clinical symptoms [4]. Newer techniques in vestibular rehabilitation utilize dual tasking, virtual reality, electrotactile stimulation, aquatic physiotherapy, and Tai Chi [9]. Standardized tests such as computerized dynamic posturography (CDP), dynamic visual acuity test (DVA), and gaze stabilization test (GST) are tools to document changes in postural control before, during, and after vestibular rehabilitation.

In cases of prolonged poor compensation of unilateral vestibular loss, vestibular rehabilitation can help by first identifying maladaptive strategies the patients have learned. Behaviors such as head and body movement restriction impede vestibular compensation. With vestibular rehabilitation, the patient is encouraged to abandon the maladaptive strategies and learn to use appropriate compensatory strategies [1, 22, 29]. In some cases, over-reliance on sensory substitution also impairs the recovery of balance control. Patients experience imbalance because visual or proprioceptive triggered responses were too large [5, 35]. Some patients report significant visual triggers, such as worsening dizziness in busy supermarkets or with scrolling of computer screen. Treatment of these cases requires detailed questioning of the patient's symptom triggers and developing vestibular rehabilitation protocols that incorporate desensitizing maneuvers to target those triggers. In addition, decompensation is a known phenomenon induced by stressful situations. Partially or even completely compensated patients can have recurrence of vertigo and instability when stressed. This is worsened by alcohol consumption and use of sedative drugs [22]. Counseling the patients in the recognition and repeat rehabilitation for decompensation episodes can contribute to more stable long-term vestibular recovery.

References

1. Balaban CD, Hoffer ME, Gottshall KR. Top-down approach to vestibular compensation: translational lessons from vestibular rehabilitation. Brain Res. 2012;1482:101–11.
2. Becker-Bense S, Dieterich M, Buchholz HG, Bartenstein P, Schreckenberger M, Brandt T. The differential effects of acute right- vs left-sided vestibular failure on brain metabolism. Brain Struct Funct. 2014;219:1355–67.
3. Bense S, Bartenstein P, Lochmann M, Schlindwein P, Brandt T, Dieterich M. Metabolic changes in vestibular and visual cortices in acute vestibular neuritis. Ann Neurol. 2004;56:624–30.
4. Brandt T, Daroff RB. Physical therapy for benign paroxysmal positional vertigo. Arch Otolaryngol. 1980;106:484–5.
5. Bronstein AM, Golding FJ, Gresty MA. Vertigo and dizziness from environmental motion: visual vertigo, motion sickness, and drivers' disorientation. Semin Neurol. 2013;33:219–30.
6. Chang WC, Yang YR, Hsu LC, Chern CM, Wang RY. Balance improvement in patients with benign paroxysmal positional vertigo. Clin Rehabil. 2008;22:338–47.
7. Darlington CL, Smith PF. Molecular mechanisms of recovery from vestibular damage in mammals: recent advances. Prog Neurobiol. 2000;62:313–25.
8. Deutschlander A, Hofner K, Kalla R, Stephan T, Dera T, Glausauer S. Unilateral vestibular failure suppresses cortical visual motion processing. Brain. 2008;131:1025–34.
9. Deveze A, Bernard-Demanze L, Xavier F, Lavieille JP, Elziere M. Vestibular compensation and vestibular rehabilitation. Current concepts and new trends. Neurophysiol Clin. 2014;44(1):49–57.
10. Dutheil S, Brezun M, Leonard J, Lacour M, Tighilet B. Neurogenesis and astrogenesis contribution to recovery of vestibular functions in the adult cat following unilateral vestibular neurectomy: cellular and behavioral evidence. Neuroscience. 2009;164:1444–56.
11. Dutheil S, Lacour M, Tighilet B. Neurogenic potential of the vestibular nuclei and behavioural recovery time course in the adult cat are governed by the nature of the vestibular damage. PLoS One. 2011;6(8):e22262.
12. Eckhard-Henn A, Best C, Bense S, Breuer P, Diener G, Tschan R, Dieterich M. Psychiatric comorbidity in different organic vertigo syndromes. J Neurol. 2008;255:420–8.
13. Gliddon CM, Darlington CL, Smith PF. Activation of the hypothalamic-pituitary-adrenal axis following vestibular deafferentation in pigmented Guinea-pigs. Brain Res. 2003;964:306–10.
14. Helmchen C, Klinkenstein J, Machner B, Rambold H, Mohr C, Sander T. Structural changes in the human brain following vestibular neuritis indicate central vestibular compensation. Ann N Y Acad Sci. 2009;1164:104–15.
15. Helmchen C, Klinkenstein JC, Kruger A, Gliemroth J, Mohr C, Sander T. Structural brain changes following peripheral vestibulo-cochlear lesion may indicate multisensory compensation. J Neurol Neurosurg Psychiatry. 2011;82:309–16.
16. Helmchen C, Ye Z, Sprenger A, Munte TF. Changes in resting-state fMRI in vestibular neuritis. Brain Struct Funct. 2014;219:1889–900.
17. Hong SK, Kim JH, Kim HJ, Lee HJ. Changes in the gray matter volume during compensation after vestibular neuritis: a longitudinal VBM study. Restor Neurol Neurosci. 2014;32:663–73.
18. Horak FB. Postural compensation for vestibular loss. Restor Neurol Neurosci. 2010;28:57–68.
19. Horii A, Masumura C, Smith PF, Darlington CL, Kitahara T, Uno A. Microarray of gene expression in the rat vestibular nucleus complex following unilateral vestibular deafferentation. J Neurochem. 2004;91:975–82.
20. Horner KC, Cazals Y. Stress hormones in Meniere's disease and acoustic neuroma. Brain Res Bull. 2005;66:1–8.
21. Lacour M, Barthelemy J, Borel L, Magnan J, Xerri C, Chays A, Ouaknine M. Sensory strategies in human postural control before and after unilateral vestibular neurectomy. Exp Brain Res. 1997;115:300–10.
22. Lacour M, Bernard-Demanze L. Interactions between vestibular compensation mechanisms and vestibular rehabilitation therapy: ten recommendations for optimal functional recovery. Front Neurol. 2014;5:285–97.

23. Lacour M, Helmchen C, Vidal PP. Vestibular compensation: the neuro-otologist's best friend. J Neurol. 2016;263(Suppl 1):S54–64.
24. Lacour M, Roll JP, Appaix M. Modifications and development of spinal reflexes in the alert baboon (Papio papio) following a unilateral vestibular neurotomy. Brain Res. 1976;113:255–69.
25. Lacour M. Restoration of vestibular function: basic aspects and practical advances for rehabilitation. Curr Med Res Opin. 2010;22:1651–9.
26. Liberge M, Manrique C, Bernard-Demanze L, Lacour M. Changes in TNFa, NFkB and MnSOD protein in the vestibular nuclei after unilateral deafferentation. J Neuroinflammation. 2010;7:91–102.
27. Lopez C, Lacour M, Magnan J, Borel L. Visual field dependence-independence before and after unilateral vestibular loss. Neuroreport. 2006;17:797–803.
28. MacDougall HG, Curthoys IS. Plasticity during vestibular compensation: the role of saccades. Front Neurol. 2012;3:21.
29. Mijovic T, Carriot J, Zeitouni A, Cullen KE. Head movements in patients with vestibular lesion: a novel approach to functional assessment in daily life setting. Otol Neurotol. 2014;35(10):348–57.
30. Nyabenda A, Briart C, Deggouj N, Gersdorff M. Benefit of rotational exercises for patients with Meniere's syndrome, method used by the ENT department of St-Luc university clinic. Ann Readapt Med Phys. 2003;46:607–14.
31. Olabi B, Bergquist F, Dutia MB. Rebalancing the commissural system: mechanisms of vestibular compensation. J Vestib Res. 2009;19:201–7.
32. Paterson JM, Short D, Flatman PW, Seckl JR, Aitken A, Dutia MB. Changes in protein expression in the rat medial vestibular nuclei during vestibular compensation. J Neurophysiol. 2006;575:777–88.
33. Ris L, de Waele C, Serafin M, Vidal PP, Godaux E. Neuronal activity in the ipsilateral vestibular nucleus following unilateral labyrinthectomy in the alert Guinea pig. J Neurophysiol. 1995;74:2087–99.
34. Saman Y, Bamiou DE, Gleeson M, Dutia MB. Interaction between stress and vestibular compensation: a review. Front Neurol. 2012;3:116.
35. Shumway-Cook A, Horak FB. Rehabilitation strategies for patients with vestibular deficits. Neurol Clin. 1990 May;8(2):441–57. PMID: 2193221.
36. Smith PF, Curthoys IS. Neuronal activity in the ipsilateral medial vestibular nucleus of the Guinea pig following unilateral labyrinthectomy. Brain Res. 1988;444:308–19.
37. Tighilet B, Brezun M, Dit Duflo Sylvie G, Gaubert C, Lacour M. New neurons in the vestibular nuclei complex after unilateral vestibular neurectomy in the adult cat. Eur J Neurosci. 2007;25:47–58.
38. Tighilet B, Manrique C, Lacour M. Stress axis plasticity during vestibular compensation in the cat. Neuroscience. 2009;160:716–30.
39. Vibert N, Beraneck CAM, Bantikyan A, Vidal PP. Vestibular compensation modifies the sensitivity of vestibular neurons to inhibitory amino-acids. Neuroreport. 2000;11:1921–7.
40. Zwergal A, Schlichtiger J, Xiong G, Beck R, Gunther L, Schniepp R, Schoberl F, Jahn K, Brandt T, et al. Sequential [^{18}F] FDG lPET whole-brain imaging of central vestibular compensation: a model of deafferentation-induced brain plasticity. Brain Struct Funct. 2016;221(1):159–70.

Part II
Evaluation of the Dizzy Patient

Chapter 3
History and Physical Examination of the Dizzy Patient

Rance J. T. Fujiwara, Brandon Isaacson, J. Walter Kutz Jr., and Daniel E. Killeen

History

A thorough and structured history is especially important in the evaluation of the dizzy patient. History alone can correctly diagnose patients with vertigo in over 60% of cases, and the diagnostic criteria for many vestibular disorders are via history and clinical examination alone [1]. A thorough history may reduce or eliminate unnecessary vestibular testing or imaging, as vestibular disorders and vestibular testing been associated with increasing healthcare expenditures and significant variability in recent years [2, 3].

The character of the dizziness is important to establish. Vertigo is the sensation of self-motion, either linearly or rotating while stationary, or the sensation that the room or objects are moving. The presence of vertigo is concerning for vestibular dysfunction, either from a central, or more commonly, a peripheral source [2]. This is different from other sensations of dizziness that may be described as imbalance, disequilibrium, lightheadedness, or near-syncope. Vertigo is usually caused by a peripheral vestibular disorder such as Meniere's disease, benign paroxysmal positional vertigo (BPPV), or vestibular neuritis. Disequilibrium, lightheadedness, imbalance, or near-syncope is associated with a much broader differential diagnosis and is often caused by a central vestibular disorder [4]. However, uncompensated vestibulopathy or other peripheral vestibular disorders will present with chronic imbalance and disequilibrium, but with careful questioning, these patients will often recall an initial event that was characterized by true vertigo. In peripheral pathology, patients are usually able to recall a sudden, acute first episode of dizziness. In those

R. J. T. Fujiwara · B. Isaacson · J. W. Kutz Jr. · D. E. Killeen (✉)
Department of Otolaryngology–Head and Neck Surgery, University of Texas Southwestern Medical Center, Dallas, TX, USA
e-mail: rance.fujiwara@utsouthwestern.edu; brandon.isaacson@utsouthwestern.edu; walter.kutz@utsouthwestern.edu; Daniel.Killeen@utsouthwestern.edu

J. C. Lucas et al. (eds.), *Diagnosis and Treatment of Vestibular Disorders*,
https://doi.org/10.1007/978-3-032-11740-3_3

with central pathology, they are often unable to recall an initial episode, as symptom onset is usually insidious and gradual.

The severity of the episodes is helpful to differentiate peripheral versus central causes of dizziness. Peripheral causes of vertigo are discrete and intense, and can be characterized by diaphoresis, nausea, and sometimes vomiting. The symptoms are usually severe enough that the patient cannot continue normal function until the episode subsides. In contrast, patients with central causes of dizziness or uncompensated vestibulopathy are bothered by the symptoms but can usually continue with daily activities.

For patients with severe vertigo, two questions can lead to the correct diagnosis in 61.4% of patients [1]. The first important distinguishing factor is if the vertigo is constant or episodic. Constant vertigo may point to labyrinthitis or vestibular neuritis. Episodic vertigo is concerning for Meniere's disease or benign positional paroxysmal vertigo. The additional presence or absence of hearing loss further leads to the correct diagnosis. The presence of hearing loss with true rotary vertigo is concerning for Meniere's disease or viral labyrinthitis. The absence of hearing loss combined with room spinning vertigo is concerning for vestibular neuritis, vestibular migraine, or benign positional paroxysmal vertigo.

The length of vertigo episodes is also an important detail in distinguishing between central and peripheral pathology, and in diagnosing various peripheral pathologies. Benign paroxysmal positional vertigo has reproducible episodes of vertigo associated with head movement that last less than a minute [4]. The diagnostic criteria for definite Meniere's disease requires two or more spontaneous vertigo attacks lasting 20 min to 12 h, or 20 min to 24 h for probable Meniere's disease. [5] Vertigo episodes related to vestibular migraines, per the Committee for Classification of Vestibular Disorders of the Bárány Society and the Migraine Classification Subcommittee of the International Headache Society (IHS), are limited to a window of 5 min to 72 h [6]. Viral labyrinthitis and vestibular neuritis have sudden onsets with room-spinning vertigo that is constant for several days with gradually improving disequilibrium for days to weeks after the inciting event [4]. PICA and AICA cerebrovascular accidents can have an onset similar to vestibular neuritis and viral labyrinthitis with sudden onset of vertigo with or without hearing loss lasting for days [7].

Inciting events should be recognized to narrow the differential diagnosis. Vertigo with loud sounds and/or changes in pressure such as picking up a heavy object or nose blowing is consistent with superior semicircular canal dehiscence (SSCD), and is associated with a history of head trauma in roughly half of patients diagnosed with SSCD [8–11]. Noise or pressure induced vertigo may also be concerning for perilymph fistula, Meniere's disease, or syphilis [10]. Patients with SSCD will often complain of hearing bodily noises such as eye or neck movement or hearing their heel strike the ground. Brief episodes of vertigo with a specific head movement suggest BPPV, though patients with unilateral vestibular weakness will also have vertigo with head movement [4]. The inability to walk in the dark or on uneven surfaces may suggest bilateral vestibulopathy, such as may occur with ototoxicity or other causes that result in bilateral loss of the peripheral vestibular function [12].

The interviewer should ask about associated symptoms. Audiometrically confirmed low to mid-frequency hearing loss, fluctuating aural symptoms (tinnitus, aural fullness, hearing loss), with discrete episodes of vertigo lasting 20 min to 12 h are diagnostic for Meniere's disease [5]. Sudden hearing loss and vertigo lasting for greater than a day is likely viral labyrinthitis [1]. Patients with a history of migraine headaches or headaches associated with dizziness suggest vestibular migraines as the cause of their dizziness, though the headaches may be remote from the dizziness [6, 13]. Patients with vestibular migraines often complain of motion intolerance and worsening of symptoms with visual stimuli. Dizziness with associated neurologic deficits such as dysarthria, hoarseness, or diplopia suggests a brainstem stroke and require prompt identification so appropriate treatment can be given [7]. Near-syncope, shortness of breath, and palpitations suggest a cardiovascular cause. Diaphoresis, dyspnea, and a sense of impending doom is consistent with a panic attack, and generalized anxiety disorder has been associated with aggravating the degree of vertigo [14].

Once the character, onset, and length of dizziness have been established, obtaining an accurate past medical history is important. Past medical history that could suggest a peripheral cause of vertigo include a history of cholesteatoma, otologic surgery, temporal bone trauma, and history of ototoxic medications. Cholesteatoma may result in a labyrinthine fistula that would be characterized by vertigo with pressure changes, with a recent meta-analysis suggesting that 54% of patients with labyrinthine fistulas report some dizziness [15]. Head trauma may result in labyrinthine concussion or fractures extending through the otic capsule and are accompanied by profound sensorineural hearing loss. Whiplash injuries have also been associated with chronic imbalance and disequilibrium [4]. Neurologic disorders such as multiple sclerosis, migraines, cerebrovascular disorders, seizure disorder, and peripheral neuropathies can also present with dizziness [16, 17]. Central etiology may be responsible for up to 25% of cases of vertigo [17]. For instance, 5% of patients with multiple sclerosis present with vertigo as the initial presenting symptom, and 50% of patients with multiple sclerosis have vertigo at some point in the disease course [16]. PICA and AICA cerebrovascular accidents can have an onset similar to vestibular neuritis and labyrinthitis with sudden onset of vertigo with or without hearing loss lasting for days [7].

Cardiovascular disease can present as dizziness but is often associated with palpitations, arrhythmias, or near-syncope. Orthostatic hypotension is a common cause of dizziness that is characterized by dizziness and near-syncope when standing from sitting or lying down. Vision problems can result in imbalance and disequilibrium. Changes in prescription lenses or the use of bi- or trifocals should be elicited since these may cause imbalance and disequilibrium.

History should include a review of medications, particularly if there were any changes in medication prior to the onset of symptoms. Common medications that cause imbalance and dizziness include antihypertensives, quinolones, neuroleptics, antidepressants, sedatives, and anticonvulsants [18]. A less recognized cause of chronic dizziness is polypharmacy, especially in elderly patients that already have age-related decrease in vestibular dysfunction; as such, coordination of care with a geriatrician to decrease the number of medications may be warranted. Aminoglycoside use is one of the most common drug-related cause of chronic dizziness and bilateral vestibulopathy. Damage to the peripheral vestibular system is dependent on drug concentration, length of treatment, and renal clearance [19, 20].

Physical Examination

Following an accurate and structured history with focused questions as demonstrated above, the next step in the clinical evaluation of the dizzy patient is a focused physical examination based on the presenting history.

General Physical Exam

A complete physical exam begins by overall assessment of general nutrition status, alertness, orientation, and vital signs. Physical exam includes testing blood pressure while supine compared to blood pressure when standing. A difference in systolic blood pressure of 20 mm Hg may indicate orthostatic hypotension [4].

Assessment of Eye Movements

Assessing eye movements in relationship to the vestibulo-ocular reflex (VOR) is crucial in the evaluation of the dizzy patient. When a unilateral vestibular weakness is present, the contralateral (normal) vestibular system remains active. The VOR interprets head movement to the normal side, resulting in slow phase eye movement toward the side of weakness [9]. The central processing system compensates for this eye movement with a fast saccade toward the normal side to correct eye deviation and keep focus on the subject, resulting in nystagmus [21].

Nystagmus can occur spontaneously or evoked by maneuvers (i.e., Dix–Hallpike maneuver). The direction of the nystagmus is also important, as this can point to the source of the deficit. Direction is denoted by the fast phase of the nystagmus, and in the case of unilateral vestibular weakness, the fast-phase nystagmus will be directed away from the affected ear, as explained above. Nystagmus can be described as horizontal, vertical, or torsional geotropic (beating toward ground) or apogeotropic (beating away from the ground) [22]. As stated by Alexander's law, nystagmus will be significantly more noticeable when the gaze is directed toward the normal side relative to the unilateral weakness. The intensity of the nystagmus, reflecting the asymmetry of the difference in vestibular system signal, is denoted by degree. First-degree nystagmus entails nystagmus that is only present when gaze is toward the fast phase of the nystagmus. Second degree describes nystagmus at mid-gaze and gaze in the direction of the fast phase. Third degree describes nystagmus occurring in all horizontal directions including toward the slow-phase side. Additionally, nystagmus may be direction fixed or direction changing, the latter of which is suggestive of central pathology. Purely vertical nystagmus is also highly suggestive of central pathology [22]. Frenzel lenses are magnifying lenses that prevent fixation, which can make the nystagmus more pronounced and may aid in diagnosis. Formal vestibular testing with recording devices in the form of electronystagmography or videonystagmography provides an objective evaluation of vestibular function.

Fistula Test

The fistula test is performed by applying pressure to the tympanic membrane using pneumatic otoscopy. Patients may then have subjective vertigo (subjectively positive fistula test) or eye deviation (objective positive fistula test). A positive fistula test suggests oval or round window fistulae, post-stapedectomy perilymph fistula, semicircular canal dehiscence, labyrinthitis, and rarely in otosyphilis [23, 24]. Patients with a positive fistula test may also demonstrate nystagmus with the application of tragal pressure, which may serve as an alternative to pneumatic otoscopy.

Dix–Hallpike Maneuver

The Dix–Hallpike maneuver is used to detect benign positional paroxysmal vertigo, with the posterior canal representing the most common variant [25]. The maneuver, as demonstrated in Fig. 3.1, is performed by turning the patient's head 45° in the direction of the side being tested. The patient starts in a seated position and is rapidly laid supine while the head remains turned with slight neck extension. A subjective positive test is denoted when this maneuver elicits subjective vertigo. An objectively positive result is observed when torsional nystagmus in the direction of the affected ear occurs with the maneuver.

Lateral canal benign positional paroxysmal vertigo can be assessed with a supine roll test, in which a supine patient's head is rotated to right ear down and left ear down positions (the test ear is whichever ear is closest to the ground). A positive result occurs when geotropic nystagmus is elicited [26].

Head Thrust Test

The head thrust test evaluates for vestibular hypofunction. The test, as demonstrated by Fig. 3.2, is performed by rapidly rotating the head to the left or right with the chin inclined 30° downward while the patient is asked to keep their eyes focused on the

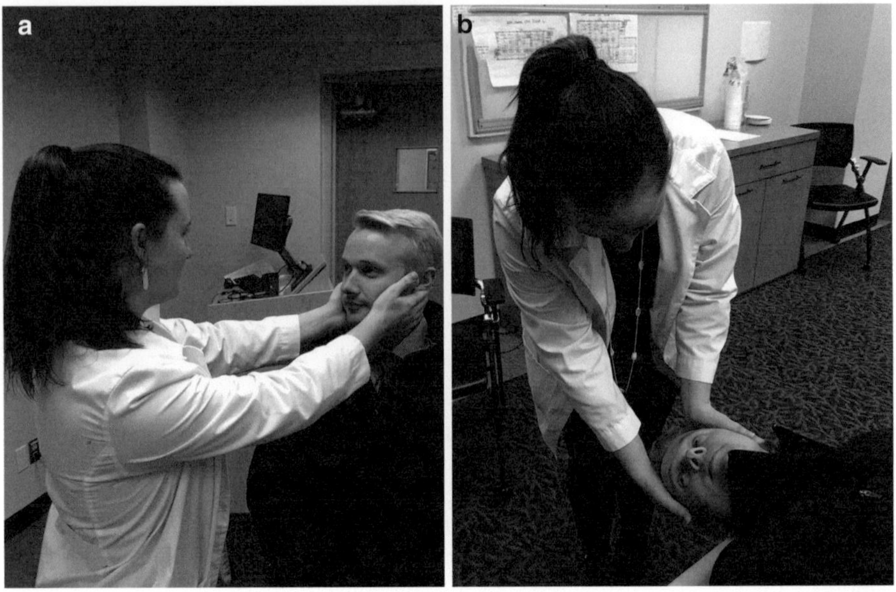

Fig. 3.1 Demonstration of the Dix–Hallpike maneuver. (**a**) Patient starts in the sitting position with their head held 45° in the direction of the examiner. (**b**) Patient is then rapidly laid supine with head turned and with slight neck extension

examiner. A normal response shows normal eye fixation or 1–2 beats of catch-up saccades. A notable contralateral catch-up saccade will appear immediately following the rapid head turn in the direction of the weak ear [27]. Interestingly, this test may be most important if it is negative than if it is positive. In patients presenting with acute onset vertigo, nausea, and vomiting with nystagmus and unsteady gait, 91% with a negative head thrust test had a stroke, while 100% of patients with labyrinthitis or vestibular neuritis had a positive head thrust test [28]. However, 30% with a positive head thrust test had a stroke. Therefore, a negative head thrust test is highly concerning for the presence of a stroke, but a positive head thrust test does not rule out a stroke and further testing would be needed to ensure that the vertigo is not central in origin. While the head thrust exam is a clinical exam able to recognize overt saccades, additional testing of the vestibulo-ocular reflex can be tested using video head impulse testing (VHIT), which is able to detect covert saccades and minimize spontaneous nystagmus, which may interfere with bedside head thrust exams [29, 30].

Head Shaking Test

The head shaking test is performed by rotating the head 20–30 times at a rate of 1–2 hertz 45° to either side with the head tilted forward 30°. Following this examination, nystagmus not present at rest may be elicited and is usually associated with

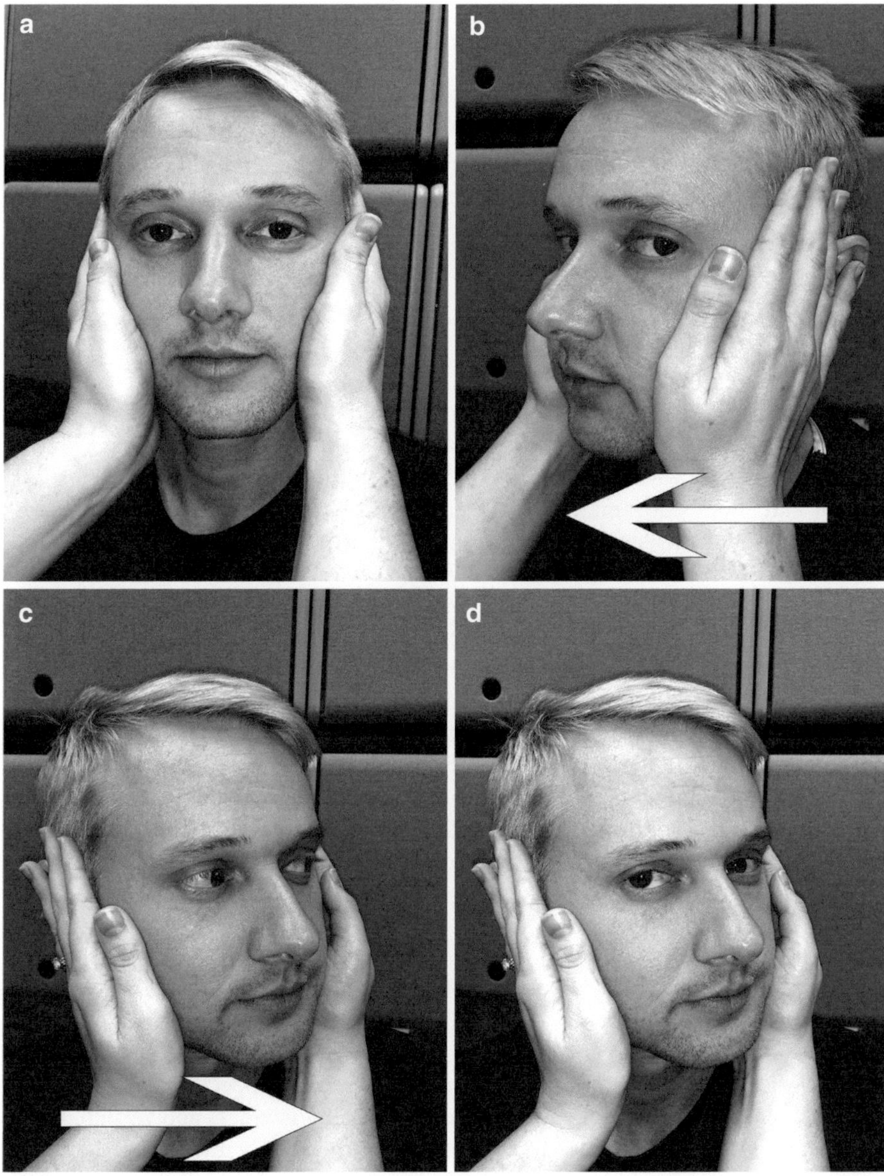

Fig. 3.2 Demonstration of the head thrust test, in which a patient's head is moved from neutral position (**a**) rapidly to the right (**b**) with fixation on the target. The head is then moved rapidly to the left (**c**), and in the case of vestibular weakness, the gaze loses focus on the examiner, resulting in a catch-up saccade (**d**)

unilateral vestibular hypofunction. This examination predicts unilateral vestibular hypofunction with sensitivity of 31%, specificity of 96%, and positive predictive value of 97% [31]. Head shaking nystagmus is associated with higher scores on the dizziness handicap index and functional level scale.

Dynamic Visual Acuity Testing

Dynamic visual acuity is tested by having patients read the lowest level on the Snellen chart with the head at rest followed by reading the lowest level on the chart while moving the head from side to side at 2 Hz rotation; the ability to read the chart should not differ by more than one line. Abnormal dynamic visual testing is concerning for bilateral vestibular hypofunction [32].

Cerebellar Testing

Cerebellar testing is important to perform in all patients with dizziness to better assess possible central causes. Examination may involve, but is not limited to, finger–nose–finger testing, heel-to-toe testing, rapid alternating movements, and tandem gait. Poor coordination on these exercises may point to cerebellar dysfunction, though consistently falling to one side may indicate a unilateral vestibular loss. In Romberg's test, patients stand still with closed eyes—falling to one side can be indicative of cerebellar disease, cerebellar stroke, or by uncompensated unilateral vestibular loss. Romberg test can be made more sensitive for vestibular hypofunction by having the patient stand in a tandem stance or on a foam pad, which alters proprioceptive sensation and leads to further dependence on the vestibular system. In the Fukuda step test, patients march in place with eyes closed and arms extended anteriorly. Deviation of greater than 30° after 50 steps may indicate a vestibular lesion on the side of deviation. Of note, several studies have found that the Fukuda test provides little benefit in detecting mild-to-moderate levels of vestibular weakness, with abnormal deviation occurring reliably in 50% of cases [33, 34].

Test of Skew

The test of skew examines for central causes of dizziness, specifically cerebrovascular accidents in the cases of sudden onset of constant dizziness and vertigo. In this test, one eye is covered for several seconds and then is quickly uncovered. Normally, the uncovered eye should be aligned with the contralateral eye. If the eye is vertically misaligned with the contralateral eye, which then starts to realigned once uncovered, this is indicative of a possible central cause of dizziness and possible cerebrovascular accident [35].

Tympanic Membrane

As with all otologic patients, careful inspection of the tympanic membrane (TM) and the scutum is necessary for a thorough evaluation of the dizzy patient. With regard to dizziness, examination should focus on identification of signs concerning for possible cholesteatoma, which could in turn raise suspicion for labyrinthine fistula, most commonly of the horizontal semicircular canal [36]. Tympanic membrane perforation should be noted, as these can lead to secondary cholesteatoma. Erosion of the scutum associated with an attic retraction pocket raises concern for the development of and epitympanic cholesteatoma [36].

Tuning Fork Exam

The tuning fork exam is a simple and effective means for the assessment of hearing loss, which can help to narrow the differential diagnosis, as evidence of sensorineural hearing loss is more concerning for labyrinthitis or Meniere's disease, though audiometry is the preferred method for assessing hearing loss. The first test using a tuning fork is the Weber test, which assesses for laterality. This is performed by placing the vibrating tuning fork on the glabella or the central incisor and assessing patient sound localization. The normal response is midline. Lateralization to one side indicates possible conductive hearing loss in the ipsilateral ear or sensorineural hearing loss in the contralateral ear. A Rinne test is then performed, which compares the patient's ability to hear a tuning fork through bone and air conduction. The tuning fork is first firmly placed against mastoid bone and the patient subjectively compares it to that of air conduction with the tuning fork placed lateral to the entrance of the auricle. The ability to hear the tuning fork more readily behind the ear points to the presence of a conductive loss.

Cranial Nerve Exam

A thorough cranial nerve examination is indicated in all dizzy patients. Examination begins with assessment of visual fields for cranial nerve 2. Cranial nerves 3, 4, and 6 are then assessed with gaze testing to evaluate extraocular motion. Cranial nerve 5 is then examined by light touch or pinprick of the skin along the forehead, cheek, chin, and preauricular areas corresponding to V1, V2, and V3, respectively. Comparing contraction of the masseter and temporalis muscles bilaterally provides an assessment of the motor division of cranial nerve 5.

Cranial nerve 7 is assessed by evaluating facial function in all distal branch muscle groups. Facial nerve deficits are commonly graded with the House–Brackmann scale [37]. Cranial nerve 8 is examined with the tuning fork exam. Cranial nerve 9 is evaluated on gag reflex and palatal elevation. Cranial nerve 10 is determined by flexible laryngoscopy with examination for vocal cord mobility. Cranial nerve XI is examined by abduction of arms above head, shoulder shrug, and head turn. Cranial nerve XII is assessed by tongue protrusion with deviation of the mobile tongue toward the side of the deficit.

Specific Disorders

The above section serves as an overview to review the general history and physical exam of a patient with dizziness in order to narrow down the differential diagnosis. Once a certain clinical entity is suspected, more specific questioning and testing tailored to the suspected disorder is needed to determine the correct diagnosis. The rest of this chapter summarizes some important clinical entities that cause vertigo with elements of the history and physical exam that can help confirm a diagnosis (Tables 3.1 and 3.2).

Benign Paroxysmal Positional Vertigo

Benign paroxysmal positional vertigo is a condition caused by otoconia dislodged from the otolith macula beds into a semicircular canal [26]. Subsequent position changes cause otoconia movement and abnormal endolymph flow with deflection of the cupula, leading to brief vertiginous attacks with position changes and nystagmus, most commonly in the posterior semicircular canal. The cumulative incidence of the disorder over the course of life is 10% with spontaneous resolutions, and roughly 50% of all primary care visits for dizziness are attributed to benign paroxysmal positional vertigo [38]. Even after treatment, recurrence rates may be as high at 24.5% within the first year according to a recent meta-analysis [39]. With regard to history, patients typically have recurrent attacks of vertigo lasting less than 1 min triggered by position changes such as lying down, turning over in the supine position, or looking upward. Physical exam is focused on utilizing certain movements in an attempt to elicit vertigo or nystagmus, specifically the Dix–Hallpike maneuver, as described above, to examine the posterior semicircular canals, which are the most commonly affected semicircular canals, or the supine roll test, also described above, to examine the lateral semicircular canal [26]. The criteria for diagnosis are listed in Table 3.3.

Table 3.1 Differentiating characteristics of conditions causing dizziness

Condition	Episodic	Time course	Hearing loss	Exacerbating factors	Associated symptoms
Benign positional paroxysmal vertigo	Yes	<1 min	No	Position changes such as lying down, turning over in the supine position, or looking upward	None
Labyrinthitis	No	Constant, lasting days to weeks	Yes	Head movement	Nausea/vomiting
Vestibular neuritis	No	Constant, lasting days to weeks	No	Head movement	Nausea/vomiting
Meniere's disease	Yes	20 min –12 h	Yes, fluctuating	None	Aural fullness, hearing loss, roaring tinnitus
Persistent postural–perceptual dizziness	Yes	Hours for most days over 3 months	No	Upright posture, active or passive motion, and exposure to moving visual stimuli or complex visual patterns	None
Vestibular migraine	Yes	Minutes to days	No	Stress, sleep deprivation, visual stimuli, motion	Headache, photophobia, phonophobia, visual aura
Superior semicircular canal dehiscence	Yes	Chronic with <1 min episodes	Yes, conductive with normal acoustic reflexes and suprathreshold bone line	Sound and/or pressure induced	Hearing loss, autophony, noise avoidance, hearing bodily sounds such as eye movement
Orthostatic hypotension	Yes	<1 min	No	Standing up, bending over	Nausea, tachycardia, presyncope
Cerebral ischemia	No	Constant, lasting days to weeks	Variable	None	Nausea/vomiting, dysarthria, facial anesthesia, hemiparesis, headache, diplopia, visual field defects, blindness, dysphagia, ataxia

Table 3.2 Differentiating physical exam findings with conditions causing dizziness

Finding	Possible diagnosis
Torsional/horizontal nystagmus	Peripheral vestibular injury
Vertical nystagmus	Central dizziness
Corrective saccades on head thrust	Unilateral vestibular hypofunction
Abnormal finger to nose testing	Cerebellar dysfunction
Blood pressure reduction of 20 mm Hg when moving from supine to standing	Orthostatic hypotension
Negative head thrust test with sudden onset of constant vertigo	Stroke
Hearing 256 Hz tuning fork on extremity	Superior semicircular canal dehiscence
Positive fistula test (Hennebert sign)	Superior semicircular canal dehiscence, labyrinthine fistula, perilymph fistula
Geotropic nystagmus on Dix–Hallpike	Benign positional paroxysmal vertigo
Abnormal dynamic visual acuity	Bilateral vestibular hypofunction

Table 3.3 Barany Society diagnostic criteria for benign paroxysmal positional vertigo [20]

Diagnostic criteria for posterior semicircular canalolithiasis	
A	Recurrent attacks of positional vertigo elicited by lying down or turning over in the supine position
B	Duration of attacks is less than 1 min
C	Positional nystagmus after a latency of a few seconds provoked by the Dix–Hallpike maneuver
D	Not attributable to another cause

Labyrinthitis/Vestibular Neuritis

Labyrinthitis and vestibular neuritis have the same vestibular presentation—sudden onset of intense vertigo that is constant for several days with gradual and slow improvement over the next few weeks and months. If there is no hearing loss, patients with this history are diagnosed with vestibular neuritis, instead of viral labyrinthitis, which includes hearing loss. Diagnosis is usually made through history with exclusion of other possible etiologies. On physical exam, patients may have nystagmus at rest or demonstrate a corrective saccade on head thrust test when the head is turned toward the affected side.

Meniere's Disease

Meniere's disease is a syndrome that is thought to be caused at least in part by the increased endolymph pressure in the cochlear duct and/or vestibular organs [5]. As previously mentioned, the diagnostic criteria for Meniere's disease include at least two discrete episodes of vertigo, audiometrically documented low- to mid-frequency hearing loss, and fluctuating aural symptoms, including tinnitus, aural fullness, or hearing loss [40]. In definite Meniere's disease, the vertigo episodes can last 20 min to 12 h, and can last 20 min to 24 h in probable Meniere's disease. The major criteria for diagnosis are described in Table 3.4. Of note, the vertiginous episodes tend to be severe and can be accompanied by nausea, vomiting, and diaphoresis [4]. In the early years of the disease, increases in tinnitus and aural fullness typically precede the vertiginous attacks. Additionally, hearing loss can fluctuate, but typically worsens within 24 h of an attack. Meniere's disease typically affects only one ear, but may be bilateral in up to 30% of cases; however, Pang et al. performed a chart review of all patients who had undergone labyrinthectomy for the treatment of Meniere's disease, with 12% of these patients subsequently developing contralateral disease [41, 42]. With regard to physical exam, patients with Meniere's disease may have normal bedside vestibular exams, but they may have positive fistula test or signs of unilateral vestibulopathy such as a positive head thrust test or head shaking nystagmus.

Persistent Postural–Perceptual Dizziness

Persistent postural–perceptual dizziness (PPPD) describes a chronic functional vestibular disorder that encompasses the previous diagnoses of phobic postural vertigo, space motion discomfort, visual vertigo, and chronic subjective dizziness [43]. This condition is characterized by symptoms of dizziness, unsteadiness, or non-spinning vertigo that are present on most days (more than 15 of 30 days), which are exacerbated by position changes or visual stimuli. This condition is often precipitated with an initial event that disrupts balance, either centrally or peripherally, such as labyrinthitis, vestibular migraines, or concussive injuries, but can also occur as a result of other medical conditions or psychological stress. The major criteria for diagnosis are listed in Table 3.5.

Table 3.4 Barany Society diagnostic criteria for Meniere's disease [4]

Definite Meniere's disease	
A	Two or more spontaneous episodes of vertigo lasting 20 min to 12 h
B	Audiometrically documented low- to mid-range sensorineural hearing loss in the one ear, defining the affected ear on at least one occasion before, during, or after a vertiginous attack
C	Fluctuating symptoms of hearing loss, tinnitus, or aural fullness in the affected ear
D	Not attributable to another cause
Probable Meniere's disease	
A	Two or more episodes of vertigo or dizziness lasting 20 min to 24 h
B	Fluctuating symptoms of hearing loss, tinnitus, or aural fullness in the affected ear
C	Not attributable to another cause

Table 3.5 Barany Society diagnostic criteria for persistent postural–perceptual dizziness [33]

Persistent postural-perceptual dizziness	
A	One or more symptoms of dizziness, unsteadiness, or non-spinning vertigo are present on most days for 3 months or more. Symptoms last prolonged periods (hours) and wax and wane in severity, but do not need to be present continuously throughout the day
B	Persistent symptoms occur without specific provocation, but are exacerbated by three factors: Upright posture, active or passive motion without regard to direction or position, and exposure to moving visual stimuli or complex visual patterns
C	The disorder is precipitated by conditions that cause vertigo, unsteadiness, dizziness, or problems with balance including acute, episodic, or chronic vestibular syndromes, other neurologic or medical illnesses, or psychological distress. If precipitant is acute, then symptoms settle into criteria A after the condition resolves. If precipitant is a chronic condition, symptoms develop gradually
D	Symptoms cause significant distress or functional impairment
E	Not attributable to another cause

Table 3.6 Barany Society diagnostic criteria for vestibular migraine [10]

Definite vestibular migraine	
A	At least 5 episodes with vestibular symptoms of moderate or severe intensity, lasting 5 min to 72 h
B	Current or previous history of migraine with or without aura
C	One or more migraine features with at least 50% of the vestibular episodes: headache with at least two of the following characteristics: one sided location, pulsating quality, moderate or severe pain intensity, aggravation by routine physical activity photophobia and phonophobia visual aura
D	Not attributable to another cause
Probable vestibular migraine	
A	At least 5 episodes with vestibular symptoms of moderate or severe intensity, lasting 5 min to 72 h
B	Only one of the criteria B and C for vestibular migraine is fulfilled
C	Not attributable to another cause

Vestibular Migraine

Vestibular migraine is a condition that affects 2.7% of the population [6, 44]. This condition is characterized by vertiginous symptoms of moderate-to-severe intensity that lasts 5 min to 72 h. Patients with disorder typically have other accompanying symptoms such as headache, photophobia, phonophobia, or visual auras. It more commonly occurs in patients who are female, younger, and with a history of head trauma, anxiety, or depression [44]. The Barany Society has diagnostic guidelines for vestibular and likely vestibular migraine, as demonstrated in Table 3.6. Recently, the Vestibular Migraine Patient Assessment Tool and Handicap Inventory (VM-PATHI) was developed and validated in 2020 to assess disease severity and disease burden for patients with vestibular migraine diagnoses [45].

Mal de debarquement

Mal de debarquement syndrome is characterized by an oscillatory perception of rocking or bobbing [46]. It tends to occur in people following boat, air, or car travel; per the Classification Committee of the Barany society, diagnosis is made if symptoms occur within 48 h after the end of exposure and last more than 48 h, and symptoms typically improve with exposure to passive motion such as driving a car. While a different entity from vestibular migraines, patients with a history of migraines are more susceptible to this entity; mal de debarquement has also been associated with patients who are female and younger in age [47].

Orthostatic Hypotension/Presyncope

Patients with orthostatic hypotension may experience a sensation of non-vertiginous dizziness and light-headedness with changes in position, particularly when moving from sitting to standing [4]. Physical exam may include testing blood pressure while supine compared to blood pressure when standing—patients with orthostatic hypotension may have a difference in systolic blood pressure of 20 mm Hg. Additionally, orthostatic hypotension may present with the sensation that the patient is about to lose consciousness, termed presyncope. Presyncope may be related to neural factors as in the case of vasovagal syncope or may be related to cardiovascular system, but usually, presyncope is not otologic in origin.

Cervical Vertigo

Cervical vertigo, which results from strain of the cervical muscles, is characterized by constant disequilibrium and restricted neck movement [4]. It often occurs after trauma with involvement of cervical muscles, such as whiplash injury [4]. Palpation of the cervical muscles may replicate the sensation in cervical vertigo [4]. Cervical vertigo is a controversial disorder and should be a diagnosis of exclusion.

Superior Semicircular Canal Dehiscence

Superior semicircular canal dehiscence syndrome was initially described by Minor in 1998, which occurs with dehiscence of the superior semicircular canal [10]. Patients with this condition present with vertigo induced by sound and/or pressure, hearing loss, chronic disequilibrium, autophony, and noise avoidance. Physical exam is concerning for nystagmus induced by pressure to the tragus or with air pressure in the ear canal near tympanic membrane. Loud sounds can also induce tilting of the head in the plane of the superior semicircular canal. Tuning fork test may demonstrate a conductive hearing loss with lateralization to the affected ear with weber and bone conduction greater than air conduction on Rinne [48]. Patients may also hear a 256 Hz tuning fork when placed on the lateral malleolus or other extremities [49]. Several studies have shown that superior canal dehiscence is often an incidental finding, with a large fraction of patients being asymptomatic [50]. Diagnosis is made by a combination of clinical presentation, CT scans revealing dehiscence of the superior semicircular canal to the floor of the middle fossa, as well as objective findings including vestibular-evoked myogenic potential testing. Some studies have suggested a correlation with head trauma as an inciting event for the development of superior semicircular canal dehiscence symptomatology [11, 51].

Central Ischemia

AICA and PICA strokes can present in a similar fashion to labyrinthitis or vestibular neuritis with sudden onset of nausea, vomiting, and vertigo with or without hearing loss lasting days [7]. The presence of dysarthria, numbness of the face, hemiparesis, headache, diplopia, visual field defects, blindness, dysphagia, and ataxia often aids in the diagnosis by raising further concern for a central cause [4]. However, 10.4% of patients with CVA can present with solely vestibular symptoms similar to vestibular neuritis [7]. Physical exam can reveal abnormalities on finger–nose–finger testing, heel-to-toe testing, rapid alternating movements, and tandem gait. Additionally, vertical nystagmus is suggestive of a central cause. The combination of negative head thrust test, direction changing nystagmus, and positive test of skew may be used as an effective battery for early diagnosis of stroke [35]. The presence of one of these factors in patients presenting with acute-onset vertigo, nausea, and vomiting predicts stroke with 100% sensitivity and 96% specificity [35].

Conclusion

A thorough and structured history and physical examination can significantly narrow the differential diagnosis when evaluating the dizzy patient. The clinician can pursue appropriate confirmatory studies, including audiological, vestibular, and radiological tests, but the narrowed scope of possible diagnoses from a thorough history and physical exam can limit unnecessary testing. An effective history and physical exam can thereby allow one to work through the differential diagnosis of dizziness in both a time-efficient and a cost-effective manner.

References

1. Kentala E, Rauch SD. A practical assessment algorithm for diagnosis of dizziness. Otolaryngol Head Neck Surg. 2003;128(1):54–9.
2. Adams ME, Yueh B, Marmor S. Clinician use and payments by medical specialty for audiometric and vestibular testing among US medicare beneficiaries. JAMA Otolaryngol Head Neck Surg. 2020;146(2):143–9.
3. Jeong SS, Simpson KN, Johnson JM, Rizk HG. Assessment of the cost burden of episodic recurrent vestibular vertigo in the US. JAMA Otolaryngol Head Neck Surg. 2022;148(12):1103–10.
4. Kutz JW Jr. The dizzy patient. Med Clin. 2010;94(5):989–1002.
5. Basura GJ, Adams ME, Monfared A, Schwartz SR, Antonelli PJ, Burkard R, et al. Clinical practice guideline: Ménière's disease. Otolaryngol Head Neck Surg. 2020;162(S2):S1–S55.
6. Lempert T, Olesen J, Furman J, Waterston J, Seemungal B, Carey J, et al. Vestibular migraine: diagnostic criteria1. J Vestib Res. 2022;32(1):1–6.
7. Lee H, Sohn S-I, Cho Y-W, Lee S-R, Ahn B-H, Park B-R, et al. Cerebellar infarction presenting isolated vertigo. Neurology. 2006;67(7):1178–83.
8. Minor LB. Superior canal dehiscence syndrome. Am J Otol. 2000;21(1):9–19.
9. Minor LB. Clinical manifestations of superior semicircular canal dehiscence. Laryngoscope. 2005;115(10):1717–27.
10. Minor LB, Solomon D, Zinreich JS, Zee DS. Sound- and/or pressure-induced vertigo due to bone dehiscence of the superior semicircular canal. Arch Otolaryngol Head Neck Surg. 1998;124(3):249–58.
11. Formeister EJ, Krishnan PS, Schoo DP, Andresen N, Sayyid Z, Wei O, et al. Traumatic events preceding the development of superior canal dehiscence syndrome. Otolaryngol Head Neck Surg. 2024;171(1):212–7.
12. Strupp M, Feil K, Dieterich M, Brandt T. Chapter 17 - Bilateral vestibulopathy. In: Furman JM, Lempert T, editors. Handbook of clinical neurology, vol. 137. Elsevier; 2016. p. 235–40.
13. O'Connell Ferster AP, Priesol AJ, Isildak H. The clinical manifestations of vestibular migraine: a review. Auris Nasus Larynx. 2017;44(3):249–52.
14. Feng S, Zang J. The effect of accompanying anxiety and depression on patients with different vestibular syndromes. Front Aging Neurosci. 2023;15:1208392.
15. Tomasoni M, Arcuri M, Dohin I, Zorzi S, Borsetto D, Piazza C, et al. Presentation, management, and hearing outcomes of labyrinthine fistula secondary to cholesteatoma: a systematic review and meta-analysis. Otol Neurotol. 2022;43(10):e1058–e68.
16. Karatas M. Central vertigo and dizziness: epidemiology, differential diagnosis, and common causes. Neurologist. 2008;14(6):355–64.
17. Brandt T, Dieterich M. The dizzy patient: don't forget disorders of the central vestibular system. Nat Rev Neurol. 2017;13(6):352–62.
18. Shoair OA, Nyandege AN, Slattum PW. Medication-related dizziness in the older adult. Otolaryngol Clin N Am. 2011;44(2):455–71. x
19. Schwartz FD. Vestibular toxicity of gentamicin in the presence of renal disease. Arch Intern Med. 1978;138(11):1612–3.
20. Black FO, Pesznecker S, Stallings V. Permanent gentamicin vestibulotoxicity. Otol Neurotol. 2004;25(4):559–69.
21. Navari E, Cerchiai N, Casani AP. Assessment of vestibulo-ocular reflex gain and catch-up saccades during vestibular rehabilitation. Otol Neurotol. 2018;39(10):e1111–e7.
22. Tarnutzer AA, Straumann D. Nystagmus. Curr Opin Neurol. 2018;31(1):74–80.
23. Nadol JB Jr. Positive "fistula sign" with an intact tympanic membrane: clinical report of three cases and histopathological description of vestibulofibrosis as the probable cause. Arch Otolaryngol. 1974;100(4):273–8.
24. Nadol JB Jr. Positive Hennebert's sign in Meniere's disease. Arch Otolaryngol. 1977;103(9):524–30.

25. Dix MR, Hallpike CS. The pathology symptomatology and diagnosis of certain common disorders of the vestibular system. Proc R Soc Med. 1952;45(6):341–54.
26. Imai T, Takeda N, Ikezono T, Shigeno K, Asai M, Watanabe Y, et al. Classification, diagnostic criteria and management of benign paroxysmal positional vertigo. Auris Nasus Larynx. 2017;44(1):1–6.
27. Hain TC, Fetter M, Zee DS. Head-shaking nystagmus in patients with unilateral peripheral vestibular lesions. Am J Otolaryngol. 1987;8(1):36–47.
28. Newman-Toker DE, Kattah JC, Alvernia JE, Wang DZ. Normal head impulse test differentiates acute cerebellar strokes from vestibular neuritis. Neurology. 2008;70(24 Pt 2):2378–85.
29. MacDougall HG, Weber KP, McGarvie LA, Halmagyi GM, Curthoys IS. The video head impulse test. Neurology. 2009;73(14):1134–41.
30. Du Y, Liu X, Wang Y, Xu Z, Ji F, Ren L, et al. Comparing saccades in visually enhanced vestibular-ocular reflex and video head impulse test in vestibular assessment. J Otol. 2024;19(3):148–57.
31. Angeli SI, Velandia S, Snapp H. Head-shaking nystagmus predicts greater disability in unilateral peripheral vestibulopathy. Am J Otolaryngol. 2011;32(6):522–7.
32. Goebel JA. The ten-minute examination of the dizzy patient. Semin Neurol. 2001;21(4):391–8.
33. Honaker JA, Shepard NT. Performance of Fukuda stepping test as a function of the severity of caloric weakness in chronic dizzy patients. J Am Acad Audiol. 2012;23(8):616–22.
34. Zhang YB, Wang WQ. Reliability of the Fukuda stepping test to determine the side of vestibular dysfunction. J Int Med Res. 2011;39(4):1432–7.
35. Kattah JC, Talkad AV, Wang DZ, Hsieh YH, Newman-Toker DE. HINTS to diagnose stroke in the acute vestibular syndrome: three-step bedside oculomotor examination more sensitive than early MRI diffusion-weighted imaging. Stroke. 2009;40(11):3504–10.
36. Hura N, Choo D, Santa Maria PL. Complications of cholesteatoma. Otolaryngol Clin N Am. 2025;58(1):51–64.
37. House JW, Brackmann DE. Facial nerve grading system. Otolaryngol Head Neck Surg. 1985;93(2):146–7.
38. von Brevern M, Bertholon P, Brandt T, Fife T, Imai T, Nuti D, et al. Benign paroxysmal positional vertigo: diagnostic criteria. J Vestib Res. 2015;25:105–17.
39. Chen J, Zhang S, Cui K, Liu C. Risk factors for benign paroxysmal positional vertigo recurrence: a systematic review and meta-analysis. J Neurol. 2021;268(11):4117–27.
40. Lopez-Escamez JA, Carey J, Chung WH, Goebel JA, Magnusson M, Mandalà M, et al. Diagnostic criteria for Menière's disease. J Vestib Res. 2015;25(1):1–7.
41. House JW, Doherty JK, Fisher LM, Derebery MJ, Berliner KI. Meniere's disease: prevalence of contralateral ear involvement. Otol Neurotol. 2006;27(3):355–61.
42. Pang B, Costeloe A, Jackson NM, Babu S. Incidence of developing contralateral Ménière's disease in patients undergoing transmastoid labyrinthectomy for unilateral Ménière's disease. Ear Nose Throat J. 2021;100(2):86–9.
43. Staab JP, Eckhardt-Henn A, Horii A, Jacob R, Strupp M, Brandt T, et al. Diagnostic criteria for persistent postural-perceptual dizziness (PPPD): consensus document of the committee for the classification of vestibular disorders of the Bárány society. J Vestib Res. 2017;27(4):191–208.
44. Formeister EJ, Rizk HG, Kohn MA, Sharon JD. The epidemiology of vestibular migraine: a population-based survey study. Otol Neurotol. 2018;39(8):1037–44.
45. Kim EK, Hum M, Sharon JD. Correlating vestibular migraine patient assessment tool and handicap inventory to daily dizziness symptoms. Otol Neurotol. 2023;44(10):1052–6.
46. Cha YH, Baloh RW, Cho C, Magnusson M, Song JJ, Strupp M, et al. Mal de débarquement syndrome diagnostic criteria: consensus document of the classification Committee of the Bárány Society. J Vestib Res. 2020;30(5):285–93.
47. Van Ombergen A, Van Rompaey V, Maes LK, Van de Heyning PH, Wuyts FL. Mal de debarquement syndrome: a systematic review. J Neurol. 2016;263(5):843–54.
48. Suzuki M, Ota Y, Takanami T, Yoshino R, Masuda H. Superior canal dehiscence syndrome: a review. Auris Nasus Larynx. 2024;51(1):113–9.

49. Yew A, Zarinkhou G, Spasic M, Trang A, Gopen Q, Yang I. Characteristics and management of superior semicircular canal dehiscence. J Neurol Surg B Skull Base. 2012;73(6):365–70.
50. Williamson RA, Vrabec JT, Coker NJ, Sandlin M. Coronal computed tomography prevalence of superior semicircular canal dehiscence. Otolaryngol Head Neck Surg. 2003;129(5):481–9.
51. McCrary HC, Babajanian E, Patel N, Yang S, Kircher M, Carlson ML, et al. Superior semicircular canal dehiscence syndrome following head trauma: a multi-institutional review. Laryngoscope. 2021;131(11):E2810–e8.

Chapter 4
Electronystagmography and Videonystagmography

Dennis Bojrab II, Wanda Lai, and Dennis I. Bojrab

Introduction

Vestibular function tests are clinical techniques used to evaluate part of the vestibular system. Stimulation of the inner ear results in specific eye movement termed "nystagmus," which are integral in the evaluation of the vestibular system. Nystagmus has a fast-phase and a slow-phase component and is named based on the fast phase. Electronystagmography (ENG), videonystagmography (VNG), and rotation testing measure nystagmus to provide objective assessment of the function of the vestibular system.

The interaction of the vestibular system with other organ systems helps to maintain balance and posture. The brain acts as the central processor to produce motor reflexes that maintain posture and equilibrium and to stabilize gaze based on information it receives from the inner ear (vestibular) system, the eyes (visual), and muscle and joint receptors (proprioception). These systems are connected within the central nervous system (CNS) and are reflex pathways providing continuous information. The most important reflex pathways are the vestibulo-ocular reflex (VOR), which integrates information between the inner ear and the eyes (the extraocular muscles) and the vestibulospinal reflex (VSR), which integrates information from the skeletal system. One system may be more dominant and override the other in certain situations. All eye movements are aimed at ensuring optimal visual acuity. Vestibular and optokinetic eye movements work to hold eye position in space (gaze) constant by producing compensatory eye movements that keep images stable on the retina during head movements. Vestibulo-ocular reflexes (VORs) are responsible for maintaining binocular fixation and stabilizing binocular foveal images during head movements. The VORs are divided into two types: angular acceleration and gravitation acceleration. Angular

D. Bojrab II (✉) · W. Lai · D. I. Bojrab
Department of Otology and Neurotology, Michigan Ear Institute,
Farmington Hills, MI, USA

J. C. Lucas et al. (eds.), *Diagnosis and Treatment of Vestibular Disorders*,
https://doi.org/10.1007/978-3-032-11740-3_4

reflexes are initiated by activation of the semicircular canals. The canals are aligned with the pulling directions of the three pairs of extraocular muscles. Activation of a single semicircular canal leads to motion of the eyes about an axis that aligns with the axis of the semicircular canal. Gravitational VORs are driven by otolith afferents and can be grouped into two categories: tilt responses that compensate for lateral head tilt with respect to gravity, and translational responses, which produce eye movements compensatory for linear movements of the head [1, 2]. Saccadic, pursuit and vergence eye movements change gaze so that images of objects of interest are brought to or kept on the fovea where visual resolution is highest. Saccades rotate the eye to bring an image onto the fovea. Pursuit maintains that image on the fovea as it moves across the visual field. Vergence movements are disjunctive, causing the eyes to move in the opposite directions to place the image of an object simultaneously on both fovea during movements of the head or object.

Electronystagmography and Videonystagmography

Electronystagmography is the oldest method of monitoring eye movements and has been in clinical use for over 50 years. It has been widely used as a diagnostic tool to evaluate patients with dizziness or unsteadiness. The ENG is based on the fact that there are steady direct current (DC) potentials between the cornea and the retina, called cornea-retinal potentials (CRP). The retina possesses a negative charge relative to the cornea, due to its high metabolic requirements. These potentials create an electric field in the front of the head that rotates as the eyes rotate in their orbits. Rotation of this electric field produces a roughly linear change in the voltage between electrodes attached to the skin on either side of the eyes. Horizontal eye position is monitored by electrodes placed on the patient's temples. Vertical eye position is monitored by electrodes placed above and below on of the patient's eyes. Eye movement causes deflection in the ENG recording that produces a characteristic tracing (Fig. 4.1a, b). Nystagmus has a fast phase and a slow phase and is an involuntary movement. The velocity of the slow phase provides a sensitive and accurate measure of intensity. In the past, recordings were made with polygraph tracer. In the 1980s, computerized ENG recording became available and provided the advantages of efficient storage and retrieval of actual eye movement tracings, eliminating cutting and pasting of strip chart recordings. Computerization also provided greater sophistication of analysis for saccade, tracking and caloric tests, and allowed automatic comparison of individual eye movement recordings with statistical norms at a variety of different frequencies [3].

There are other methods of recording eye movements that do not use skin surface electrodes. The most common and cost-effective manner is use of video infrared recording goggles. Direct infrared oculography involves an array of tiny infrared lights reflected off the surface of the eye and uses the differential reflection between the iris and the sclera to track eye movement. Other research-oriented methods include scleral search coils, which are often limited by patient discomfort and cost.

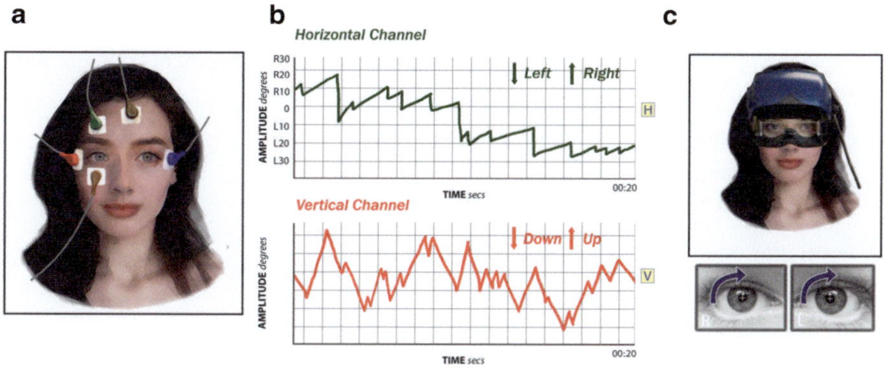

Fig. 4.1 Electro-oculography (EOG) and videonystagmography (VNG). A-VNG. (**a**) Corneal retinal potential with recording. In electro-oculography (EOG), the cornea has a relatively positive charge signal in comparison to the retina. An electric potential exists between the two. Electrodes are placed around the eyes, the movement of the eye brings the cornea closer to one electrode and the negatively charged retina closer to the other. (**b**) The relative voltage difference provides the basis for the tracing. Results are charted digitally with time plotted on the horizontal axis and eye movements recorded on the vertical axis. By convention, rightward eye movement is recorded as an upward deflection, and leftward eye motion is shown as a downward deflection. (**c**) Videonystagmography goggles contain video cameras that allow the patient's eye movements to be recorded for viewing analysis. This allows for superior documentation of torsional nystagmus when compared with traditional EOG

One current trend in many vestibular laboratories is toward the use of computer-based video-recorded nystagmography (VNG) (Fig. 4.1c). This VNG technique determines eye position by locating the pupil and tracking its center. The internal computer program plots, measures, and analyzes the eye movement similar to traditional ENG. An additional benefit of the technique is the ability to record eye images. This feature is helpful for later study and for teaching personnel and patients. Videonystagmographic tracings are clean with no drift, improving the accuracy of analysis and interpretation. This technique is also easier and quicker than using electrodes and only one calibration is necessary. Limitations of VNG include the expense of testing equipment, sense of confinement experienced by some patients with claustrophobia, and difficulty in testing patients with ptosis, pupil-obscuring eyelashes, or other eye abnormalities [3].

Electronystagmography/Videonystagmography Test Battery

The ENG/VNG test battery generally consists of eight tests in most clinical setting though some centers may choose to use fewer. Five tests are primarily tests of vestibular function, although they sometimes also reveal non-vestibular eye movement abnormalities as well. Three are tests of non-vestibular eye movements [4].

Vestibular Function Tests

1. Presence of abnormal eye movements and whether the movements change with head position
   (a) Positioning test (Dix–Hallpike maneuver)
   (b) Positional test
   (c) Gaze test
2. Vestibular oculomotor function
   (a) Bithermal caloric test
   (b) Head shake test

Non-vestibular Tests

1. Visual oculomotor function or non-vestibular (tracking) eye movements
   (a) Saccade test
   (b) Tracking test
   (c) Optokinetic test

Vestibular Function Tests

Positioning Test (Dix–Hallpike Maneuver)

The patient is tested for two brisk movements, both beginning with the patient in the sitting position. The patient's head is turned 45° toward one side. Then the examiner, standing behind the patient, pulls them briskly backward so that the patient is lying supine with their head still turned to that side and hanging over the end of the examining table. The examiner holds the patient's head in that position for at least 20–30 s and monitors the patient's eye movements. The patient is then returned to the sitting position. If a response was elicited, the examiner repeats the same maneuver to determine if the response fatigues. The examiner performs the maneuver with the patient's head turned 45° to the other side and repeats the maneuver sequence (Fig. 4.2a, b). For some patients with neck disease where the head hanging position is not available, the Bojrab maneuver may be employed placing the posterior semicircular canal in the same position for testing (Fig. 4.2f).

During the backward movement, the Dix–Hallpike maneuver may induce a few beats of nystagmus. After the head has reached the hanging position, normal individuals do not have nystagmus. Some patients with benign positional vertigo display a burst of intense paroxysmal positioning nystagmus that is the hallmark of the disorder (Fig. 4.2c, d). Paroxysmal positioning nystagmus has three characteristics:

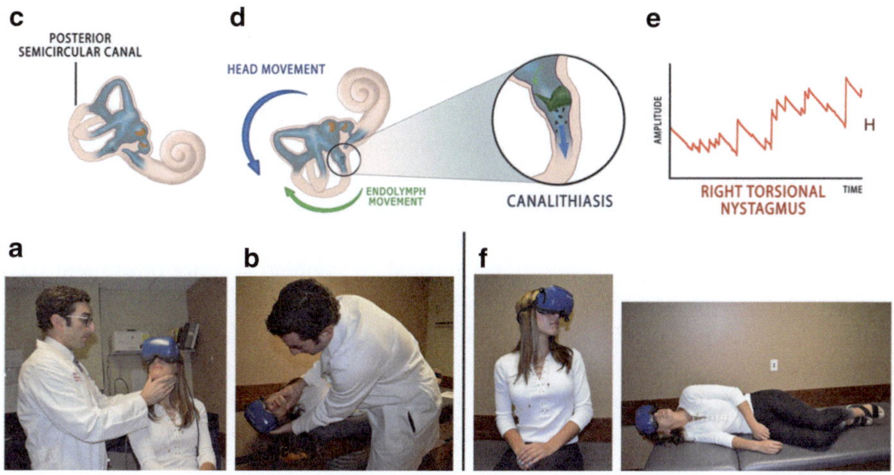

Fig. 4.2 Positioning testing. (**a**, **b**) Dix–Hallpike positioning maneuver demonstrated. The patient's head is first turned to the right. The patient is then rapidly brought into the head-hanging position. Patients with benign paroxysmal positional vertigo typically demonstrate a geotropic, torsional nystagmus with the affected ear down. (**c**) Corresponding labyrinth position that results in ampullofugal endolymphatic flow in the right posterior canal. (**d**) Stimulatory cupula deflection by right posterior canalithiasis. (**e**) VNG tracing representing right lateral canal electrode showing right beating nystagmus, which is seen with right posterior canal BPPV. (**f**) The Bojrab maneuver demonstrated as an alternative method for positional testing of the right posterior canal. The head is turned 45° to the left so that the pinna is perpendicular to the table surface. The examiner holds the head in that position as the patient is briskly lowered onto his/her shoulder with the head resting on the table. This position is held for at least 20 s, while eye movements are monitored. The patient is then returned to the sitting position. If nystagmus was elicited, the examiner repeats the same maneuver to determine if the nystagmus is fatigable

1. Usually (but not always) delayed in onset by at least a few seconds. Some patients may have a delay of up to 30–45 s before onset.
2. The nystagmus is transient being present for a number of seconds and then subsiding but may continue for 30–45 s.
3. The nystagmus is accompanied by vertigo, which is often intense and follows the same time course as the nystagmus.

The response usually fatigues upon repetition of the maneuver. The direction frequently reverses when the person sits up. If the nystagmus lasts longer than 1 min, a possible explanation is by cupulolithiasis in which the cupula remains deflected as long as the position is held. Positioning nystagmus that lasts longer than 1 min, nystagmus that does not fatigue with repeated positioning, actively beating positional nystagmus not associated with vertigo, and conjugate vertical positioning nystagmus are signs of central nervous system disease [5, 6].

Paroxysmal positional nystagmus can be readily appreciated by visual observation with the patient's eyes open or with the patient wearing Frenzel's lenses in a darkened room. The examiner sees primarily the torsional component of the nystagmus, with counter clockwise fast phases when the right ear is involved and clockwise fast phases when the left ear is involved. Another way to think of this is torsional nystagmus that is geotropic of turning toward the downward labyrinth or ear. Traditional ENG is insensitive to the torsional component of the nystagmus, but does record the horizontal and vertical components. The horizontal component generally has fast phases away from the undermost ear and the vertical component has upward fast phases. Paroxysmal positional nystagmus changes somewhat with the direction of the patient's gaze. The torsional component is more prominent during gaze toward the undermost ear and the vertical component is more prominent during gaze toward the uppermost ear (Fig. 4.2e).

In 1985, McClure described a variant of BPPV that affects the horizontal or lateral semicircular canal. In this condition, which has been called horizontal canal BPPV, the positioning maneuver results in horizontal nystagmus that displays some of the characteristics as that of posterior canal BPPV (paroxysmal, accompanied by vertigo) [7, 8].

Positional Test

The purpose of the positional test is to determine whether different head positions, not head movements, induce or modify vestibular nystagmus. The patient's eye movements are monitored while the head is located in at least in four positions: sitting, supine, right head turn, and left head turn. Eye movements are recorded for at least 30 s eyes open and eyes closed in each of these positions. If nystagmus appears or is modified in either of the latter two positions, the patent is tested again while lying on that side to determine if the effect was due to neck rotation. If this disappears in the lateral position, then it was caused at least partly by neck rotation (Fig. 4.3).

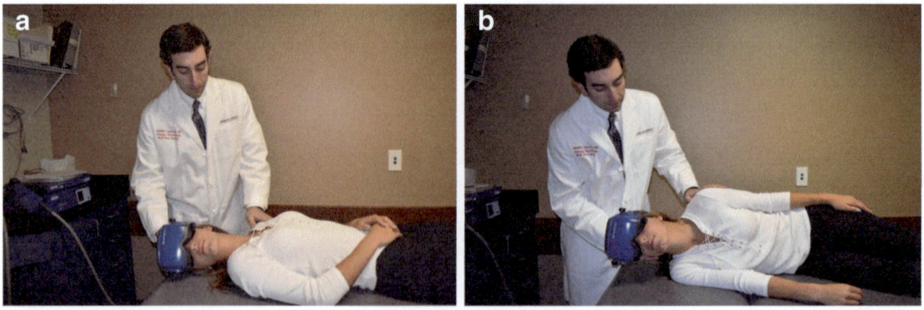

Fig. 4.3 Drawing of positional test: Positional test is to determine if different head positions induce or modify nystagmus. Nystagmus induced by positional testing is referred to as positional nystagmus or static positional nystagmus. During the positional tests, the patient's eye movements are monitored while the head is in at least four positions: sitting, supine, head right, and head left. If nystagmus appears or is modified in either of the latter two positions, the patient is tested again while lying on that side to determine if the effect is caused by neck rotation

Positional nystagmus may be intermittent or persistent unlike positioning nystagmus, which disappears if the head is still. Persistent positional nystagmus is sustained as long as the head position is held and may reflect the effect of changing otolithic influence. As with positioning nystagmus, the terms "geotropic" and "ageotropic" may be used to describe the direction of the nystagmus. The nystagmus may be direction fixed (beating in the same direction in different head positions) of direction changing (beating in a different direction in different head positions). Both of these types of nystagmus occur most commonly with peripheral vestibular disorders, but can also be a sign of a central lesion. Peripheral vestibular nystagmus usually stops with visual fixation. Positional nystagmus has little localizing value but is a valuable indicator of vestibular system dysfunction. Other signs and clinical data must be used to localize the lesion. The most common abnormality seen with the positional test is spontaneous nystagmus. When persistent nystagmus is found, it is important to observe it for at least 2 min because certain types of direction-changing nystagmus reverse direction every 2 min (acquired periodic alternating nystagmus). This type of nystagmus usually is caused by a central nervous system lesions, but vestibular stimulation can reset the oscillation [9, 10].

Gaze Test

The gaze test discloses nystagmus in the absence of vestibular stimulation. It may be the first step in identification of vestibular, central, or congenital disorders that present with nystagmus. The test is performed by recording the patient's eye movements first in the primary position with gaze straight ahead. Then, eye movements are recorded while looking 30° to the right, to the left, up, and down. Eye positions should be held for at least 30 s. Vestibular spontaneous nystagmus occurs when there is an imbalance in the tonic input from the vestibular system. It is typically seen during and directly after unilateral vestibular dysfunction. The nystagmus usually has a fast phase away from the site of the diseased labyrinth or nerve. An exception would be in Meniere's disease when there could be in hyperactive or irritative response causing nystagmus to beat toward the disease side. Vestibular spontaneous nystagmus is seen at ENG as a horizontal nystagmus. The intensity of the spontaneous nystagmus may change with change in eye position, being stronger when the gaze is directed toward the direction of the nystagmus (Alexander's law). Gaze deviation beyond 40° may cause end-point nystagmus even among healthy persons. Spontaneous nystagmus that does not lessen or increases with visual fixation suggests a central lesion (failure of fixation suppression) (Fig. 4.4) [11].

Alternatively, gaze-evoked nystagmus may be a side effect of a variety of medications including anticonvulsants, sedatives, and alcohol. It can also occur in such diverse conditions as myasthenia gravis, multiple sclerosis, and cerebellar atrophy. Dysconjugate gaze nystagmus is commonly present with medial longitudinal fasciculus lesions, such as internuclear ophthalmoplegia [12, 13].

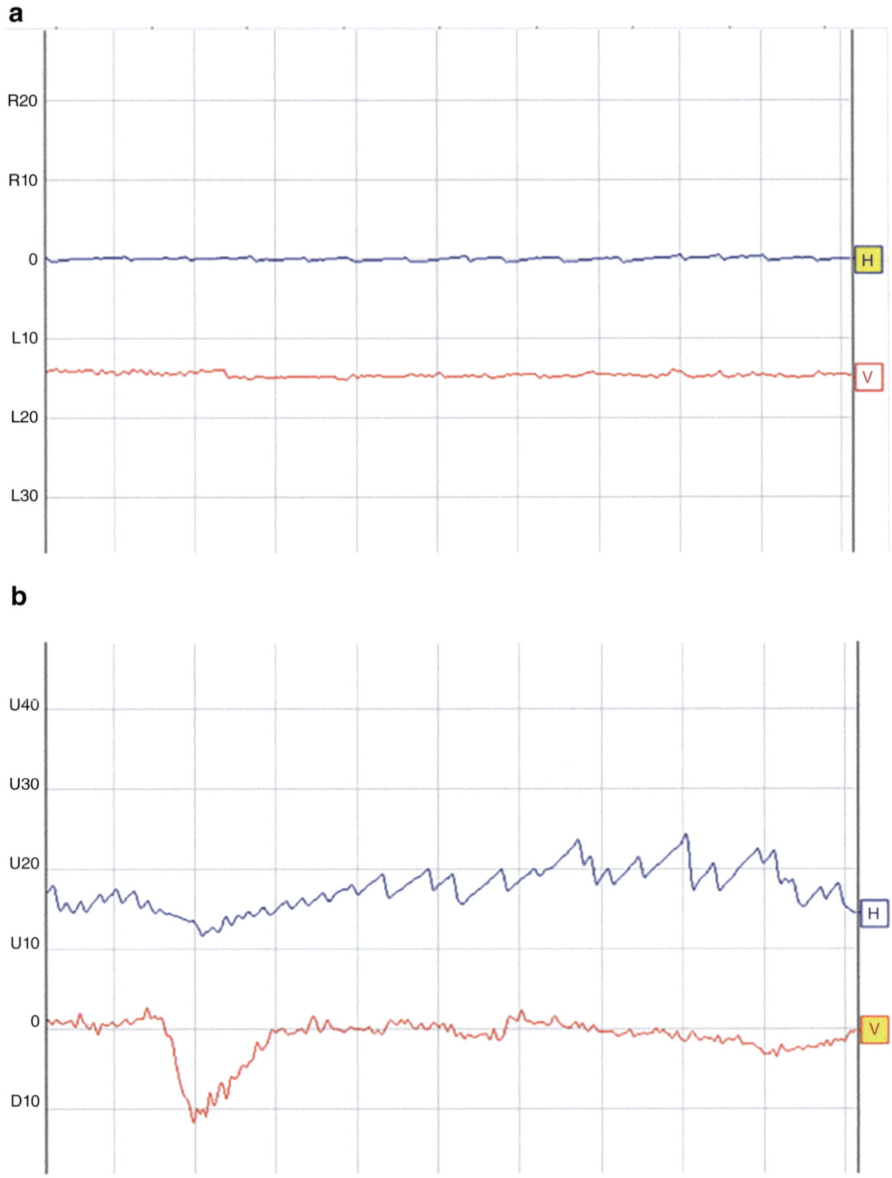

Fig. 4.4 Gaze testing: The gaze test detects nystagmus that occurs without active vestibular stimulation. (**a**) Demonstrates left gaze with fixation which suppresses the nystagmus. (**b**) Demonstrates left gaze without fixation, such as when Frenzel glasses are worn, unmasking left beating nystagmus

Vestibular Oculomotor Function

Bithermal Caloric Test

The caloric test is the most difficult, the most time-consuming and the most important test in the VNG test battery. This test is useful in lateralizing a vestibular lesion or identifying disorders of the labyrinth and vestibular nerve. It is an invaluable aid in the diagnosis of peripheral vestibular disorders such as Meniere's disease, vestibular neuronitis, labyrinthitis, and ototoxicity. It is the only test that allows stimulation of each ear separately.

The theory of the caloric stimulation was created by Viennese scientist, Robert Barany, who received the Nobel Prize for Medicine in 1914 for his work on the vestibular system. Barany proposed that caloric irrigation induces endolymphatic flow in the lateral semicircular canal by producing a temperature gradient from one side of the canal to the other. The temperature change alters the density of the endolymph on the lateral aspect of the canal closest to the temperature source. Gravity causes fluid to move, deflect the cupula, and stimulate or inhibit the vestibular nerve and the afferent pathway. Cold stimuli produce ampullofugal (away from the cupula) deviation and warm stimuli cause ampullopetal deviation (toward the cupula). We now know that this theory is incomplete because caloric responses are seen, though diminished, in monkeys even after occlusion of the horizontal semicircular canal and in humans tested in microgravity (outer space) [14, 15]. The mechanism of caloric stimulation probably involves endolymphatic convection and a direct effect of temperature change on the discharge rate of the superior vestibular nerve and end organ (cold temperature depresses the firing rate and warm temperature elevates the firing rate [16].

Many vestibular labs have changed to the usage of air. Caloric stimuli are uncalibrated, that is, stimulus strength varies from person to person, depending on the size and shape of the external ear canal and other uncontrollable variables. The basic assumption is that the two ears receive equal caloric stimuli. If both ears are normal and or similar, then the response from the two ears should be equal intensity. Therefore, the strength of the caloric responses of the two ears is compared. This current standard caloric test evolved from the bithermal caloric test introduced by Fitzgerald and Hallpike in 1942.

The patient is placed in the supine position with the head elevated 30°, thereby placing the lateral semicircular canal in the vertical plane. Each ear is irrigated twice: once with air (or water) at 7° above body temperature (44 °C) and then with air (or water) at 7° below body temperature (30 °C). In a healthy patient, irrigation with a warm stimulus provokes nystagmus with the fast phase directed toward the stimulated ear; irrigation with a cool stimulus evokes nystagmus with the fast phase directed away from the stimulated ear (Fig. 4.5a).

The caloric data are analyzed, and five characteristics of the nystagmus are calculated: duration, latency, amplitude, frequency, and velocity. Of these parameters, the most important variable is the peak slow-phase eye velocity. In normal individuals, the slow-phase eye velocity should be equally strong in both directions as

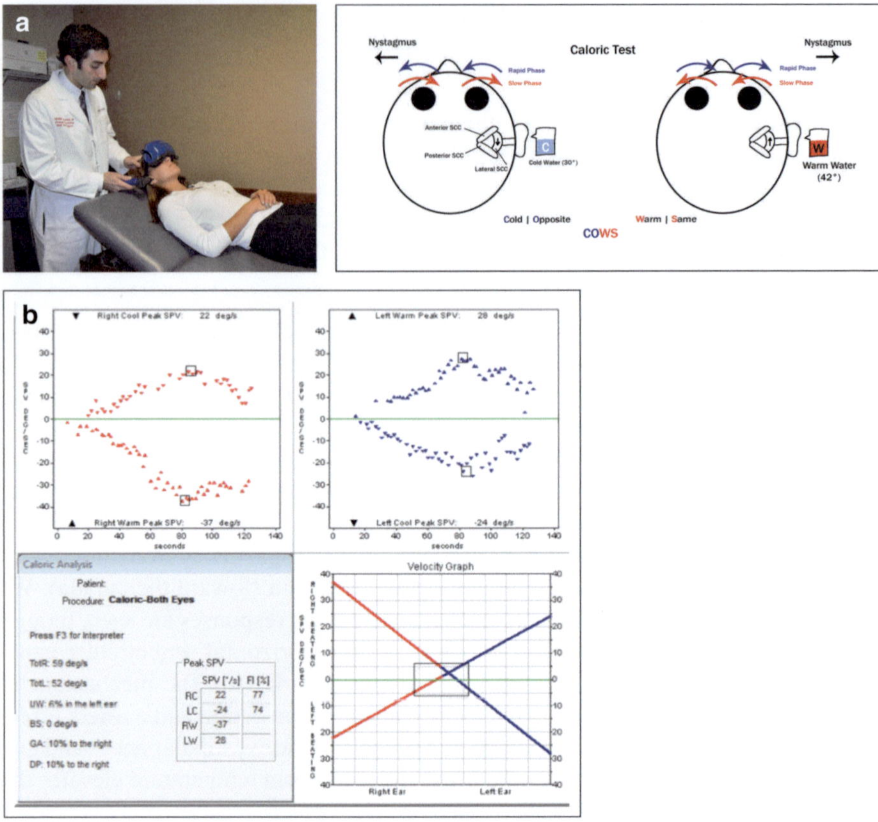

Fig. 4.5 Caloric testing: (**a**) The patient is positioned so that the head is elevated 30°, aligning the lateral canal in a vertical position, perpendicular to the ground. Cold air/water is introduced into the right ear causing ampullofugal endolymph flow and corresponding nystagmus with the fast phase toward the opposite ear. (**b**) VNG tracing of caloric evaluation to cool and warm stimulation demonstrating normal bilateral responses. The upper panels plot the growth and decay of the right and left ears' caloric responses over time. The lower right panel plots the peak velocity of the slow component of nystagmus for the right ear and left ear. respectively. The lower left panel reveals a unilateral weakness (UW) of 6%, which is less than the 20–25% seen in unilateral weakness and therefore in the range of normal

measured with VNG (Fig. 4.5b). Comparing the peak slow-phase eye velocity of the cool and warm caloric responses of the right ear with those of the left ear, using the following formula, allows the examiner to determine whether a unilateral vestibular weakness exists [17].

$$\frac{(\mathrm{RW}+\mathrm{RC})-(\mathrm{LW}+\mathrm{LC})}{\mathrm{RW}+\mathrm{RC}+\mathrm{LW}+\mathrm{LC}}\times 100\% = \mathrm{UW}$$

where RW, RC, LW, and LC are peak slow-phase eye velocities of the responses to right warm, right cool, left warm, and left cool responses, respectively, and UW is unilateral weakness. In general, a unilateral caloric weakness (CW) of greater than 20–25% indicates peripheral vestibular dysfunction on the side of the weaker response.

Patients with labyrinthine hypofunction may demonstrate reduced or absent caloric responses to the initial bithermal stimuli. In this case, the test is repeated with ice water (approximately 0 °C) irrigations. However, one should keep in mind that the absence of a caloric response does not always imply absent peripheral function, as the stimulus levels are below the level which the VOR generally functions.

The most common abnormality seen with caloric responses would be a unilateral lesion. Patients may also have both a unilateral weakness and spontaneous nystagmus. This pattern is typical of patients with acute sudden unilateral peripheral vestibular lesions. Such a lesion causes a reduction in the resting input coming from the damaged ear, producing an asymmetry that induces nystagmus with slow phases toward the damaged ear (Fig. 4.6a).

Whereas the bithermal caloric test is highly sensitive to unilateral peripheral vestibular dysfunction, it is relatively insensitive to bilateral dysfunction. Even though the stimulus at the entrance to the external ear canal is the same for everyone, the stimulus reaching the inner ear shows great interindividual variability owing to differences in the size and shape of the ear canal and the status of the middle ear. Therefore, the range of normal absolute response intensities is extremely wide, and bilateral caloric weaknesses must be severe to fall below them. The usual rule of thumb is that a bilateral weakness exists if the caloric responses of both ears fall below 12 degrees/s, per side (Fig. 4.6b) [1, 18–23].

Head Shake Test

A head shake test should also be included as part of the VNG battery. The test is performed with the patient in the seated position. The patient's head is rapidly rotated in the horizontal plane with the head down about 30° for maximal stimulation of the lateral canals. The rotation must be performed at approximately 1–2 Hz for about 30 cycles and then abruptly stopped. The patient may shake their own head as directed (autorotational) or may be assisted by the examiner, who grasps the head firmly and rotates it side to side (Fig. 4.7). If the head is rotated side to side in the horizontal plane in normal subjects, the velocity storage is charged equally on both sides. There is no post rotatory nystagmus as the stored velocities decay at the same rate on either side. However, nystagmus does occur after head shaking in subjects with unilateral vestibular hypofunction. This may persist for 5–30 s. This pattern may even reverse after several seconds presumably because neurons affected by velocity storage adapt to the prolonged change in firing from their baseline rates [24–26].

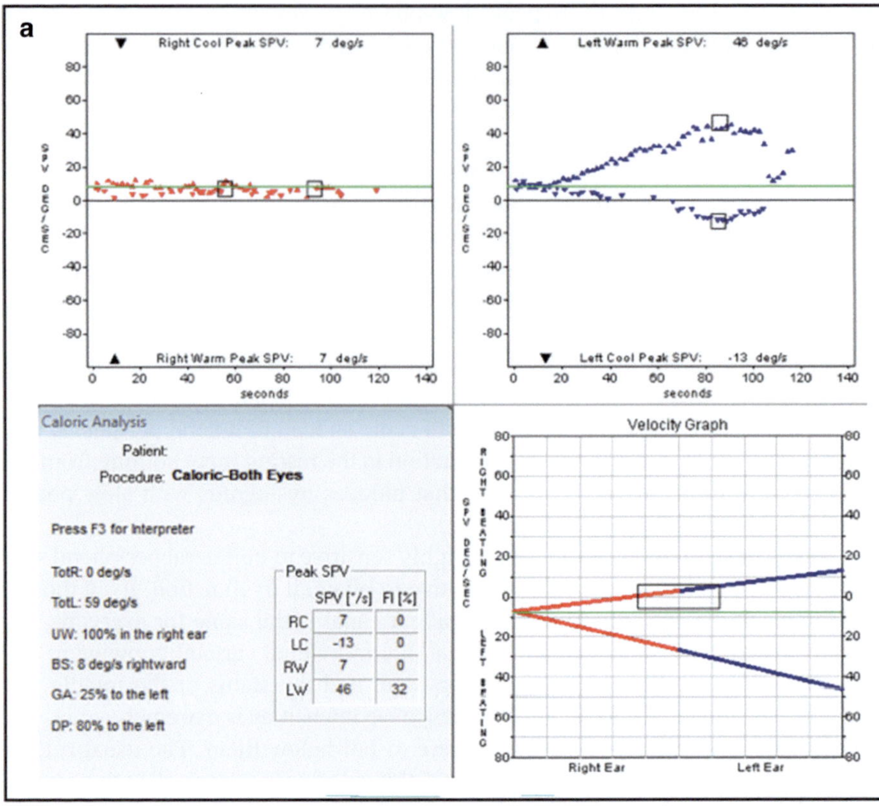

Fig. 4.6 Unilateral and bilateral weakness. (**a**) A unilateral caloric weakness (CW) of greater than 20–25% indicates peripheral vestibular dysfunction on the side of the weaker response. This is an example of a right-sided unilateral weakness, with no response in the right ear and the calculated unilateral weakness (UW) is 100%. (**b**)This is an example of bilateral CW. It is important to pay attention to the scale on the *x*-axis. Caloric responses of both ears fall below 12 degrees/s per side which is consistent with bilateral CW

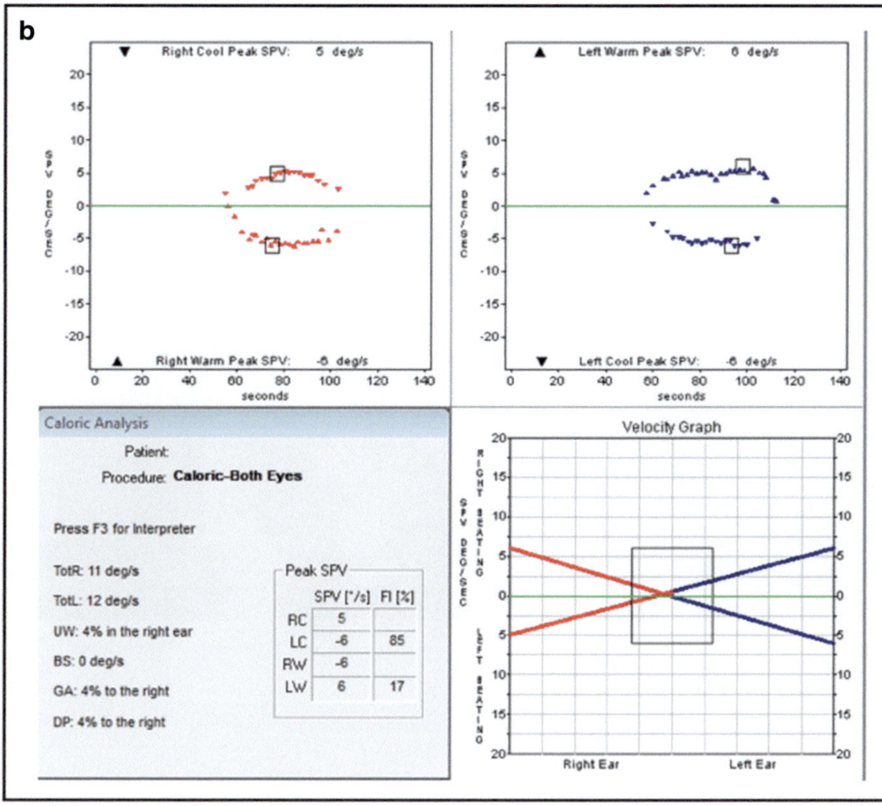

Fig. 4.6 (continued)

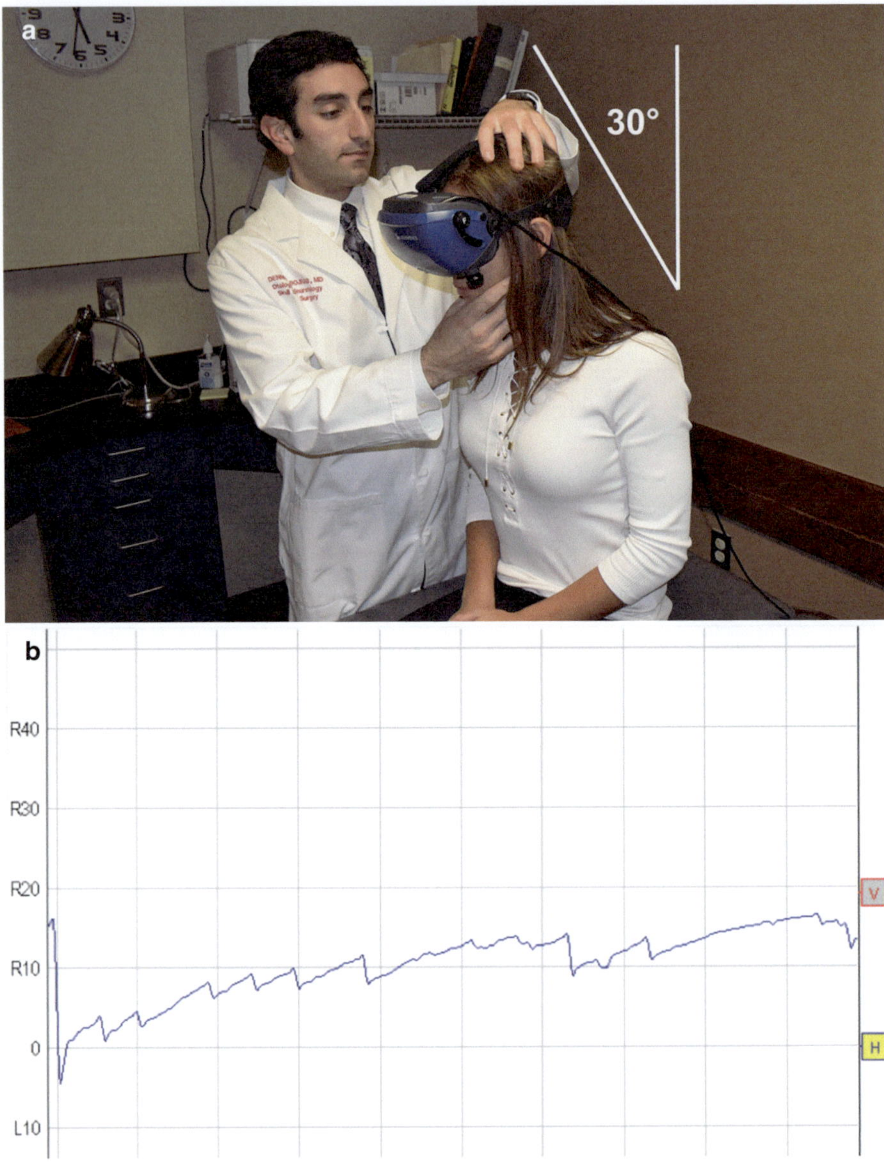

Fig. 4.7 Head shake nystagmus. (**a**) The head is held tilted down roughly 30° to bring the lateral canal into the horizontal plane. Rotation laterally 30–45° side to side at 1–2 hz is done for 10–15 s. The patient's head is abruptly stopped and the patient's eyes are observed. (**b**) If peripheral vestibular dysfunction is present, then, a few beats of nystagmus are usually seen, typically away from the affected side. In this case, there is left beating nystagmus after the head shake

Non-vestibular Tests

1. Visual oculomotor function or non-vestibular (tracking) eye movements
    (a) Saccade test
    (b) Tracking or pursuit test
    (c) Optokinetic test

Saccade Test

The saccade control system generates all voluntary and involuntary fast eye movements. The purpose of the saccade system is to be able to capture visual targets in the periphery of the visual field and focus them onto the fovea. Saccade testing is performed at the beginning of the VNG while calibrating eye movements. The patient's eye movements are compared to the target stimuli and the analysis typically yields measurements of saccade accuracy, latency, and velocity. A variety of saccade paradigms exist from the various manufacturers. The most common test is of horizontal and vertical eye movements during fixation on a computer-controlled visual target that goes back and forth in the horizontal plane in a random sequence (Fig. 4.8). The interpretation of saccade data must take into account patient variabilities such as age, cognitive status, attention to task, visual acuity, sedation, sleep deprivation, comprehension level, and medications. Symmetrically inaccurate or slow saccades are often attributable to one or more of those variables. Characteristic saccade abnormalities can suggest relatively specific sites of lesion and can provide for differentiating between brainstem and posterior cerebellar vermis involvement. The conditions such as internuclear ophthalmoplegia (INO) result from a lesion in the medial longitudinal fasciculus that causes a reduction in the neural signal to the ipsilateral medial rectus muscle (adduction) and preserved lateral rectus-mediated movements (abduction). The resulting saccades in the INO demonstrate slow velocity of adduction eye movements and overshoot for the abduction eye movements. Errors of saccade accuracy include hypometric and hypermetric saccades and may suggest a cerebellar disorder, whereas abnormal saccade slowing may suggest an abnormality of the parapontine reticular formation of the brainstem [12].

Tracking Test

The smooth pursuit testing is conducted by having a patient follow a computer-controlled visual target that typically moves in a sinusoidal pattern that varies in frequency over time (Fig. 4.9). Patients' variables can negatively impact performance and interfere with interpretation. The most common abnormality is the presence of "catch-up" saccades. Smooth pursuit is the most sensitive of ocular motor tests, but it provides poor lesion site localization with the multiple pathways involved

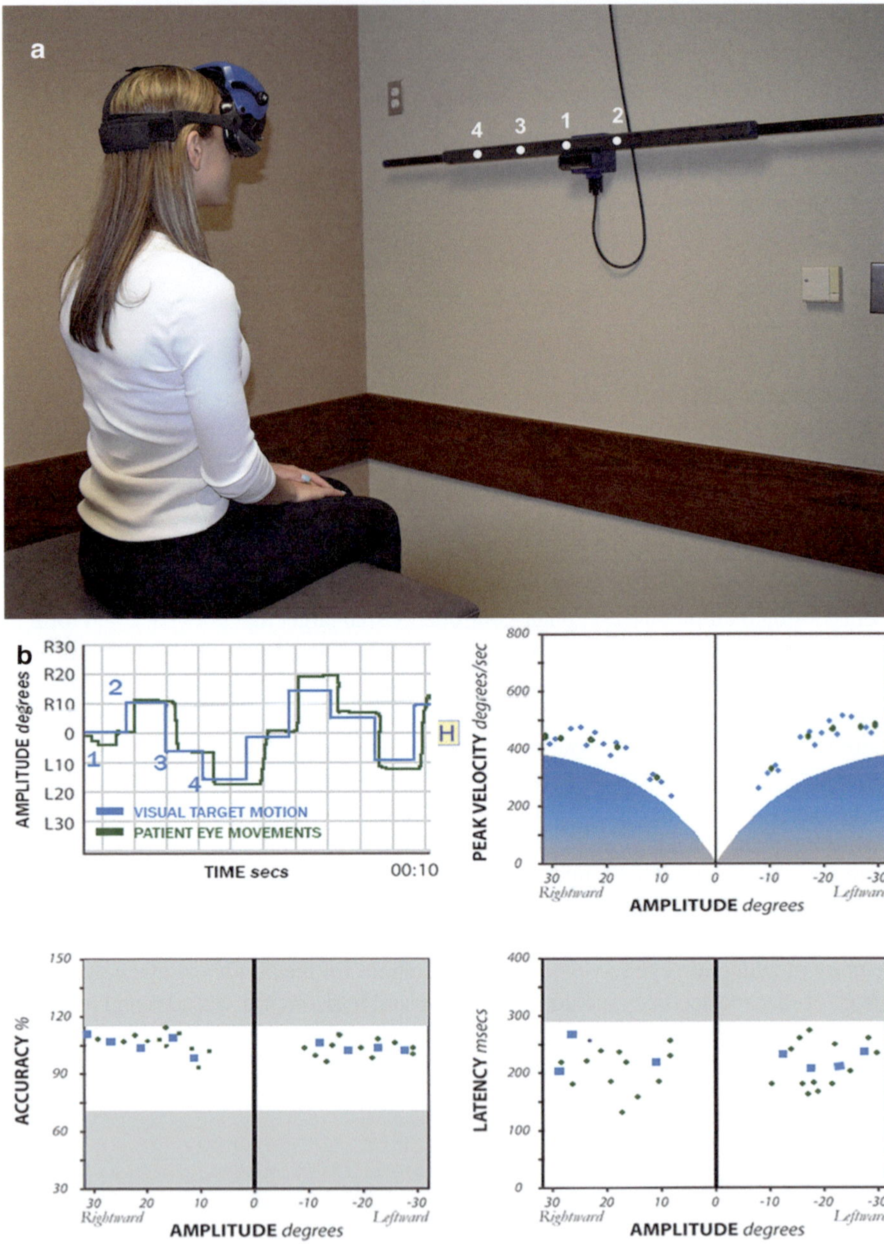

Fig. 4.8 Saccade test simulation. (**a**) Light targets are presented in random locations along the strip in a sequential manner, which results in a step configuration on horizontal oculography. (**b**) The patient's eyes peak velocity, accuracy, and latency are plotted as seen above

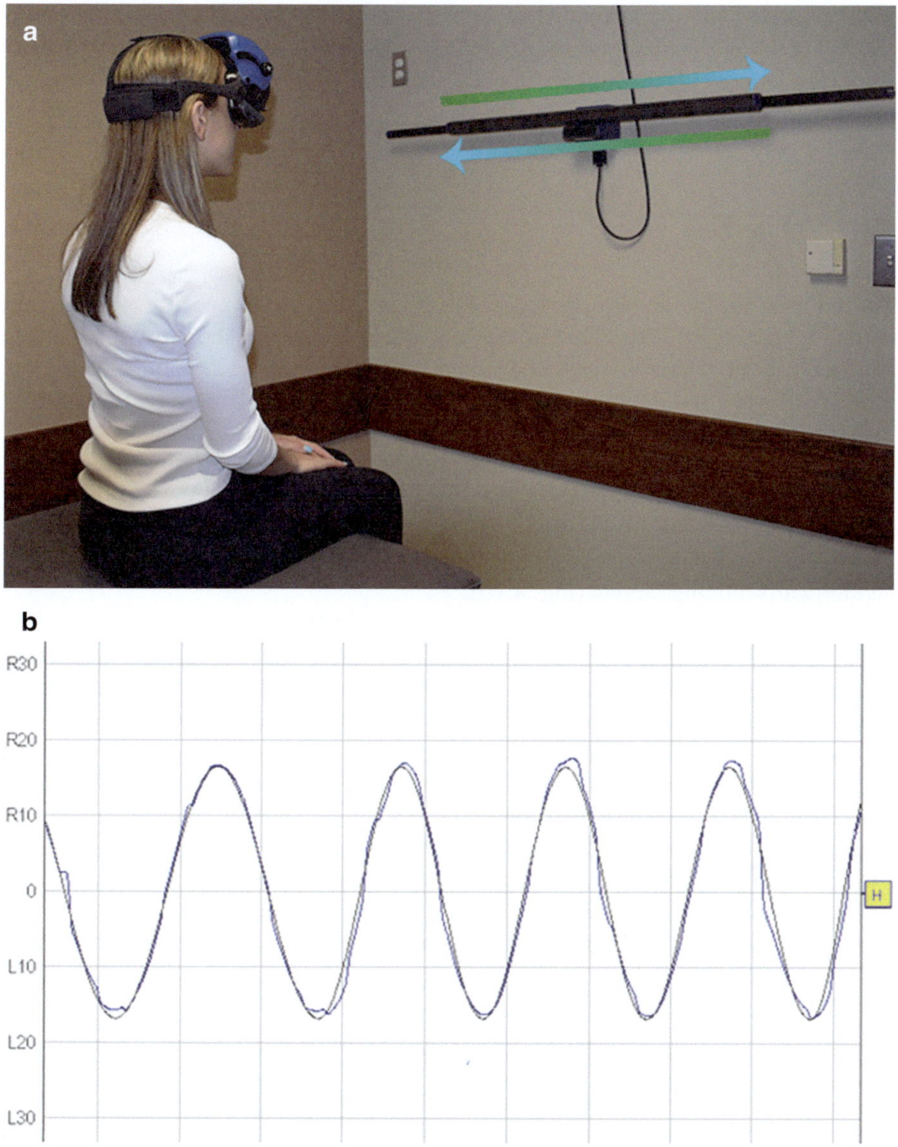

Fig. 4.9 (**a**) Standard setup for smooth pursuit. (**b**) Oculographic recording of smooth pursuit

in the pursuit generation. Abnormalities with pursuit are typically taken as an indication of possible vestibulocerebellar region involvement. Asymmetrically impaired pursuit is a more specific finding and suggest a unilateral hemispheric or asymmetrical posterior fossa lesion [3, 27].

Optokinetic Test

The stimulus for the optokinetic test varies by laboratory. The specific methods and stimuli used in the optokinetic test vary according to testing laboratory. In one version, the patient's horizontal eye movements are monitored while following a series of visual targets that move to the right and then to the left. This stimulus evokes a nystagmus with the slow phase in the direction of target motion, periodically interrupted by fast phases in the opposite direction. The optokinetic test, like the tracking test, is a test of eye pursuit pathways, and the results of the tracking and optokinetic tests show concordance with tasks of similar difficulty. In normal individuals, the slow-phase eye velocities approximately match target velocities for both rightward- and leftward-moving targets (Fig. 4.10).

The production of true optokinetic nystagmus (OKN) involves a combination of the neurologic substrate involved with smooth pursuit tracking together with areas that respond to moving visual stimuli in a full-field format but do not respond to head movement, the so-called optokinetic areas. When viewing a full-field stimulus, the initiation of the nystagmus is dominantly a result of smooth pursuit tracking with the OKN component added as the stimulus is continued requiring seconds to fully develop. The response then continues as a combination of both smooth pursuit tracking and optokinetics. Therefore, to evaluate OKN function in the isolation from smooth pursuit, one must take advantage of a perseveration of nystagmus caused by stimulation of the optokinetic system when the person is suddenly put into the dark after a minimum of 30 s worth of stimulation, called optokinetic after nystagmus (OKAN). As soon as the target has been extinguished for 1 s, the smooth

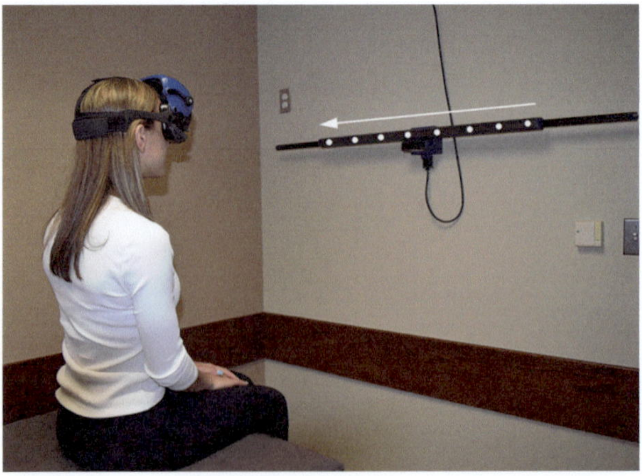

Fig. 4.10 Optokinetic test setup from our laboratory. A train of dots is passed across the strip while the patient is asked to count the number of dots

pursuit system no longer has any influence and the OKAN is a direct result of the activity of the optokinetic system reflected through the area of the brainstem referred to as the velocity storage system. Abnormal responses can reflect abnormal fast-phase velocity or abnormal slow-phase velocity. Abnormal OKN has a localizing value that is similar to smooth pursuit, although the sensitivity is poorer [1].

Benefits of ENG/VNG

Although ENG has correlates with many portions of the physical examination, it is an important part of the evaluation of many patients with complaints of dizziness or balance disturbance. Electronystagmographic testing has a number of advantages: [1] the results of the test are quantified, and there are well-defined normal limits; [2] the bithermal caloric test cannot be done as accurately without the precise stimulus control and response quantification provided by ENG; [3] because ENG provides accurate documentation of results, it can be used to follow up the patient with known vestibular disease; [4] standardized documentation is helpful in medical–legal and workers' compensation cases; and [5] it is the only test that assesses each ear separately and can give side-of-lesion localizing information.

Limitations of ENG/VNG

It is important to recognize that caloric stimulation tests only the lateral semicircular canal and provides little information about the status of the posterior or superior semicircular canals, utricle, or saccule. Traditional ENG testing using electro-oculography is also relatively insensitive to torsional nystagmus because rotational movement of the eye about the axis of the pupil does not move the cornea with respect to any of the skin electrodes. However, this limitation is easily overcome using VNG.

The results of ENG testing may fluctuate in concordance with the patient's disease process. Two of the more common illnesses seen in vestibular clinics are BPPV and Meniere's disease. Both illnesses can be associated with a normal ENG despite "classic" symptomatology. For example, on the day of testing a patient with complaints consistent with BPPV, the response may have been fatigued or the disease may have gone into remission. For that patient, the test results may be normal or indicate a unilateral vestibular weakness on the suspected side. Nevertheless, we maintain clinical suspicion of BPPV and ask the patient to return for retesting on a particularly "dizzy day." Similarly, the patient suspected of having Meniere's disease may have a normal ENG early in the course of the illness, and only later, will the caloric evaluation demonstrate a unilateral peripheral weakness, gaze-evoked nystagmus, or even spontaneous nystagmus. It is best to have patients abstain from vestibular suppressant medications (e.g., diazepam) for at least 48–72 h prior to

ENG testing, as they can also cause a "false-negative" test or show abnormal central vestibular function.

Some patients may present with dizziness not related to vestibular system dysfunction, e.g., syncope or presyncope, vertebral-basilar insufficiency, migraine-associated dizziness, multiple sclerosis, ocular dizziness, motion sickness syndrome, or cardiovascular disease. In these patients, a unilateral weakness found on ENG does not necessarily implicate vestibular dysfunction as the cause of their symptoms. The ENG finding may be incidental and must be considered in light of the clinical history and physical examination.

Summary

Electronystagmography testing is an important tool in the management of the patient with dizziness. It is by no means a substitute for a thorough neurotologic history and physical examination, and the results should be interpreted in light of the clinical evaluation. Those who use ENG testing should have a thorough understanding of how the test is performed, what its components are, and the significance of the results. When used properly, ENG/VNG is the single most valuable test currently available in the vestibular laboratory.

Acknowledgements We would like to personally thank our amazing audiology colleagues, specifically Jaclyn Ranker Au.D. and Rachel Beckley Au.D, for all their help with both the compiling of images for our figures and the descriptions of these figures.

Bibliography

1. Baloh RW, Honrubia V. Clinical neurophysiology of the vestibular system. Philadelphia: FA Davis; 1990.
2. Leigh RJ, Zee DS. The neurology of eye movements. Philadelphia: FA Davis; 1991.
3. Stockwell CW. Vestibular testing: past, present, future. Br J Audiol. 1997;31:387–98.
4. Bhansali SA, Honrubia V. Current status of electronystagmography testing. Otolaryngol Head Neck Surg. 1999;120:419–26.
5. Bhansali SA, Stockwell CW, Bojrab DI. Oscillopsia in patients with loss of vestibular function. Otolaryngol Head Neck Surg. 1993;109:120–5.
6. Stockwell CW, Bojrab DI. Background and technique of rotational testing. In: Jacobson GP, Newman CW, Kartush JM, editors. Handbook of balance function testing. St. Louis: Mosby-Year Book; 1993. p. 237–48.
7. McClure JA. Horizontal canal benign positional vertigo. J Otolaryngol. 1985;14:30–5.
8. Pagnini P, Nuti D, Vannucchi P. Benign positional vertigo of the horizontal canal. ORL J Otorhinolaryngol Relat Spec. 1989;51:161–70.
9. Stockwell CW, Bojrab DI. Vestibular function tests. In: Paparella MM, et al., editors. Otolaryngology. 3rd ed. Philadelphia: WB Saunders; 1991. p. 921–48.
10. Leigh RJ, Robinson DA, Zee DS. A hypothetical explanation for periodic alternating nystagmus: instability in the optokinetic-vestibular system. Ann N Y Acad Sci. 1981;374:619–35.

11. Barber HO, Stockwell CW. Annual of electronystagmography. St Louis: Mosby; 1980.
12. Leigh RJ, Zee DS. The neurology of eye movements, vol. 393. 2nd ed. Philadelphia: FA Davis; 1991. p. 416–8.
13. Highstein SM, Baker R. Excitatory termination of abducens internuclear neurons on medial rectus motoneurons: relationship to syndrome of internuclear ophthalmoplegia. J Neurophysiol. 1978;41:1647–61.
14. Paige G. Caloric vestibular responses despite canal inactivation. Invest Ophthalmol Vis Sci. 1984;25(Suppl):229–32.
15. Scherer H, Brandt U, Clarke AH, et al. European vestibular experiments on the spacelab I mission, III: caloric nystagmus in microgravity. Exp Brain Res. 1986;64:255.
16. Bhansali SA. Other caloric tests. In: Arenberg JK, editor. Dizziness and balance disorders. New York: Kugler; 1993. p. 283–7.
17. Jongkees LBW, Philipszoon AJ. Electronystagmography. Acta Otolaryngol. 1964;198(Suppl 189):55.
18. Ford CR, Stockwell CW. Reliabilities of air and water caloric responses. Arch Otolaryngol. 1978;104:380.
19. Baloh RW, Solingen L, Sills AW, Honrubia V. Caloric testing I: effect of different conditions of ocular fixation. Ann Otol Rhinol Laryngol. 1977;86(Suppl 43):1–6.
20. Custer DD, Black FO, Hemenway WG, Thorby JI. The sequential bithermal caloric test, I: a statistical analysis of normal subject responses. Ann Otol Rhinol Laryngol. 1973;83(Suppl 6):3–9.
21. Hamersma H. The caloric test: a nystagmographical study (thesis). Amsterdam: University of Amsterdam; 1957.
22. Mehra YG. Electronystagmography: a study of caloric tests in normal subjects. J Laryngol Otol. 1964;78:520.
23. Betnitez JT, Bouchard KR, Choe YK. Air calorics: a technique and results. Ann Otol Rhinol Laryngol. 1978;87:216.
24. Hain TC, Fretter M, Zee DS. Head shaking nystagmus in patients with unilateral peripheral vestibular lesions. Am J Otolaryngol. 1987;8:36–47.
25. Takahashi S, Fetter M, Koenig E, et al. The clinical significance of head shaking nystagmus in the dizzy patient. Acta Oto-Laryngol. 1990;109:8–14.
26. Kamei T, Kornhuber HH. Spontaneous and head shaking nystagmus in normal and in patients with central lesions. Can J Otolaryngol. 1979;3:372–80.
27. Waldorf RA. Observations of eye movements related to vestibular and other neurological problems using the house infrared/video ENG system. In: Arenberg IK, editor. Dizziness and balance disorders. New York: Kugler; 1993. p. 277–81.

Chapter 5
The Vestibulo-Ocular Reflex and Head Impulse Testing

Erika McCarty Walsh and Dennis I. Bojrab

Eye movements resulting from low-frequency rotational testing are composed of slow and fast phases of nystagmus. The slow phase is directed by VOR and the fast phase is a result of compensation by the paramedian pontine reticular formation, which causes the saccadic eye movements. Linear analysis of the VOR cumulative eye position results in relatively accurate gain and phase because of the apparent linearity of the system. Phase and gain change abnormalities are the basis of the testing paradigm.

Vestibulo-Ocular Reflex

The vestibulo-ocular reflex (VOR) is a vestigial reflex that serves to maintain visual focus on a target during head movement. The reflex arc includes the end organs of balance—the 3 paired semicircular canals and 2 paired otolith organs—the vestibular and oculomotor nuclei, and extraocular muscles; it is also under modulatory control by the cerebellum [1, 2]. VOR can be suppressed when desired, such as when reading in a moving vehicle, and it is most active with high-frequency head movements greater than 2 Hz. In fact, at slower frequencies, eye movements are under the control of a variety of reflexes, including optokinetics, smooth pursuit, and the cervico-ocular reflex. Therefore, high-frequency head movements specifically test VOR and, by proxy, the peripheral vestibular system [3].

E. M. Walsh
Department of Otolaryngology, University of Alabama, Birmingham, AL, USA

D. I. Bojrab (✉)
Department of Otolaryngology - Head and Neck Surgery, The University of Alabama at Birmingham, Birmingham, AL, USA

J. C. Lucas et al. (eds.), *Diagnosis and Treatment of Vestibular Disorders*,
https://doi.org/10.1007/978-3-032-11740-3_5

Head movement stimulates the semicircular canal (or canals) ipsilateral and in the plane of the head movement; simultaneously, the contralateral semicircular canals are inhibited. First, this afferent signal travels to the ipsilateral vestibular nucleus. The signal then decussates, traveling to and stimulating the contralateral abducens nucleus. Internuclear neurons travel via the medial longitudinal fasciculus to the ipsilateral oculomotor nucleus. The sum of these signals is a slow eye movement opposite the head movement. For example, head movement to the left would result in an excitatory impulse to the right abducens nucleus and left oculomotor nucleus, creating contraction of the right lateral rectus and left medial rectus with resultant movement of both eyes to the right. The eyes remain focused on their target, and the visual scene is not disturbed by head motion [3]. The particular set of semicircular canals and otolithic end organs stimulated by a head motion is determined by the location of the head relative to gravity, the rotation in x, y, and z axes, and the amount of pitch (rotation around an axis through the external auditory canals), yaw (rotation around a cranial caudal axis), and roll (rotation around an anterior to posterior axis) [2, 4]. Results of VOR testing are often expressed in terms of gain—a numeric value derived from the ratio of the area under the curve of eye velocity and the area under the curve of head velocity [3]. Gain of 1 suggests perfect compensation of eye movements with head movement. When VOR fails, corrective saccades re-center the point of interest on the gaze; they are typically contralateral to the direction of stimulation. The movement of the target in the visual scene, known as retinal slip, targets visual refixation on the target [5]. Overt saccades are easily visible by an observer testing the vestibular system, and are the basis of bedside head impulse testing (see below) [6]. In contrast, covert saccades are not readily detectable by a clinician and require objective, precise measurement of eye movement and head movement [7].

Described by Barany in his work on the vestibular system that ultimately won the Nobel Prize in 1914, caloric testing was long the gold standard test of peripheral vestibular function [8]. However, caloric testing is generally a specific testing of the horizontal semicircular canals and, by extension, the superior vestibular nerve. Therefore, interest grew in provocative tests that evaluate the VOR and, by extension, the function of any of the 3 paired semicircular canals and otolith end organs. In general, these provocative tests can be divided into whole-body or head-only impulse testing. Whole-body impulse testing in the form of rotary chair gained popularity in the 1980s as a way to evaluate the VOR. However, rotary chair testing is limited by the frequency a rotary chair can produce and the velocity patients can tolerate. Frequencies more than 1 Hz are technically infeasible, which confounds results given the non-vestibular reflexes that dominate eye movements at these frequencies [9]. In contrast, the head alone can be rotated rapidly to reach VOR-specific frequencies of greater than 2 Hz; this is referred to as head-only impulse testing. Head-only impulse testing can be classified into active and passive testing. In active testing, patients are in control of head motion; in passive testing, the examiner controls the patient's head movements.

Halmagyi and Curthoys first described passive head impulse testing in 1988. In this testing paradigm, the head is rapidly turned by the examiner 15–20° from neutral in one direction while the patient is instructed to fix their gaze on a central midpoint. The patient is observed for overt catch-up saccades, suggestive of vestibular dysfunction ipsilateral to the direction of the head turn [6]. If the vestibular end organs in the plane of head thrust on the ipsilateral side are hypofunctioning, the VOR will fail and eyes will drift with head movement; therefore, a corrective saccade to the contralateral side will be necessary to re-center the visual scene. Scleral search coils have been used with this paradigm to provide objective data about eye movements; however, comfort and expense make this technique of limited clinical utility [3]. While bedside head thrust testing is appealing for its simplicity, its sensitivity is too low to function independently as a test of peripheral vestibular function; it is, however, highly specific [10]. The position of the head during head thrust can be altered to more specifically test particular semicircular canals or otolithic end organs. Clinical evaluation of catch-up saccades has provided quick, simple bedside testing of peripheral vestibular function and can provide valuable evaluation about the semicircular canals and otolithic end organs [11].

In active head thrust or autorotational testing, subjects rotate their heads while fixing their gaze on a central target. They are directed to rapidly rotate their heads in response to auditory stimulation in the form of clicks or beeps; these sound cues result in head shake in the range of 2–6 Hz. Electro-oculography with electrodes at the lateral canthi bilaterally is used to obtain objective measurements of eye movement [12]. The gain measured in autorotational testing has proven valuable in a number of clinical scenarios. Use of this testing has revealed a significant decrease in gain with cisplatin (vestibulotoxic chemotherapy) [13], increased gain in Meniere's disease [14], and decreased gain in acoustic neuroma that positively correlates in many cases to the size of the tumor [15]. Similarly, autorotational testing has been shown to pick up peripheral vestibular pathology that caloric testing may miss when compared head to head [16]. However, volitional head movements can still be confounded by secondary reflexes, such as the cervico-ocular reflex, even at high frequencies [2]. Therefore, autorotational testing has fallen out of favor.

Passive head-only impulse testing has taken a modern form in video head impulse testing (vHIT). The vHIT testing involves high-impulse head movements combined with video software that measures pupil velocity. For patients, it is a relatively simple and non-invasive test; instead of electro-oculography or scleral coils, a set of goggles that precisely track pupil movements are worn (Fig. 5.1). Data suggest that this tracking technology is equivalent to the precision seen with scleral search coils, while being more comfortable and cost-effective [17]. Two sets of data can be collected with the vHIT technology. In head impulse testing or HIMP testing, the patient fixes their gaze on a set target while an examiner performs head thrust maneuvers. Eye and head velocities, along with overt and covert catch-up saccades, are recorded. Secondary data can be obtained with suppression head impulse or SHIMP testing. In this paradigm, the stimulus of rapid, passive, unpredictable head turns is unchanged; however, the visual target moves with the patient's head. In contrast to HIMP testing, patients with normal vestibular function make the catch-up saccade as they overcome VOR to fix on the visual target [18]. In contrast, patients with vestibular dysfunction are able to track the moving target freely with rapid head thrust. SHIMP testing eliminates the need to monitor for overt saccades in patients with peripheral vestibular pathology, with easy interpretation of results

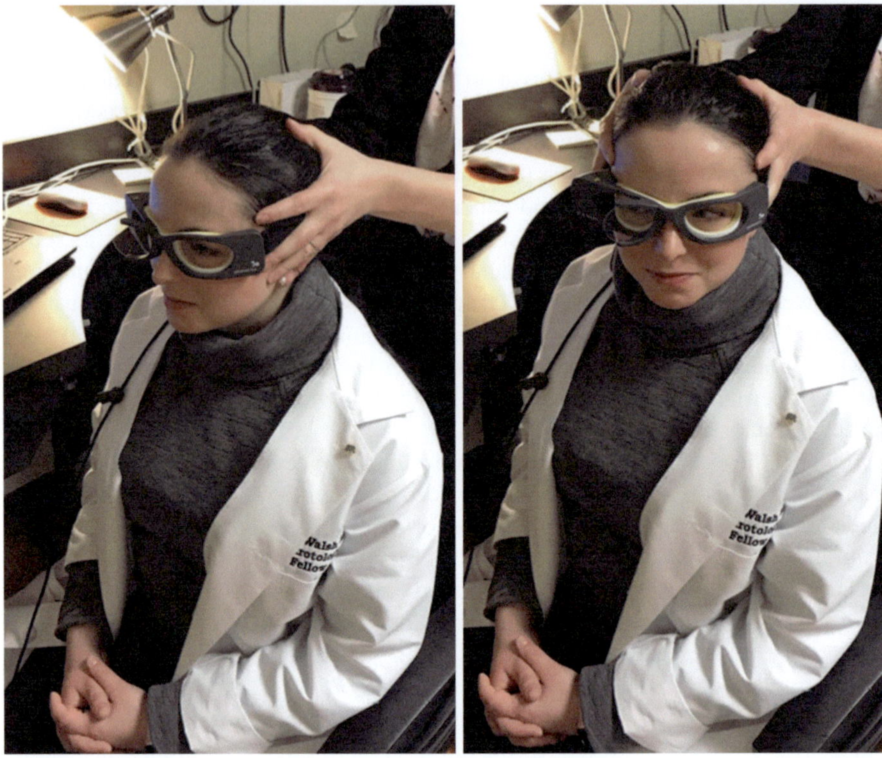

Fig. 5.1 The testing setup for video head impulse test. At left, neutral head position with video goggles in place. Right: after thrust 15–20° lateral, patient continues to fix their eyes on a midline target

[3, 19]. As with bedside head thrust testing, the position of the head during the examination can be manipulated to provide information more specific to certain portion of the peripheral vestibular system. These datasets are complementary and can provide significant information for the examiner about the function of the peripheral vestibular system.

Some authors have suggested that vHIT may replace caloric testing as the gold standard screen for peripheral vestibular system function, and it has shown significant promise (Figs. 5.2 and 5.3). vHIT has shown value in a number of clinical scenarios. In acoustic neuroma, vHIT shows ipsilesional decreased gain and presence of catch-up saccades. Similarly, decreases in gain have been shown to positively correlate with tumor size [20]. In acute vestibular neuritis, vHIT

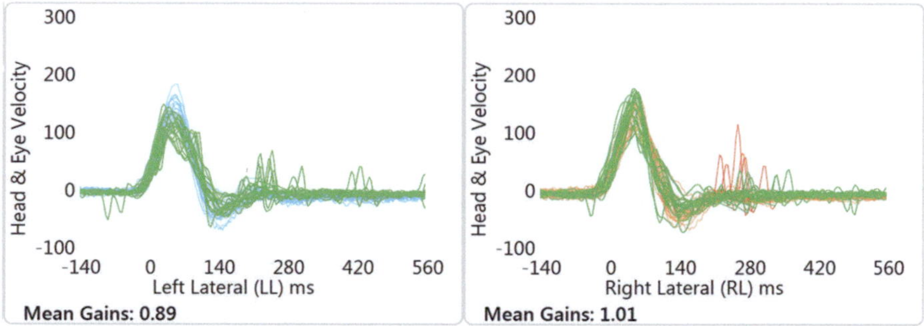

Fig. 5.2 Normal vHIT tracing. Blue represents head thrust to the left (in this case, in the plane of the lateral semicircular canal); orange represents head thrust to the right. The green tracing is calculated vestibulo-ocular reflex activity during head thrust. In normal patients, there is excellent compensation for head thrust by the VOR

both can show unilateral weakness in terms of ipsilesional reduced gain and presence of catch-up saccades and improvement in ipsilesional gain that correlates with clinical recovery [21] (Fig. 5.4). In Meniere's disease, outside of active vertigo, vHIT testing can be variable and may be normal or gain may be decreased [22]. In Meniere's disease, significant decrease in vHIT gain after ablative intratympanic gentamicin injection has been shown to correlate with symptom control [23]. Additionally, vHIT provides two complementary forms of data in calculations of gain and presence of saccades, and the presence of catch-up saccades in the presence of normal calculated gain may still be of significant clinical importance in some scenarios [24, 25]. However, McCaslin et al. found that mild unilateral peripheral weakness (<40% UW) detectable on caloric testing may be missed with measurement of vHIT gain [26]. Others have found that caloric testing is more sensitive than vHIT in detecting unilateral weakness associated with acoustic neuroma [27]. vHIT continues to grow in clinical use and is a valuable complementary test in the peripheral vestibular test battery, but further research is needed to determine its utility in various clinical scenarios.

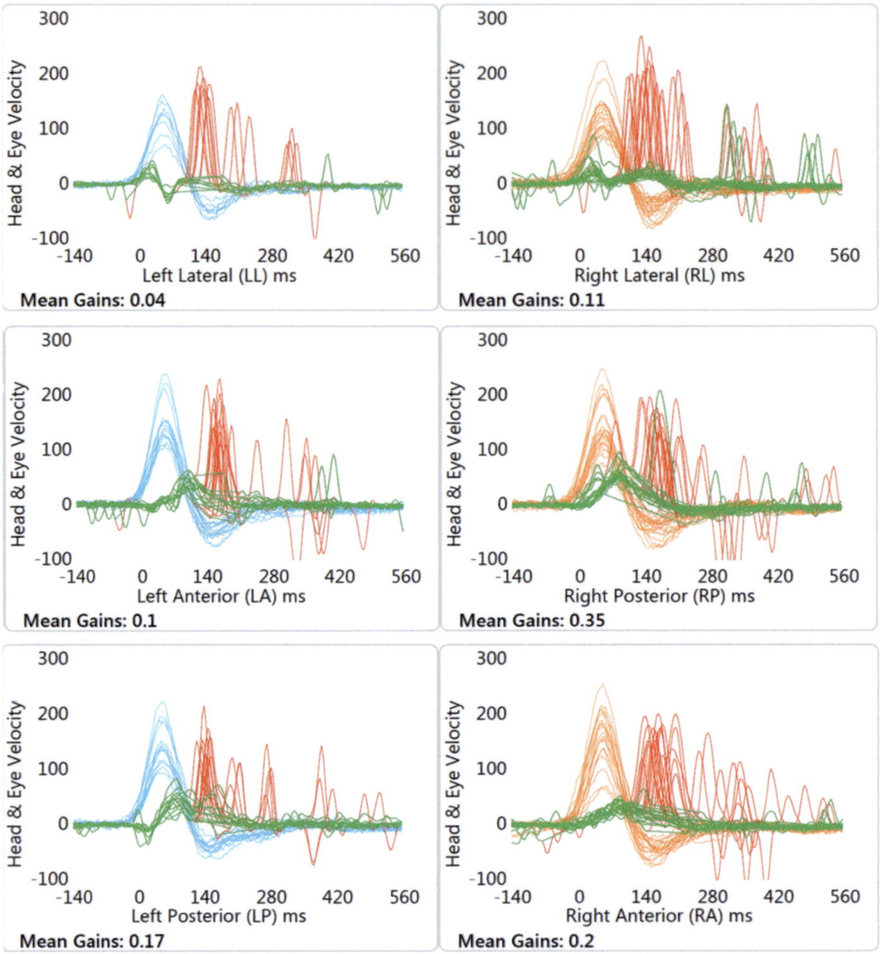

Fig. 5.3 vHIT in bilateral vestibular loss. Blue represents head thrust to the left; orange represents head thrust to the right. The green tracing is calculated vestibulo-ocular reflex activity during head thrust. Red represents compensatory saccades. Head thrust in either direction in the planes of all semicircular canals shows decreased VOR activity compared to head thrust with catch-up saccades noted. Note that for testing of the anterior and posterior canals, the contralateral thrust is to the appropriate LARP or RALP pairing. Top panel: lateral canal testing, middle panel: LARP testing, bottom panel: RALP testing

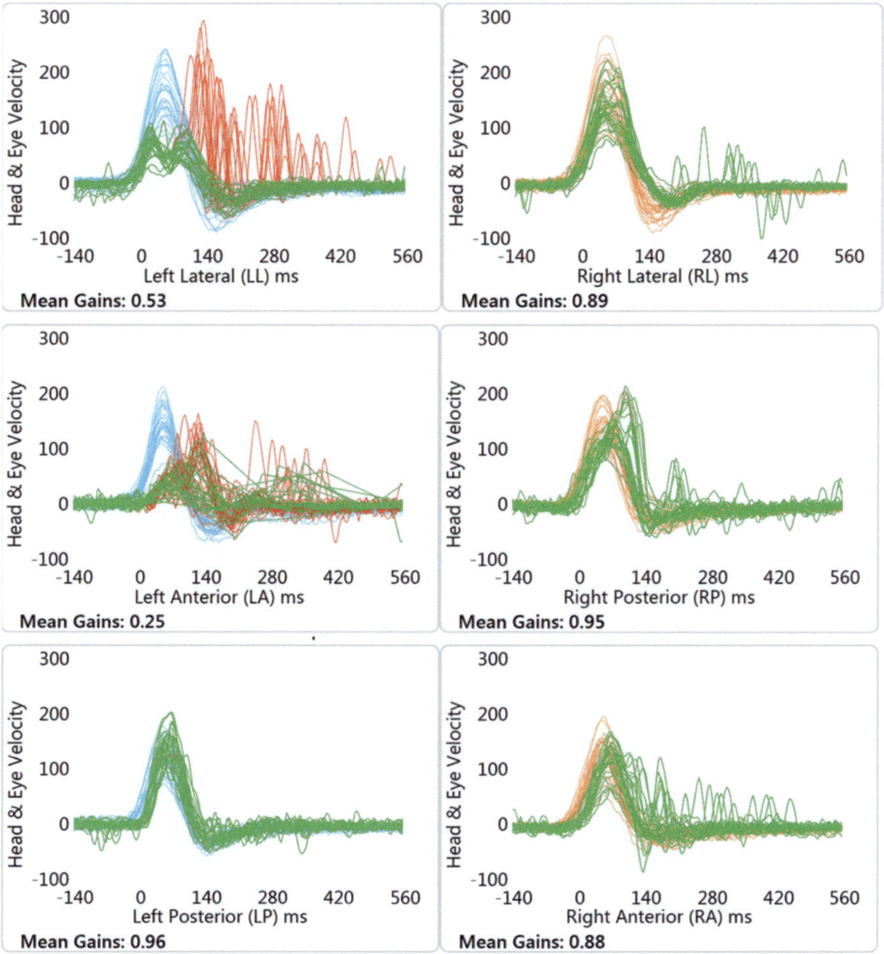

Fig. 5.4 vHIT in acute left superior vestibular neuritis. Blue represents head thrust to the left; orange represents head thrust to the right. The green tracing is calculated vestibulo-ocular reflex activity during head thrust. Red represents compensatory saccades. On head thrust to the ipsilesional side for the lateral and anterior semicircular canals, VOR activity is decreased compared to head thrust and catch-up saccades are noted (top and middle panels). vHIT tracings, in contrast, for the ipsilesional posterior semicircular canal are expectedly normal (bottom panel). Note that for testing of the anterior and posterior canals, the contralateral thrust is to the appropriate LARP or RALP pairing

References

1. Beh SC, Frohman TC, Frohman EM. Cerebellar control of eye movements. J Neuro-Ophthalmol. 2017;37(1):87–98. https://doi.org/10.1097/WNO.0000000000000456.
2. Furman JM. Rotational testing. Handb Clin Neurol. 2016;137:177–86. https://doi.org/10.1016/B978-0-444-63437-5.00012-1.
3. Halmagyi GM, Chen L, MacDougall HG, Weber KP, McGarvie LA, Curthoys IS. The video head impulse test. Front Neurol. 2017;8:258. https://doi.org/10.3389/fneur.2017.00258.
4. Kheradmand A, Zee DS. The bedside examination of the vestibulo-ocular reflex (VOR): an update. Rev Neurol (Paris). 2012;168(10):710–9. https://doi.org/10.1016/j.neurol.2012.07.011.
5. Schubert MC, Hall CD, Das V, Tusa RJ, Herdman SJ. Oculomotor strategies and their effect on reducing gaze position error. Otol Neurotol. 2010;31(2):228–31. https://doi.org/10.1097/MAO.0b013e3181c2dbae.
6. Halmagyi GM, Curthoys IS. A clinical sign of canal paresis. Arch Neurol. 1988;45(7):737–9.
7. Weber KP, Aw ST, Todd MJ, McGarvie LA, Curthoys IS, Halmagyi GM. Head impulse test in unilateral vestibular loss: vestibulo-ocular reflex and catch-up saccades. Neurology. 2008;70(6):454–63. https://doi.org/10.1212/01.wnl.0000299117.48935.2e.
8. Robert Barany (1876–1936). Investigator of labyrinthine function. JAMA. 1965;191:132–3.
9. Jenkins HA, Honrubia V, Baloh RH. Evaluation of multiple-frequency rotatory testing in patients with peripheral labyrinthine weakness. Am J Otolaryngol. 1982;3(3):182–8.
10. Harvey SA, Wood DJ, Feroah TR. Relationship of the head impulse test and head-shake nystagmus in reference to caloric testing. Am J Otol. 1997;18(2):207–13.
11. Kessler P, Tomlinson D, Blakeman A, Rutka J, Ranalli P, Wong A. The high-frequency/acceleration head heave test in detecting otolith diseases. Otol Neurotol. 2007;28(7):896–904.
12. Fineberg R, O'Leary DP, Davis LL. Use of active head movements for computerized vestibular testing. Arch Otolaryngol Head Neck Surg. 1987;113(10):1063–5.
13. Kitsigianis GA, O'Leary DP, Davis LL. Active head-movement analysis of cisplatin-induced vestibulotoxicity. Otolaryngol Head Neck Surg. 1988;98(1):82–7. https://doi.org/10.1177/019459988809800114.
14. O'Leary DP, Davis LL. Vestibular autorotation testing of Menière's disease. Otolaryngol Head Neck Surg. 1990;103(1):66–71. https://doi.org/10.1177/019459989010300110.
15. O'Leary DP, Davis LL, Maceri DR. Vestibular autorotation test asymmetry analysis of acoustic neuromas. Otolaryngol Head Neck Surg. 1991;104(1):103–9. https://doi.org/10.1177/019459989110400119.
16. Saadat D, O'Leary DP, Pulec JL, Kitano H. Comparison of vestibular autorotation and caloric testing. Otolaryngol Head Neck Surg. 1995;113(3):215–22. https://doi.org/10.1016/S0194-5998(95)70109-5.
17. Macdougall HG, McGarvie LA, Halmagyi GM, Curthoys IS, Weber KP. The video head impulse test (vHIT) detects vertical semicircular canal dysfunction. PLoS One. 2013;8(4):e61488. https://doi.org/10.1371/journal.pone.0061488.
18. Crane BT, Demer JL. Latency of voluntary cancellation of the human vestibulo-ocular reflex during transient yaw rotation. Exp Brain Res. 1999;127(1):67–74.
19. Shen Q, Magnani C, Sterkers O, et al. Saccadic velocity in the new suppression head impulse test: a new indicator of horizontal Vestibular canal paresis and of vestibular compensation. Front Neurol. 2016;7:160. https://doi.org/10.3389/fneur.2016.00160.
20. Tranter-Entwistle I, Dawes P, Darlington CL, Smith PF, Cutfield N. Video head impulse in comparison to caloric testing in unilateral vestibular schwannoma. Acta Otolaryngol (Stockh). 2016;136(11):1110–4. https://doi.org/10.1080/00016489.2016.1185540.
21. Palla A, Straumann D. Recovery of the high-acceleration vestibulo-ocular reflex after vestibular neuritis. J Assoc Res Otolaryngol. 2004;5(4):427–35.
22. Cordero-Yanza JA, Arrieta Vázquez EV, Hernaiz Leonardo JC, Mancera Sánchez J, Hernández Palestina MS, Pérez-Fernández N. Comparative study between the caloric vestibular and

the video-head impulse tests in unilateral Menière's disease. Acta Otolaryngol (Stockh). 2017;137(11):1178–82. https://doi.org/10.1080/00016489.2017.1354395.
23. Nguyen KD, Minor LB, Della Santina CC, Carey JP. Vestibular function and vertigo control after intratympanic gentamicin for Ménière's disease. Audiol Neurootol. 2009;14(6):361–72. https://doi.org/10.1159/000241893.
24. Perez-Fernandez N, Eza-Nuñez P. Normal gain of VOR with refixation saccades in patients with unilateral Vestibulopathy. J Int Adv Otol. 2015;11(2):133–7. https://doi.org/10.5152/iao.2015.1087.
25. Pérez-Fernández N, Gallegos-Constantino V, Barona-Lleo L, Manrique-Huarte R. Clinical and video-assisted examination of the vestibulo-ocular reflex: a comparative study. Acta Otorrinolaringol Esp. 2012;63(6):429–35. https://doi.org/10.1016/j.otorri.2012.04.010.
26. McCaslin DL, Jacobson GP, Bennett ML, Gruenwald JM, Green AP. Predictive properties of the video head impulse test: measures of caloric symmetry and self-report dizziness handicap. Ear Hear. 2014;35(5):e185–91. https://doi.org/10.1097/AUD.0000000000000047.
27. Blödow A, Blödow J, Bloching MB, Helbig R, Walther LE. Horizontal VOR function shows frequency dynamics in vestibular schwannoma. Eur Arch Otorhinolaryngol. 2015;272(9):2143–8. https://doi.org/10.1007/s00405-014-3042-2.

Chapter 6
Rotary Chair Testing

Christopher K. Zalewski, Devin L. McCaslin, and Matthew L. Carlson

Introduction to Rotational Testing

Similar to the auditory system, the vestibular system's sensitivity range is significantly broader than what is needed for daily life activities. Specifically, the vestibular system's response characteristics are principally efficient and effective for a narrow range between 0.05 and 6 Hz. Figure 6.1 highlights the vestibular system's effectiveness for the narrow frequency range where natural head movements occur. Within the frequency range of natural head movements, the responsiveness of the vestibular system can be characterized as linear, capable of operating with nearly perfect vestibular ocular reflex (VOR) gain and phase [9, 14]. This is ideal, insomuch that the operating range of the VOR is functionally matched to those activities that are most common during ambulation, and particularly those active head movements that are associated with daily life activities.

Figure 6.1 also depicts the nonlinearity and lack of response unity (i.e., perfect gain) of the VOR for frequencies that occur above and below those associated with natural head movements. As can be seen, the efficiency of VOR gain and phase is significantly poorer for these frequencies. Unfortunately, the test stimulus that is most commonly used to clinically evaluate the vestibular system, the caloric stimulus, falls within this highly inefficient range and is, therefore, neither truly

C. K. Zalewski
Auditory and Vestibular Clinical Research Section (AVCRS), Neurotology Branch, National Institute on Deafness and Other Communication Disorders (NIDCD), National Institutes of Health (NIH), Bethesda, MD, USA
e-mail: zalewski@nidcd.nih.gov

D. L. McCaslin · M. L. Carlson (✉)
Department of Otolaryngology-Head and Neck Surgery, Mayo Clinic School of Medicine, Rochester, MN, USA
e-mail: mccaslin@med.umich.edu; carlson.matthew@mayo.edu

J. C. Lucas et al. (eds.), *Diagnosis and Treatment of Vestibular Disorders*,
https://doi.org/10.1007/978-3-032-11740-3_6

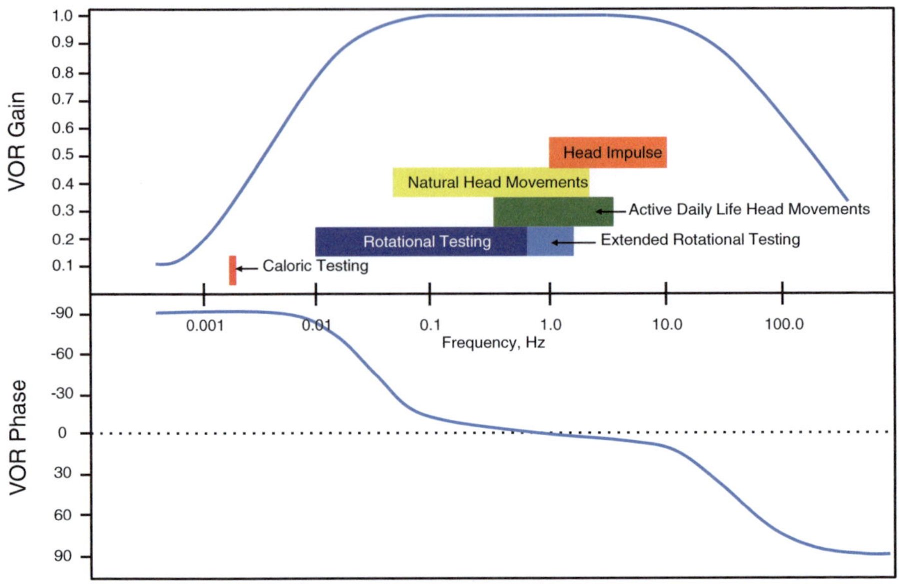

Fig. 6.1 Distribution of tests and head movements by frequency. Traditional rotational frequency range is from 0.01 to 0.64 Hz. Extended rotational frequency range can, at times, include through 2.0 Hz. Caloric test frequency is plotted at 0.003 Hz. Head impulse testing is between 1 and 10 Hz [5]. Response characteristics for gain and phase of the vestibular system (VOR) are superimposed on the frequency range. (Adapted from Wilson and Jones [14] and Goldberg et al. [9]). Note the linear response and near perfect phase of the VOR for natural and active head movements of daily life between 0.05 and 5 Hz

ideal nor representative of daily life activities. Moreover, the caloric stimulus is a relatively non-functional stimulus, being one of thermal convection rather than one of true motion. Rotational testing is uniquely situated to address both of these clinical shortcomings. First, the rotational stimuli are significantly closer in frequency to those encountered during daily life activities, and second, the rotational nature of the stimulus is more *natural*, being one of angular rotation. That being said, rotational testing may be best suited to evaluate vestibular physiology, and subsequently best suited to identify vestibular pathology.

Principles of Rotational Testing

Rotational testing delivers a repeatable, reliable, consistent, precise, and tolerable stimulus, which makes it an excellent clinical test for investigating the physiological response of the vestibular system. Because rotational stimuli are so precisely delivered across a broad frequency range, it has been suggested that rotational assessment should be the primary test of vestibular function, with videonystagmography (VNG) reserved as a complementary test [1].

In response to angular rotations in the yaw plane, the VOR is precisely recorded through electrooculography (EOG) or via high sampling-rate videographic (VOG) methods. Testing is conducted using a rotational chair housed in a lightproof enclosure, or at least conducted under vision-denied conditions, so as not to allow for any visual or optokinetic contributions when measuring the VOR (Fig. 6.2). Precise rotational paradigms have been well established and are applicable to a wide range of populations from very young patients to nonagenarians. Most commonly, rotational testing is usually comprised of a series of back-and-forth accelerations (oscillations), in addition to a series of abrupt, step-wise, accelerations followed by persistent rotations. Rotations are delivered to a seated patient via a computer-controlled torque-driven chair that can be finely tuned to apply exacting accelerations and velocities. With the head tilted downward by approximately 30° so as to place the horizontal semicircular canal in the horizontal plane for maximal stimulation (Fig. 6.3), the body and head can be precisely rotated at exacting frequencies from as slow as 0.003 Hz (that of the caloric stimulus) to as quick as 2.0 Hz. In addition, constant velocity stimuli as fast as 400–600°/s and accelerations as quick as 1000°/s^2 can also be delivered [7].

Fig. 6.2 Earth-vertical axis rotational chair

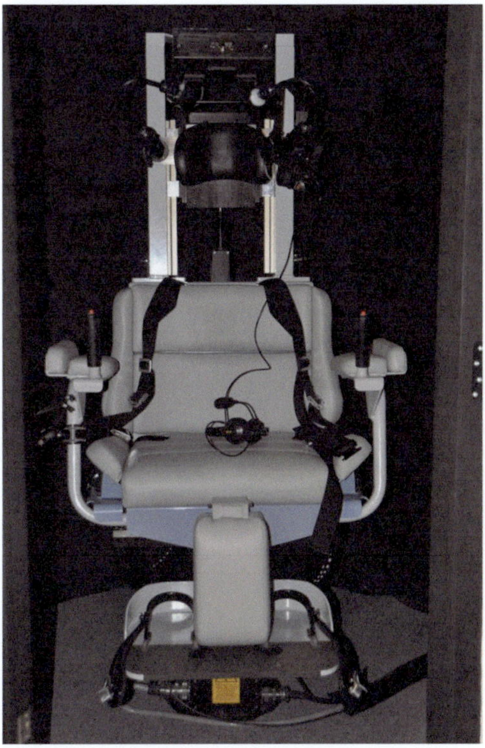

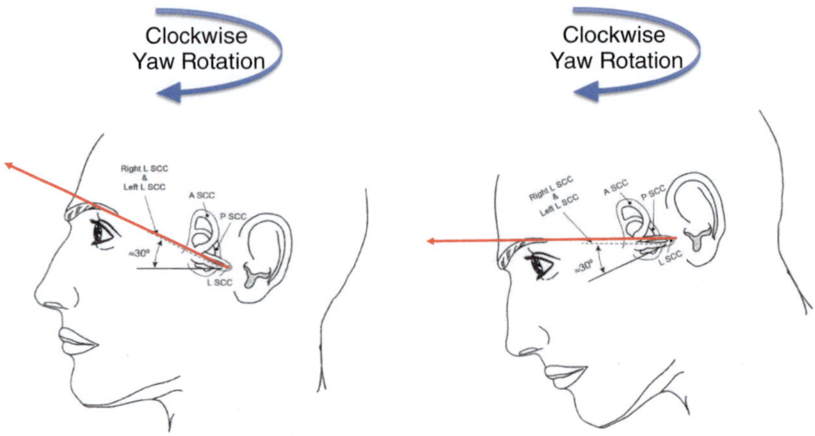

Fig. 6.3 Rotation around the earth-vertical axis is performed with the head tilted downward by 30° so as to align the horizontal semicircular canal in the optimal plane of [yaw] rotation (red arrow), thus maximizing excitation and inhibition in accordance with Ewald's law. (Adapted and reprinted with permission from Canalis and Lambert ([6], p. 120)

Rotational Test Protocols

There are two principal test protocols that are essential to a basic, or routine, clinical rotational vestibular assessment: sinusoidal harmonic acceleration (SHA) testing and velocity step testing (VST). Additional rotational tests are available, but may not be routinely performed during a standard clinical assessment. Such additional tests include fixation suppression, visual–vestibular enhancement, subjective visual vertical, subjective visual horizontal, unilateral centrifugation (UCF), off vertical axis rotation (OVAR), and chair head impulse testing (crHIT) (Table 6.1).

Table 6.1 Rotational test protocols

Test	Protocol	Stimuli parameters
Calibration	10° gaze right, left, up, and down.	Smooth pursuit between gaze positions or saccades.
Ocular motor	Routinely performed	Saccades, smooth pursuit, gaze, optokinetic pursuit, spontaneous testing
Sinusoidal harmonic acceleration (SHA)	Routinely performed	0.01, 0.02, 0.04, 0.08, 0.16, 0.32, 0.64 Hz[a] (higher frequencies optional)
Velocity (trapezoidal) step (VST)	Routinely performed	Low (60°) velocity step testing High (240°) velocity step testing
VOR suppression	Routine performed	0.08, 0.16, 0.32, 0.64 Hz (no higher than 1.0 Hz)
Visual–vestibular enhancement	Perform when clinically indicated (central/cerebellar/migraine)	0.08, 0.16, 0.32, 0.64 Hz (no higher than 1.0 Hz)
Unilateral centrifugation	Perform when clinically indicated (otolith)	SVV or SVH during static, On-center rotation, UCF-R, and UCF-L eccentric rotations; Generally high velocity 300°/s.
Off-vertical axis rotation (OVAR)	Perform when clinically indicated (otolith)[b]	VOR gain, VOR phase, VOR symmetry

[a]Minimum of 2 cycles performed for 0.01–0.02 Hz, 4 cycles for 0.04–0.08 Hz, and 8–10 cycles for 0.16–0.64 Hz

[b] Currently limited by the FDA to IRB-approved research only

Sinusoidal Harmonic Acceleration

When performing rotational testing, the primary test most often performed is SHA testing. Sinusoidal acceleration testing provides critical data regarding the responsiveness of the vestibular system across a broad frequency range (Fig. 6.1). This is essential when considering the role of the rotational testing in a comprehensive vestibular assessment, insomuch that vestibular lesions often impact the effectiveness of the vestibular system for detecting and transducing *low-frequency* movements (<0.1 Hz). Because of this, a bilateral vestibular lesion will often yield absent caloric responses (0.003 Hz), even though residual and even normal vestibular reactivity can objectively be measured for higher frequency stimuli (>0.1 Hz) like those conducted during SHA testing.

During SHA testing, a vertically upright individual is rotated (or oscillated) back and forth in the horizontal (or yaw) plane, while the responsiveness of the vestibular system to such rotations (i.e., the VOR) is determined across a known frequency range of stimuli. Rotational stimuli are most commonly presented as sinusoids, with the chair first accelerating in one direction until a peak target velocity is achieved (usually 50°/s or more commonly 60°/s), after which the chair slows and reverses to the same peak velocity in the opposite direction. This periodic motion, whereby the chair (head) oscillates about a centric position, is known as sinusoidal acceleration testing. Provided the rotational frequencies being administered are simple harmonics of one another, this form of stimulation is known as SHA testing [13]. The frequencies most commonly administered are harmonic or octave frequencies between 0.01 and 0.64 Hz, specifically, 0.01, 0.02, 0.04, 0.08, 0.16, 0.32, and 0.64 Hz.

Due to the constant varying acceleration and deceleration stimuli during SHA testing, the cupulae are subjected to omnipresent (acceleration and deceleration) deflection forces that are commensurate with the target velocity stimulus. This is eloquently described by the pendulum model of cupular deflection, which offers the reasoning for the alternating nystagmus provoked during SHA testing (Fig. 6.4). According to the pendulum model, the degree of cupular deflection is dependent upon the frequency of angular rotation (acceleration force), and the resulting VOR nystagmus will similarly crescendo and decrescendo in relation to the acceleration and deceleration of the angular stimulus.

Sinusoidal Harmonic Acceleration Analysis Parameters

Analysis of the VOR in response to sinusoidal chair rotations produces three salient response parameters: gain, phase, and symmetry [8, 12] (Fig. 6.5). Comparison of the peak ocular response to that of peak chair rotational velocity can be easily determined. This ratio of peak eye velocity to peak chair velocity is known as the sensitivity, or gain, of the vestibular system and, through a series of rotations

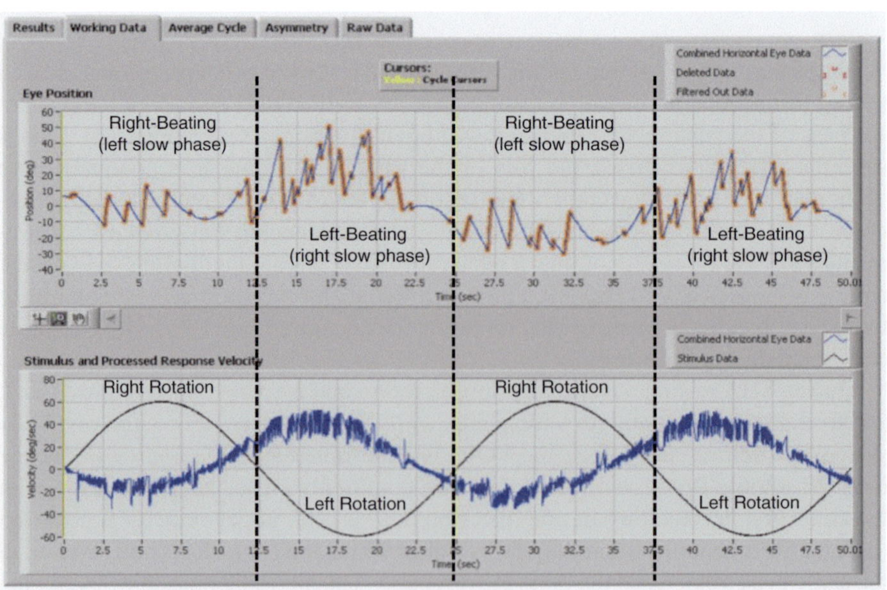

Fig. 6.4 Relationship between direction of chair rotation versus slow and fast phase of nystagmus. Raw tracing of nystagmus (top plot) shows right-beating and left-beating nystagmus in relation to rightward and leftward chair rotation, respectively

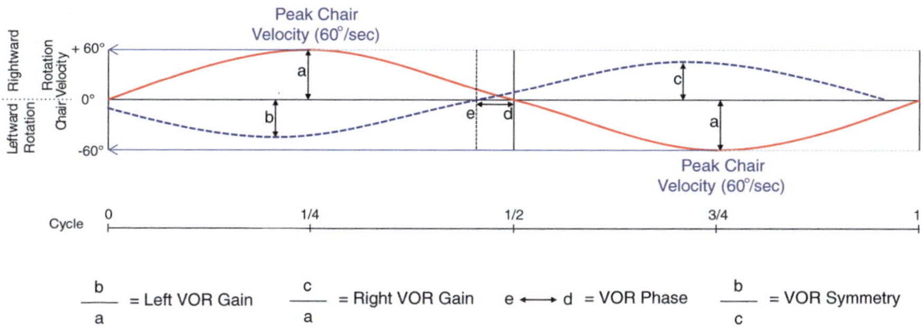

Fig. 6.5 Single cycle of chair rotation illustrating how the various analysis parameters of SHA testing (gain, phase, and symmetry) are determined

(accelerations), the gain of the vestibular system can be effectively determined across a wide range of frequencies during SHA testing.

In addition, as the chair begins to accelerate in one direction and the eyes begin to slowly deviate in the opposite direction due to the vestibular response, the timing relationship between the exact moment chair rotation begins and the exact moment the eyes begin to move in the opposite direction can also be determined. This timing relationship is known as the phase of the VOR response, and describes the temporal movement of the eyes in relation to the movement of the chair (Fig. 6.5).

Finally, the degree of peak eye response can be compared from rotations in the clockwise direction to those from the counter-clockwise direction. The ratio between these two peak responses is known as the symmetry of the VOR. Therefore, three primary measures are specifically analyzed during rotational testing: VOR gain, phase, and symmetry (Fig. 6.5). Each parameter has unique characteristics, strengths, and limitations [15].

Sinusoidal Harmonic Acceleration Interpretation

Normal Sinusoidal Harmonic Acceleration Response

Although VOR gain in the absence of any visual stimuli is not perfectly compensatory or is VOR phase for frequencies below 1.0 Hz, responses can be compared against normative reference ranges for the determination of vestibular function in association with the rotational stimulus frequency range delivered. Figure 6.6 illustrates VOR response parameters from a patient during a normal rotational examination.

Unilateral Peripheral Impairments

Unilateral peripheral labyrinthine disorders can generate a varied pattern of SHA results, depending on the severity and acute nature of the impairment. In cases where a lesioned end organ is only mildly impaired, the results of rotational testing may be

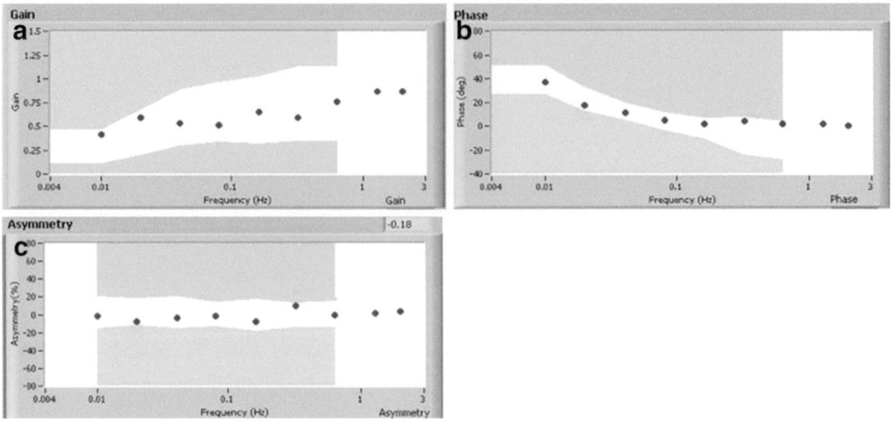

Fig. 6.6 Normal sinusoidal harmonic acceleration (SHA) results for VOR gain (**a**), VOR phase (**b**), and VOR symmetry (**c**) from 0.01 through 2.0 Hz. Abnormal response regions are indicated by the gray regions for each results graph

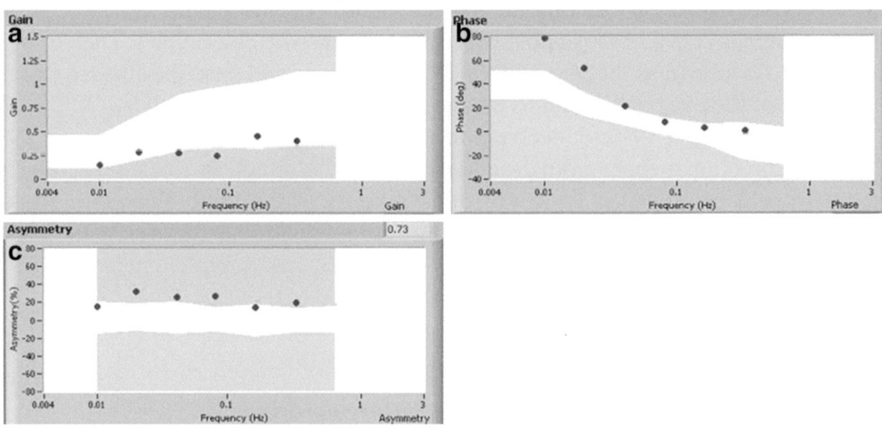

Fig. 6.7 Common sinusoidal harmonic acceleration (SHA) results for an acute unilateral labyrinthine hypofunction. Results for VOR gain (**a**), VOR phase (**b**), and VOR symmetry (**c**) from 0.01 through 0.32 Hz. Abnormal response regions are indicated by the gray regions for each results graph

completely normal due to central compensation. In instances where there is more severe dysfunction in one of the labyrinths, the most commonly observed abnormality is increased phase in lower frequencies. Results can, therefore, vary depending on the severity and acute nature of the unilateral peripheral vestibulopathy.

When assessing patients who have incurred an *acute* peripheral vestibulopathy, there are a number of characteristic findings that can be expected. Figure 6.7 illustrates such an example. First, VOR gain is often reduced and phase prolonged immediately after the event. Secondly, findings often reveal a significant asymmetry that is biased in the direction of the spontaneous nystagmus. Symmetry is calculated using the slow-phase eye velocities and indicates a bias in VOR responses during

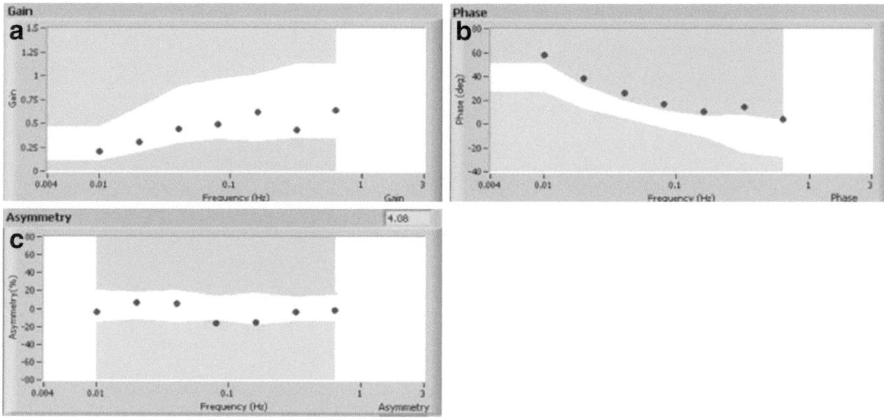

Fig. 6.8 Common sinusoidal harmonic acceleration (SHA) results for unilateral labyrinthine hypofunction. Results for VOR gain (**a**), VOR phase (**b**), and VOR symmetry (**c**) from 0.01 through 0.64 Hz. Normal VOR gain and symmetry in the presence of abnormal low-HZ VOR phase provides good evidence for effective compensation

rotation. A right asymmetry corresponds to left-beating nystagmus and a left asymmetry corresponds to right-beating nystagmus. A significant asymmetry is a non-localizing finding that can be indicative of central or peripheral dysfunction. Asymmetry measures can be isolated and also found in the presence of phase and gain abnormalities. Significant asymmetries are commonly found in patients with acute or uncompensated unilateral vestibular dysfunction. In rare cases, significant asymmetry may indicate the presence of a lesion in the central pathways.

Figure 6.8 illustrates rotational findings from a patient with a compensated complete unilateral peripheral vestibulopathy. In patients such as this, vestibular gain has been centrally compensated; however, phase abnormalities continue to persist. The persistence of phase abnormalities is a result of impairment in the velocity storage mechanism. This centrally distributed system acts as a neural integrator to enhance the low-frequency performance of the vestibular system beyond what would be expected based on cupular mechanics. Significant unilateral vestibular impairments disrupt the normal functioning of the velocity storage mechanism and consequently reduce the efficiency of the VOR for low frequencies [9]. This loss of velocity storage has the effect of increasing VOR phase leads, generally for low-frequency stimuli below 1.0 Hz. In cases where the unilateral peripheral vestibulopathy is severe or complete, VOR phase abnormalities may be more inclusive of frequencies greater than 1.0 Hz.

Bilateral Peripheral Impairments

SHA testing is extremely useful in describing and quantifying the severity of bilateral vestibular loss. Figure 6.9 shows rotational results from a patient with partial bilateral vestibular dysfunction. As can be seen, there is significantly reduced gain at 0.01 Hz and 0.02 Hz with recovery of function at higher frequencies. At the

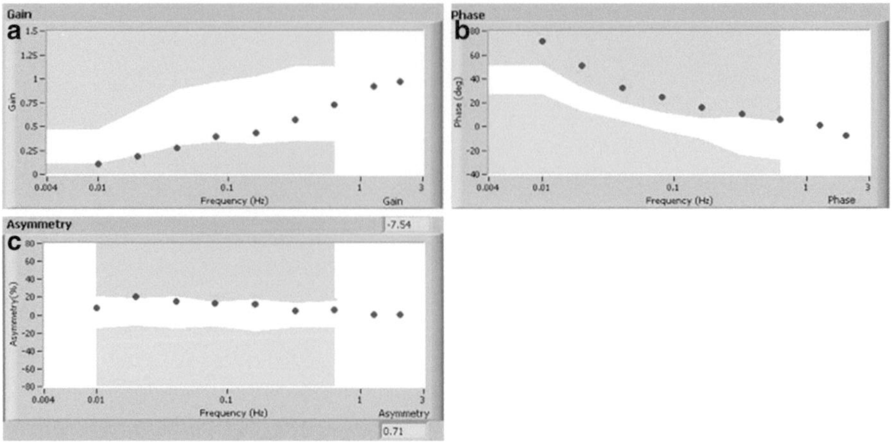

Fig. 6.9 Common sinusoidal harmonic acceleration (SHA) results for bilateral labyrinthine hypofunction. Results for VOR gain (**a**), VOR phase (**b**), and VOR symmetry (**c**) from 0.01 through 2.0 Hz. Abnormal response regions are indicated by the gray regions for each results graph

frequencies where gain is significantly low, phase and symmetry measures should be interpreted with caution. This pattern of partial bilateral loss at low frequencies is a relatively common finding and will often be accompanied by reduced caloric responses. In these cases, abnormally low but measurable VOR responses are often accompanied by corresponding prolonged phase at the same frequencies. Symmetry measures obtained from patients with bilateral peripheral impairments in the absence of spontaneous nystagmus are typically within normal limits. Patients manifesting a complete vestibular loss or labyrinthine areflexia (i.e., no response at any frequency) are relatively uncommon (Fig. 6.10). Finally, it is important to keep in mind that, because VOR phase and symmetry measures are calculated from VOR gain, in cases where VOR phase is below 10–15%, such measures of phase and symmetry should be performed with caution.

Central Impairments

Pure central lesions are often difficult to isolate using SHA testing. More commonly, mixed lesions will be suggested, as both a reduction of peripheral afferent vestibular input and central lesions can produce the more common SHA abnormalities of abnormal VOR phase lead and VOR asymmetry. Mixed lesions are often suggested when concomitant central findings are identified, such as abnormal ocular motor findings. There are, however, specific SHA response patterns that have a greater proclivity secondary to a central lesion. First, abnormal VOR phase leads that are isolated to the mid- to high frequencies suggest an inappropriate recruitment of the central neural integrator mechanism (velocity storage) that would

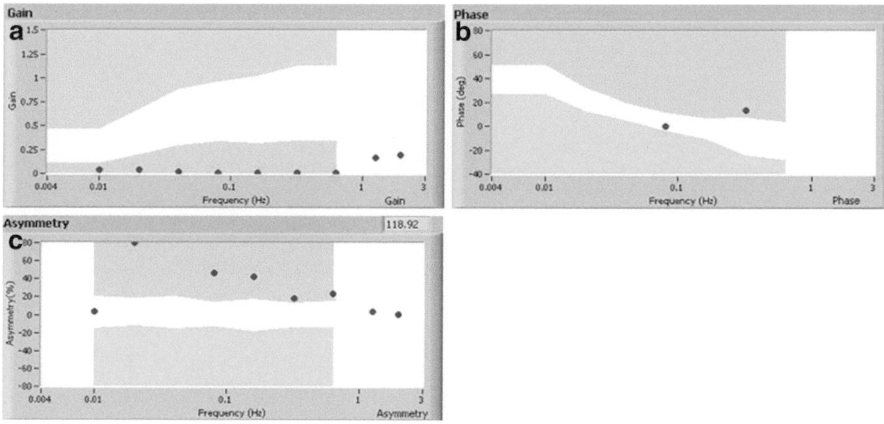

Fig. 6.10 Common sinusoidal harmonic acceleration (SHA) results for bilateral labyrinthine areflexia. Results for VOR gain (**a**), VOR phase (**b**), and VOR symmetry (**c**) from 0.01 through 2.0 Hz. Since VOR phase and symmetry are calculated form VOR, these parameters should be interpreted with caution under such conditions

normally not require recruitment of such processes during higher frequency head movements. Second, VOR asymmetries in the absence of any peripherally induced spontaneous nystagmus may suggest a central pathology, similar to that of an isolated caloric directional preponderance. Such a SHA result may suggest a lack of central compensation mechanisms for a unilateral peripheral vestibular insult, particularly when VOR gain remains uncompensated. Finally, significantly increased VOR gain, most commonly for low rotational frequencies, may be associated with a central lesion, similar to that of hyper-reactive caloric responses. Although not ubiquitously present with increased VOR gain, a *decrease* in VOR phase lead, or even a phase lag, may be present in such cases, as problems involving uncontrolled cerebellar modulation of VOR gain cause concomitant problems with central velocity storage mechanisms and tend to shorten low-frequency VOR phase leads (Fig. 6.11).

Sinusoidal Harmonic Acceleration Clinical Summary

Overall, the SHA provides the examiner with a number of useful applications. This includes documenting the degree of bilateral vestibular loss, tracking compensation when caloric testing is impossible, monitoring vestibular function in patients being administered vestibulotoxic medications, and assessing young children. However, SHA is best utilized in the context of other tests, including ocular motor and velocity step testing, as well as other vestibular function testing (e.g., videonystagmography, vestibular-evoked myogenic potentials, video head impulse test, and/or dynamic posturography).

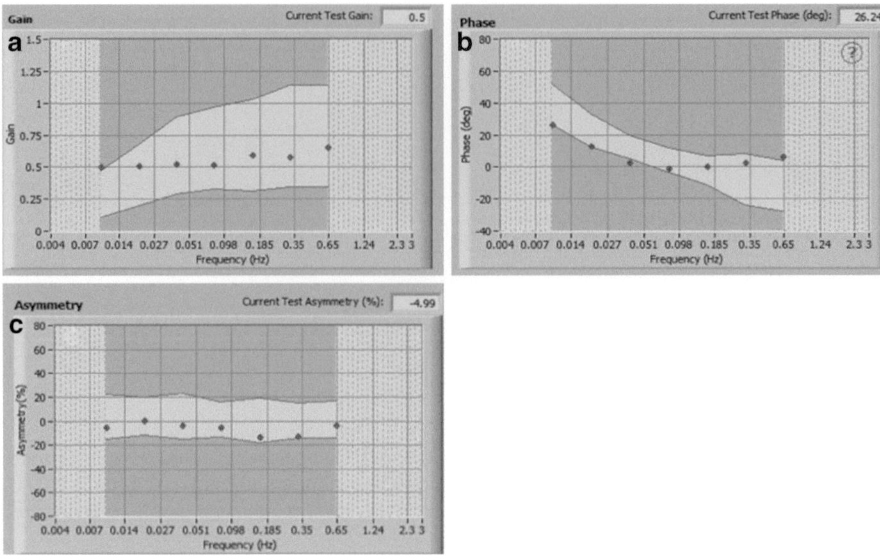

Fig. 6.11 Central sinusoidal harmonic acceleration (SHA) pattern for VOR gain (**a**), VOR phase (**b**), and VOR symmetry (**c**) from 0.01 through 0.64 Hz. Borderline hyper-labyrinthine VOR gain for 0.01 Hz with a concomitant decrease in VOR phase is identified

Velocity Step Testing

Velocity step testing is one the oldest of all clinical vestibular tests, initially introduced to the vestibular clinic by Róbert Bárány in 1907. It consists of a quick acceleration of the chair to a sustained constant velocity rotation before an equally quick deceleration of the chair brings the chair back to a full stop. The test is then repeated in the opposite direction. Depending on the intensity of the target angular velocity, the velocity step test can either give unique insights into the central functioning of the vestibular system or can offer valuable insights into lateralizing a peripheral vestibular lesion.

Velocity Step Stimuli

During velocity step testing, abrupt computer-controlled accelerations of 120–200°/s^2 are precisely delivered to an upright seated patient in the yaw (horizontal) plane until a predetermined constant velocity is achieved and can be subsequently maintained for a given period of time. Sustained step target velocities usually fall into one of two categories: low-velocity target step stimuli and high-velocity target step stimuli. Low-velocity step stimuli are usually performed at 60° per second, while high-velocity step stimuli are performed at 240–300° per second [7, 8].

Physiologic Vestibular Ocular Reflex Response

The pendular model of cupular dynamics once again predicts the degree of cupular deflection during VST, which is in direct relationship to the degree of acceleration in accordance with the target angular velocity [2]. During such time of acceleration step stimuli, afferent neural asymmetry and subsequent VOR response can be expected as long as the horizontal cupulae remain deflected. In short, the longer the cupulae remain under the influence of an acceleration or deceleration force, the greater the deflection of the cupulae and the stronger the resultant afferent neural response. The duration of acceleration force is, therefore, dependent upon the target angular velocity, with higher target velocities producing a longer period of acceleration and a subsequent greater afferent vestibular response than lower target velocities. As a result of the step stimuli, a right-beating nystagmus is generated in response to rightward acceleration and post leftward deceleration. Conversely, a left-beating nystagmus is generated in response to leftward acceleration and post rightward deceleration (Fig. 6.12). In general, VST is performed using both a low and high target velocity.

Low-Velocity Step Testing

The primary purpose of a low VST is to measure the rate of nystagmus decay in response to an abrupt angular acceleration and deceleration to the right (clockwise) and left (counterclockwise) [8]. Target step velocities of 60° per second are often considered standard for low VST, largely because normative reference data for nystagmus decay have been determined for this velocity. Figure 6.12 depicts a 60° per second test rotational paradigm. A step velocity to the right is followed by a step

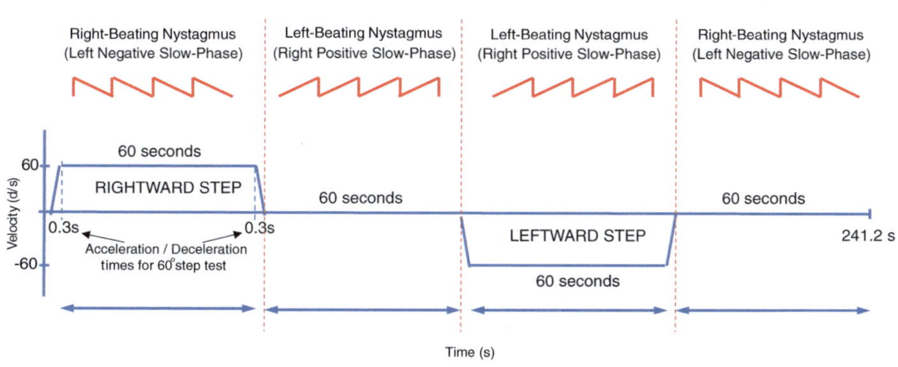

Fig. 6.12 60°/s step velocity paradigm showing each 60-s per and post, rightward and leftward step stimuli. Time (in seconds) is plotted on the *x*-axis and velocity (in degrees/second) is on the *y*-axis. Acceleration and deceleration stimuli are held constant at 200°/s^2, which produce an acceleration and deceleration period equal to 0.3 s. Total test time including the acceleration, deceleration, and constant velocity stimuli periods of 60 s each, equals 241.2 s. Resulting nystagmus from each acceleration/deceleration is shown for each segment

velocity to the left. Each period of per-rotation and post rotation contains a 60-s interval during which the nystagmus response is recorded. The low VST is primarily concerned with the rate of nystagmus decay, specifically the time, in seconds, for the nystagmus response to deteriorate by 63% from the peak slow-phase eye velocity (or alternatively said, the time, in seconds, for the response to decline to 37% of its peak value) [13]. This is referred to as the VOR time decay constant.

The cupular pendulum model would dictate an afferent neural response and resultant VOR nystagmus by as much as 6–7 s due to cupular mechanics alone. However, the central vestibular velocity storage mechanism extends the enduring nystagmus VOR response well beyond the 6–7 s [10] (Fig. 6.13). The persistence of the VOR response is dependent upon a sufficient peripheral afferent drive as well as an intact commissural pathway between vestibular nuclei. The persistence and decaying of the VOR response beyond cupular mechanics alone (i.e., VOR time

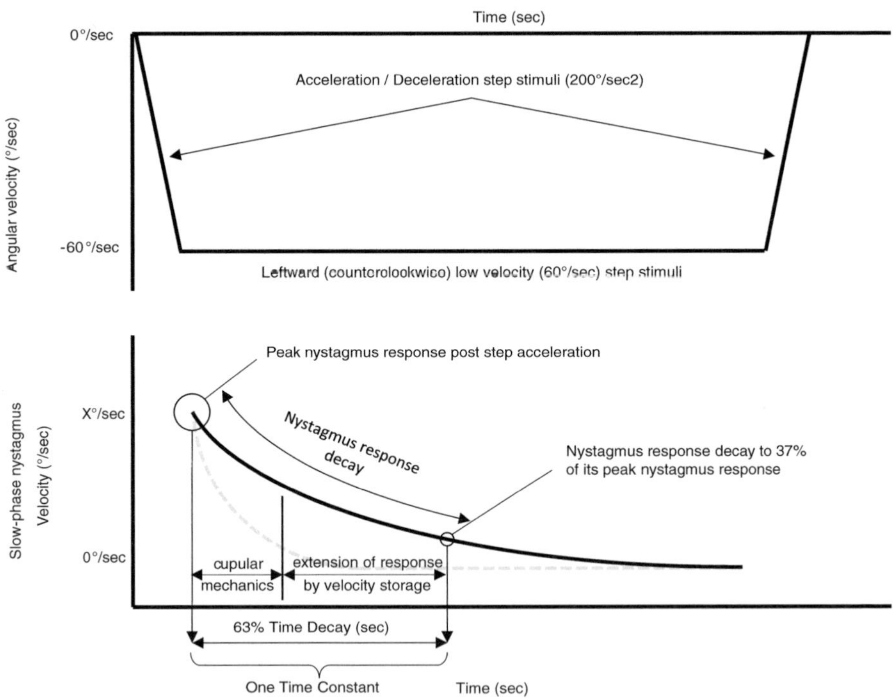

Fig. 6.13 Illustration of a 60°/s step velocity stimulus and theoretical VOR response to a leftward acceleration and constant velocity angular step rotation. Top chart depicts a 60°/s step velocity stimulus. Bottom graph depicts the theoretical plotting of a progressively decreasing (decaying) slow-phase eye velocity (SPEV) nystagmus response over time. Response is parsed and identified by the peak response and by one time constant, or TC (i.e., depiction of the cupular response and extension of the nystagmus response by the velocity storage mechanisms). One VOR TC is equal to the decaying of the SPEV nystagmus response to 37% of its peak eye velocity response. Light gray dashed line represents the decay of the nystagmus response in the event of a loss of velocity storage, where the propagation of the VOR response is lost, and the VOR TC is essentially no longer than what is provided by cupular mechanics alone (see Fig. 6.18)

decay constant) are of significant clinical interest. The general consensus for a normal time decay reference range (±2SD from the mean) across studies is between 10 and 30 s [11]. A normal propagation of VOR nystagmus in response to both acceleration and deceleration stimuli to the right and left is shown in Fig. 6.14. VOR time decay constants that are below 10 s are usually considered abnormal.

High-Velocity Step Testing

The primary purpose of high VST is to lateralize unilateral vestibular lesions. This directly addresses the primary limitation of rotational testing. Administration procedures for high VST are equivalent to the 60° step test with the exception of selecting a higher target step velocity (Fig. 6.15). As opposed to the low-velocity step stimulus, use of a high target velocity stimulus can now effectively saturate the inhibitory response of the trailing ear due to maximal cupular displacement and subsequent saturation of the afferent response to 0 spikes/s. Concomitantly, the ipsiversive cupulae have a similar maximal cupular displacement and theoretical maximal

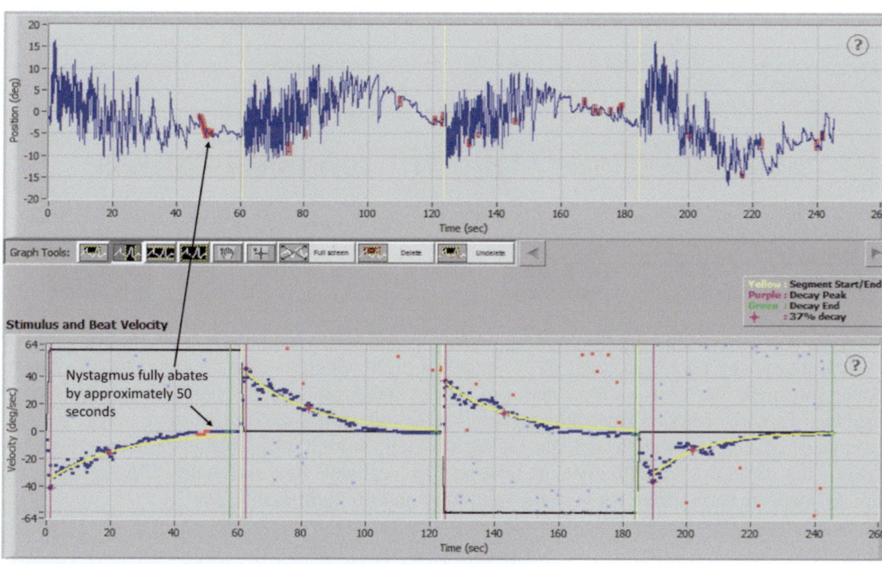

	Per-Rotary Right	Post-Rotary Right	Per-Rotary Left	Post-Rotary Left
Peak Vel. (deg/sec)	-41.67	46.13	37.60	-36.91
Decay Time(sec)	18.46	19.70	18.34	12.53
Validity	88.00	90.99	92.63	89.26
Gain	0.69	0.77	0.63	0.62

Fig. 6.14 Normal 60°/s velocity step test. Top chart shows raw nystagmus VOR response and plot of decaying nystagmus. Bottom chart shows relative response parameters (e.g., peak slow phase eye velocity, decay time constants, and VOR gain) for each stimulus condition

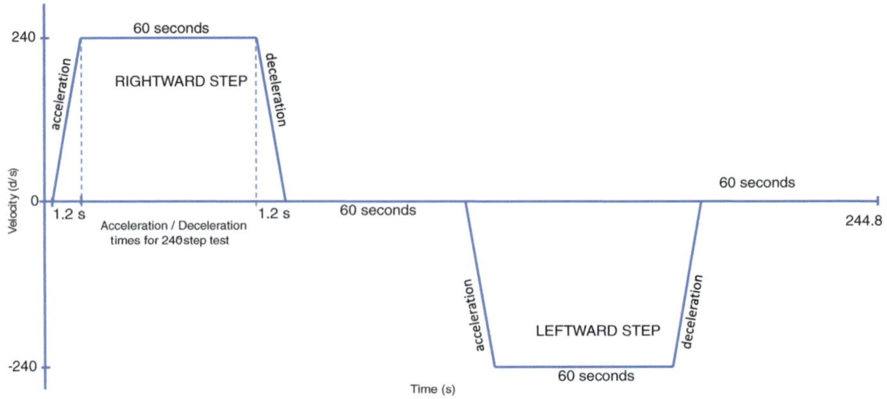

Fig. 6.15 240°/s step velocity paradigm showing each 60-s per and post, rightward and leftward step stimuli. Time (in seconds) is plotted on the *x*-axis and velocity (in degrees/second) is on the *y*-axis. Acceleration and deceleration stimuli are held constant at 200°/s^2, which produce an acceleration and deceleration period equal to 1.2 s. Total test time including the acceleration, deceleration, and constant velocity stimuli periods of 60 s each, equals 244.8 s

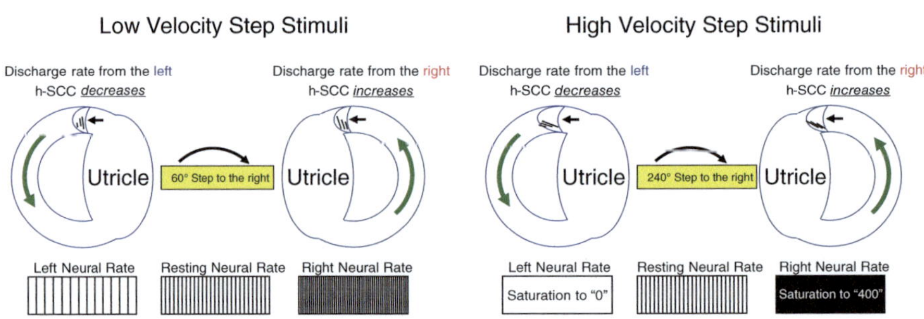

Fig. 6.16 Cartoon comparing the cupular mechanics and subsequent afferent neural firing rate of a low velocity step paradigm (e.g., 60°/s) versus a high velocity step paradigm (240°/s). Green arrows and small black arrows represent direction of endolymph force against the cupulae during a rightward angular rotation like a step stimuli. Degree of cupular deflection is commensurate with the velocity of angular rotation such that the high velocity stimuli (right image) depict the displacement of the cupular stereocillia near maximum displacement. Respective neural firing rates are depicted beneath each image for both the inhibitory and excitatory labyrinth

afferent excitatory response of the leading ear (Fig. 6.16). Consequently, the resultant VOR response is, theoretically, a reflection of the excitatory response from the leading ear, although the trailing ear provides the excitatory response during abrupt decelerations. In theory, such high-velocity step stimuli allow for identification and quantification of the excitatory response from each labyrinth, and subsequently offers a measure of labyrinthine symmetry, much like that of the caloric stimulus.

A response symmetry ratio is calculated from the peak VOR response produced during each acceleration and deceleration stimulus, much like the Jongkees' formula applied during caloric irrigations. Specifically, the equation for high VST is written as such:

$$\frac{\left(\text{Per rotation right} + \text{post rotation left}\right) - \left(\text{Per rotation left post rotation right}\right)}{\left(\text{Per rotation right} + \text{post rotation left}\right) + (\text{Per rotation left} + \text{post rotation right}} \times 100$$

Figure 6.17 depicts an example of a normal high-velocity step response pattern and corresponding VOR peak eye responses to each of the step stimuli.

Clinical Response Patterns for Velocity Step Testing

The VST can offer valuable insights into a patient's underlying vestibular impairment, particularly when used in conjunction with SHA testing. The horizontal VOR, neural integrator, and the velocity storage mechanisms can all be effectively evaluated during velocity step testing, thereby making it possible to identify peripheral asymmetries (i.e., lateralize peripheral lesions), as well as monitor or confirm vestibular central compensation.

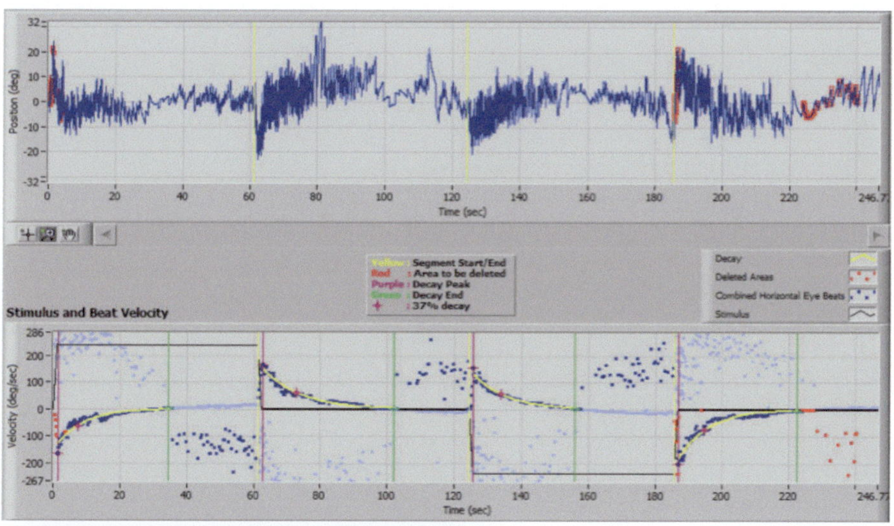

	Per-Rotary Right	Post-Rotary Right	Per-Rotary Left	Post-Rotary Left
Peak Vel. (deg/sec)	-166.87	166.95	154.90	-201.87
Decay Time(sec)	5.97	9.88	8.04	7.79
Validity	92.44	91.14	90.00	88.72
Gain	0.70	0.70	0.65	0.84

Asymmetry 6.79 %

Right Excitation
166.87+ 201.87= 368.74

Left Excitation
166.95+ 154.90= 321.85

$$\frac{368.74-321.85}{368.74+321.85} = \frac{46.89}{690.59} = 0.0679\ (6.79\%)$$

Fig. 6.17 Normal 240°/s velocity step test (after correcting/deleting for noise). Asymmetry calculation is shown

Low-Velocity Step Response Interpretation

Abnormalities from low VST are manifested as reduced VOR time constants and interpreted in association with other vestibular test abnormalities when lateralizing and differentiating site of lesion. In isolation, a reduced VOR time constant is a non-localizing finding as both peripheral and central lesions can deleteriously impact the functioning of the neural integrator and the velocity storage mechanisms. That is, a reduction in peripheral afferent drive, or a damaging impact on the central neural integrator, can reduce the effectiveness and efficiency of the velocity storage mechanism. Time constants below 10 s are generally considered abnormal. Figure 6.18 depicts an example of an abnormal low VST. In general, reduced VOR time constants, in association with concomitant peripheral vestibular pathology, can lateralize to the affected side, although exceptions to this can exist. Therefore, using abnormal low VST results to definitively lateralize peripheral vestibulopathies should be performed cautiously.

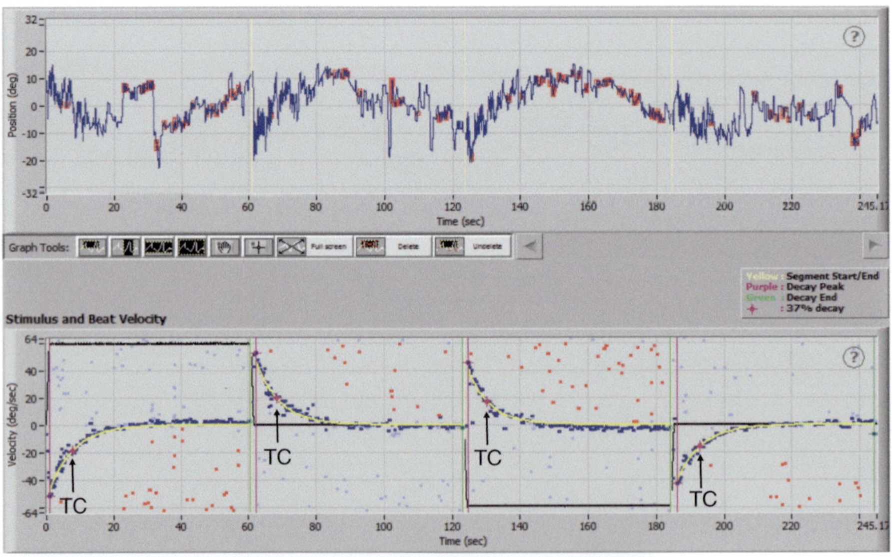

	Per-Rotary Right	Post-Rotary Right	Per-Rotary Left	Post-Rotary Left
Peak Vel. (deg/sec)	-51.96	53.27	45.65	43.13
Decay Time(sec)	6.49	6.04	5.69	6.72
Validity	71.31	68.53	82.36	72.67
Gain	0.87	0.89	0.76	0.72
Asymmetry	-1.97 %			

Fig. 6.18 Abnormal corrected 60°/s velocity step test results. Abnormally shortened decay time constants are identified for each stimulus interval. Notice the sharp decline of each decaying nystagmus in the slow phase eye velocity plots. TC One time constant

High-Velocity Step Response Interpretation

Abnormalities from high VST are manifested as reduced peak VOR eye velocity and interpreted similarly to that of the Jongkees' formula during caloric irrigations. A comparison of peak eye velocity response secondary to rightward cupular deflection is compared against peak eye velocity response secondary to leftward cupular deflection. Labyrinthine asymmetry is determined from the asymmetry peak eye velocity ratio. A VOR asymmetry greater than 20%, similar to a significant caloric asymmetry, is generally agreed upon as significant for unilateral dysfunction [3], with the weaker labyrinthine response appropriately assigned by the weaker peak eye velocity response. Figure 6.19 depicts an example of an abnormal high VST. In general, greater sensitivity and specificity for identifying labyrinthine asymmetry are often commensurate with higher step stimuli and greater unilateral labyrinthine damage [4]. Therefore, in the presence of normal high VST symmetries, the presence of a slight or mild unilateral labyrinthine lesion may not also be ruled out, which may require a more comprehensive vestibular assessment.

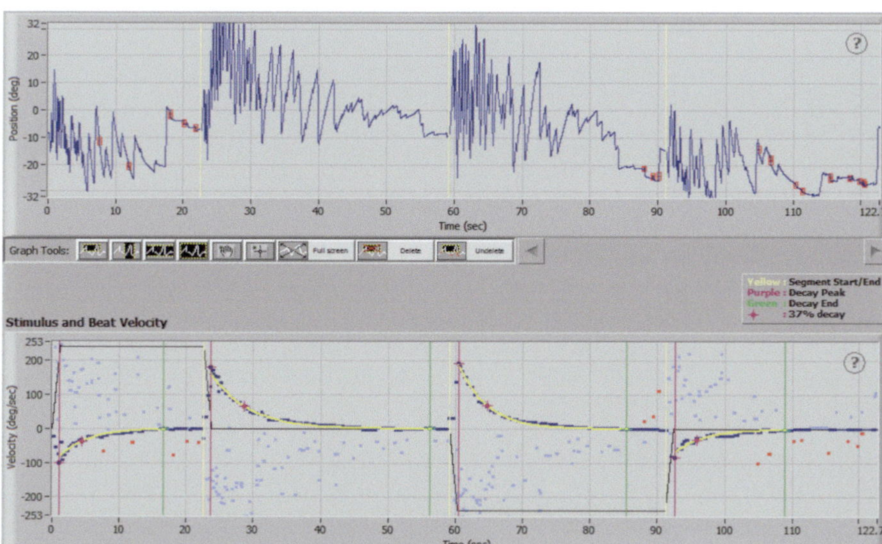

	Per-Rotary Right	Post-Rotary Right	Per-Rotary Left	Post-Rotary Left
Peak Vel. (deg/sec)	-99.82	178.58	190.63	-83.10
Decay Time(sec)	3.33	5.03	4.27	3.28
Validity	85.71	87.04	83.99	86.49
Gain	0.42	0.74	0.79	0.35
Asymmetry -33.74 %				

Right Excitation
99.82+ 83.10= 182.92

Left Excitation
178.58 + 190.63= 369.21

$$\frac{182.92-369.21}{182.92+369.92} = \frac{-186.29}{552.13} = -0.3374\ (-33.74\%)$$

Fig. 6.19 Abnormal 240°/s velocity step test (after correcting/deleting for noise). Asymmetry calculation is shown. VOR gain in greater than 20%. Labyrinthine hypofunction is assigned to the weaker excitation conditions (right ear)

Chapter Summary

Collectively, SHA and VST are often performed together during rotational assessments. Jointly, their data can provide invaluable diagnostic insights into peripheral and central vestibular function that no other test can equally deliver. Table 6.1 details the clinical test protocols that should be performed during a standard or routine rotational assessment, as well as the typical stimuli that should be conducted for each test. In addition, various specialized rotational test protocols are listed, which should be performed when clinically indicated. A clinical summary of abnormal results during SHA testing is detailed in Tables 6.2 and 6.3. Finally, a clinical summary of abnormal results during VST is detailed in Table 6.4.

Table 6.2 Abnormalities associated with SHA testing

Sinusoidal harmonic acceleration (SHA) test abnormalities			
Parameter	Abnormal result	Possible interpretation	Rule out
Gain	Low VOR gain for low Hzs (<0.04–0.08 Hz)	1. With concomitant abnormal phase lead at low Hzs and asymmetry—uncompensated UVL on side of asymmetry 2. With no phase abnormalities but abnormal symmetry, possible irritative or stable lesion (side uncertain) 3. No other abnormalities and normal spectral purity, compensated UVL is likely	Insufficient alerting
	Low VOR gain for all Hzs	1. BVL given eyes open during test (symmetry and phase cannot be interpreted) 2. Vestibulotoxic medication, aging (usually >65–70 years), rare degenerative disorders of the brainstem and/or cerebellum (especially if caloric data are normal)	Insufficient altering, restricted EOM, fixation
	High VOR gain for all or most	1. Cerebellar lesion (associated ocular motor abnormalities) 2. Has been observed in migraine and hydrops	Medications; stimulants
Phase	↑ Low Hz Phase lead	1. Peripheral vestibular end-organ lesion/vestibular nuclei lesion 2. With concomitant asymmetry, uncompensated UVL (on side of asymmetry) 3. Acute vestibular end organ lesion; vestibular hydrops	Compare with step tests and calorics
	↑ High Hz Phase lead	1. CNS lesion; (look for associated ocular motor abnormalities)	Lateral medullary syndrome
	↓ Low/High Hz Phase lead/lag	1. CNS lesion; (associated ocular motor abnormalities); consider lesions involving brainstem or posterior cerebellum; cerebellar nodulus	
Symmetry	Asymmetric SPV	1. Two or more consecutive abnormal Hzs; similar to DP on caloric testing (non-localizing with respect to site-of-lesion unless secondary to spontaneous nystagmus) 2. With low Hz phase lead, uncompensated peripheral lesion on side of asymmetry	Unstable lesion with normal phase findings

Table 6.3 SHA abnormalities associated with site of lesion

Sinusoidal harmonic acceleration (SHA) test abnormalities			
Site of lesion		Possible response	Rule out
Peripheral	Unilateral	1. Initial loss of VOR gain can involve low, mid, and high frequencies with a greater impact towards the lower frequencies. 2. VOR gain can return to normal and often does for the higher frequencies over days or months. 3. Increased low frequency phase leads that remain even following compensation (secondary to a permanent change in central integrator processing). 4. Asymmetrical "bias" often is present due to afferent asymmetry. At first, fast-phase components of the vestibular nystagmus are ipsilesional but may change over time and are, therefore, poor indicators of laterality of the lesion. 5. The severity of the abnormal response will often co-vary with the severity of the peripheral lesion. 6. SHA gain and symmetry may be entirely within normal limits with an isolated low-frequency VOR phase lead suggesting a compensated unilateral pathology.	Decreased spectral purity is often associated with the onset of a unilateral lesion, which may contribute to the initial decrease in overall gain; rule out anti-dizziness medication effects if patients remain on pharmacology treatment.
	Bilateral	1. Low, mid, and high frequency gain is reduced below normal limits. 2. When gain is within normal limits, it almost is always confined to the higher frequencies suggesting an incomplete bilateral vestibular loss. 3. Phase leads are often randomly distributed, particularly at low frequencies. 4. Phase and symmetry data should be interpreted with caution when gain falls below 0.15 (15%). 5. Spectral purity is often poor, particularly for frequencies where gain is poor.	Insufficient altering, restricted EOM, fixation; differentiate peripheral and central with concomitant results (ocular motor, etc.)

(continued)

Table 6.3 (continued)

Sinusoidal harmonic acceleration (SHA) test abnormalities		
Site of lesion	Possible response	Rule out
Central	1. Hyperactive gain may involve any frequency but often occurs in the low frequencies where central control (velocity storage) is in higher demand (i.e., cerebellar site of lesion). 2. Hypoactive gain with no concomitant peripheral indicators (rare). 3. Isolated mid-to-low frequency phase leads (or sometimes involving the entire frequency range), suggesting an inappropriate processing of central velocity storage mechanisms for frequencies where the neural integrator is not required. 4. Bias (asymmetry) may or may not be present	Compare with step test and caloric data; central pathologies rarely cause abnormalities isolated to a single test—identify concomitant abnormalities across tests (ocular motor, etc.).

Adapted from Wall (1990)

Table 6.4 Common abnormalities from 60°/s and 240°/s velocity step testing

Velocity step testing			
	Abnormality	Possible interpretation	Rule out
60°/s	Low time constant (<10 s)	1. Peripheral UVL if oculomotor testing is normal, likely labyrinth or VIII nerve 2. At 60° or 100°/s, information is from both labyrinths 3. Non-localizing cupular time constants plus velocity storage—gains should be >0.3; if not, consider migraine	Inattention; too much blinking; bilat loss; fixation
	If 3 of 4 time constants are abnormal	1. Abnormal study; non-localizing	Inattention; too much blinking
240°/s	Consider peak slow phase velocity; >20% difference between CW and CCW directions	1. Significant asymmetric results in peak SPV indicate peripheral UVL and side of loss	Eye closure (eyes must be open when chair starts and stops)

References

1. Arriaga MA, Chen DA, Cenci KA. Rotational chair (ROTO) instead of electronystagmography (ENG) as the primary vestibular test. Otolaryngol Head Neck Surg. 2005;133(3):329–33.
2. Baloh RW, Honrubia V. Clinical neurophysiology of the vestibular system. 2nd ed. Philadelphia: F.A. Davis Company; 1990.
3. Baloh RW, Honrubia V. Clinical neurophysiology of the vestibular system. 3rd ed. Philadelphia: F.A. Davis Company; 2001.
4. Baloh RW, Sills AW, Honrubia V. Impulsive and sinusoidal rotatory testing: a comparison with results of caloric testing. Laryngoscope. 1979;89:646–54.
5. Barin K. New tests for diagnoses of peripheral vestibular disorders. Proceedings from the Illinois academy of audiology, Jan 30–Feb 1, 2013.
6. Barin K, Durrant JD. Applied physiology of the vestibular system. In: Canalis RF, Lempert PR, editors. The ear: comprehensive otology. Philadelphia: Lippincott Williams & Wilkins; 2000. p. 113–40.
7. Brey RH, McPherson JH, Lynch RM. Background and introduction to whole body rotational testing. In: Jacobson GP, Shepard NT, editors. Balance function assessment and management. San Diego: Plural Publishing; 2008. p. 253–80.
8. Brey RH, McPherson JH, Lynch RM. Technique, interpretation, and usefulness of whole body rotational testing. In: Jacobson GP, Shepard NT, editors. Balance function assessment and management. San Diego: Plural Publishing; 2008. p. 281–317.
9. Goldberg JM, Wilson VJ, Cullen KE, Angelaki DE, Broussard DM, Bütner-Ennever JA, et al. The vestibular system: a sixth sense. New York: Oxford University Press; 2012.
10. Goulson AM, McPherson JH, Shepard NT. Background and introduction to whole-body rotational testing. In: Jacobson GP, Shepard NT, editors. Balance function assessment and management. San Diego: Plural Publishing; 2016. p. 347–64.
11. Shepard NT, Goulson AM, McPherson JH. Clinical utility and interpretation of whole-body rotation. In: Jacobson GP, Shepard NT, editors. Balance function assessment and management. San Diego: Plural Publishing; 2016. p. 365–90.
12. Shepard NT, Telian SA. Practical management of the balanced disordered patient. San Diego: Singular Publishing Group; 1996.
13. Stockwell CW, Bojrab DI. Background and technique of rotational testing. In: Jacobson GP, Newman CW, Kartush JM, editors. Handbook of balance function testing. San Diego: Singular Publishing Group; 1997. p. 237–48.
14. Wilson VJ, Jones JG. Mammalian vestibular physiology. New York: Plenum Press; 1979.
15. Zalewski C. Rotational vestibular assessment. San Diego: Plural Publishing; 2018.

Chapter 7
Computerized Dynamic Posturography

Tristan J. Allsopp and John L. Dornhoffer

Introduction

Postural response and subsequent balance have always been difficult to analyze and isolate. Initial attempts involved testing somatosensory input under eyes-closed and eyes-open conditions to look for postural sway [1]. This involves the patient standing on a forceplate to quantitatively measure the center of vertical forces exhibited by the patient and, thereby, the patient's center of gravity (COG). Using the COG and the center of vertical force, characteristics of the patient's sway and functional compensation can be examined to look for postural disturbance [2]. However, testing via this method can be consciously manipulated and is highly dependent on patient cooperation.

Further attempts have aimed to provide diagnostic information independent of the patient's willingness by measuring discrete evoked postural responses. This is usually achieved by causing periods of stability alteration by rotating the standing surface. Measurements from these toes-up or toes-down positions give valuable information about the latency, strength, and pattern of the neurological response.

Computerized dynamic posturography (CDP) is a method that aims to combine the results from the static conditions of performance testing with those from the dynamic postural responses. Typically, CDP has four main functional protocols: the posture-evoked response (PER), the motor control test (MCT), the adaptive protocol (ADP), and the sensory organization test (SOT).

T. J. Allsopp (✉) · J. L. Dornhoffer
Otolaryngology Department, The University of Arkansas for Medical Sciences, Little Rock, AR, USA
e-mail: TAllsopp@uams.edu; DornhofferJohnL@uams.edu

J. C. Lucas et al. (eds.), *Diagnosis and Treatment of Vestibular Disorders*,
https://doi.org/10.1007/978-3-032-11740-3_7

Posture-Evoked Response (PER)

Description of Test

The PER utilizes support-surface rotations to cause gastrocnemius and anterior tibialis muscle stretch bilaterally [3]. Muscle response to these actions is then measured via surface electromyography (EMG). With rapid dorsiflexion of the ankle (toes up), the gastrocnemius muscle is stretched, stimulating an EMG response. When rapid plantar flexion occurs (toes down), the anterior tibialis muscle provides a response [1]. Testing with toes-up and -down movements occur randomly at high velocity and are usually repeated up to 20 times.

Under normal circumstances, after a support-surface rotation, short-latency and medium-latency responses in the above muscles initially exaggerate the sway disturbance. In a non-dizzy patient, loss of balance is then prevented by the stabilizing long-latency component. EMG readings can identify the presence of these responses and be analyzed. PER testing gives qualitative leg- and muscle-dependent information about the presence, duration, and onset of each of these responses.

Depiction of Results

Averaged responses from multiple attempts will usually be shown as a graph with SL, ML, and LL marked, corresponding to the short latency, medium latency, and long latency responses, respectively. In addition, the responses will often be annotated with the numbers 1 (onset of the response) and 2 (the end of the response). Abnormal responses will be illustrated by delayed onset or absence.

1. SL: This corresponds to the monosynaptic stretch reflex system [4] and are not seen after stretching the anterior tibialis muscles [1]. Normal latencies of the SL response are 32 msec [1].
2. ML: This can be absent in non-dizzy patients but, when present, will represent the polysynaptic segmental reflex mechanisms [5]. These are present in both muscles and typically activate around 80 msec [1].
3. LL: The origin remains controversial but the response usually occurs at 110 msec in both muscles [1, 6, 7].

Motor Control Test (MCT)

Description of Test

The MCT involves a patient standing on a forceplate that is displaced anteriorly or posteriorly at different velocities to elicit autonomic postural responses. Under normal conditions, when the standing surface is moved horizontally, the patient's COG will initially be stationary and the patient will rotate at the ankles, (i.e., the patient will lean forward or backward) [7]. Stretch of the gastrocnemius muscle (when the base plate is moved backwards and the patient leans forward) or anterior tibialis muscle (when the forceplate moves forward and the patient leans backwards) [1] elicits compensation to remain upright [7].

Autonomic postural responses are examined by testing a range of conditions by varying the velocity, displacement of the footplate, and timing. This random testing decreases the chances of biasing the results. Each specific condition is repeated three times for an average result. Typically, responses of both legs to movement forward and backward are analyzed separately to localize which part of the individual pathways may be affected. Compensatory forces and the proportion of total body weight distributed by each foot can also be recorded.

Depiction of Results

Graphical results such as those in Fig. 7.1 will be seen for backward and forward movement in addition to each leg, typically COG sway, horizontal shear force, and left and right center of vertical force responses. Three plots for each of the above conditions are provided, with normal results falling in the unshaded areas. Typical results include the following:

1. Weight symmetry: This indicates the percentage of total body weight on each leg during the postural response. A score of 100 means the weight is distributed equally between both legs while a score of 0 or 200 means none or all of the weight is borne by that leg, respectively [1].
2. Active force latency: This measures the time it takes for the postural responses to be enacted after medium or large displacements of the support surface. Typically, a latency score [2–4] will also be displayed, with 4 representing the most consistent results. Latency increases with age and during the medium displacement [1].
3. Active force strength: This measures the force exerted to restore the patient to an upright position. Typically, each leg will be measured separately and results between the two legs and anterior and posterior direction will be similar.

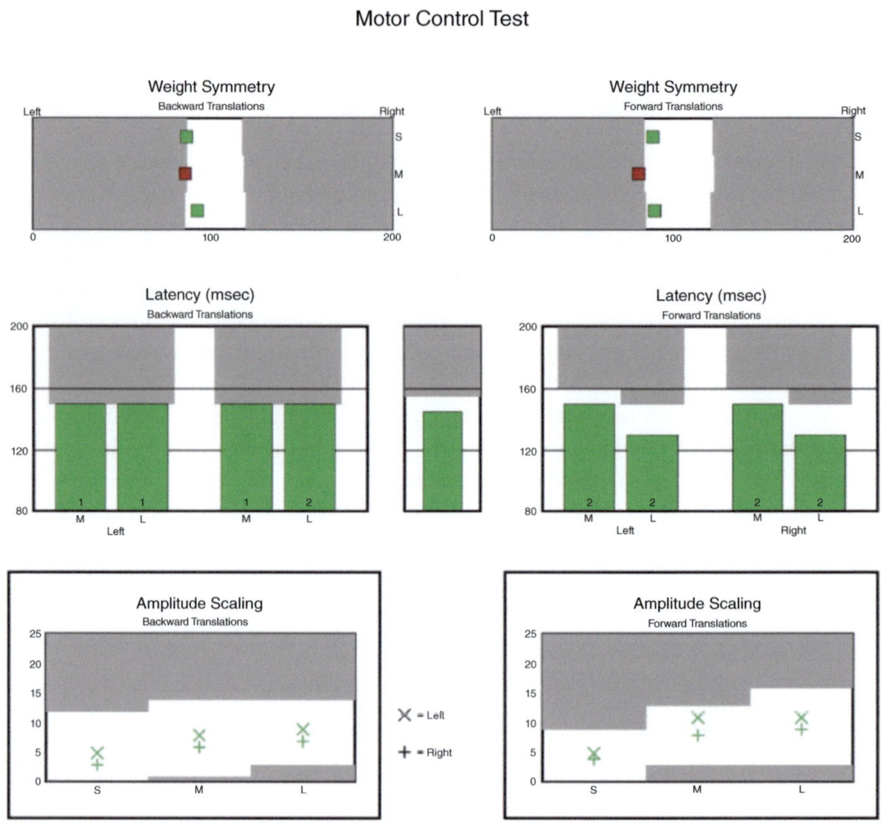

Fig. 7.1 Typical motor control test

Adaptive Protocol (ADP)

Description of Test

The ADP is similar to PER testing except that the toes-up and toes-down movement of the support surface is at a much slower rate. The slower velocities enable the autonomic nervous system to enact adaptive responses that are not witnessed during the MCT. Response testing is repeated five times to look for adaption. Initially, the patient is not expecting the first toes-up/toes-down rotation and is unable to stabilize the COG by swaying at the ankle. Patients with normal postural control may show large variances in COG sway during this first displacing movement but will usually not fall over. By the fifth toes-up/toes-down movement, non-dizzy patients will be able to anticipate the rotation [8]. During these last rotations, autonomic responses are enacted to increase the resistance of the ankles and overall stability.

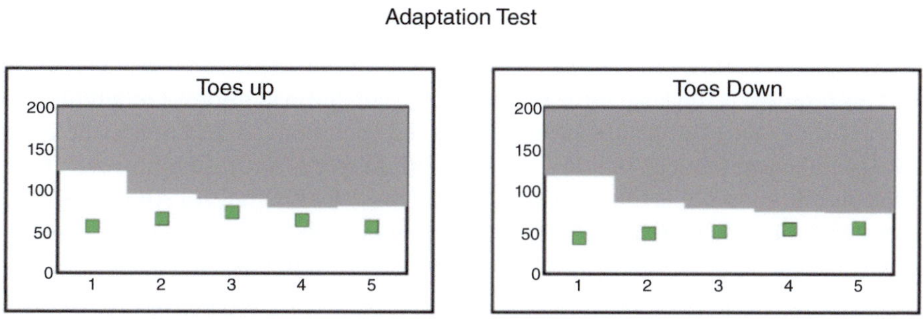

Fig. 7.2 Adaptive test

Depiction of Results

The COG is expressed as sway energy scores during the adaptive periods following a rotation. Scores typically decrease from the first to the fifth rotation as can be seen in the example in Fig. 7.2. Graphs of sway energy will also illustrate shaded areas, which represent responses outside the normal distribution. Impairment of central processing, reduced muscle strength, or limited mobility at the ankles may be responsible for abnormal adaptive responses.

Sensory Organization Testing (SOT)

Description of Test

SOT aims to evaluate the patient's ability to utilize information provided by the visual, vestibular, and somatosensory systems to maintain posture. Testing is performed by a method called sway referencing, where somatosensory and/or visual inputs are disrupted. Sway referencing is accomplished by tilting the support surface and/or visual surround to follow the anteroposterior (AP) sway of the patient [9]. Although information is still received from these senses, the body perceives no change in position relative to gravity due to the altered conditions and inputs. The non-dizzy patient ignores this "inaccurate" information provided by the sway-reference sense and maintains balance via other senses [1].

During the testing protocol, patients are exposed to the following six sensory conditions with increasing difficulty for adaptation [9]:

1. Eyes open and support surface fixed.
2. Eyes closed and support surface fixed.
   (Both of the above conditions provide baseline measurements.)
3. Visual input is sway referenced and support surface is fixed.
4. Eyes open and support surface is sway referenced.

5. Eyes closed and support surface is sway referenced.
6. Both visual input and support structure are sway referenced.

This protocol is repeated three times for each condition to improve reliability and identify if the patient can compensate for altered conditions. In addition to the COG sway, another measure of stability, the equilibrium score, is measured for each trial. The equilibrium score is found by comparing the peak amplitude of AP sway to that experienced by the matched non-dizzy population. This is expressed as a percentage, with 100 representing perfect balance and 0 indicating loss of balance.

Depiction of Results (Fig. 7.3)

The first graph typically shows the equilibrium scores for each trial under the six sensory conditions. Results that are below the fifth centile of an age-matched sample are seen as the notched aspect of the graph. The final column in the graph shows the composite equilibrium score, which is the best representation of a patient's performance. This composite score places more emphasis on the results of conditions 3 through 6 than 1 and 2.

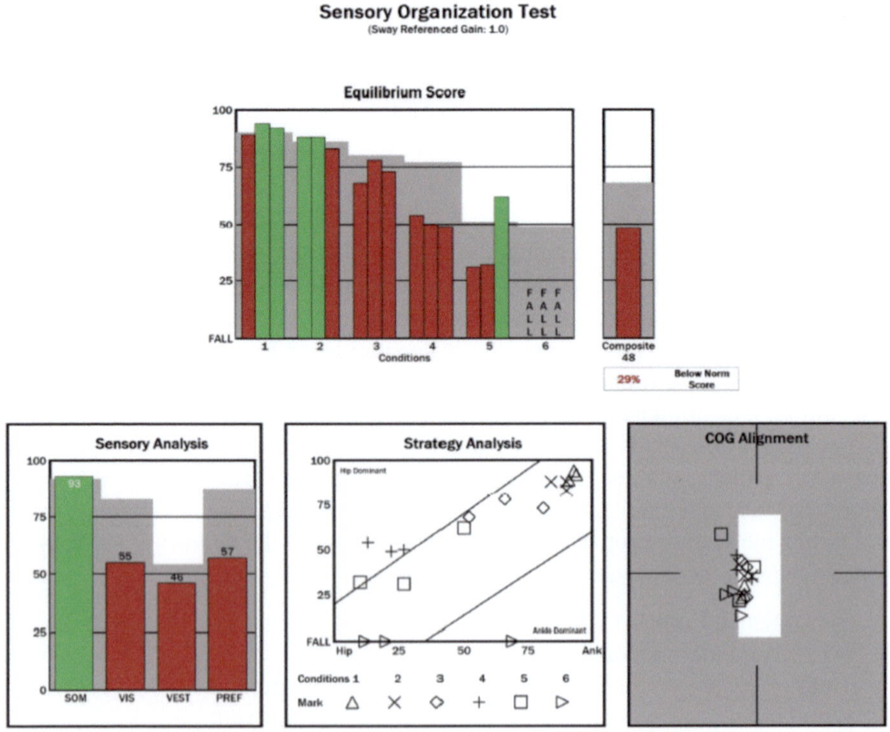

Fig. 7.3 Example of sensory organization testing

Sensory organization analysis characterizes the specific cause of the patient's balance disturbance, with results indicating the contribution of particular senses. This is identified by analyzing the averaged equilibrium scores of one condition compared to that of another condition.

1. The somatosensory ratio quantifies the effect of balance when eyes are closed on a stationary platform by comparing conditions 1–2.
2. The visual ratio compares conditions 4 and 1 by removing the somatosensory input.

(For both of the above ratios, if the vestibular input is used, instead of the somatosensory or visual input, the sway ratio would remain large. Therefore, an abnormal [lower than normal] ratio would indicate an abnormality of the mentioned senses [1].

3. The vestibular ratio compares conditions 5 and 1 and occurs when both the visual and somatosensory inputs are disrupted.
4. The vision preference compares conditions 3 and 6 with the sum of conditions 2 and 5. This compares the balance with eyes open and closed when the visual input and platform are sway referenced.

Strategy analysis examines the contribution of the hip and ankle to the sway and movement of the patient. Normal results are found within a diagonal area of the graph. Typically, when the sway is small, ankle movement will be used to compensate, with hip movement used prior to loss of balance.

The COG is also illustrated by plotting the AP and lateral COG positions of all trials. Points located superior to the center of the plot indicate a COG forward on the support structure, while those inferior reflect a more posterior position on the platform. Points left or right correspond to lateral displacement of the COG.

Conclusion

CDP can give the physician objective information about a patient's postural control by examining their motor control, sensory input, and adaption. Results can be used to examine a patient's functional impairment or localize the areas contributing to loss of balance. Together with clinical acumen, they may help diagnose postural instability and tailor treatments for individual patients.

References

1. Nasher L. Computerized dynamic posturography. In: Jacobson GP, Shepard NT, editors. Balance function assessment and management. 2nd ed. San Diego: Plural Publishing; 2014. p. 451–76.
2. Blaszczyk JW. The use of force-plate posturography in the assessment of postural instability. Gait Posture. 2016;44:1–6.

3. Diener HC, Horak FB, Nasher LM. Influence of stimulus parameters on human postural responses. J Neurophysiol. 1988;59(6):1888–905.
4. Jacobs JV, Horak FB. Cortical control of postural responses. J Neural Transm. 2007;114(10):1339–48.
5. Dietz V, Quintern J, Berger W. Cerebral evoked potential associated with the compensatory reactions following stance and gait disturbance. Neurosci Lett. 1984;50(1–3):181–6.
6. Berger W, Dietz V, Quintern J. Corrective reactions to stumbling in man: neuronal co-ordination of bilateral leg muscle activity during gait. J Physiol. 1984;357:109–25.
7. Nasher LM. Fixed patterns of rapid postural responses among leg muscles during stance. Exp Brain Res. 1977;150:403–7.
8. Nasher LM. Adapting reflexes controlling the human posture. Exp Brain Res. 1976;26(1):59–72.
9. Nasher LM, Black FO, Wall C. Adaption to altered support and visual conditions during stance: patients with vestibular deficits. J Neurosci. 1992;2(5):536–44.

Chapter 8
Vestibular-Evoked Myogenic Potentials

Robert J. Macielak, Saul Strieb, Oliver F. Adunka, and Desi P. Schoo

Vestibular-Evoked Potentials

The use of evoked potentials plays an important role in diagnosing certain types of vestibular impairments. The most commonly used forms of vestibular-evoked potentials are vestibular-evoked myogenic potentials (VEMPs). Testing is relatively easy to perform and is highly reproducible. VEMPs are part of the standard vestibular test battery at most institutions, and when combined with other vestibular procedures, such as bithermal caloric testing or video head-impulse testing (vHIT), are thought to allow for assessment of the entire peripheral vestibular system. Of greatest import, their use has become paramount in the diagnosis of conditions involving active third mobile window phenomena such as superior canal dehiscence syndrome (SCDS).

Cervical VEMPS (cVEMPs)

cVEMPs are inhibitory (relaxation) myogenic responses measured via surface electrodes from the sternocleidomastoid (SCM) muscle ipsilateral to the stimulated ear and are used to assess the integrity of the vestibulocollic reflex (VCR) pathway [1]. Based on results from human neurectomy [1–4], vestibular schwannoma removal [4, 5], and vestibular neuritis [6–10] studies, as well as neurophysiologic studies in animals, [11, 12] the cVEMP response is generally attributed to saccular

R. J. Macielak · S. Strieb · O. F. Adunka · D. P. Schoo (✉)
Department of Otolaryngology-Head and Neck Surgery, The Ohio State University Wexner Medical Center, Columbus, OH, USA
e-mail: robert.macielak@osumc.edu; saul.strieb@osumc.edu; oliver.adunka@osumc.edu; desi.schoo@osumc.edu

J. C. Lucas et al. (eds.), *Diagnosis and Treatment of Vestibular Disorders*,
https://doi.org/10.1007/978-3-032-11740-3_8

stimulation, with the afferent signal transmitted through the inferior vestibular nerve; and to a lesser extent stimulation from the utricular traveling through the superior vestibular nerve. [13, 14] Other evidence suggests that the cVEMP may actually reflect a common pathway response that includes input of varying degree from all of the semicircular canals and otolith organs. [15–17]

Clinically, cVEMP testing most commonly employs air conduction sound stimuli using either tone bursts or clicks. Additionally, bone conduction stimuli via a bone oscillator or through skull taps using a hand-held Bruel and Kjaer mini-shaker device or specially adapted tendon hammer may also be used, [3, 9, 18] particularly in cases of conductive hearing loss due to middle ear dysfunction where an air conduction stimuli may not reach the inner ear to trigger the VEMP response [19–22]. Lastly, galvanic stimulation also produces VEMP responses, [23–25] but this method is rarely used in clinical practice.

The electrode montage for cVEMP testing places the recording electrodes at the midpoint of the belly of the SCM muscles and the shared reference electrode approximately 1 inch below the sternal notch (Fig. 8.1). During testing, the patient is asked to contract the targeted SCM by turning their head contralaterally while seated, or lifting their head, with or without turning their head to the contralateral side while recumbent. These actions produce myogenic activity in the ipsilateral

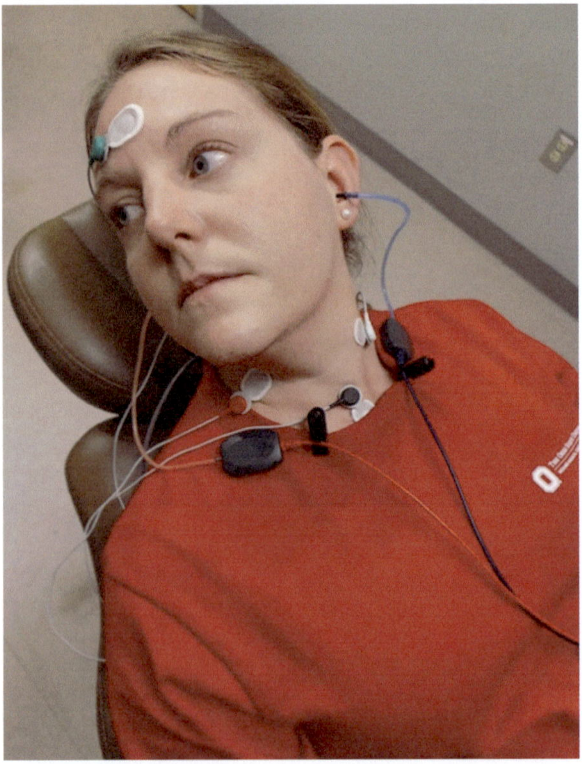

Fig. 8.1 Head position for left cVEMP testing and cVEMP electrode montage

SCM muscle which is measured using electromyography (EMG). Stimulation then evokes a signal through the VCR pathway that briefly and repeatedly inhibits this baseline myogenic activity, [26, 27] in turn producing a biphasic electrical potential response. The normal response (Fig. 8.2) displays a positive peak labeled P13 followed by a negative peak labeled N23, so named because their *peak latencies* are measured at approximately 13 ms and 23 ms, respectively, following stimulus onset. [1] Other pertinent cVEMP measures include *threshold*, defined as the lowest stimulus level producing a response, *interpeak amplitude*, the voltage difference between the P13 and N23 peaks, and the *interaural interpeak amplitude asymmetry ratio (AAR)*, which is calculated as the difference between amplitudes divided by their sum and expressed as a percentage, to quantify the degree of amplitude asymmetry between ears.

The cVEMP P13-N23 interpeak amplitude scales with increasing muscle contraction and is associated with increasing EMG activity. While some studies [1, 28] describe a linear relationship between the interpeak amplitude and EMG activity, others [29, 30] have observed non-proportional growth in the responses, in part due to saturation of the response amplitude above a certain EMG level. As a result, clinicians must ensure that patients undergoing cVEMP testing produce stable and equivalent baseline EMG levels that are well below the saturation point during each test run, optimally between 30 and 50 μV [31], although 60 μV is also often used. This is accomplished through biofeedback, either with instruction from the clinician or having the patient viewing and adjusting their baseline EMG levels to a target as displayed on a monitor and may be used in combination with response *amplitude correction* (also termed *amplitude normalization*). Amplitude correction is performed by dividing the raw response amplitude by the average rectified baseline EMG level measured within an interval of approximately 20–100 μsec prior to stimulus onset. [1, 30, 32] The aim of these methods—biofeedback and amplitude correction—is to promote consistency of responses, ensuring that both symmetrical and asymmetrical

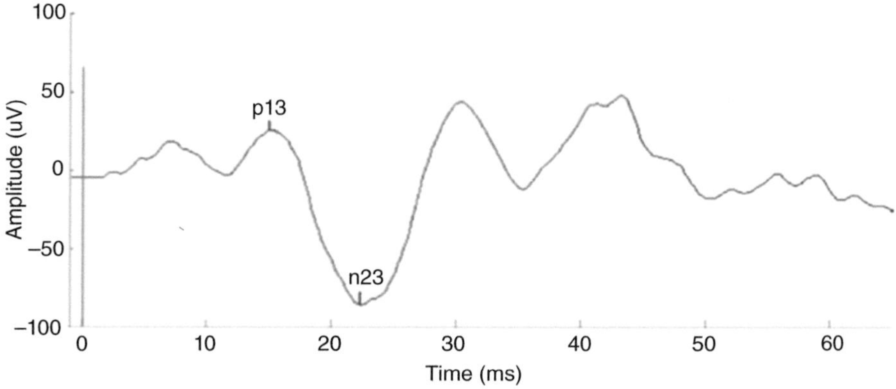

Fig. 8.2 cVEMP response recorded from the left sternocleidomastoid muscle of an adult patient in response to a 500 Hz air conduction tone burst stimulus at 90 dB nHL

responses are correctly identified, quantified, and interpreted, rather than artificially produced by variation in baseline EMG levels between sides or individual runs.

Ocular VEMPS (oVEMPs)

oVEMPs are excitatory (contraction) myogenic responses evoked bilaterally and recorded from the inferior oblique (IO) muscle via surface electrodes in response to contralateral inner ear stimulation, including air conduction sound stimulation, bone conduction stimulation (i.e., using a bone oscillator or skull taps via a mini-shaker or tendon hammer), or galvanic stimulation. [18, 33–36] oVEMP testing assesses the integrity of the crossed vestibulo-ocular reflex (VOR) pathway. The oVEMP response is mediated by the superior vestibular nerve, [37–39] which contains nerve fibers from both otolith organs. [9] These responses appear to predominantly encode utricular stimulation, [13, 35, 40] which is greater when evoked by bone conduction than air conduction stimulation, and to a lesser extent saccular stimulation. [13] Of note, in SCDS, in addition to the enlarged oVEMP responses, the pattern of oVEMP-evoked eye movements (i.e., VOR) suggests a significant stimulation of the superior semicircular canal in addition to the saccular activation. [41, 42]

The standard electrode montage for oVEMP testing places the active electrodes approximately 1 cm inferior to the lower eyelid, with the reference electrodes 2 cm below the active electrodes (Fig. 8.3). Other electrode montages have been promoted to further magnify responses and reduce reference contamination by relocating the reference electrodes; these include reference placement over the IO tendon ("belly-tendon" montage) [43] and on the chin. [44] During oVEMP testing, the patient gazes upward, which magnifies the responses through increased tonic IO muscle activation as well as bringing the muscle closer to the recording electrode. [45] Stimulation produces a biphasic response (Fig. 8.4) with an initial negative peak (n1 or n10) displaying *latency* normally measured at approximately 10–11 ms, followed by a positive peak (p1 or p15) with latency measured at approximately 15 ms post-stimulus. Additional oVEMP measures include *n1 amplitude* measured from baseline *n1-p1 interpeak amplitude, threshold, and interaural interpeak amplitude asymmetry ratio (AAR).*

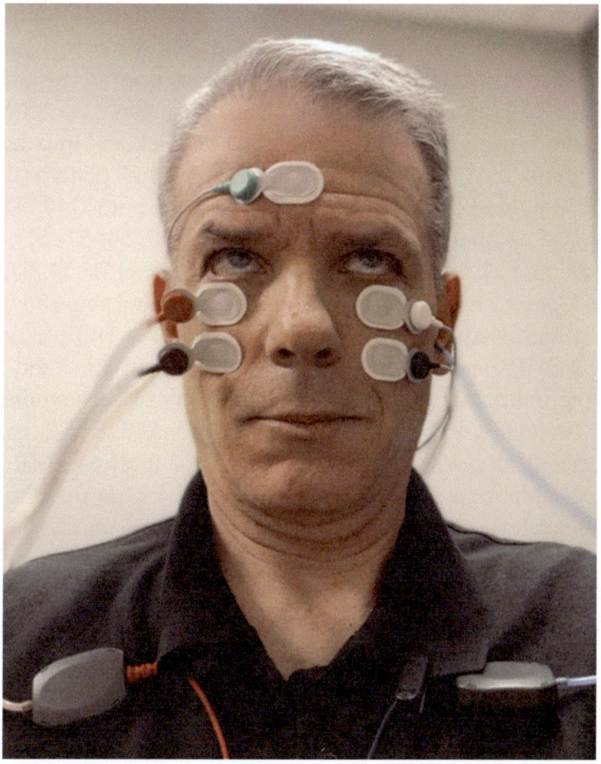

Fig. 8.3 Traditional electrode montage and gaze direction for oVEMP testing

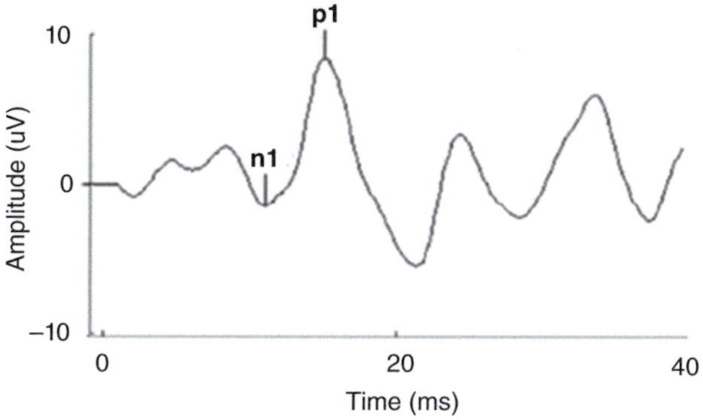

Fig. 8.4 oVEMP response recorded from an adult patient using a 500 Hz air conduction tone burst stimulus at 90 dB nHL

Clinical Use of VEMPs

The primary use of both cVEMPs and oVEMPs is to aid in the diagnosis of SCDS. SCDS is a disorder variably characterized by vertigo and oscillopsia to loud sounds or acute changes in intracranial or inner ear pressure, along with other auditory and otologic symptoms (e.g., autophony, ear fullness). The pathologic third mobile window in SCDS is thought to create a low impedance system resulting in enhanced transmission of sound and pressure energy through the vestibular portions of the inner ear, which causes them to become responsive to sound and pressure changes [46, 47] as well as to display abnormal VEMP response patterns. Prior studies using air and bone conduction click and low- and high-frequency tone burst stimuli have demonstrated these abnormal patterns to include reduced cVEMP thresholds [22, 48–58] and oVEMP thresholds [49, 51, 52, 54]; enlarged cVEMP n13-P23 interpeak amplitudes [41, 51, 52, 54, 57–61], oVEMP n1 amplitudes [41, 49, 53, 62], and n1-p1 interpeak amplitudes [51–54, 57, 60, 63]; prolonged oVEMP n1 latency when using skull taps [64, 65]; and abnormally present oVEMP responses to high-frequency stimuli. [56, 60, 66] Overall, as a diagnostic test for SCDS, cVEMPs and oVEMPs demonstrate sensitivities and specificities in the range of approximately 70–100% in the majority of such studies. To this effect, the Barany Society consensus diagnostic criteria for SCDS [67] list enhanced VEMP responses, specifically, low cVEMP thresholds or high oVEMP amplitudes, as one of three possible signs or test results required for its diagnosis. Similarly, the American Academy of Neurology practice guideline on cVEMP and oVEMP testing [68] indicates that both cVEMP and oVEMP responses, including low thresholds and increased response amplitudes (i.e., uncorrected oVEMP and corrected cVEMP amplitudes) may be used in the identification and diagnosis of SCDS. Following successful SCDS repair surgery, abnormal VEMP responses have been found to return to their normal ranges in most of these studied measures. [22, 48, 49, 51] It should be noted that other third mobile window disorders, including enlarged vestibular aqueduct and lateral and posterior semicircular canal dehiscence, produce similar abnormal VEMP responses patterns. [22, 69]

The cVEMP and oVEMP peak latencies and AAR are useful in assessing the integrity of the VCR and VOR pathways. Abnormally prolonged latencies have been proposed as indicators of slowed neural conduction along these pathways due to retrolabyrinthine disorders such as demyelinating disease, neuropathy, and tumors. Supporting examples include (1) unilateral or bilateral delays in one or both peak latencies, with or without interpeak interval enlargement, for cVEMP [70–76] and/or oVEMP [74] [75], [77], responses in cases of multiple sclerosis, (2) prolonged latencies of both peaks in cVEMP [78] and oVEMP [78, 79] responses in patients with diabetic neuropathy, and (3) delayed cVEMP and oVEMP peaks occasionally observed in patients with vestibular schwannomas. [70, 80] The pattern of such abnormalities obtained when combining oVEMP and cVEMP results has the potential to localize involvement within the ascending (i.e., VOR) and descending (i.e., VCR) brainstem pathways. [81]

Asymmetric vestibular function may also be identified by measuring the interaural interpeak AARs using air conduction tone burst stimuli. AARs greater than 31–46% for cVEMPs [82–84] and 34–43% for oVEMPs [44] [85–87], are generally considered abnormal, suggesting an asymmetric vestibular loss on the side of the ear generating weaker response, and thus the involved VCR or VOR pathway. These interpretations assume that other potential causes of asymmetry have been ruled out, such as unilateral middle ear dysfunction with conductive hearing loss abolishing the VEMP responses [19, 20, 22], or SCDS enlarging them. Many sources [88–93] go further, promoting cVEMPs as an effective test of saccular and inferior vestibular nerve integrity and oVEMPs as a test of utricular and superior vestibular nerve integrity, with weak or absent responses indicating dysfunction of the respective otolith organ, vestibular nerve, or their afferent central pathways. However, the validity of using VEMPs for these purposes is debated, with contesting sources citing issues including the following:

1. The absence of another quantitative test of saccular and utricular function in humans against which to compare and validate VEMP measurements. [17, 68]
2. Concerns [17, 39] regarding test design flaws, incorporation bias, and other circular logic apparent in various publications concluding that VEMP tests can be used in these ways.
3. Ongoing concern regarding which of the vestibular end organs actually serve as the generators of the VEMP responses, that may well be common pathway responses generated by several or all of the end organs. In addition to the overall complexity of the central processing of vestibular signals, some of the other factors raised for this particular concern recently by Kjaersgaard, Hougaard, and Kingma [17] include the following:

   - Stimulation by air conduction at the levels used in clinical VEMP testing activates afferents in each of the five vestibular end organs. [15, 16]
   - Second-order vestibular neurons ("convergent neurons"), especially those within the VCR pathway, receive input from more than one end organ, most commonly a combination of both otolith and semicircular canal input. [94]
   - Stimulation of the afferents from each end organ individually produces an inhibitory response in the ipsilateral SCM muscle. [95, 96]

Studies on VEMP responses in vestibular migraine patients further complicate the interpretation of response amplitude asymmetries and peak latency prolongation by revealing a variety of somewhat inconsistent abnormalities and conflicting results in such patients. These include increased incidence of enlarged AAR due to unilaterally reduced amplitude or absent oVEMP [91] [97–100], or cVEMP [100] responses, bilaterally reduced amplitude and absent oVEMP [97, 98] or cVEMP [100–102] responses, and delayed oVEMP [100, 102] and cVEMP [99, 100, 102, 103] peaks.

Despite the concerns noted above, VEMP testing, when combined with a more comprehensive vestibular testing battery, is likely to provide greater clarity regarding site of lesion within the vestibular end organs and nerves and central vestibular pathways. Examples include the following:

- Inferior vestibular nerve involvement suggested in an ear with both a weak or absent cVEMP response and a concurrent abnormal posterior vHIT response.
- Superior nerve involvement indicated by reduced/absent oVEMP response concurrent with abnormal caloric and lateral and anterior vHIT responses.

Considerations/Limitations

Constraints involved in VEMP testing are usually specific to the type of VEMP performed. However, both cVEMP and oVEMP responses are elicited by high-intensity acoustic signals and as stated above, are typically abolished when conductive hearing loss exists. It should be noted that VEMPs are unaffected by cochlear hearing loss and can be evoked in patients with severe to profound sensorineural hearing loss, contrary to the effect of conductive hearing losses. [1, 104, 105]

Additional limitations include the need to actively contract the various muscles during testing, specifically related to cVEMPs. Patients who are restricted physically due to cervical injury or cannot cause a SCM contraction for an extended period of time have limited ability to complete cVEMP testing. This limitation becomes a particular concern when evaluating the elderly population. Constraints for oVEMPs are in general far fewer compared to cVEMPs. The main limitation includes any condition that prevents the patient from being able to move the eye in the vertical direction for an extended period of time. Congenital nystagmus, although an issue for other vestibular testing, does not appear to affect the oVEMP procedure. [106]

It is important to keep in mind that both VEMP pathways involve the central nervous system tracts, and thus, various neurologic disorders can influence VEMP results, including the latency amplitude of the response. Caution should be taken when testing patients with hyperacusis, as the stimulation intensity is at the equipment's maximum and can cause extreme discomfort in these patients. Finally, although rare, sudden hearing loss has been reported following VEMP testing, possibly because of loud stimulus intensity [107].

Summary

Cervical and ocular vestibular-evoked potentials complement the traditional vestibular test battery. Although previously considered in a number of different pathologies, its main clinical utility remains in the assessment of patients with suspected SCDS.

References

1. Colebatch JG, Halmagyi GM, Skuse NF. Myogenic potentials generated by a click-evoked vestibulocollic reflex. J Neurol Neurosurg Psychiatry. 1994;57(2):190–7. https://doi.org/10.1136/jnnp.57.2.190.
2. Colebatch JG, Halmagyi GM. Vestibular evoked potentials in human neck muscles before and after unilateral vestibular deafferentation. Neurology. 1992;42(8):1635–6. https://doi.org/10.1212/WNL.42.8.1635.

3. Halmagyi GM, Yavor RA, Colebatch JG. Tapping the head activates the vestibular system. Neurology. 1995;45(10):1927–9. https://doi.org/10.1212/WNL.45.10.1927.
4. Brantberg K, Mathiesen T. Preservation of tap vestibular evoked myogenic potentials despite resection of the inferior vestibular nerve. J Vestib Res. 2004;14(4):347–51. http://www.ncbi.nlm.nih.gov/pubmed/15328448
5. Magliulo G, Gagliardi M, Appiani GC, D'Amico R. Preservation of the saccular nerve and of the vestibular evoked myogenic potential during vestibular schwannoma surgery. Otol Neurotol. 2003;24(2):308–11. https://doi.org/10.1097/00129492-200303000-00029.
6. Magliulo G, Gagliardi S, Appiani MC, Iannella G, Re M. Vestibular Neurolabyrinthitis. Ann Otol Rhinol Laryngol. 2014;123(3):162–73. https://doi.org/10.1177/0003489414522974.
7. Murofushi T, Halmagyi GM, Yavor RA, Colebatch JG. Absent vestibular evoked myogenic potentials in vestibular neurolabyrinthitis: an indicator of inferior vestibular nerve involvement? Arch Otolaryngol Head Neck Surg. 1996;122(8):845–8. https://doi.org/10.1001/archotol.1996.01890200035008.
8. Brantberg K, Tribukait A, Fransson PA. Vestibular evoked myogenic potentials in response to skull taps for patients with vestibular neuritis. J Vestib Res. 2003;13(2–3):121–30. http://www.ncbi.nlm.nih.gov/pubmed/14757915
9. Govender S, Rosengren SM, Colebatch JG. Vestibular neuritis has selective effects on air- and bone-conducted cervical and ocular vestibular evoked myogenic potentials. Clin Neurophysiol. 2011;122(6):1246–55. https://doi.org/10.1016/j.clinph.2010.12.040.
10. Shin BS, Oh SY, Kim JS, et al. Cervical and ocular vestibular-evoked myogenic potentials in acute vestibular neuritis. Clin Neurophysiol. 2012;123(2):369–75. https://doi.org/10.1016/j.clinph.2011.05.029.
11. Murofushi T, Curthoys IS, Gilchrist DP. Response of Guinea pig vestibular nucleus neurons to clicks. Exp Brain Res. 1996;111(1):149–52. https://doi.org/10.1007/BF00229565.
12. Murofushi T, Curthoys IS. Physiological and anatomical study of click-sensitive primary vestibular afferents in the Guinea pig. Acta Otolaryngol. 1997;117(1):66–72. https://doi.org/10.3109/00016489709117994.
13. Govender S, Dennis DL, Colebatch JG. Vestibular evoked myogenic potentials (VEMPs) evoked by air- and bone-conducted stimuli in vestibular neuritis. Clin Neurophysiol. 2015;126(10):2004–13. https://doi.org/10.1016/j.clinph.2014.12.029.
14. Kushiro K, Zakir M, Ogawa Y, Sato H, Uchino Y. Saccular and utricular inputs to sternocleidomastoid motoneurons of decerebrate cats. Exp Brain Res. 1999;126(3):410–6. https://doi.org/10.1007/s002210050747.
15. Zhu H, Tang X, Wei W, et al. Input–output functions of vestibular afferent responses to air-conducted clicks in rats. J Assoc Res Otolaryngol. 2014;15(1):73–86. https://doi.org/10.1007/s10162-013-0428-6.
16. Huang J, Tang X, Xu Y, et al. Differential activation of canal and otolith afferents by acoustic tone bursts in rats. J Assoc Res Otolaryngol. 2022;23(3):435–53. https://doi.org/10.1007/s10162-022-00839-1.
17. Kjærsgaard JB, Hougaard DD, Kingma H. Thirty years with cervical vestibular myogenic potentials: a critical review on its origin. Front Neurol. 2025;15:1502093. https://doi.org/10.3389/fneur.2024.1502093.
18. Greenwalt NL, Patterson JN, Rodriguez AI, Fitzpatrick D, Gordon KR, Janky KL. Bone conduction vibration Vestibular Evoked Myogenic Potential (VEMP) testing: reliability in children, adolescents, and Young adults. Ear Hear. 2021;42(2):355–63. https://doi.org/10.1097/AUD.0000000000000925.
19. Bath AP, Harris N, Mcewan J, Yardley MP. Effect of conductive hearing loss on the vestibulo-collic reflex. Clin Otolaryngol Allied Sci. 1999;24(3):181–3. https://doi.org/10.1046/j.1365-2273.1999.00234.x.
20. Yang TL, Young YH. Comparison of tone burst and tapping evocation of myogenic potentials in patients with chronic otitis media. Ear Hear. 2003;24(3):191–4. https://doi.org/10.1097/01.AUD.0000069224.02224.4C.

21. Sheykholeslami K, Murofushi T, Kermany M, Kaga K. Bone-conducted evoked myogenic potentials from the sternocleidomastoid muscle. Acta Otolaryngol. 2000;120(6):731–4. https://doi.org/10.1080/000164800750000252.
22. Zhou G, Poe D, Gopen Q. Clinical use of vestibular evoked myogenic potentials in the evaluation of patients with air-bone gaps. Otol Neurotol. 2012;33(8):1368–74. https://doi.org/10.1097/MAO.0b013e31826a542f.
23. Watson SRD, Colebatch JG. Vestibulocollic reflexes evoked by short-duration galvanic stimulation in man. J Physiol. 1998;513(2):587–97. https://doi.org/10.1111/j.1469-7793.1998.587bb.x.
24. Murofushi T, Monobe H, Ochiai A, Ozeki H. The site of lesion in "vestibular neuritis": study by galvanic VEMP. Neurology. 2003;61(3):417–8. https://doi.org/10.1212/01.WNL.0000076480.11463.17.
25. Chang C, Cheng P, Young Y. Aging effect on galvanic vestibular-evoked myogenic potentials. Otolaryngol Head Neck Surg. 2010;143(3):418–21. https://doi.org/10.1016/j.otohns.2010.04.269.
26. Colebatch JG, Rothwell JC. Motor unit excitability changes mediating vestibulocollic reflexes in the sternocleidomastoid muscle. Clin Neurophysiol. 2004;115(11):2567–73. https://doi.org/10.1016/j.clinph.2004.06.012.
27. Wit HP, Kingma CM. A simple model for the generation of the vestibular evoked myogenic potential (VEMP). Clin Neurophysiol. 2006;117(6):1354–8. https://doi.org/10.1016/j.clinph.2006.03.014.
28. Lee Lim C, Clouston P, Sheean G, Yiannnikas C. The influence of voluntary EMG activity and click intensity on the vestibular click evoked myogenic potential. Muscle Nerve. 1995;18(10):1210–3. https://doi.org/10.1002/mus.880181021.
29. Bogle JM, Zapala DA, Criter R, Burkard R. The effect of muscle contraction level on the cervical vestibular evoked myogenic potential (cVEMP): usefulness of amplitude normalization. J Am Acad Audiol. 2013;24(2):77–88. https://doi.org/10.3766/jaaa.24.2.2.
30. McCaslin DL, Fowler A, Jacobson GP. Amplitude normalization reduces cervical vestibular evoked myogenic potential (cVEMP) amplitude asymmetries in Normal subjects: proof of concept. J Am Acad Audiol. 2014;25(3):268–77. https://doi.org/10.3766/jaaa.25.3.6.
31. Akin FW, Murnane OD, Panus PC, Caruthers SK, Wilkinson AE, Proffitt TM. The influence of voluntary tonic EMG level on the vestibular-evoked myogenic potential. J Rehabil Res Dev. 2004;41(3b):473. https://doi.org/10.1682/JRRD.2003.04.0060.
32. McCaslin DL, Jacobson GP, Hatton K, Fowler AP, DeLong AP. The effects of amplitude normalization and EMG targets on cVEMP Interaural amplitude asymmetry. Ear Hear. 2013;34(4):482–90. https://doi.org/10.1097/AUD.0b013e31827ad792.
33. Rosengren SM, McAngus Todd NP, Colebatch JG. Vestibular-evoked extraocular potentials produced by stimulation with bone-conducted sound. Clin Neurophysiol. 2005;116(8):1938–48. https://doi.org/10.1016/j.clinph.2005.03.019.
34. Iwasaki S, McGarvie LA, Halmagyi GM, et al. Head taps evoke a crossed vestibulo-ocular reflex. Neurology. 2007;68(15):1227–9. https://doi.org/10.1212/01.wnl.0000259064.80564.21.
35. Todd NPM, Rosengren SM, Colebatch JG. Ocular vestibular evoked myogenic potentials (OVEMPs) produced by impulsive transmastoid accelerations. Clin Neurophysiol. 2008;119(7):1638–51. https://doi.org/10.1016/j.clinph.2008.03.009.
36. Cheng PW, Chen CC, Wang SJ, Young YH. Acoustic, mechanical and galvanic stimulation modes elicit ocular vestibular-evoked myogenic potentials. Clin Neurophysiol. 2009;120(10):1841–4. https://doi.org/10.1016/j.clinph.2009.08.002.
37. Iwasaki S, Chihara Y, Smulders YE, et al. The role of the superior vestibular nerve in generating ocular vestibular-evoked myogenic potentials to bone conducted vibration at Fz. Clin Neurophysiol. 2009;120(3):588–93. https://doi.org/10.1016/j.clinph.2008.12.036.
38. Curthoys IS, Iwasaki S, Chihara Y, Ushio M, McGarvie LA, Burgess AM. The ocular vestibular-evoked myogenic potential to air-conducted sound; probable superior ves-

tibular nerve origin. Clin Neurophysiol. 2011;122(3):611–6. https://doi.org/10.1016/j.clinph.2010.07.018.
39. Todd NPM. The 'double dissociation' is based on a circular logic. Clin Neurophysiol. 2014;125(12):2448–51. https://doi.org/10.1016/j.clinph.2014.03.009.
40. Curthoys IS, Vulovic V, Manzari L. Ocular vestibular-evoked myogenic potential (oVEMP) to test utricular function: neural and oculomotor evidence. Acta Otorhinolaryngol Ital. 2012;32(1):41–5. http://www.ncbi.nlm.nih.gov/pubmed/22500066
41. Rosengren SM, Aw ST, Halmagyi GM, McAngus Todd NP, Colebatch JG. Ocular vestibular evoked myogenic potentials in superior canal dehiscence. J Neurol Neurosurg Psychiatry. 2008;79(5):559–66. https://doi.org/10.1136/jnnp.2007.126730.
42. Cremer PD, Minor LB, Carey JP, Della Santina CC. Eye movements in patients with superior canal dehiscence syndrome align with the abnormal canal. Neurology. 2000;55(12):1833–41. https://doi.org/10.1212/WNL.55.12.1833.
43. Sandhu JS, George SR, Rea PA. The effect of electrode positioning on the ocular vestibular evoked myogenic potential to air-conducted sound. Clin Neurophysiol. 2013;124(6):1232–6. https://doi.org/10.1016/j.clinph.2012.11.019.
44. Piker EG, Jacobson GP, McCaslin DL, Hood LJ. Normal characteristics of the ocular vestibular evoked myogenic potential. J Am Acad Audiol. 2011;22(4):222–30. https://doi.org/10.3766/jaaa.22.4.5.
45. Rosengren SM, Colebatch JG, Straumann D, Weber KP. Why do oVEMPs become larger when you look up? Explaining the effect of gaze elevation on the ocular vestibular evoked myogenic potential. Clin Neurophysiol. 2013;124(4):785–91. https://doi.org/10.1016/j.clinph.2012.10.012.
46. Minor LB, Solomon D, Zinreich JS, Zee DS. Sound- and/or pressure-induced vertigo due to bone dehiscence of the superior Semicircular Canal. Arch Otolaryngol Head Neck Surg. 1998;124(3):249. https://doi.org/10.1001/archotol.124.3.249.
47. Minor LB. Superior canal dehiscence syndrome. Am J Otol. 2000;21(1):9–19. http://www.ncbi.nlm.nih.gov/pubmed/10651428
48. Zhou G, Gopen Q, Poe S. Clinical and diagnostic characterization of canal dehiscence syndrome: a great Otologic mimicker. Otol Neurotol. 2007;28:920–6. https://doi.org/10.1097/MAO.0b013e31814b25f2.
49. Janky KL, Nguyen KD, Welgampola M, Zuniga MG, Carey JP. Air-conducted oVEMPs provide the best separation between intact and superior canal dehiscent labyrinths. Otol Neurotol. 2013;34(1):127–34. https://doi.org/10.1097/MAO.0b013e318271c32a.
50. Kim DH, Kim SW, Kim SH, Jung J h, Hwang SH. Usefulness of cervical vestibular-evoked myogenic potentials for diagnosing patients with Superior Canal dehiscence syndrome: a meta-analysis. Otol Neurotol. 2022;43(2):146–52. https://doi.org/10.1097/MAO.0000000000003430.
51. Welgampola MS, Myrie OA, Minor LB, Carey JP. Vestibular-evoked myogenic potential thresholds normalize on plugging superior canal dehiscence. Neurology. 2008;70:464–72. https://doi.org/10.1212/01.wnl.0000299084.76250.4a.
52. Maheu M, Elblidi A, Saliba I. Investigating performance of cVEMP and oVEMP in the identification of superior canal dehiscence in relation to dehiscence location and size. Audiol Res. 2021;11(3):452–62. https://doi.org/10.3390/audiolres11030042.
53. Zuniga MG, Janky KL, Nguyen KD, Welgampola MS, Carey JP. Ocular versus cervical VEMPs in the diagnosis of superior semicircular canal dehiscence syndrome. Otol Neurotol. 2013;34(1):121–6. https://doi.org/10.1097/MAO.0b013e31827136b0.
54. Govender S, Fernando T, Dennis DL, Welgampola MS, Colebatch JG. Properties of 500 Hz air- and bone-conducted vestibular evoked myogenic potentials (VEMPs) in superior canal dehiscence. Clin Neurophysiol. 2016;127(6):2522–31. https://doi.org/10.1016/j.clinph.2016.02.019.
55. Streubel S-O, Cremer PD, Carey JP. Vestibular-evoked myogenic potentials in the diagnosis of Superior Canal dehiscence syndrome. Acta Otolaryngol. 2001;121(545):41–9. https://doi.org/10.1080/000164801750388090.

56. Lin K, Lahey R, Beckley R, et al. Validating the utility of high frequency ocular vestibular evoked myogenic potential testing in the diagnosis of superior Semicircular Canal dehiscence. Otol Neurotol. 2019;40(10):1353–8. https://doi.org/10.1097/MAO.0000000000002388.
57. Hunter JB, Patel NS, O'Connell BP, et al. Cervical and ocular VEMP testing in diagnosing superior Semicircular Canal dehiscence. Otolaryngol Head Neck Surg. 2017;156(5):917–23. https://doi.org/10.1177/0194599817690720.
58. Noij KS, Herrmann BS, Guinan JJ Jr, Rauch SD. Toward optimizing cVEMP: 2,000-Hz tone bursts improve the detection of Superior Canal dehiscence. Audiol Neurotol. 2018;23(6):335–44. https://doi.org/10.1159/000493721.
59. Noij KS, Remenschneider AK, Herrmann BS, Guinan JJ, Rauch SD. Optimized diagnostic approach to patients suspected of superior Semicircular Canal dehiscence. Ear Hear. 2021;42(5):1295–305. https://doi.org/10.1097/AUD.0000000000001015.
60. Tran ED, Swanson A, Sharon JD, et al. Ocular vestibular-evoked myogenic potential amplitudes elicited at 4 kHz optimize detection of superior Semicircular Canal dehiscence. Front Neurol. 2020;11:879. https://doi.org/10.3389/fneur.2020.00879.
61. Brantberg K, Verrecchia L. Testing vestibular-evoked myogenic potentials with 90-dB clicks is effective in the diagnosis of superior canal dehiscence syndrome. Audiol Neurotol. 2008;14(1):54–8. https://doi.org/10.1159/000153435.
62. Manzari L, Burgess AM, McGarvie LA, Curthoys IS. Ocular and cervical vestibular evoked myogenic potentials to 500 Hz Fz bone-conducted vibration in superior Semicircular Canal dehiscence. Ear Hear. 2012;33(4):508–20. https://doi.org/10.1097/AUD.0b013e3182498c09.
63. Verrecchia L, Brantberg K, Tawfique Z, Maoli D. Diagnostic accuracy of ocular vestibular evoked myogenic potentials for Superior Canal dehiscence syndrome in a large cohort of dizzy patients. Ear Hear. 2019;40(2):287–94. https://doi.org/10.1097/AUD.0000000000000613.
64. Taylor RL, Magnussen JS, Kwok B, et al. Bone-conducted oVEMP latency delays assist in the differential diagnosis of large air-conducted oVEMP amplitudes. Front Neurol. 2020;11:580184. https://doi.org/10.3389/fneur.2020.580184.
65. Taylor RL, Blaivie C, Bom AP, et al. Ocular vestibular-evoked myogenic potentials (oVEMP) to skull taps in normal and dehiscent ears: mechanisms and markers of superior canal dehiscence. Exp Brain Res. 2014;232(4):1073–84. https://doi.org/10.1007/s00221-013-3782-z.
66. Manzari L, Burgess AM, McGarvie LA, Curthoys IS. An indicator of probable semicircular canal dehiscence: ocular vestibular evoked myogenic potentials to high frequencies. Otolaryngol Head Neck Surg. 2013;149(1):142–5. https://doi.org/10.1177/0194599813489494.
67. Ward BK, Van De Berg R, Van Rompaey V, et al. Superior semicircular canal dehiscence syndrome: diagnostic criteria consensus document of the committee for the classification of vestibular disorders of the Bárány society. J Vestib Res. 2021;31(3):131–41. https://doi.org/10.3233/VES-200004.
68. Fife TD, Colebatch JG, Kevin Kerber DA, et al. Practice guideline: cervical and ocular vestibular evoked myogenic potential testing: report of the guideline development, dissemination, and implementation Subcommittee of the American Academy of neurology. Neurology. 2017;89:2288–96. https://doi.org/10.1212/WNL.0000000000004690.
69. Sheykholeslami K, Schmerber S, Kermany MH, Kaga K. Vestibular-evoked myogenic potentials in three patients with large vestibular aqueduct. Hear Res. 2004;190(1–2):161–8. https://doi.org/10.1016/S0378-5955(04)00018-8.
70. Murofushi T, Shimizu K, Takegoshi H, Cheng PW. Diagnostic value of prolonged latencies in the vestibular evoked myogenic potential. Arch Otolaryngol Head Neck Surg. 2001;127(9):1069. https://doi.org/10.1001/archotol.127.9.1069.
71. Alpini D, Pugnetti L, Caputo D, Cornelio F, Capobianco S, Cesarani A. Vestibular evoked myogenic potentials in multiple sclerosis: clinical and imaging correlations. Mult Scler J. 2004;10(3):316–21. https://doi.org/10.1191/1352458504ms1041oa.
72. Bandini F, Beronio A, Ghiglione E, Solaro C, Parodi RC, Mazzella L. The diagnostic value of vestibular evoked myogenic potentials in multiple sclerosis. J Neurol. 2004;251(5):617–21. https://doi.org/10.1007/s00415-004-0378-3.

73. Sartucci F, Logi F. Vestibular-evoked myogenic potentials: a method to assess vestibulo-spinal conduction in multiple sclerosis patients. Brain Res Bull. 2002;59(1):59–63. https://doi.org/10.1016/S0361-9230(02)00842-0.
74. Tutar B, Berkiten G, Salturk Z, et al. Evaluation of vestibular system using c-VEMP and o-VEMP in patients with relapsing-remitting multiple sclerosis. Tr-ENT. 2019;29(3):119–25. https://doi.org/10.5606/Tr-ENG.2019.51423.
75. Gazioglu S, Boz C. Ocular and cervical vestibular evoked myogenic potentials in multiple sclerosis patients. Clin Neurophysiol. 2012;123(9):1872–9. https://doi.org/10.1016/j.clinph.2012.01.022.
76. Di Stadio A, Dipietro L, Ralli M, Greco A, Ricci G, Bernitsas E. The role of vestibular evoked myogenic potentials in multiple sclerosis-related vertigo. A systematic review of the literature. Mult Scler Relat Disord. 2019;28:159–64. https://doi.org/10.1016/j.msard.2018.12.031.
77. Sangu Srinivasan V, Rangappan Munirathinam B, Singh NK, Rajalakshmi K. Usefulness of masseter vestibular evoked myogenic potentials in identifying brainstem dysfunction among individuals with multiple sclerosis. Int J Audiol. 2023;62(7):635–43. https://doi.org/10.1080/14992027.2022.2065548.
78. Zhang J, Ye L, Bai X, Huang Y, Lin J, Huang H. Cervical and ocular vestibular evoked myogenic potentials in patients with diabetic peripheral neuropathy. Diabetol Metab Syndr. 2023;15(1):100. https://doi.org/10.1186/s13098-023-01068-z.
79. El-seady IY, Abd El-Tawab MM, El-Shawaf WI, El-Sehrawy AA. Role of vestibular evoked myogenic potential (VEMP) in diagnosis of vestibular abnormalities in patients with type 2 diabetes mellitus. Egypt J Intern Med. 2022;34(1):36. https://doi.org/10.1186/s43162-022-00103-1.
80. Taylor RL, Kong J, Flanagan S, et al. Prevalence of vestibular dysfunction in patients with vestibular schwannoma using video head-impulses and vestibular-evoked potentials. J Neurol. 2015;262(5):1228–37. https://doi.org/10.1007/s00415-015-7697-4.
81. Rosengren SM, Nogajski JH, Cremer PD, Colebatch JG. Delayed vestibular evoked responses to the eyes and neck in a patient with an isolated brainstem lesion. Clin Neurophysiol. 2007;118(9):2112–6. https://doi.org/10.1016/j.clinph.2007.05.068.
82. Wiener-Vacher SR, Campi M, Boizeau P, Thai-Van H. Cervical vestibular evoked myogenic potentials in healthy children: normative values for bone and air conduction. Front Neurol. 2023;14:1157975. https://doi.org/10.3389/fneur.2023.1157975.
83. Blakley BW, Wong V. Normal values for cervical vestibular-evoked myogenic potentials. Otol Neurotol. 2015;36(6):1069–73. https://doi.org/10.1097/MAO.0000000000000752.
84. McCaslin DL, Jacobson GP. Vestibular-evoked myogenic potentials (VEMPs). In: Jacobson GP, Shepard NT, Barin K, Burkard RF, Janky K, McCaslin DL, editors. Balance function assessment and management. 3rd ed. Plural Publishing, Inc.; 2021. p. 399–438.
85. Murnane OD, Akin FW, Kelly JK, Byrd S. Effects of stimulus and recording parameters on the air conduction ocular vestibular evoked myogenic potential. J Am Acad Audiol. 2011;22(7):469–80. https://doi.org/10.3766/jaaa.22.7.7.
86. Chihara Y, Iwasaki S, Ushio M, Murofushi T. Vestibular-evoked extraocular potentials by air-conducted sound: another clinical test for vestibular function. Clin Neurophysiol. 2007;118(12):2745–51. https://doi.org/10.1016/j.clinph.2007.08.005.
87. Park HJ, Lee IS, Shin JE, Lee YJ, Park MS. Frequency-tuning characteristics of cervical and ocular vestibular evoked myogenic potentials induced by air-conducted tone bursts. Clin Neurophysiol. 2010;121(1):85–9. https://doi.org/10.1016/j.clinph.2009.10.003.
88. Curthoys IS. The interpretation of clinical tests of peripheral vestibular function. Laryngoscope. 2012;122(6):1342–52. https://doi.org/10.1002/lary.23258.
89. Dlugaiczyk J. Evidence-based diagnostic use of VEMPs: from neurophysiological principles to clinical application. HNO. 2020;68(S2):69–78. https://doi.org/10.1007/s00106-019-00767-2.
90. Choi JY. Vestibular-evoked myogenic potentials: principle and clinical findings. Ann Clin Neurophysiol. 2020;22(2):67–74. https://doi.org/10.14253/acn.2020.22.2.67.

91. Makowiec KF, Piker EG, Jacobson GP, Ramadan NM, Roberts RA. Ocular and cervical vestibular evoked myogenic potentials in patients with vestibular migraine. Otol Neurotol. 2018;39(7):e561–7. https://doi.org/10.1097/MAO.0000000000001880.
92. Murofushi T, Suh MW, Manzari L. Editorial: isolated otolith dysfunction and vertigo. Front Neurol. 2022;13:1030513. https://doi.org/10.3389/fneur.2022.1030513.
93. Rosengren SM, Young AS, Taylor RL, Welgampola MS. Vestibular function testing in the 21st century: video head impulse test, vestibular evoked myogenic potential, video nystagmography; which tests will provide answers? Curr Opin Neurol. 2022;35(1):64–74. https://doi.org/10.1097/WCO.0000000000001023.
94. Uchino Y, Sasaki M, Sato H, Bai R, Kawamoto E. Otolith and canal integration on single vestibular neurons in cats. Exp Brain Res. 2005;164(3):271–85. https://doi.org/10.1007/s00221-005-2341-7.
95. Wilson VJ, Schor RH. The neural substrate of the vestibulocollic reflex. Exp Brain Res. 1999;129(4):0483–93. https://doi.org/10.1007/s002210050918.
96. Uchino Y, Kushiro K. Differences between otolith- and semicircular canal-activated neural circuitry in the vestibular system. Neurosci Res. 2011;71(4):315–27. https://doi.org/10.1016/j.neures.2011.09.001.
97. Zaleski A, Bogle J, Starling A, et al. Vestibular evoked myogenic potentials in patients with vestibular migraine. Otol Neurotol. 2015;36(2):295–302. https://doi.org/10.1097/MAO.0000000000000665.
98. Goto F, Wasano K, Kaneda S, Okami K. Prognostic significance vestibular examination results in patients with vestibular migraine. Front Neurol. 2024;15:1370940. https://doi.org/10.3389/fneur.2024.1370940.
99. Tutar B, Berkiten G, Akan O, et al. Analysis of vestibular-evoked myogenic potentials in the vestibular migraine. Neurol Sci Neurophysiol. 2020;37(2):63–9. https://doi.org/10.4103/NSN.NSN_4_20.
100. Sanitha AS, Sinha SK. Cervical and ocular vestibular-evoked myogenic potentials test results and its relation to vestibular signs and symptoms in individuals with vestibular migraine. Egypt J Otolaryngol. 2024;40(1):63. https://doi.org/10.1186/s43163-024-00610-8.
101. Baier B, Stieber N, Dieterich M. Vestibular-evoked myogenic potentials in vestibular migraine. J Neurol. 2009;256(9):1447–54. https://doi.org/10.1007/s00415-009-5132-4.
102. Khalil LH, Hazzaa NM, Nour AA. Vestibular migraine: a correlation study between clinical findings and vestibular evoked myogenic potentials (VEMPs). Egypt J Ear Nose Throat Allied Sci. 2016;17(1):11–6. https://doi.org/10.1016/j.ejenta.2015.05.005.
103. Elmoazen D, Kozou H, Mekky J, Ghanem D. Assessment of cervical and ocular vestibular evoked myogenic potentials in migraine patients. Egypt J Otolaryngol. 2020;36(1):19. https://doi.org/10.1186/s43163-020-00017-1.
104. Bickford RG, Jacobson JL, Cody D. Nature of average evoked potentials to sound and other stimuli in man. Ann N Y Acad Sci. 1964;112(1):204–18. https://doi.org/10.1111/j.1749-6632.1964.tb26749.x.
105. Wu CC, Young YH. Vestibular evoked myogenic potentials are intact after sudden deafness. Ear Hear. 2002;23(3):235–8. https://doi.org/10.1097/00003446-200206000-00007.
106. Manzari L, Burgess AM, Curthoys IS. Is it possible to measure peripheral vestibular function in a patient with congenital nystagmus? Eur Arch Otorrinolaringol. 2012;269(1):349–52. https://doi.org/10.1007/s00405-011-1760-2.
107. Mattingly JK, Portnuff CDF, Hondorp BM, Cass SP. Sudden bilateral hearing loss after cervical and ocular vestibular evoked myogenic potentials. Otol Neurotol. 2015;36(6):961–4. https://doi.org/10.1097/MAO.0000000000000764.

Chapter 9
Electrocochleography

Alexander L. Luryi and Christopher A. Schutt

Introduction

In response to acoustic stimuli, cochlear inner and outer hair cells produce electrical impulses, which propagate through the cochlear nerve to the central nervous system, resulting in perception of sound. The integrity and characteristics of these impulses provide valuable information about cochlear functioning in patients with hearing loss. The first measurements of cochlear electrical activity were obtained in 1930, from the ear of a cat [1]. Five years later, these impulses were observed in a human patient during ear surgery [2]. In 1947, the first clinical application for these measurements was described: to assess cochlear reserve in patients with otosclerosis.[3] As clinical interest continued to increase over the following decades, measurement methods improved, yielding increasingly favorable signal-to-noise ratios. The development of computer averaging algorithms led to further improvements in signal quality and clinical viability, and the first measurements of cochlear electrical activity in awake patients were accomplished in the 1960s and 1970s [4].

Electrocochleography (ECOG) is the measurement of the electrical responses of the cochlea and acoustic nerves to acoustic stimuli. Three primary electrical signals are detected: the cochlear microphonics (CM), thought to represent instantaneous deflection of the cochlear partition in response to noise; the summating potential (SP), thought to represent overall distortion of the basilar membrane; and the

[Alexander L. Luryi] has died before the publication of this book.

A. L. Luryi (Deceased)
Camden, NJ, USA

C. A. Schutt (✉)
Department of Otology and Neurotology, Michigan Ear Institute, Farmington Hills, MI, USA

J. C. Lucas et al. (eds.), *Diagnosis and Treatment of Vestibular Disorders*,
https://doi.org/10.1007/978-3-032-11740-3_9

compound action potential (AP), thought to represent currents produced by simultaneous firing of auditory nerve fibers [5].

Currently, ECOG is most often used as an adjunct tool in the diagnosis of Meniere's disease [6]. However, other indications, including real-time intraoperative monitoring in cochlear implantation [7–9] and diagnosis of superior semicircular canal dehiscence,[10] have been described, and additional applications continue to develop. This chapter describes the technical aspects of ECOG, its relevant electrophysiology, and its clinical applications with emphasis on supporting evidence.

ECOG Procedure

Electrode Placement and Design

Electrode location is a critical variable in ECOG. For comparison, a stimulus at 90 dB sound pressure level (SPL) signal generates an AP signal of approximately 1 μV to the ear canal, 3 μV to the tympanic membrane, and 10 μV to a trans-tympanic electrode on the promontory [11]. For three decades following its inception, ECOG was exclusively measured intraoperatively with electrodes on the round window or promontory [4]. Trans-tympanic measurement using a needle electrode was first proposed in 1947 but was not accomplished until 1960 [3, 12] (Fig. 9.1). As measurement techniques continued to improve, extra-tympanic approaches, including electrodes in the external auditory canal [13, 14] and later on the tympanic membrane [15], were developed. Measurements from more distal locations, including the lobule and the occipital scalp, failed to detect CM and SP signals but did reveal higher latency waveforms originating in the central nervous system, which

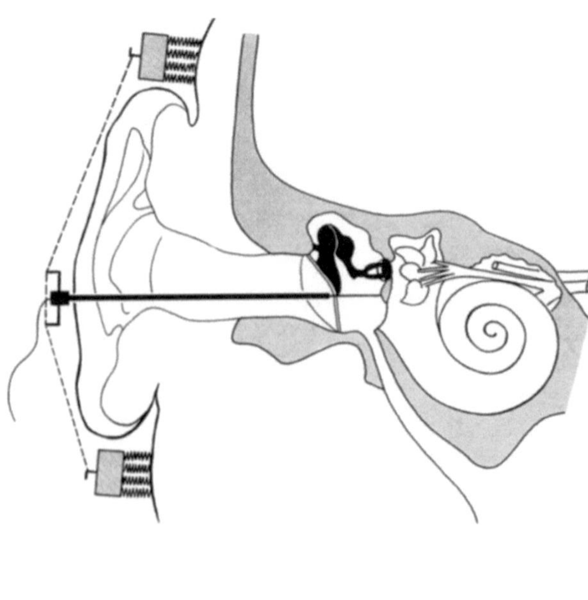

Fig. 9.1 Trans-tympanic electrocochleography. A needle electrode is affixed to the patient and inserted through the tympanic membrane onto the promontory. Adapted with permission from Eggermont, 1976 [4]

formed the basis for auditory brainstem response (ABR) testing [16, 17]. More recently, ECOG measurements have been obtained through cochlear implants; these have very high fidelity as they are measured directly from the inner ear.

Despite its higher fidelity, trans-tympanic ECOG has largely fallen out of favor due to patient discomfort and the potential for complications, including tympanic membrane perforation and otitis media [18, 19]. ECOG measured from the surface of the tympanic membrane is typically accomplished using an insulated wire with a bare tip, which is inserted into the external auditory canal until the patient reports the tip touching the tympanic membrane [20]. Other authors perform a similar procedure with a probe against the external auditory canal skin or free in the canal [21].

Stimuli

ECOG measurements are taken immediately following acoustic stimuli. The first ECOG measurements were obtained following wide-band "clicks," which incorporate a wide range of frequencies simultaneously. This method is a rapid and simple evaluation of cochlear functioning and can yield a reasonable threshold estimation for flat hearing loss. [22] Additionally, some authors argue that click stimuli generate the best synchronization of AP firing [23]. Narrow-band stimuli, including filtered clicks or pure tones, were developed later and carry the advantage of frequency specificity [24, 25]. Nevertheless, wide-band 100 millisecond clicks remain the most popular stimuli in current practice [20]. Extended-duration wide-band tone burst stimuli are sometimes used for improved resolution of the CM and SP, which last for the duration of the stimulus [26].

Measurements

Cochlear Microphonics

In the normal cochlea, the CM is directly proportional to the instantaneous displacement of the basilar membrane [27]. This signal occurs immediately at the onset of stimulus and is generated by the outer hair cells, although the inner hair cells do produce a similar signal of approximately 30–40 dB lower intensity [28]. Due to proximity, the hair cells at the base of the cochlea are primarily represented [29]. The CM is an alternating current signal in phase with the stimulus. It can be difficult to distinguish from stimulus artifact and has limited clinical utility [11]. As a result, early authors strove to silence the CM to better reveal the AP and SP; this was accomplished using stimuli of successively alternating polarity, leading to destructive interference [30] (Fig. 9.2). The CM has recently been shown to be useful in the diagnosis of auditory neuropathy [31].

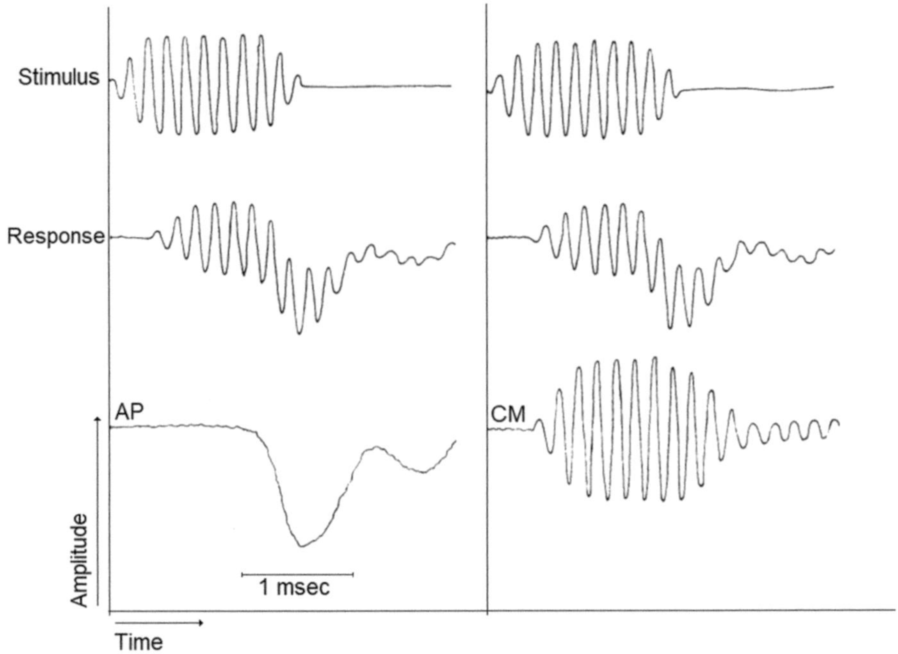

Fig. 9.2 Elimination of cochlear microphonics. Stimuli are presented in opposite phase (top), yielding responses with similar AP but CM of opposite phase (middle). Averaging these responses eliminates the CM, yielding the AP (bottom left), whereas subtraction eliminates the AP, yielding the CM (bottom right). Summating potentials are not visible in this example. AP, compound action potential; CM, cochlear microphonics. Adapted with permission from Eggermont, 1976 [4]

Summating Potential

The SP, also generated by the outer hair cells, represents the baseline shift in position of the basilar membrane during an acoustic stimulus [28]. Complex non-linear relationships govern the movement of the basilar membrane in response to stimulus, leading to an overall displacement of the average position of the membrane independent of the phase of the stimulus [32]. This shift generates a direct current potential beginning approximately 0.8 msec following stimulus onset (at 90 dB HL; this varies with stimulus intensity) and lasting the duration of the stimulus (Fig. 9.3). The direction of this potential (positive or negative) is inconsistent and is based on the stimulus and the position of the electrode.

Compound Action Potential

The AP represents the combined firing of cochlear nerve fibers. This produces a short alternating current signal, which occurs only at the onset of the stimulus. The AP consists of peaks N1 and N2 (Fig. 9.3), which correspond to peaks I and

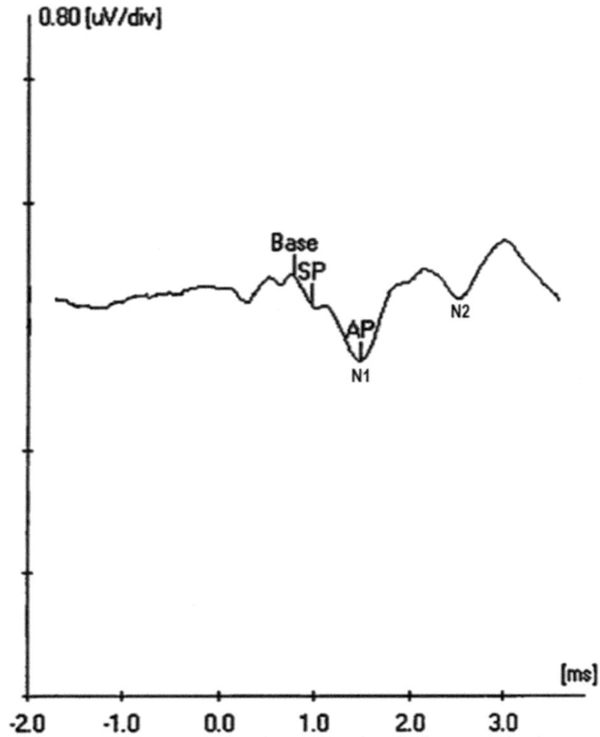

Fig. 9.3 Normal ECOG tracing in response to broadband click stimulus (0.0 ms) with SP/AP ratio of 0.35

II in ABR testing, thought to represent the firing of distal and proximal auditory nerve fibers. The N1 latency, measured from stimulus onset to the N1 peak, ranges from approximately 1 to 2 msec and depends on the stimulus as well as the measurement hardware. The amplitude of the AP (measured by the N1 peak) increases with increasing stimulus intensity, while its latency decreases with increasing stimulus intensity (Fig. 9.4) [11]. The AP N2 peak has limited clinical use.

SP/AP Ratio

The ratio between the intensity of the SP and the AP N1 peak is the most utilized measure obtained from ECOG. Normal values for this ratio vary between institutions but range from approximately 0.1 to between 0.35 and 0.5 for stimuli between 125 and 8000 Hz [21, 32, 33]. Levels higher than 0.5 are abnormal and typically represent inner ear pathology. A normal ECOG tracing is shown in Fig. 9.3, and abnormal ECOG tracings with elevated SP/AP ratios are shown in Fig. 9.5. Significant inter-interpreter variability exists for ECOG interpretation, complicating attempts at standardization [34].

Fig. 9.4 Variation of AP latency with stimulus intensity (wide band click stimulus, normal ear). Adapted with permission from Eggermont, 1976 [4]

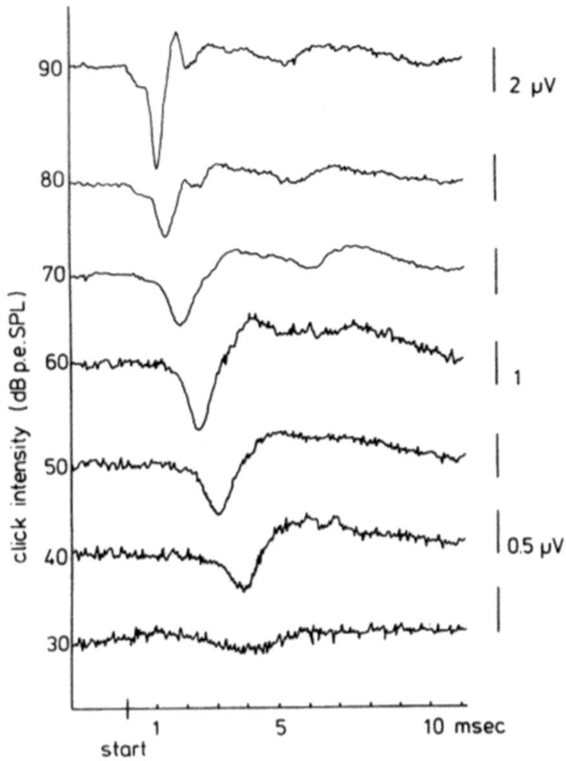

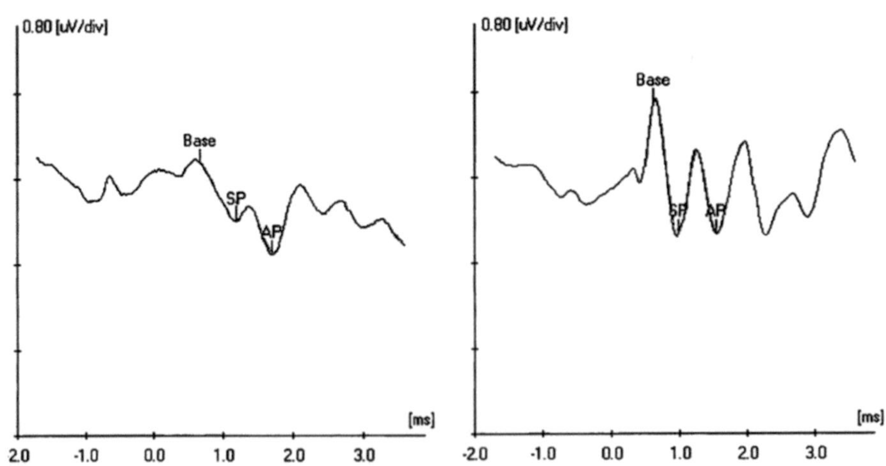

Fig. 9.5 Abnormal ECOG tracings in response to broadband click stimuli (0.1 ms) in patients with Meniere's disease. Left: SP/AP = 0.65; right: SP/AP = 1.00

Applications of ECOG

Many uses have been proposed for ECOG since its inception, although no strict indications exist for its use in any condition. Endolymphatic hydrops is by far the most studied application. However, over recent years, ECOG has been found to be useful in the evaluation of other inner ear disorders as well as in certain intraoperative scenarios.

Meniere's Disease /Endolymphatic Hydrops.

Endolymphatic hydrops is associated with an elevated SP, and more specifically, an increased SP/AP ratio [35–42]. These findings are conserved in the presence and absence of clinical Meniere's disease. SP elevation is thought to be due to the dilation of the scala media in the hydropic cochlear apex, leading to thinning of the basilar membrane and increased displacement in response to stimuli [28, 42]. However, the exact mechanism is unknown, and various mechanical, electrical, biochemical, and ischemic/vascular mechanisms have been proposed [39, 43, 44].

With adequate clinical suspicion, an elevated SP/AP ratio is specific but not sensitive for the diagnosis of Meniere's disease. Reported specificities of ECOG for Meniere's disease range from 92% to 100%, whereas sensitivities range from 30% to 70% [21, 32, 33, 40, 42, 45]. Higher sensitivities have been achieved in more recent studies by using other measurements obtained from ECOG (such as SP/AP area ratio or total SP/AP area; sensitivity 80%) [38, 41] or by combining ECOG measurements with pure tone audiometry findings. One report demonstrated sensitivity and specificity of 94% and 98%, respectively, by combining the SP amplitude at 4000 Hz with air conduction thresholds at 125 and 8000 Hz in binary logistic regression [46]. Elevated SP alone is neither sensitive nor specific for Meniere's disease.

Debate exists regarding the reliability of ECOG in patients with severe hearing loss, with some authors arguing that the integrity of SP and AP waveforms deteriorates in patients with hearing loss greater than 60 dB [6]. These authors advocate ECOG use only in early Meniere's disease. However, more recent data suggest that ECOG findings are conserved in severe hearing loss, with some data suggesting that the sensitivity of ECOG improves for more advanced Meniere's disease [44, 47, 48]. Recent consensus is that ECOG is applicable to Meniere's disease in all stages.

ECOG can be useful to confirm a diagnosis of Meniere's disease or to distinguish it from other possible diagnoses, including benign positional vertigo or vestibular migraine. However, it is a poor screening tool in patients with nonspecific symptoms. Despite its favorable and improving reliability, there is currently no role for ECOG in routine diagnosis of Meniere's disease by American Academy of Otolaryngology-Head and Neck Surgery guidelines [49].

Use in Cochlear Implantation

Speech perception following cochlear implantation is a critical outcome and is highly variable. Intraoperative ECOG immediately prior to cochlear implantation has been shown to predict postoperative word recognition scores with higher accuracy than common clinical factors, such as duration of deafness or degree of residual hearing [8, 50]. Although these data were obtained using electrodes on the round window, they suggest that extra-tympanic ECOG could be used in a clinical setting to assess candidacy for cochlear implants and to set realistic expectations for hearing outcomes. This remains an area of active study.

Furthermore, most modern cochlear implants allow for direct intra-cochlear electrocochleography [51]. This ability confers several notable advantages. As measurements are taken directly from the inner ear, the signal fidelity is significantly improved compared with all other measurement methods. In addition, the need for invasive trans-tympanic monitoring is completely eliminated. Finally, this allows for real-time monitoring of ECOG during cochlear implantation. This can be used to direct surgical technique, both in guiding implant insertion and in monitoring residual hearing for hybrid implants or "soft" cochlear implantation [52, 53]. Postoperative monitoring of cochlear function is also possible and has generated valuable information concerning the pattern of loss of native hearing following cochlear implantation [54].

Other Surgical Applications

ECOG can be used for intraoperative monitoring of hearing during hearing-preservation surgery for tumors of the cerebellopontine angle [9, 55, 56]. This is usually accomplished using a trans-tympanic electrode and the AP signal is monitored, reflecting the function of the eighth cranial nerve. The primary disadvantages of this approach are the invasiveness and technical difficulty involved in placement of the electrode and the instability of the trans-tympanic probe. To address the latter issue, stabilized probes placed through the tragus or extratympanically in the ear canal have been used [57, 58].

Alternative methods of intraoperative nerve monitoring include ABRs and direct nerve measurement (using recording electrodes placed directly on the exposed eighth cranial nerve). Because it is non-invasive, ABR is the most widely used method. However, several studies have shown ECOG to be more reliable in monitoring eighth nerve integrity, which is expected as ECOG measures the same electrophysiologic signals at closer range [57, 59]. Direct nerve measurement is very reliable when properly executed, but requires identification of the eighth nerve and placement of electrodes intraoperatively, increasing operative time. Furthermore, the electrode must be placed on the nerve at the proximal extent of the surgical field, as it will not detect more proximal injuries. This may be difficult in the setting of very large tumors or unfavorable anatomy [60, 61].

ECOG has also been used during stapedectomy to monitor for cochlear damage and to fine-tune ossicular reconstruction. However, it was not found to prevent sensorineural hearing loss during stapedectomy, but only to predict it postoperatively [62, 63]. Monitoring of hearing during vestibular nerve section using ECOG has also been reported [64].

Superior Semicircular Canal Dehiscence and Perilymph Fistula

Because ECOG measures electrical signals created by physical deflections within the cochlea, changes in the fluid dynamics of the scala media have profound impact on the measured potentials. In the case of superior semicircular canal dehiscence, an elevated SP/AP ratio is a specific but insensitive finding, with sensitivity and specificity of approximately 70% and 90%, respectively [10, 65]. This finding likely reflects the increased deformability of the scala media compartment, similar to the changes seen in endolymphatic hydrops. These changes are reversed when the dehiscence is surgically corrected [65].

Likewise, the SP/AP ratio is elevated in some patients with perilymph fistula. This elevation does not occur with the creation of a fistula, but only when significant volume of endolymph is lost [66–68]. ECOG may be useful in intraoperative monitoring for perilymph fistula, or as an adjunct test in the evaluation of patients with signs or symptoms concerning for perilymph fistula or superior semicircular canal dehiscence, particularly in concert with vestibular-evoked myogenic potential testing (see Chap. 8).

Evaluation of Auditory Neuropathy /Dyssynchrony/ Synaptopathy

Auditory neuropathy/auditory dyssynchrony (AN/AD) is a relatively newly described disorder, which is broadly defined by normal cochlear outer hair cell function and abnormal brainstem responses. It occurs in all age groups and has a wide range of etiologies, including hereditary, infectious, metabolic, immune, and developmental [69]. AN/AD is traditionally diagnosed using three criteria: absent or seriously impaired ABRs, normal otoacoustic emissions, and absent or reduced stapedial reflexes [70].

Several ECOG patterns have been identified in patients with AN/AD, corresponding to theoretical sites of dysfunction. Patients with normal SP and absent AP signals likely have pre-synaptic dysfunction of inner hair cells. Those with intact SP and AP likely have post-synaptic dysfunction of the proximal auditory nerve. Finally, those with no distinct SP or AP but an overall prolonged neural potential may have dysfunction in producing action potential ("synaptopathy") [71]. However, some authors have been unable to reliably isolate these groups [72].

Apart from these findings, ECOG in AN/AD typically reveals a greatly increased CM and an abnormal positive SP, at least at higher frequency [73]. CM and SP thresholds are frequently low, in comparison both to CM and SP thresholds in healthy ears and to AP thresholds in affected ears. Furthermore, the SP/AP ratio is significantly higher in patients with AN/AD when compared with patients with comparable SNHL of other origin, which is a sensitive and specific finding [72]. ECOG can be used as an adjunct test for AN/AD in patients meeting diagnostic criteria, and future study may reveal a role for ECOG in the determination of specific subtypes of AN/AD.

Conclusions

ECOG has been of considerable and evolving interest to otologists and neurotologists for over 80 years. Its utility in the diagnosis of Meniere's disease is well known and continues to develop. At the same time, novel intraoperative and diagnostic applications of ECOG continue to be discovered. Further study of ECOG in the context of various inner ear conditions will likely yield more powerful applications in coming years.

References

1. Wever EG, Bray CW. Action currents in the auditory nerve in response to acoustical stimulation. Proc Natl Acad Sci U S A. 1930;16:344–50.
2. Fromm B, Nylen C, Zotterman Y. Studies in the mechanism of the Wever and Bray effect. Acta Otolaryngol (Stockh). 1935;22:477–86.
3. Lempert J, Wever EG, Lawrence M. The cochleogram and its clinical application; a preliminary report. Arch Otolaryngol. 1947;45:61–7.
4. Eggermont J. Electrocochleography. In: Auditory system. Springer; 1976. p. 625–705.
5. Coats AC. The summating potential and Meniere's disease. I. Summating potential amplitude in Meniere and non-Meniere ears. Arch Otolaryngol. 1981;107:199–208.
6. Ferraro JA. Electrocochleography: a review of recording approaches, clinical applications, and new findings in adults and children. J Am Acad Audiol. 2010;21:145–52.
7. Adunka OF, Giardina CK, Formeister EJ, et al. Round window electrocochleography before and after cochlear implant electrode insertion. Laryngoscope. 2016;126:1193–200.
8. Fitzpatrick DC, Campbell AP, Choudhury B, et al. Round window electrocochleography just before cochlear implantation: relationship to word recognition outcomes in adults. Otol Neurotol. 2014;35:64–71.
9. Attias J, Nageris B, Ralph J, et al. Hearing preservation using combined monitoring of extra-tympanic electrocochleography and auditory brainstem responses during acoustic neuroma surgery. Int J Audiol. 2008;47:178–84.
10. Adams ME, Kileny PR, Telian SA, et al. Electrocochleography as a diagnostic and intra-operative adjunct in superior semicircular canal dehiscence syndrome. Otol Neurotol. 2011;32:1506–12.
11. Eggermont JJ. Basic principles for electrocochleography. Acta Otolaryngol Suppl. 1974;316:7–16.
12. Ruben RJ, Bordley JE, Nager GT, et al. Human cochlea responses to sound stimuli. Ann Otol Rhinol Laryngol. 1960;69:459–79.
13. Yoshie N, Ohashi T, Suzuki T. Non-surgical recording of auditory nerve action potentials in man. Laryngoscope. 1967;77:76–85.
14. Humphries KN, Ashcroft PB, Douek EE. Extra-tympanic electrocochleography. Acta Otolaryngol. 1977;83:303–9.
15. Ferraro JA, Ferguson R. Tympanic ECochG and conventional ABR: a combined approach for the identification of wave I and the I-V interwave interval. Ear Hear. 1989;10:161–6.
16. Thornton AR, Coleman MJ. The adaptation of cochlear and brainstem auditory evoked potentials in humans. Electroencephalogr Clin Neurophysiol. 1975;39:399–406.
17. Terkildsen K, Osterhammel P, Huis In't Veld F. Far-Field Electrocochleography, Adaptation. Scand Audiol. 1975;4:215–20.
18. Ng M, Srireddy S, Horlbeck DM, et al. Safety and patient experience with transtympanic electrocochleography. Laryngoscope. 2001;111:792–5.

19. Bonucci AS, Hyppolito MA. Comparison of the use of tympanic and extratympanic electrodes for electrocochleography. Laryngoscope. 2009;119:563–6.
20. Ferraro JA. Clinical electrocochleography: overview of theories, techniques and applications. University of Kansas.
21. Chung WH, Cho DY, Choi JY, et al. Clinical usefulness of extratympanic electrocochleography in the diagnosis of Meniere's disease. Otol Neurotol. 2004;25:144–9.
22. Yoshie N. Clinical cochlear response audiometry by means of an average response computer: non-surgical technique and clinical use. Rev Laryngol Otol Rhinol (Bord). 1971;92(Suppl):646–72.
23. Lev A, Sohmer H. Sources of averaged neural responses recorded in animal and human subjects during cochlear audiometry (electro-cochleogram). Arch Klin Exp Ohren Nasen Kehlkopfheilkd. 1972;201:79–90.
24. Coats AC, Martin JL, Kidder HR. Normal short-latency electrophysiological filtered click responses recorded from vertex and external auditory meatus. J Acoust Soc Am. 1979;65:747–58.
25. Montandon PB, Shepard NT, Marr EM, et al. Auditory-nerve potentials from ear canals of patients with otologic problems. Ann Otol Rhinol Laryngol. 1975;84:164–73.
26. Durrant JD, Ferraro JA. Analog model of human click-elicited SP and effects of high-pass filtering. Ear Hear. 1991;12:144–8.
27. Von Békésy G. Experiments in hearing. McGraw-Hill Inc. p. 1960.
28. Dallos P. Electrical correlates of mechanical events in the cochlea. Audiology. 1975;14:408–18.
29. Spoendlin H, Baumgartner H. Electrocochleography and cochlear pathology. Acta Otolaryngol. 1977;83:130–5.
30. Gibson WP, Beagley HA. Electrocochleography in the diagnosis of acoustic neuroma. J Laryngol Otol. 1976;90:127–39.
31. Shi W, Ji F, Lan L, et al. Characteristics of cochlear microphonics in infants and young children with auditory neuropathy. Acta Otolaryngol. 2012;132:188–96.
32. Ruth RA, Lambert PR, Ferraro JA. Electrocochleography: methods and clinical applications. Am J Otol. 1988;9(Suppl):1–11.
33. Ferraro JA, Arenberg IK, Hassanein RS. Electrocochleography and symptoms of inner ear dysfunction. Arch Otolaryngol. 1985;111:71–4.
34. Roland PS, Roth L. Interinterpreter variability in determining the SP/AP ratio in clinical electrocochleography. Laryngoscope. 1997;107:1357–61.
35. Conlon BJ, Gibson WP. Electrocochleography in the diagnosis of Meniere's disease. Acta Otolaryngol. 2000;120:480–3.
36. Goin DW, Staller SJ, Asher DL, et al. Summating potential in Meniere's disease. Laryngoscope. 1982;92:1383–9.
37. Sass K. Sensitivity and specificity of transtympanic electrocochleography in Meniere's disease. Acta Otolaryngol. 1998;118:150–6.
38. Mammarella F, Zelli M, Varakliotis T, et al. Is electrocochleography still helpful in early diagnosis of meniere disease? J Audiol Otol. 2017;21:72–6.
39. Gibson WP, Moffat DA, Ramsden RT. Clinical electrocochleography in the diagnosis and management of Meneere's disorder. Audiology. 1977;16:389–401.
40. Kim HH, Kumar A, Battista RA, et al. Electrocochleography in patients with Meniere's disease. Am J Otolaryngol. 2005;26:128–31.
41. Al-momani MO, Ferraro JA, Gajewski BJ, et al. Improved sensitivity of electrocochleography in the diagnosis of Meniere's disease. Int J Audiol. 2009;48:811–9.
42. Levine S, Margolis RH, Daly KA. Use of electrocochleography in the diagnosis of Meniere's disease. Laryngoscope. 1998;108:993–1000.
43. Durrant JD, Gans D. Biasing of the summating potentials. Acta Otolaryngol. 1975;80:13–8.
44. Takeda T, Kakigi A. The clinical value of extratympanic electrocochleography in the diagnosis of Meniere's disease. ORL J Otorhinolaryngol Relat Spec. 2010;72:196–204.
45. Ge X, Shea JJ Jr. Transtympanic electrocochleography: a 10-year experience. Otol Neurotol. 2002;23:799–805.

46. Claes GM, De Valck CF, Van de Heyning P, et al. The Meniere's Disease index: an objective correlate of Meniere's disease, based on audiometric and electrocochleographic data. Otol Neurotol. 2011;32:887–92.
47. Oh KH, Kim KW, Chang J, et al. Can we use electrocochleography as a clinical tool in the diagnosis of Meniere's disease during the early symptomatic period? Acta Otolaryngol. 2014;134:771–5.
48. Noguchi Y, Nishida H, Tokano H, et al. Comparison of acute low-tone sensorineural hearing loss versus Meniere's disease by electrocochleography. Ann Otol Rhinol Laryngol. 2004;113:194–9.
49. Goebel JA. 2015 Equilibrium Committee Amendment to the 1995 AAO-HNS guidelines for the definition of Meniere's disease. Otolaryngol Head Neck Surg. 2016;154:403–4.
50. McClellan JH, Formeister EJ, Merwin WH 3rd, et al. Round window electrocochleography and speech perception outcomes in adult cochlear implant subjects: comparison with audiometric and biographical information. Otol Neurotol. 2014;35:e245–52.
51. Calloway NH, Fitzpatrick DC, Campbell AP, et al. Intracochlear electrocochleography during cochlear implantation. Otol Neurotol. 2014;35:1451–7.
52. Campbell L, Kaicer A, Sly D, et al. Intraoperative Real-time Cochlear Response Telemetry Predicts Hearing Preservation in Cochlear Implantation. Otol Neurotol. 2016;37:332–8.
53. Mandala M, Colletti L, Tonoli G, et al. Electrocochleography during cochlear implantation for hearing preservation. Otolaryngol Head Neck Surg. 2012;146:774–81.
54. Campbell L, Kaicer A, Briggs R, et al. Cochlear response telemetry: intracochlear electrocochleography via cochlear implant neural response telemetry pilot study results. Otol Neurotol. 2015;36:399–405.
55. Morawski KF, Niemczyk K, Bohorquez J, et al. Intraoperative monitoring of hearing during cerebellopontine angle tumor surgery using transtympanic electrocochleography. Otol Neurotol. 2007;28:541–5.
56. Schlake HP, Milewski C, Goldbrunner RH, et al. Combined intra-operative monitoring of hearing by means of auditory brainstem responses (ABR) and transtympanic electrocochleography (ECochG) during surgery of intra- and extrameatal acoustic neurinomas. Acta Neurochir (Wien). 2001;143:985–95. discussion 95–6
57. Lenarz T, Ernst A. Intraoperative monitoring by transtympanic electrocochleography and brainstem electrical response audiometry in acoustic neuroma surgery. Eur Arch Otorhinolaryngol. 1992;249:257–62.
58. Prass RL, Kinney SE, Luders H. Transtragal, transtympanic electrode placement for intraoperative electrocochleographic monitoring. Otolaryngol Head Neck Surg. 1987;97:343–50.
59. Mullatti N, Coakham HB, Maw AR, et al. Intraoperative monitoring during surgery for acoustic neuroma: benefits of an extratympanic intrameatal electrode. J Neurol Neurosurg Psychiatry. 1999;66:591–9.
60. Moller AR. Monitoring auditory function during operations to remove acoustic tumors. Am J Otol. 1996;17:452–60.
61. Youssef AS, Downes AE. Intraoperative neurophysiological monitoring in vestibular schwannoma surgery: advances and clinical implications. Neurosurg Focus. 2009;27:E9.
62. Freeman SR, Sanli H, Gibson WP. Intraoperative electrocochleography for monitoring during stapes surgery. J Int Adv Otol. 2009;5(2)
63. Wazen JJ, Emerson R, Foyt D. Intra-operative electrocochleography in stapedectomy and ossicular reconstruction. Am J Otol. 1997;18:707–13.
64. Silverstein H, Wazen J, Norrell H, et al. Retrolabyrinthine vestibular neurectomy with simultaneous monitoring of eighth nerve action potentials and electrocochleography. Am J Otol. 1984;5:552–5.
65. Arts HA, Adams ME, Telian SA, et al. Reversible electrocochleographic abnormalities in superior canal dehiscence. Otol Neurotol. 2009;30:79–86.
66. Meyerhoff WL, Yellin MW. Summating potential/action potential ratio in perilymph fistula. Otolaryngol Head Neck Surg. 1990;102:678–82.

67. Gibson WP. Electrocochleography in the diagnosis of perilymphatic fistula: intraoperative observations and assessment of a new diagnostic office procedure. Am J Otol. 1992;13:146–51.
68. Campbell KC, Savage MM, Harker LA. Electrocochleography in the presence and absence of perilymphatic fistula. Ann Otol Rhinol Laryngol. 1992;101:403–7.
69. Starr A, Picton TW, Sininger Y, et al. Auditory neuropathy. Brain. 1996;119(Pt 3):741–53.
70. Berlin CI, Hood LJ, Morlet T, et al. Absent or elevated middle ear muscle reflexes in the presence of normal otoacoustic emissions: a universal finding in 136 cases of auditory neuropathy/dys-synchrony. J Am Acad Audiol. 2005;16:546–53.
71. Santarelli R, Starr A, Michalewski HJ, et al. Neural and receptor cochlear potentials obtained by transtympanic electrocochleography in auditory neuropathy. Clin Neurophysiol. 2008;119:1028–41.
72. Stuermer KJ, Beutner D, Foerst A, et al. Electrocochleography in children with auditory synaptopathy/neuropathy: diagnostic findings and characteristic parameters. Int J Pediatr Otorhinolaryngol. 2015;79:139–45.
73. Gibson WP. The Clinical Uses of Electrocochleography. Front Neurosci. 2017;11:274.

Chapter 10
Repositioning Chairs in Management of BPPV

Bora Agabigum, Heather D. Balon, and Jacob C. Lucas

Introduction

Benign paroxysmal positional vertigo (BPPV) is the most common peripheral vestibular disorder with a lifetime prevalence of 2.4% [1]. BPPV has a mean onset around the fourth to fifth decade of life, and there is a 2:1 female to male predilection [1, 2]. The clinical presentation of BPPV is classically described as a transient vertigo triggered by head movements, lasting seconds up to a minute in duration. The underlying pathophysiology is due to dislodged otoconia within the semicircular canals, with diagnosis of the condition being clinical and first-line treatment relying on repositioning of these loosened particles [2–4]. The episodes are "benign" in nature, but due to the severity of an active episode, BPPV can be debilitating to the affected individual and can lead to falls or serious injury. Particle repositioning maneuvers (PRMs) are effective in the treatment of BPPV, but studies have shown a high recurrence rate approaching 30% [4, 5]. The recurrence can be attributed to several factors, including, but not limited to, sub-optimal repositioning of the offending otoconia, poor adherence to post-restriction movements, or conversion of BPPV to another ipsilateral or contralateral semicircular canal [2]. Thus, clinicians may have a difficult time treating patients with recalcitrant BPPV. As a result, several mechanical apparatuses have been developed with the intent to diagnose and treat BPPV for these select patient populations [5–7].

B. Agabigum · J. C. Lucas (✉)
Department of Otology and Neurotology, Michigan Ear Institute, Farmington Hills, MI, USA

H. D. Balon
Department of Audiology, Michigan Ear Institute, Farmington Hills, MI, USA
e-mail: hbalon@michiganear.com

J. C. Lucas et al. (eds.), *Diagnosis and Treatment of Vestibular Disorders*, https://doi.org/10.1007/978-3-032-11740-3_10

Background

Initially described by Dr. Bárány in 1921, BPPV is the most common cause of vertigo, present in around 17–40% of patients with a peripheral vestibular disorder [2]. The classic presentation of BPPV is a transient episodic room-spinning dizziness that is elicited by head movement. There are two primary theories that explain the pathophysiology of BPPV: cupulolithiasis and canalithiasis. The former theory, pioneered by Dr. Schuknecht, explains that otoconia attached to the cupula cause it to deflect with certain head positions, leading to aberrant vestibular activity. However, the canalithiasis theory states that free moving otoconia within the semicircular canal shifts with certain head positions, leading to deflection of the cupula [2, 5]. Regardless of the underlying mechanism, the patient experiences episodes which can last generally from seconds up to a minute, and most commonly affect the posterior semicircular canal (SCC). Cupulolithiasis can be characterized by an episode that lasts for greater than 1 min due to the offending otoconia weighing down the cupula for the length of time that the patient is in a triggering position.

The diagnosis of BPPV is through clinical evaluation. The Dix–Hallpike maneuver, developed in 1952, is used to identify BPPV, especially BPPV related to the posterior SCC (p-BPPV). The first-line treatment for BPPV is through a series of physical maneuvers to reposition the offending otoconia, termed particle repositioning maneuvers (PRMs). Though several methods have been described in the literature, the Epley maneuver is most common and readily utilized [3, 4, 8]. First described by Dr. Epley in 1992, the Epley maneuver is used to treat BPPV, with efficacy ranging from 80% to 90% [4–6]. However, several factors can limit the ability to diagnose and treat BPPV.

The recurrence rate of p-BPPV following PRM is approximately 30–40%, and this rate can significantly increase if the BPPV is related to head trauma [4, 5, 9]. Additionally, less frequent variants of BPPV affecting the superior (s-BPPV) or horizontal (h-BPPV) SCC, and BPPV affecting multiple ipsilateral or contralateral SCCs lead to inadequate diagnosis in up to 10–20% of cases [6, 8, 9]. Patients over the age of 50 and those with osteoporosis also pose a similar challenge in treatment of BPPV due to the inability to adequately perform the PRM, leading to higher failure rates compared to more agile and younger patients [5, 6].

In order to manage this subset of challenging BPPV cases, particle repositioning chairs (PRC) were developed with a dual function in both diagnosis and treatment of BPPV based on the affected semicircular canal(s). Although several chairs have been developed over the past 30 years, the most prominent include the Omniax System, developed under Dr. Epley in 1996, and the TRV chair developed by Dr. Thomas Richard-Vitton in 2005 [6–8]. The availability of these chairs is limited, and in the case of the Omniax System, only a handful exist across the world as it is no longer commercially available. Though an exact number of the Omniax system is unknown, it is speculated that there are at least six in use across the world.

Equipment Overview

Although several different automated repositioning chairs exist, the Omniax system is currently used at the authors' institution and will therefore be the focus of this section. Based on the specifications set forth by Nakayama et al., the Omniax system is an automated two-axis chair capable of positioning in any angle relative to gravity, such that a patient can undergo full 360-degree rotation of any of the six SCCs while oriented in the true vertical plane [6]. Patients are secured within the chair with shoulder, waist, and ankle harnesses, and the head and neck are supported with an adjustable head rest. The patient is fitted with goggles containing an infrared camera that records eye movements and nystagmus throughout testing.

The chair apparatus is connected to a computer and monitor displaying simultaneous live feedback of the infrared camera and chair orientation. The system can be automated and is designed to recognize nystagmus. The software can then help correlate body/head positioning to identify the affected SCC and subsequently perform the appropriate repositioning maneuver. At the conclusion of testing, all data are recorded and can be reviewed by the operator with patients or other practitioners. The TRV system is similar in concept to the Omniax, with both utilizing infrared goggles to track eye movements during maneuvers. However, the TRV chair is manually operated by a provider, while the Omniax moves by way of mechanical assembly controlled by the computer software [8]. Additionally, the TRV chair is less costly compared to the Omniax [10].

In our institutional experience, the system can effectively identify and treat patients with either a singular or multiple affected SCCs. Patients are advised to keep an empty stomach prior to testing due to the vertigo elicited and extreme positioning adopted for treatments during testing, where patients can be inverted for a period of time. Additionally, although the chair can support the weight of most patients, the weight limit is set at 350 lbs. and the smaller frame of the chair may not accommodate patients of a larger body habitus.

Testing Process

As there are very few machines in operation across the world, our institution in Michigan, the Midwest United States, receives referrals from outside practices within the state and other states across the country. On a weekly basis, our institution treats 35 patients. The following section will detail a step-by-step process of the Omniax test.

First, the patient is seated within the Omniax chair (Fig. 10.1). The patient is secured within the seat with adjustable shoulder, waist/lap, and ankle straps. The head rest is adjusted to firmly stabilize the crown and occiput of the head, which provides patient support during maneuvers, especially when inverted. The infrared goggles are placed on the patient's head and adjusted to fit firmly. Depending on the

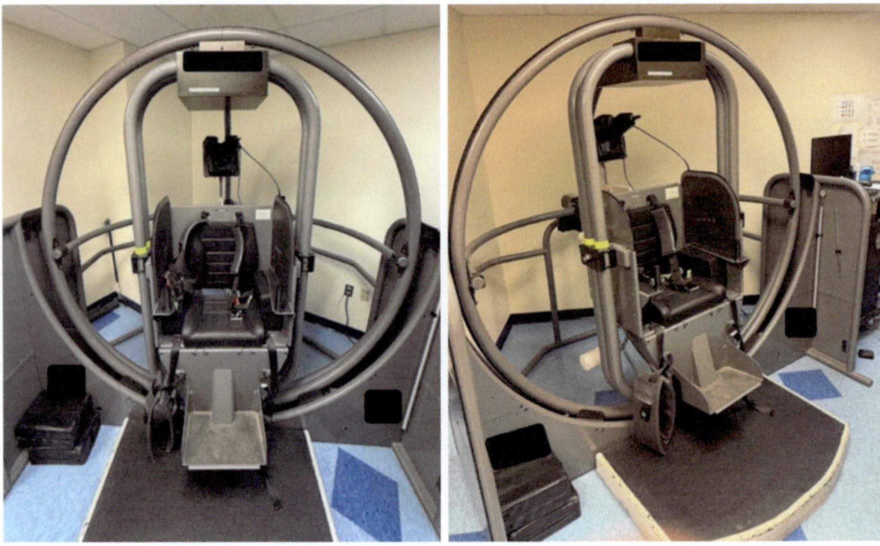

Fig. 10.1 The Omniax system, including chair and computer module. The chair is able to secure the patient with adjustable headrest, shoulder, waist, and ankle straps

preference of the provider performing the test, each lens on the goggle can be interchanged with an eye shield or infrared lens, which can also be adjusted throughout the test.

Second, the software interface allows the provider to input angle adjustments for each axis of rotation, which is also displayed with pictorial representation of each SCC in the current axis orientation and final orientation after the axes are adjusted (Fig. 10.2). Additionally, the interface displays the infrared camera, which tracks movement of the eye with focus centered on the pupil. Throughout the test, the camera output is recorded and can be reviewed at test completion. During testing, the provider instructs the patient which direction they will be moving prior to the onset of the chair rotation. The provider then adjusts the axes angles to test each semicircular canal oriented in the plane of gravity dependence. After each rotation, the chair is held in position and the provider monitors for any nystagmus recorded by the infrared goggles.

Once the offending SCC is identified, the provider performs the appropriate PRM by adjusting the angles on the software interface, allowing the chair to rotate through each step of the PRM. As an aside, from the patient perspective, the chair rotation is smooth. Most positions are well tolerated, but during complete inversion, there is increased head pressure and fullness, which can be mildly discomforting to the patient. The provider frequently checks on patient status during testing due to the nature of the uncomfortable positioning inherent to the test.

After completion of the maneuver, the patient is returned back to starting position. Typically, two to three maneuvers are performed consecutively for each patient, depending on the response achieved by the initial PRM. Once all testing is done, the

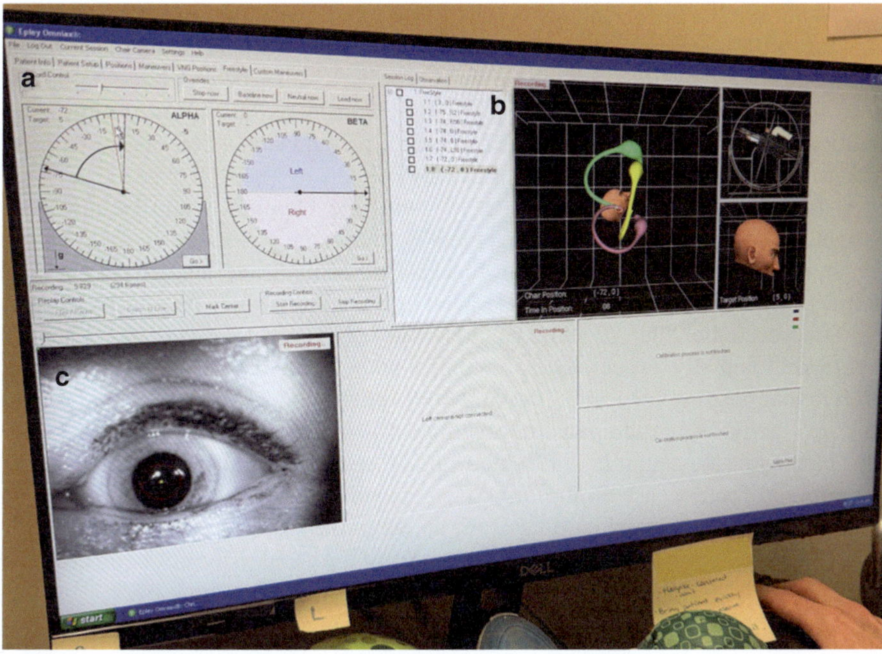

Fig. 10.2 Software user interface for the Omniax system. Individual axes are adjustable (**a**), and the before and after position of the semicircular canals with respect to the axes is also displayed (**b**). Eye movements captured from the infrared goggles are monitored and recorded for review (**c**)

patient is instructed to only move out of the chair apparatus when they feel comfortable. At our institution, repeat Omniax testing is typically performed 2 weeks later if symptoms recur.

Multiple and Atypical Maneuvers

The Omniax and related multi-axial chair devices are well suited for complex pathology involving multiple SCCs, or in cases where otoconia are displaced into other canals. One such maneuver is the "Backflip." In cases where the patient has bilateral p-BPPV, it is near impossible to treat both canals during the same appointment using manual maneuvers. The reason for this is that after PRM resolves the p-BPPV for side A, completing the PRM to resolve p-BPPV for side B would be likely to undo what was fixed for side A given that each maneuver is equal and opposite to each other. By completing a 360-degree rotation backwards, the otoconia are able to travel through the posterior SCCs and away from the ampulla to resolve p-BPPV on both sides at the same time. Therefore, in the case of bilateral s-BPPV, a 360-degree "Forward Flip" could be completed.

Another treatment for unilateral p-BPPV would be a Right or Left Backflip. In this case, a 360-degree backwards rotation would be completed in the plane of the right or left posterior SCCs. Due to the discomfort of the patient hanging upside down from the straps, this treatment would be considered a last resort after more traditional maneuvers fail. The same type of "flip" but using a 360-degree forward rotation could be used to treat unilateral s-BPPV.

A more typical treatment for s-BPPV with the Omniax would be the Deep Hallpike. The Deep Hallpike is performed by laying the patient down in either the left or right Hallpike position except that instead of maneuvering the patient with their head down at a 120-degree angle from upright, their whole body is reclined to a 150-degree angle. Such an angle would be very difficult for patients and clinicians to perform manually, especially as flexibility tends to be lost with age. The patient is left in that position for 1 min, if tolerated by the patient, and then they are brought back up slowly. When the patient is reclined 150 degrees, the part of the superior SCC closest to the ampulla is oriented purely vertical, which allows the greatest gravitational force to act on the offending otoconia and pull them away from the ampulla. Once the otoconia are far from the ampulla, sitting the patient up slowly gives them time to move through the remainder of the canal to the common crus and then the utricle.

Outcomes

Previous studies examining the outcomes of PRCs show similar rates of BPPV symptom relief comparing the chair to manual PRMs [6, 10–12]. The resolution rates depending on study range from approximately 86% to 100% with a mean number of treatments ranging from 2 to 3. In a study by Tan et al., there was a significantly greater number of patients with symptom resolution after 1 week, determined by negative Dix–Hallpike response, for the PRC treatment group (85.2%) compared to the PRM treatment group (72.6%) [13]. However, both groups showed similar resolution rates at 1–6 months' follow-up. These studies indicated that the PRC is equally effective and non-inferior to the conventional PRM treatment for BPPV.

The experience of the Omniax system at our institution with data from 610 patients showed a mean number of 2.6 and median of 2 treatment visits prior to symptom resolution [14, 15]. Although prior reports indicated poorer outcomes in variants of BPPV outside of p-BPPV, our data found no significant difference in resolution and recurrence rates between traditional p-BPPV (68.8%, 27.9%) and other BPPV variants (66.4%, 27.3%), respectively. This has suggested that the Omniax system is efficacious in identification and management of BPPV, regardless of the affected SCC. As a diagnostic tool, we found approximately 81% of patients with p-BPPV alone, 12.6% with h-BPPV alone, 6.7% with s-BPPV alone, and 6.6% of patient with multiple SCCs involved. These rates are comparable to prior data [5, 6]. Additionally, in Omniax treatment of patients with severe immobility ($n = 34$),

68% achieved resolution of symptoms with a 13% recurrence [14]. This further illustrates the efficacy of the Omniax system in the management of challenging BPPV cases.

Future Directions

The Omniax system is capable of effectively and safely treating patients with recalcitrant or complicated cases of BPPV that would not tolerate traditional PRMs. While the system has shown comparable success to other PRCs, the automation of the Omniax program is unique and is capable of removing variables such as user error in application. The downside to all PRCs is availability and especially with the Omniax system, this is a concern. Since the discontinuation of the Omniax system production, maintenance and replacement of system components has been the biggest challenge. However, the utility of systems such as Omniax and TRV have shown such success that it is still recognized in the overall treatment paradigm for BPPV. Newer automated PRCs are reported in the literature and initial results indicate similar success in management of refractory BPPV [16]. These systems include the Rotundum R1 and VertiChair, which similarly use a multi-axial rotary chair system compared to the TRV and Omniax [8]. Regardless of the system, over the past 30 years, PRCs remained relevant in the management of complicated or refractory cases of BPPV worldwide. Although the Omniax system is less prevalent, its methodology and success carry on in existing and newer technology.

References

1. von Brevern M, Radtke A, Lezius F, Feldmann M, Ziese T, Lempert T, Neuhauser H. Epidemiology of benign paroxysmal positional vertigo: a population based study. J Neurol Neurosurg Psychiatry. 2007;78(7):710–5. https://doi.org/10.1136/jnnp.2006.100420.
2. Flint PW, Cummings CW. Chapter 167 peripheral vestibular disorders. In: Cummings otolaryngology: head and neck surgery, vol. 3. 7th ed. Philadelphia: Elsevier; 2021. p. 2517–35.
3. Bhattacharyya N, Gubbels SP, Schwartz SR, Edlow JA, El-Kashlan H, Fife T, Holmberg JM, Mahoney K, Hollingsworth DB, Roberts R, Seidman MD, Steiner RW, Do BT, Voelker CC, Waguespack RW, Corrigan MD. Clinical practice guideline: benign paroxysmal positional vertigo (Update). Otolaryngol Head Neck Surg. 2017;156(3_suppl):S1–S47. https://doi.org/10.1177/0194599816689667.
4. Hilton MP, Pinder DK. The Epley (canalith repositioning) manoeuvre for benign paroxysmal positional vertigo. Cochrane Database Syst Rev. 2014;2014(12):CD003162. https://doi.org/10.1002/14651858.CD003162.pub3.
5. Epley JM. Human experience with canalith repositioning maneuvers. Ann N Y Acad Sci. 2001;942:179–91. https://doi.org/10.1111/j.1749-6632.2001.tb03744.x.
6. Nakayama M, Epley JM. BPPV and variants: improved treatment results with automated, nystagmus-based repositioning. Otolaryngol Head Neck Surg. 2005;133(1):107–12. https://doi.org/10.1016/j.otohns.2005.03.027.

7. Richard-Vitton T, Seidermann L, Fraget P, Mouillet J, Astier P, Chays A. Vertige positionnel paroxystique Bénin, un fauteuil au service du diagnostic et du traitement: description et intérêt [Benign positional vertigo, an armchair for diagnosis and for treatment: description and significance]. Revue de laryngologie – otologie – rhinologie. 2005;126(4):249–51.
8. Abdulovski S, Klokker M. Repositioning chairs in the diagnosis and treatment of benign paroxysmal positional vertigo – a systematic review. J Int Adv Otol. 2021;17(4):353–60. https://doi.org/10.5152/iao.2021.9434.
9. Babac S, Djeric D, Petrovic-Lazic M, Arsovic N, Mikic A. Why do treatment failure and recurrences of benign paroxysmal positional vertigo occur? Otol Neurotol. 2014;35(6):1105–10. https://doi.org/10.1097/MAO.0000000000000417.
10. West N, Hansen S, Møller MN, Bloch SL, Klokker M. Repositioning chairs in benign paroxysmal positional vertigo: implications and clinical outcome. Eur Arch Otorhinolaryngol. 2016;273(3):573–80. https://doi.org/10.1007/s00405-015-3583-z.
11. Schuricht A, Hougaard DD. Is a mechanical rotational chair superior to manual treatment maneuvers on an examination bed in the treatment of benign paroxysmal positional vertigo? Otol Neurotol. 2022;43(2):e235–42. https://doi.org/10.1097/MAO.0000000000003380.
12. Power L, Murray K, Szmulewicz D. Early experience with a multi-axial, whole body positioning system in the treatment of benign paroxysmal positional vertigo (BPPV). J Clin Neurosci. 2019;61:186–8. https://doi.org/10.1016/j.jocn.2018.10.039.
13. Tan J, Yu D, Feng Y, Song Q, You J, Shi H, Yin S. Comparative study of the efficacy of the canalith repositioning procedure versus the vertigo treatment and rehabilitation chair. Acta Otolaryngol. 2014;134(7):704–8. https://doi.org/10.3109/00016489.2014.899711.
14. Luryi AL, Lawrence J, LaRouere M, Babu S, Bojrab DI, Zappia J, Sargent EW, Schutt CA. Treatment of patients with benign paroxysmal positional vertigo and severe immobility using the particle repositioning chair: a retrospective cohort study. Ann Otol Rhinol Laryngol. 2018;127(6):390–4. https://doi.org/10.1177/0003489418771988.
15. Luryi AL, Wright D, Lawrence J, Babu S, LaRouere M, Bojrab DI, Sargent EW, Zappia J, Schutt CA. Analysis of non-posterior canal benign paroxysmal positional vertigo in patients treated using the particle repositioning chair: a large, single-institution series. Am J Otolaryngol. 2018;39(3):313–6. https://doi.org/10.1016/j.amjoto.2018.03.019.
16. Bayram O, Kucuk H, Karabulut B, Canturk M. The efficacy of automated repositioning chair in refractory benign paroxysmal positional vertigo-a pilot study. Auris Nasus Larynx. 2025;52(2):179–85. https://doi.org/10.1016/j.anl.2025.01.012.

Chapter 11
Cost-Effective Evaluation of the Dizzy Patient

Lauren Mueller, Brekel Kemp, and Neal M. Jackson

Introduction

As the authors have explained in great detail in the preceding chapters, evaluating the vestibular patient can be challenging, multifaceted, and complex. Evaluation can include dedicated history, extensive physical exam, electrophysiologic testing of the vestibular system, and specific imaging protocols to evaluate the anatomy of the vestibular and central nervous system.

Due to the multitude of subspecialty physicians and evaluation techniques available, there is an increased risk of high utilization and high cost associated with this patient population. The purpose of this chapter is to review current literature and expert opinions from a variety of fields of medicine to study cost-effectiveness in evaluation of the vestibular patient.

L. Mueller
Department of Otolaryngology, Washington University, St. Louis, MO, USA
e-mail: m.lauren@wustl.edu

B. Kemp
Department of Otolaryngology, Tulane University School of Medicine, New Orleans, LA, USA
e-mail: bkemp@tulane.edu

N. M. Jackson (✉)
Departments of Otolaryngology & Neurosurgery, Tulane University School of Medicine, New Orleans, LA, USA

Departments of Otology and Neurotology, Michigan Ear Institute, Farmington Hills, MI, USA

J. C. Lucas et al. (eds.), *Diagnosis and Treatment of Vestibular Disorders*, https://doi.org/10.1007/978-3-032-11740-3_11

The Challenge of the Dizzy Patient

It is well known the dizzy patient interview can be very challenging for even the most experienced clinicians. This is multifactorial as balance includes multiple organ systems and patients may describe the same sensation in various ways. The dizzy patient may have great difficulty in describing the precise feeling or details of his or her dizzy symptoms [1]. For example, in one study, when dizzy patients were asked a series of questions to classify their type of dizziness and then re-asked the same questions 10 min later, over half of the patients changed their dizziness type. Patients may often endorse multiple dizziness categories (lightheaded, room-spinning, head swimming, etc.) [2]. Even patients with confirmed benign paroxysmal positional vertigo (BPPV) with observed nystagmus and assumed room-spinning vertigo sensation may often endorse lightheadedness (and not vertigo), and over one-third of patients with cardiovascular causes may endorse vertigo (and not lightheadedness) [3].

Because of patients' difficulty in describing symptoms, primary care and acute care providers may seek consultative referral to a neurologist, cardiologist, or otolaryngologist/neurotologist. Sometimes, patients end up seeing multiple specialists for the same dizziness symptoms. When the diagnosis is unclear or potentially multifactorial, patients might be referred to a panel of specialists to "rule out" each involved organ. A recent evaluation of patient experience showed that many patients are sent to multiple specialists, experience a delay in diagnosis, incur greater costs, and are sometimes not confident in the ultimate diagnosis [4].

Rates of true vestibular pathology in patients with dizziness can vary. One particular study utilizing multimodality assessments (Dizziness Handicap Index (DHI), rotational chair, and head thrust dynamic visual acuity) examined elderly dizzy patients and concluded that only 38% of patients truly have peripheral vestibulopathy and 1% had central vestibulopathy. Of those with peripheral vestibulopathy, BPPV was the etiology in 63% [5]. Additionally, the rate of true vestibular pathology in children is substantially less frequent. One in 20 children in the United States have presented to their primary care provider for dizziness or imbalance with only 1.3% of complaints being diagnosed as BPPV [6].

Some patients experience their dizziness acutely and therefore present to acute care providers in the emergency department. In fact, annual costs of dizziness evaluations in the emergency departments in the United States are increasing; this is due to both an increased number of visits and increased rates of testing (e.g., imaging) [7]. In the United States, the combined cost of patients with peripheral vestibular diagnoses is estimated to be $151 billion [8]. Therefore, a section of this chapter will address the evaluation of acute vestibular syndrome in the emergency department and the role of neuroimaging.

Cost-Effectiveness

Cost-effectiveness in healthcare pertains to the relation of monetary expenditure to perceived health gain. This can be done utilizing various methods of analysis to answer specific questions. For example, when a new but more expensive technology occurs, a cost-effective analysis can be done to assess the measured expenditure of a new test or treatment in light of the standard practice. If the new test is more expensive and less effective, there is little reason to favor it. If the new test is less expensive and more effective, then likely it will gain favor. When the new intervention is more expensive and seems more effective, a cost-effective analysis may be done to determine if the new intervention is "worth" the added cost—and this perceived value is based on multiple factors including funds available, cultural attitudes, system priorities, etc.

Multiple formulas and philosophical approaches exist to evaluate cost effectiveness. A cost-effective ratio is typically a ratio between monetary cost (typically measured in US dollars) and some measure of health gain. Monetary costs may vary significantly based on contracts, insurance status, etc. Additionally, health gains can be very difficult to quantify.

Whereas objective outcome measures like HbA1C levels in diabetic patients may be more straightforward to calculate, health gains concerning dizziness tend to not be as objective. Given the variety of dizziness etiologies, there is no true gold standard of diagnosis or treatment outcome. Quality of life, patient satisfaction, and quality-adjusted life years (QALYs) are just a few of the measurements used to quantify effectiveness.

While cost-effectiveness is important to avoid wasteful utilization of limited resources, there are caveats to consider. First and foremost, there can be biases in cost-effectiveness evaluations as in other scientific literature. Selection bias in choosing which health gains outcomes to include may unfairly set the standard too high or too low. Second, a cost-effectiveness study referencing actual monetary costs are usually not true costs but instead assumed averages or ranges based on costs at a specific institution at a specific time for one specific test; the specific costs often vary based on complex and evolving contracts, insurance deductibles, and market forces that can modulate prices. Also, one must consider the value of the intervention to the individual patient as well as the value of the intervention to the population as a whole. Therefore, cost-effectiveness should be critically considered in clinical care and any guidelines on cost-effectiveness should be interpreted carefully [9].

With regard to specific cost-effective evaluation of dizziness, there is limited literature to guide the interested clinician. Most studies are from single institutions and examine only the cost-effectiveness of one intervention in one specific clinical scenario. However, expert opinions from Emergency Medicine, Neurology, and Otolaryngology about clinical appropriateness may be combined with a fundamental understanding of relative costs to gauge some degree of cost-effectiveness. For example, a Dix–Hallpike test has minimal costs, whereas an imaging study, such as magnetic resonance imaging (MRI), may cost thousands of dollars.

Evaluation of Dizziness in the Acute Care Setting

As mentioned previously, the presentation of dizziness in emergency departments is becoming more common and more costly in the United States. A cross-sectional survey of the National Ambulatory Medical Care Survey determined the rate of emergency room visits for dizziness to be 8.8 out of 1000 visits [10]. Most causes are not otologic, but rather cardiovascular or due to other medical pathologies. Nevertheless, in the acute care setting, dizzy patients have been found to have longer hospital stays, more resource utilization, including imaging, and yet, many patients did not receive an actual diagnosis (e.g., vestibular neuritis, BPPV) beyond their stated symptom (i.e., dizziness) [11].

In the acute care setting, it is important to determine whether the dizzy patient is experiencing acute vestibular syndrome (AVS) or another form of dizziness. The AVS can be defined as acute, sudden-onset, non-remitting and persistent dizziness that resolves over days to weeks. The use of the words like "vertigo" or "lightheadedness" is irrelevant to diagnose AVS.

For the patient with AVS, the most critical outcome of an emergency department visit is to either diagnose or confidently rule out posterior circulation stroke.

Initial evaluation begins with chief complaint and history. As discussed earlier, dizzy patients have difficulty in precisely describing their symptoms, so a clear history is not considered essential. In the elderly dizzy population in the ED, the use of the term "vertigo" as opposed to "dizziness" or "lightheadedness" does not correlate with a stroke diagnosis [2, 12]. Patients in the acute setting may have even greater difficulty in describing the exact feelings of their dizziness, as they may be experiencing extreme anxiety, nausea, or vomiting.

For the acute care provider, it is necessary to consider the differential diagnosis, which includes benign conditions (such as BPPV, vestibular neuritis, labyrinthitis, multiple sclerosis, vestibular migraine, temporal bone fracture with otic capsule injury, and Meniere's attack) and more emergent conditions (posterior circulation stroke). It is frequently necessary to evaluate for cardiac and neurologic causes of imbalance.

As opposed to classifying dizziness predominantly on the patient's descriptors, another line of thought has been to distinguish four separate vestibular syndromes based on timing and causative factors: acute vestibular syndrome, chronic vestibular syndrome, episodic vestibular syndrome, and triggered vestibular syndrome. In this paradigm, acute vestibular syndrome is sudden onset with persistent symptoms lasting days–weeks (vestibular neuritis/labyrinthitis vs. posterior circulation CVA). Chronic vestibular syndrome includes prolonged dizziness lasting weeks to months; consider medication side effects or slowly growing posterior fossa lesions. Episodic vestibular syndrome is mainly intermittent, may arise spontaneously, and can last minutes–days. Differential includes Meniere's disease, migraine-associated vertigo, or posterior circulation TIA. Finally, triggered vestibular syndrome lasts less than 1 min and is elicited by change in body/head position, suggestive of BPPV or orthostatic hypotension [13].

On physical examination, vital signs are essential to rule out orthostatic hypotension or signs of any cardiovascular disease. Next, a neurologic exam including cranial nerve exam, cerebellar, and gait testing is critical to rule out focal deficits. One study found 16% of benign paroxysmal positional vertigo (BPPV) patients to have a positive neurological exam compared to 64% of stroke patients [14]. Otoscopy can be done to investigate for less likely causes of dizziness such as suppurative otomastoiditis, erosive cholesteatoma, or recent otic capsule trauma. Neuro-otologic assessment includes examining for spontaneous nystagmus, gaze-evoked nystagmus, or ocular misalignment.

In patients without focal neurologic deficit, positional maneuvers such as the Dix–Hallpike test should be performed. For patients with sudden-onset dizziness, one of the most common etiologies is BPPV. Interestingly, the Dix–Hallpike maneuver requires no additional costs, but is surprisingly rarely performed in dizzy patients. According to one study looking at patients presenting to the ED with dizziness, in those diagnosed with BPPV, the Dix–Hallpike exam maneuver was only documented in 21.8% of cases, and the canalith repositioning maneuver (CRP) was only done in 3.9% of patients diagnosed with BPPV [15]. The HINTS (Head Impulse, Nystagmus, Tests of Skew) procedure was documented in 23% of cases, but was undiagnostic in 65% of cases [14]. This may be related to the fact that there is limited confidence among ED providers in performing the Dix–Hallpike maneuver, the Epley canalith repositioning maneuver, and HINTS compared to cranial nerve testing or ABCD2 [16]. A 2000 retrospective study of patients who ultimately underwent the Epley CRP found that delayed diagnosis caused the average patient to spend over $2000 out of pocket in medications, multiple doctor visits, and other ineffective interventions [17].

Special attention has been paid in the EM literature with regard to the importance of the physical exam in the evaluation of patients with acute vestibular syndrome. Updated guidelines for reasonable and appropriate care in the emergency department (GRACE-3) have been released in 2023, addressing adult patients presenting to the emergency room with acute dizziness or vertigo [18]. The guidelines establish use of HINTS as best practice when evaluating these patients; however, it acknowledges that few emergency medicine physicians are trained in the use of HINTS. A randomized controlled trial has shown that educational intervention pertaining to physical examination maneuvers used in vestibular diagnostics increases physicians' appropriate utilization and performance of these maneuvers [19]. An excellent primer by Edlow and Newman-Toker is recommended to understand nuances of evaluation of the vestibular system during AVS as compared to during the non-acute setting [20].

HINTS is a combination of different oculomotor exam maneuvers that includes the head impulse test (HIT); observation of nystagmus in primary, left, and right gaze; and assessment for skew deviation. The HIT relies on the vestibulo-ocular reflex (VOR) in which head movements are sensed by the inner ears and used to guide the oculomotor reactions to keep the eyes fixated on a target. The VOR requires the examiner watch the patients' eyes as the upright head is quickly rotated horizontally by the examiner and the patient is instructed to maintain gaze on the examiner's nose. In a "normal" patient without any vestibulopathy, with sudden horizontal rotation of the head, the eyes should continue to fixate on the examiner's nose. However, if the head is turned and the VOR fails, then there is a corrective saccade observed—this would indicate a peripheral vestibulopathy. It is important to understand that for patients with AVS, a "normal" HIT with intact VOR suggests that the vestibular system is intact and therefore, this clinical combination of AVS with intact VOR is concerning for central stroke. It is important to note that the HIT with an intact VOR will only be "positive" with saccades in patients with acute vestibulopathy due to peripheral causes and will be "negative" in patients with central dizziness.

Nystagmus testing involves close observation of eye motion in all 9 visual fields. Most patients with acute vestibular syndrome with nystagmus will show horizontal nystagmus with a fast phase in one direction. Nystagmus due to peripheral vestibulopathy will beat more quickly when looking in the direction of fast phase and beat more slowly when looking in the opposite direction. If the direction of the fast phase changes with eccentric gaze, this is strongly suggestive of a central lesion such as stroke.

Skew deviation refers to a disconjugate vertical gaze and is suggestive of central lesion. It results from disruption of the vestibular input, especially the otolothic inputs, to the oculomotor nuclei through the brainstem.

A recent systemic review and meta-analysis examined the diagnostic accuracy of imaging in distinguishing benign peripheral processes (vestibular neuritis or labyrinthitis) from a more treacherous posterior circulation ischemia [21]. Vertebrobasilar ischemic stroke does not always have obvious focal neurologic deficits. Non-contrast CT has poor sensitivity of 29% and MRI with diffusion-weighted imaging (DWI) will not reliably show stroke in posterior fossa in the first 24–48 h, having sensitivity around 80% [21]. In a review of vascular risk factors for patients with suspected posterior circulation ischemia who underwent computer tomography angiography (CTA) and neurology consultation, the risk factors for posterior circulation ischemia in dizzy patients were increasing age, increased blood pressure, and focal neurologic deficits. The CTA did not yield significant diagnostic information [22]. Neuroimaging alone is not sufficient to rule out stroke etiology in dizzy patients presenting to the emergency department.

The use of imaging can also lead to prolonged ED stay times due to time spent waiting for the scanner, radiologic interpretation, etc., all contributing to increased associated costs. There is low-dose but certain radiation exposure. For these reasons, patients presenting with dizziness or syncope may not benefit from CT unless they have recent evidence of head trauma, focal neurologic deficit, or advanced age [23]. In a 2015 study, Canadian physicians who ordered CT scans for stroke evaluation may have been falsely reassured by negative head CT, as patients who were discharged after a false-negative CT scan were twice as likely to have a stroke compared to patients not scanned [24].

With regard to the role of neurology consult and neuroimaging in the emergency department, there are various practice patterns that currently exist. Headache and focal neurologic deficit were associated with neurology consult and imaging, whereas age > 60 years and prior stroke predicted use of only neuroimaging [25]. Interestingly, positional symptoms prompted neurology consultation and not imaging. Twenty-one percent of neurology consultations were retrospectively associated with a serious neurologic diagnosis (stroke, tumor, MS, etc.). Seven percent of neuroimaging had significant findings pertaining to dizziness [25]. Therefore, one may conclude that neurology consults are more diagnostic and potentially less costly than MRI. However, the timeliness and availability of dedicated neurologists may be limited.

Overall, the cost-effective evaluation of the dizzy patient in the acute care setting should include history and physical examination with close attention paid to vital signs, neurologic exam, dedicated oculomotor exam, and neurotologic maneuvers (HIT, Dix–Hallpike maneuver). If focal neurologic deficits or truly positive Dix–Hallpike provocation are observed, then the diagnosis may be streamlined. HINTS does not include additional cost and may be more accurate than DWI MRI for stroke diagnosis. If imaging is pursued, head CT has a very low yield. MRI scan may help elucidate other central pathologies (CVA, MS, mass lesion, etc.), but may miss acute ischemic stroke within the first 24–28 h.

Cost-Effective Evaluation in the Otolaryngology/ Neurotology Clinic

Out of all primary care referrals to neurotology clinic, 24% of referrals are for a primary complaint of dizziness [26]. Outpatient visits account for 65% of the cost for patients with vestibular diagnoses [8]. The differential diagnosis most commonly includes peripheral causes (BPPV, Meniere's, vestibular neuritis/labyrinthitis, etc.) and central causes (migraine dizziness, multiple sclerosis, etc.); a mass of the IAC/CPA should also be considered.

Muelleman et al. recently reviewed the epidemiology of dizzy patients who visited a neurotology clinic at an academic institution [27]. Only 57% of the patients ultimately were diagnosed with a peripheral vestibular etiology. Overall, the most common causes were Meniere's (23%), vestibular migraine (19.3%), BPPV (19.1%), and non-migraine central causes (16.4%). Some patients had multiple diagnoses (migraine plus BPPV or migraine plus Meniere's).

Some institutions obtain the patient's self-reported symptoms before the clinic visit. In one interesting study, a simple question assessment asking about association of hearing loss, duration of vertigo, and if vertigo is 'true vertigo' or an alternative feeling of disequilibrium suggested a correct basic categorization of BPPV,

Meniere's, VN, and labyrinthitis in 60% of patients [28]. Another study requiring patients to complete a 37-question survey dedicated to the patient experience of dizziness was able to accurately predict the cause of dizziness about 78.5% of the time [29]. While history is not completely diagnostic, it represents an inexpensive way to categorize the dizziness and potentially initiate treatment.

The physical examination of the dizzy patient should include vital signs, otoscopy, Weber and Rinne test, cranial nerve exam, and standard neurotologic maneuvers such as Dix–Hallpike maneuver, head impulse test (HIT), Fakuda step test, Romberg balance test, and others. Frenzel goggles can aid in suppressing visual fixation and visually magnifying nystagmus for the observer.

As BPPV is one of the most common peripheral vestibulopathies and its examination maneuver is seemingly straightforward, special attention has been paid to its diagnosis. In fact, the American Academy of Otolaryngology Head & Neck Surgery (AAOHNS) recently updated its guidelines on BPPV, which is diagnosed with the Dix–Hallpike test [30]. The cost-effective management of BPPV with CRP has also been studied. As noted previously, a 2000 retrospective study of patients who ultimately underwent the Epley CRP found that delayed diagnosis caused the average patient to spend over $2000 in medications, multiple doctor visits, and other ineffective interventions [17].

Some patients whose symptoms or exam findings are not sufficiently diagnostic may undergo additional evaluation of the vestibular system. A typical vestibular battery includes close monitoring of the eyes for nystagmus using either videonystagmography (VNG) or electronystagmography (ENG). The eyes are observed at rest, tracking visual objects, when the head is in certain positions, and with caloric stimulation of the horizontal semicircular canal. Testing requires VNG goggles, a computer with software, and time with a trained audiologist. It is the most widely utilized vestibular test. It can be very effective in confirming the laterality of a vestibulopathy in cases of unilateral Meniere's disease.

Critics of the VNG may state that the only part of the inner ear it tests is the horizontal semicircular canal at a low-frequency stimulation through caloric stimulation and does not provide information about the rest of the vestibular function of the one inner ear. A recent cost-effectiveness analysis showed a cost of $870 per VNG with abnormal findings and a cost of $5455 per VNG, which led to a change in management, meaning very few VNG tests led to a change in clinical management of a patient [31]. The VNG testing may provide supplemental quantitative diagnostic data for vestibular pathology, and may be valuable in patient management and counseling. However, a thorough patient history and physical exam are sufficient and cost-effective for diagnosing and managing vestibular pathology.

Rotational chair can be helpful in evaluating both inner ears at various frequencies, including higher frequencies compared to low-frequency caloric stimulation with VNG. However, rotational chairs can be very expensive to purchase and requires space in the office.

Vestibular-evoked myogenic potential (VEMP) testing is not routinely employed for vestibular patients. One of its greatest utilities is in the diagnosis of superior semicircular canal dehiscence (SSCD), although thin-slice CT imaging with images in the plane of the canal is considered the best single test.

There can be significant variation in the use of vestibular diagnostic testing for patients presenting to otolaryngology clinics [32]. Patients report high rates of intolerance to vestibular testing due to induced dizziness and nausea. About 15% of vestibular testing is discontinued by patient request due to intolerance [33].

Other electrophysiologic tests of the inner ear, discussed in greater detail in other chapters (e.g., ABR, ECOG), are generally considered not as sensitive or specific as MRI for retrocochlear pathology.

Imaging for Dizziness

If vestibular testing is not helpful in evaluation, imaging can play a role in the evaluation of dizzy patients. Due to relatively higher costs compared to physical exam or vestibular testing, imaging is often used to confirm a suspected diagnosis (e.g., confirmation of SSCD in patients with suspected third-window disorder) or to rule out other lesions (e.g., posterior fossa mass lesion in patient with asymmetric hearing loss and vestibulopathy). Of individuals presenting with dizziness, 20% undergo imaging within the following 6-month period [34]. In a cross-sectional analysis of commercial and Medicare insurance claims, per-test individual spending ranged from $40 to $70 for CT scan and from $320 to $360 for an MRI of the brain among Medicare beneficiaries and commercially insured individuals, respectively [34].

CT imaging of the temporal bone can be helpful in the diagnosis of a fistula of the inner ear such as horizontal semicircular canal erosion due to cholesteatoma, superior semicircular canal dehiscence, or temporal bone fracture. Otherwise, CT of the head or temporal bones is typically not diagnostic in the evaluation of much more common causes of vestibulopathy (BPPV, Meniere's, migraine dizziness, or central causes). There are notable considerations including cost, radiation exposure, and limited yield; therefore, it is not very cost-effective.

MRI is a more sensitive test for dizziness. It is the imaging modality for 25% of patients with dizziness; yet, it amounts to 70% of imaging spending [34]. It is considered the gold standard for the evaluation of retrocochlear pathology, such as acoustic neuromas, which are known to cause hearing loss and dizziness. An analysis by Gandolfi et al. in 2015 assessing cost-effectiveness of MRI scans in patients with abnormal VNG/ENG demonstrated helpful insights [35]. The study examined patients with unilateral weakness >20%, abnormal oculomotor testing, or nystagmus on positional testing who underwent MRI to rule out retrocochlear pathology. The rate of positive findings on MRI for treatable conditions associated with vertigo was found to be 5.5%. Given that the average cost of an MRI is approximately $1200, this results in an average expenditure of about $15,180 for each patient diagnosed with a positive MRI result. This calculation underscores the significant financial implications of using MRI as a diagnostic tool in these cases. With regard to acoustic neuromas, there is a precedent for MRI to be more sensitive and specific over ABR. MRI demonstrates a remarkable sensitivity of 100% for accurately diagnosing acoustic schwannomas, with a specificity of 92.86%. The positive predictive value stands at 94.12%, and the overall accuracy is reported to be 96.67% [36]. The overall sensitivity of auditory brainstem response (ABR) testing for diagnosing acoustic neuromas is 90%. However, this sensitivity decreases as tumor size diminishes. In fact, ABR only detected 7 out of 12 tumors that were 1 cm or smaller, reflecting a detection rate of just 58% for these smaller tumors [37]. While MRI is a cost-intensive tool for diagnosing retrocochlear pathologies, its high sensitivity and specificity for conditions like acoustic neuromas highlight its value in clinical practice.

The American College of Radiology has published guidelines regarding expert panel recommendations on appropriateness of imaging for specific indications [38]. For isolated vertigo, MRI with and without contrast is preferred over MRI without contrast. MRI with and without contrast is more sensitive to acoustic neuroma/vestibular schwannoma, meningioma, multiple sclerosis plaques (hyperintense plaques on fluid-attenuated inversion recovery or T2 weighted images), as well as acute/chronic ischemic disease.

For patients with either episodic or persistent vertigo, MRI with and without is slightly preferred over MRI without contrast in the evaluation of the dizzy patient. However, some studies have shown low yield from MRI for audiovestibular dysfunction. One study looking at 52 consecutive patients with audiovestibular dysfunction who underwent MRI found that 0% had any pathology [39].

Due to the relatively high cost of standard MRI with contrast and relatively low yield, there has been interest in the utility of less expensive non-contrasted scans. The concept of using steady-state free precession (SSFP) sequences such as constructive interference in steady state (CISS) or fast imaging employing steady-state acquisition (FIESTA) to detect mass lesions can be done without the cost and potential allergic risk from administration of Gadolinium contrast.

The cost-effectiveness of non-contrast MRI for vestibular schwannoma in patients with asymmetric hearing loss has been recently studied [40]. In this particular study, a "screening" MRI utilizing non-contrast T1 axial and coronal images as well as axial SSFP sequence of the IACs and posterior fossa was employed. Scans with filling defect in the IACs or CPA were considered suspicious for mass and therefore received a more thorough imaging evaluation. A "full" MRI of internal auditory canals (IACs) included the same sequences as the "screening" MRI plus post-contrast axial and coronal T1 sequences of posterior fossa as well as whole-brain axial T2, FLAIR, and DWI sequences. The cost of a contrasted MRI was around $4000 (USD), and non-contrast MRI costs were around $2872 (USD). While this particular study was focused on patients with asymmetric hearing loss, further study of a "screening" MRI might be interesting for asymmetric vestibulopathy.

Treatment

For decades, vestibular rehabilitation therapy (VRT) has been the mainstay treatment for patients with vestibular disorders [41]. Through central compensation, vestibular rehabilitation improves symptoms of imbalance, dizziness, vertigo, and motion sensitivity. A Cochrane review has determined moderate-to-strong evidence for VRT as treatment for unilateral peripheral vestibular disorders. For BPPV, canalith repositioning is the first-line treatment [42]. However, studies have shown benefit of VRT following canalith repositioning to be beneficial. Treatment of dizzy patients costs $2000–$5000 more per patient than the treatment of non-dizzy patients [8]. Recent literature has explored the efficacy of online-based therapy sessions and the reduction of the amount of therapy sessions [43, 44].

Conclusion

Cost-effective evaluation of the dizzy patient begins with a dedicated cost-free history of the duration, trigger, and associated symptoms of the dizziness. For patients with vestibulopathy, a dedicated low cost (i.e., zero additional cost) physical exam including neurologic exam, oculomotor exam, Dix–Hallpike maneuver, and head impulse test is essential. The use of Frenzel goggles, which have limited up-front costs, is encouraged to enhance the observation of nystagmus. Weber and Rinne tuning fork tests are also minimally costly and can quickly suggest whether sensorineural or significant conductive hearing loss is present. Vestibular testing including videonystagmography with caloric stimulation and rotational chair requires special equipment and trained audiology personnel; testing can help detect subtle oculomotor abnormality, confirm laterality of vestibulopathy, and provide a relative degree of remaining vestibular function. CT scans of the head and temporal bones are usually low yield for dizziness, whereas MRI scan may detect some central pathologies as well as tumors of the IAC/CPA. It is unclear if the recent interest in "screening" MRIs with T2 non-contrasted CISS for IAC/CPA masses will be effective for the evaluation of vestibular patients.

In general, cost-effectiveness calculations are challenging. The costs of evaluation are difficult to capture, and the gained health from diagnosis and treatment of dizziness is difficult to quantify. A review of the expanding literature from the fields of Emergency Medicine, Neurology, Physical Therapy, Otolaryngology, and Otology/Neurotology indicates that there is a growing interest in cost-effectiveness with an emphasis on accurate physical exams and a focus on avoiding misdiagnosis of posterior circulation strokes and intracranial lesions.

References

1. Edlow JA. Diagnosing dizziness: we are teaching the wrong paradigm! Acad Emerg Med. 2013;20(10):1064–6. https://doi.org/10.1111/acem.12234.
2. Newman-Toker DE, Cannon LM, Stofferahn ME, Rothman RE, Hsieh YH, Zee DS. Imprecision in patient reports of dizziness symptom quality: a cross-sectional study conducted in an acute care setting. Mayo Clin Proc. 2007;82(11):1329–40. https://doi.org/10.4065/82.11.1329.
3. Newman-Toker DE, Dy FJ, Stanton VA, Zee DS, Calkins H, Robinson KA. How often is dizziness from primary cardiovascular disease true vertigo? A systematic review. J Gen Intern Med. 2008;23(12):2087–94. https://doi.org/10.1007/s11606-008-0801-z.
4. To-Alemanji J, Ryan C, Schubert MC. Experiences engaging healthcare when dizzy. Otol Neurotol. 2016;37(8):1122–7. https://doi.org/10.1097/mao.0000000000001145.
5. Chau AT, Menant JC, Hübner PP, Lord SR, Migliaccio AA. Prevalence of vestibular disorder in older people who experience dizziness. Front Neurol. 2015;6:268. https://doi.org/10.3389/fneur.2015.00268.
6. Brodsky JR, Lipson S, Bhattacharyya N. Prevalence of pediatric dizziness and imbalance in the United States. Otolaryngol Head Neck Surg. 2020;162(2):241–7. https://doi.org/10.1177/0194599819887375.
7. Saber Tehrani AS, Coughlan D, Hsieh YH, et al. Rising annual costs of dizziness presentations to U.S. emergency departments. Acad Emerg Med. 2013;20(7):689–96. https://doi.org/10.1111/acem.12168.
8. Jeong SS, Simpson KN, Johnson JM, Rizk HG. Assessment of the cost burden of episodic recurrent vestibular vertigo in the US. JAMA Otolaryngol Head Neck Surg. 2022;148(12):1103–10. https://doi.org/10.1001/jamaoto.2022.3247.
9. Hill SR. Cost-effectiveness analysis for clinicians. BMC Med. 2012;10(1):10. https://doi.org/10.1186/1741-7015-10-10.
10. Dunlap PM, Khoja SS, Whitney SL, Freburger JK. Assessment of health care utilization for dizziness in ambulatory care settings in the United States. Otol Neurotol. 2019;40(9):e918–24. https://doi.org/10.1097/mao.0000000000002359.
11. Newman-Toker DE, Hsieh YH, Camargo CA Jr, Pelletier AJ, Butchy GT, Edlow JA. Spectrum of dizziness visits to US emergency departments: cross-sectional analysis from a nationally representative sample. Mayo Clin Proc. 2008;83(7):765–75. https://doi.org/10.4065/83.7.765.
12. Kerber KA, Brown DL, Lisabeth LD, Smith MA, Morgenstern LB. Stroke among patients with dizziness, vertigo, and imbalance in the emergency department: a population-based study. Stroke. 2006;37(10):2484–7. https://doi.org/10.1161/01.STR.0000240329.48263.0d.
13. Edlow JA, Kerber K. Benign paroxysmal positional vertigo: a practical approach for emergency physicians. Acad Emerg Med. 2023;30(5):579–88. https://doi.org/10.1111/acem.14558.
14. Hanna J, Malhotra A, Brauer PR, Luryi A, Michaelides E. A comparison of benign positional vertigo and stroke patients presenting to the emergency department with vertigo or dizziness. Am J Otolaryngol. 2019;40(6):102263. https://doi.org/10.1016/j.amjoto.2019.07.007.
15. Kerber KA, Burke JF, Skolarus LE, et al. Use of BPPV processes in emergency department dizziness presentations: a population-based study. Otolaryngol Head Neck Surg. 2013;148(3):425–30. https://doi.org/10.1177/0194599812471633.
16. Kene MV, Ballard DW, Vinson DR, Rauchwerger AS, Iskin HR, Kim AS. Emergency physician attitudes, preferences, and risk tolerance for stroke as a potential cause of dizziness symptoms. West J Emerg Med. 2015;16(5):768–76. https://doi.org/10.5811/westjem.2015.7.26158.
17. Li JC, Li CJ, Epley J, Weinberg L. Cost-effective management of benign positional vertigo using canalith repositioning. Otolaryngol Head Neck Surg. 2000;122(3):334–9. https://doi.org/10.1016/s0194-5998(00)70043-x.
18. Edlow JA, Carpenter C, Akhter M, et al. Guidelines for reasonable and appropriate care in the emergency department 3 (GRACE-3): acute dizziness and vertigo in the emergency department. Acad Emerg Med. 2023;30(5):442–86. https://doi.org/10.1111/acem.14728.

19. Meurer WJ, Johnson P, Brown D, et al. An educational intervention for acute dizziness care: a randomized, vignette-based study. Otol Neurotol. 2019;40(8):e830–8. https://doi.org/10.1097/mao.0000000000002338.
20. Edlow JA, Newman-Toker D. Using the physical examination to diagnose patients with acute dizziness and vertigo. J Emerg Med. 2016;50(4):617–28. https://doi.org/10.1016/j.jemermed.2015.10.040.
21. Shah VP, Oliveira JESL, Farah W, et al. Diagnostic accuracy of neuroimaging in emergency department patients with acute vertigo or dizziness: a systematic review and meta-analysis for the guidelines for reasonable and appropriate care in the emergency department. Acad Emerg Med. 2023;30(5):517–30. https://doi.org/10.1111/acem.14561.
22. Chen K, Schneider AL, Llinas RH, Marsh EB. Keep it simple: vascular risk factors and focal exam findings correctly identify posterior circulation ischemia in "dizzy" patients. BMC Emerg Med. 2016;16(1):37. https://doi.org/10.1186/s12873-016-0101-6.
23. Mitsunaga MM, Yoon HC. Journal Club: head CT scans in the emergency department for syncope and dizziness. AJR Am J Roentgenol. 2015;204(1):24–8. https://doi.org/10.2214/ajr.14.12993.
24. Grewal K, Austin PC, Kapral MK, Lu H, Atzema CL. Missed strokes using computed tomography imaging in patients with vertigo: population-based cohort study. Stroke. 2015;46(1):108–13. https://doi.org/10.1161/strokeaha.114.007087.
25. Navi BB, Kamel H, Shah MP, et al. The use of neuroimaging studies and neurological consultation to evaluate dizzy patients in the emergency department. Neurohospitalist. 2013;3(1):7–14. https://doi.org/10.1177/1941874412458677.
26. Murphy C, Reinhardt C, Linehan D, Katiri R, O'Connor A. A review of primary care referrals for patients with dizziness and vertigo: prevalence and demographics. Ir J Med Sci. 2022;191(1):385–9. https://doi.org/10.1007/s11845-021-02575-6.
27. Muelleman T, Shew M, Subbarayan R, et al. Epidemiology of dizzy patient population in a Neurotology clinic and predictors of peripheral etiology. Otol Neurotol. 2017;38(6):870–5. https://doi.org/10.1097/mao.0000000000001429.
28. Kentala E, Rauch SD. A practical assessment algorithm for diagnosis of dizziness. Otolaryngol Head Neck Surg. 2003;128(1):54–9. https://doi.org/10.1067/mhn.2003.47.
29. Roland LT, Kallogjeri D, Sinks BC, et al. Utility of an abbreviated dizziness questionnaire to differentiate between causes of vertigo and guide appropriate referral: a multicenter prospective blinded study. Otol Neurotol. 2015;36(10):1687–94. https://doi.org/10.1097/mao.0000000000000884.
30. Bhattacharyya N, Gubbels SP, Schwartz SR, et al. Clinical practice guideline: benign paroxysmal positional vertigo (update). Otolaryngol Head Neck Surg. 2017;156(S3):S1–S47. https://doi.org/10.1177/0194599816689667.
31. Ni G, Kim C, Nair L, Bien AG, Yu D, Foyt D. Impact and cost effectiveness of Videonystagmography. Ann Otol Rhinol Laryngol. 2021;130(7):718–23. https://doi.org/10.1177/0003489420968873.
32. Piker EG, Schulz K, Parham K, et al. Variation in the use of vestibular diagnostic testing for patients presenting to otolaryngology clinics with dizziness. Otolaryngol Head Neck Surg. 2016;155(1):42–7. https://doi.org/10.1177/0194599816650173.
33. Kelly EA, Stocker C, Kempton CM, Dierking DM, Fehlberg HE, Adams ME. Vestibular testing: patient perceptions, morbidity, and opportunity costs. Otol Neurotol. 2018;39(10):1222–8. https://doi.org/10.1097/mao.0000000000002025.
34. Adams ME, Karaca-Mandic P, Marmor S. Use of neuroimaging for patients with dizziness who present to outpatient clinics vs emergency departments in the US. JAMA Otolaryngol Head Neck Surg. 2022;148(5):465–73. https://doi.org/10.1001/jamaoto.2022.0329.
35. Gandolfi MM, Reilly EK, Galatioto J, Judson RB, Kim AH. Cost-effective analysis of unilateral vestibular weakness investigation. Otol Neurotol. 2015;36(2):277–81. https://doi.org/10.1097/mao.0000000000000649.

36. Kabashi S, Ugurel MS, Dedushi K, Mucaj S. The role of magnetic resonance imaging (MRI) in diagnostics of acoustic Schwannoma. Acta Inform Med. 2020;28(4):287–91. https://doi.org/10.5455/aim.2020.28.287-291.
37. Schmidt RJ, Sataloff RT, Newman J, Spiegel JR, Myers DL. The sensitivity of auditory brainstem response testing for the diagnosis of acoustic neuromas. Arch Otolaryngol Head Neck Surg. 2001;127(1):19–22. https://doi.org/10.1001/archotol.127.1.19.
38. Sharma A, Kirsch CFE, Aulino JM, et al. ACR appropriateness criteria (®) hearing loss and/or vertigo. J Am Coll Radiol. 2018;15(11s):S321–s331. https://doi.org/10.1016/j.jacr.2018.09.020.
39. Al-Barki AA, Hudise JY, Malik N, Junaid M, Almothahbi A. Role of MRI in audio-vestibular dysfunction; is it cost-effective? Int J Otorhinolaryngol Head Neck Surg. 2017;4(1):80. https://doi.org/10.18203/issn.2454-5929.ijohns20175123.
40. Crowson MG, Rocke DJ, Hoang JK, Weissman JL, Kaylie DM. Cost-effectiveness analysis of a non-contrast screening MRI protocol for vestibular schwannoma in patients with asymmetric sensorineural hearing loss. Neuroradiology. 2017;59(8):727–36. https://doi.org/10.1007/s00234-017-1859-2.
41. Sulway S, Whitney SL. Advances in vestibular rehabilitation. Adv Otorhinolaryngol. 2019;82:164–9. https://doi.org/10.1159/000490285.
42. McDonnell MN, Hillier SL. Vestibular rehabilitation for unilateral peripheral vestibular dysfunction. Cochrane Database Syst Rev. 2015;1:Cd005397. https://doi.org/10.1002/14651858.CD005397.pub4.
43. van Vugt VA, Bosmans JE, Finch AP, van der Wouden JC, van der Horst HE, Maarsingh OR. Cost-effectiveness of internet-based vestibular rehabilitation with and without physiotherapy support for adults aged 50 and older with a chronic vestibular syndrome in general practice. BMJ Open. 2020;10(10):e035583. https://doi.org/10.1136/bmjopen-2019-035583.
44. Soto-Varela A, Rossi-Izquierdo M, Del-Río-Valeiras M, et al. Vestibular rehabilitation using Posturographic system in elderly patients with postural instability: can the number of sessions be reduced? Clin Interv Aging. 2020;15:991–1001. https://doi.org/10.2147/cia.S263302.

Chapter 12
Inpatient Evaluation of Dizziness and Vertigo

Hyunseo D. Jung and Jacob C. Lucas

Introduction

Despite the remarkable progress in diagnostic tools to evaluate the dizzy patient, dizziness remains a challenging problem for both the patient and the clinician. Patients often have difficulty describing their symptoms coherently, while clinicians are tasked with probing and identifying key elements of the patient's presentation. Dizziness is an exceedingly common complaint, in both outpatient and inpatient settings. It is the most common chief complaint among patients of age 75 and older who visit their primary care providers [1]. Other literature report that about 60% of patients over the age of 60 experience some degree of dizziness and imbalance [2]. As such, it is not unusual for a portion of this large population of patients to be admitted to the hospital for workup. Literatures reported across multiple clinical settings (primary care, emergency room, and specialized clinics) generally agree on the proportion of patients with various etiologies—approximately 40% with peripheral vestibular dysfunction, 10% with central dysfunction, 15% with psychiatric disorder, 25% with non-vestibular disorders (cardiac, orthopedic, etc.), and finally, the remaining 10% without a clear-cut diagnosis [3]. Admitted patients may also develop dizziness and vertigo while hospitalized, even when this is not an initial complaint.

Diagnostic testing for peripheral vestibular dysfunction may require extended visit time for history-gathering and testing using specialized equipment; it is not uncommon for evaluation of the dizzy patient to span multiple visits as test findings are reviewed, and a wide diagnostic differential is narrowed. Due to this, the goal of treatment in the inpatient setting oftentimes is *not* definitive diagnosis and treatment of the dizziness. Rather, the dizziness-aware clinician (internist, intensivist,

H. D. Jung · J. C. Lucas (✉)
Department of Otology and Neurotology, Michigan Ear Institute, Farmington Hills, MI, USA

J. C. Lucas et al. (eds.), *Diagnosis and Treatment of Vestibular Disorders*,
https://doi.org/10.1007/978-3-032-11740-3_12

otolaryngologist, neurologist, cardiologist, etc.) should focus on ruling out life-threatening causes of acute vestibular syndrome such as thromboembolic events and secondarily identifying common and easily treatable vestibular conditions. Good multidisciplinary care should also prioritize early specialty referrals in the outpatient setting to allow for more focused workup and diagnosis of complex dizziness presentations.

Appropriate management of dizziness in the inpatient setting begins with a sound understanding of the physiology of vestibular function, followed by detailed history-taking, physical examination, and an algorithmic approach to workup that will lead a clinician to the proper diagnosis and treatment paradigm. This chapter is written to reflect this stepwise approach.

Vestibular Physiology Review

Peripheral vestibular function starts from the firing of vestibular receptors located within the labyrinth, which is composed of the orthogonally oriented semicircular canals (superior, horizontal, and posterior) and the two otolith organs (utricle and saccule). The endolymph within these fluid-filled organs and the pressure differential caused by head movement is what ultimately activates the afferent nervous system, primarily via the vestibular nerve, to give us a sense of direction and motion. This afferent system is always firing at rest, maintaining a tonic rate of electrical discharge. The directional or rotational movement of the head causes specialized sensory cells called the Cupula to deflect in specific directions in the balance system of *both* ears, which then leads to differential firing rate of the afferent system. For example, during horizontal head rotation to the left, afferents in the left horizontal semicircular canal fire faster, and those on the right fire slower [4].

The eyes are the "window" into vestibular function. Examination of eye movements is the most important physical exam tool to identify the nature of the patient's vestibular dysfunction. As such, an understanding of the mechanics behind eye movements and vestibulo-ocular physiology is paramount in the bedside evaluation of dizziness. When our eyes perceive motion, the sole purpose is to enhance visual acuity, and there are specific terms that denote these *normal* eye movements. *Saccades* refer to rotational movements of the globe to bring an image to focus. *Pursuit* refers to eye movement to maintain the image in focus on the fovea as an object moves within the visual field. *Vergence* refers to eye movement in opposite directions to put objects in focus on both foveae during movement. Then, one can understand the vestibulo-ocular reflex (VOR) as our brain's efforts to maintain binocular fixation and visual acuity on both foveae during head movements.

The lesser discussed reflexes responsible for normal vestibular function are related to head movements—the vestibulo-collic reflex (VCR) as well as the cervico-collic reflex (CCR). VCR refers to the activation of neck muscles in response to vestibular input and CCR is responsible for activation of neck muscles in response to stretch receptors [5]. It is not uncommon for a patient with vestibular hypofunction from any cause to develop significant imbalance if they have pre-existing weakness of these two reflex pathways, which is commonly seen in any pathology leading to muscle atrophy.

Similarly, postural control from the proprioceptive sensory organs located in our skin and joints contributes significantly to a normal vestibular function. Our body's postural response to change in our body position and support surface on which it stands is organized in a discrete pattern centered on our ankle and hip joints specifically [6]. This explains patients having peripheral neuropathy or joint disorders presenting with imbalance that cannot be overcome by normal peripheral or central vestibular input.

Finally, our brainstem is the end organ responsible for synthesizing all vestibular inputs. The cerebellum also plays a vital role in ocular motor control. Lesions of the cerebellum thus commonly present with abnormal eye movements. For example, floccular lesions commonly present with abnormal gaze-evoked nystagmus. [7] Other lesions of the vestibulocerebellum can cause dysmetria by impairing smooth pursuit dysfunction and saccadic inaccuracies [7]. For a more detailed description of vestibular physiology, please refer to earlier chapters.

Approaching the Hospitalized Dizzy Patient

It cannot be emphasized enough how important accurate history taking is in the evaluation of the dizzy patient. Just as when seeing a dizzy patient in clinic, we recommend beginning the encounter by allowing the patient to give an uninterrupted description of the nature of their chief complaint before interjecting, as the clinician will be able to glimpse important pearls of the presentation that could be missed. While the patient is talking, the clinician should be able to form a preliminary list of differential diagnoses as well as get a sense of whether the dysfunction is related to a non-vestibular, central vestibular, or peripheral vestibular cause of dizziness.

In the authors' experience, undifferentiated "dizziness" may be categorized into either *vestibular* or *non-vestibular* causes. Non-vestibular dizziness might include presyncope, syncope, lightheadedness, postural dizziness, dysautonomia, and multisensory imbalance. It is important to distinguish early on in a patient encounter that those with non-vestibular complaints will usually not describe vertigo, which is the illusory sensation of movement triggered by inner ear or central nervous system pathology. They also will not exhibit spontaneous or evoked nystagmus, the hallmark physical exam finding of vestibular pathology. Non-vestibular dizziness will usually be elucidated and treated in the routine workup of a hospitalized patient and will resolve as the underlying pathology is treated. Typically, multi-specialty input is required to ensure that no additional workup or follow up is required. For instance, if the clinician suspects intermittent cardiac arrhythmia, then arranging a Holter monitor beyond the inpatient stay can expedite subsequent workup and treatment. The necessity to check each appropriate organ system for underlying causes of dizziness often lies in stark contrast to cost-effective care. Regardless, expense must be weighed against appropriate care and the provision of answers to an often anxious and distressed dizzy patient.

When a true vestibular pathology is suspected, effort is made to then employ a systematic approach following the initial narrative. The authors find it helpful to ask some of the same questions each time to extract the key aspects of the dizzy patients' presentations. Following is a list of those questions.

1. *How would you describe your dizziness?*

   (a) There are many words that patient use to describe their symptoms, such as unsteadiness, vertigo, light-headedness and disequilibrium. It is imperative to ask this question early on, as it will help parse out non-vestibular etiologies of dizziness, most commonly those related to vascular pathology (cerebrovascular and cardiovascular). Vertigo of peripheral etiology almost always presents with visual distortion, often described by our patients as rotary ("room-spinning") or linear ("tilting," "leaning"). It is the authors' experience that central vertigo is more commonly described as a general sense of imbalance or disequilibrium. Obviously, there are diagnoses that tend to present with a combination of these symptoms, including vestibular migraines. It is also important to recognize that many patients with peripheral vestibular disorders may initially experience true vertigo and are left with generalized imbalance, including recalcitrant BPPV patients as well as post-vestibular neuritis patients.

2. *Can you describe the first time you noticed the dizziness?*

   This is an important question to probe the duration, progression, and severity of their current symptoms. It is remarkable how the patient's initial presentation can be more telling than the ensuing accounts, as it usually is a vivid memory to many patients. Other associated temporal relationships can be helpful to know. For example, onset or worsening of dizziness that coincides with menstrual periods would suggest a potential hormonal relationship, which is very commonly seen in vestibular migraines [8]. Another good example is a BPPV patient describing head motion while waking up or recent head trauma prior to symptom onset.

3. *Are the symptoms episodic or continuous? If episodic, how long does the episode last?*

   This question allows the clinician to mainly distinguish peripheral vs. central vestibular dysfunction. Unlike central etiologies, which tend to present with a relatively vague time course with seemingly continuous symptoms, many peripheral vestibular disorders have characteristic symptom durations that the authors have found to be remarkably consistent across the thousands of patients we have evaluated in both inpatient and outpatient settings. BPPV vertigo episodes usually last only a few seconds to minutes. However, some of the aftereffects of the initial episodes may cause the patient to feel off-balance for a longer period. A Meniere's episode may be minutes to rarely hours, depending on the stages of their respective disease. A significant episode of vestibular neuritis could present with initially protracted periods of vertigo lasting from hours to 1–2 days, followed by variable duration of imbalance.

4. *Is there anything that triggers the dizziness—position, environment (temperature, pressure)?*

Movement of the head is classically described with BPPV episode onset. A more subtle trigger may be from dietary lifestyle (caffeine, certain dairy products, and salted/smoked products), as well as changes in the physical environment like temperature and humidity. Both triggers are well documented among vestibular migraine patients. On the other hand, dizziness that is triggered by barometric pressure changes can point to anatomical vertigo, including superior semicircular canal dehiscence (SSCD), perilymphatic fistula (either due to trauma or chronic infections), or Meniere's disease.

5. *Any associated ear symptoms?*

The clinician should always be alerted for inner-ear-related peripheral vestibular dysfunction when a patient presents with aural symptoms. The most important include fluctuating hearing loss, tinnitus, hyperacusis, or autophony. These aural symptoms classically are associated with certain inner ear disorders differing significantly in management.

6. *Ask yourself: does the patient have a stroke or a heart problem?*

The clinician should always suspect in mind cerebral ischemia or hemorrhage when evaluating the dizzy patient, especially because the demographics susceptible to dizziness are also those that are at risk of a stroke. As many as 15% of stroke patients present with dizziness as their first symptom [9]. Barring absence of a clear trigger in a low-risk individual, a basic set of questions assessing systemic focal neurologic deficits, including cranial neuropathies, is paramount. Often, a patient being consulted for specialist evaluation has already undergone serologic and imaging workup if there is clinical concern, but it never hurts to remind yourself to check off that box.

Cardiovascular etiologies of dizziness are also important to screen for, given the sheer prevalence of cardiovascular comorbidities among patients presenting with dizziness. Literature reports that anywhere from 20% to 50% of patients presenting to ED or inpatient evaluation have comorbid cardiovascular disease that may or may not contribute to their current chief complaint [10].

7. *Others*

A swift review of the patient's medication history as well as recent changes in medication can sometimes explain a patient's presentation.

Review of comorbid conditions is sometimes helpful characterizing patients that come in with multifactorial dizziness. Recent history of stroke, recent trauma (traumatic brain injury, post-concussive syndrome, etc.), migraines, psychiatric disorders are among the most encountered confounders when evaluating a dizzy patient. It is important to identify these associations early on, as they may alter management and prevent unnecessary use of resources for workup.

Vestibular syndromes can be broadly categorized as *continuous* or *episodic*. Continuous vertigo with constant nystagmus defines the so-called acute vestibular syndrome (AVS), which is well described in the emergency room literature [11]. Patients with true AVS are either experiencing vestibular neuritis (or the related condition with hearing loss—labyrinthitis), a posterior circulation stroke, or are in the middle of an *episode* of vertigo due to an underlying condition such as Meniere's disease or vestibular migraine (see associated chapters for further discussion of treatment for these specific conditions). *Episodes* of vertigo are either *spontaneous* (as seen in Meniere's or vestibular migraine) or *triggered* as in the case of benign paroxysmal positional vertigo (BPPV). Characterizing dizziness based on *timing* (continuous or episodic) and *triggers* (position, posture, diet, etc.) may be a more efficient way to characterize and diagnose dizziness in an inpatient setting [12], when advanced vestibular testing modalities are unavailable.

Adapting the Physical Examination

A sound understanding of eye movements is probably the most useful tool in bedside examination of the dizzy patient. As mentioned earlier, our eyes move to fix a clear image at the foveae. The pathologic eye movements seen in dizzy patients reflect this tenet, and it is sometimes possible to correctly localize and/or diagnose the cause based on a thorough, systematic bedside examination.

Nystagmus

Characterizing spontaneous or evoked nystagmus, if present, is the first step. Nystagmus has two phases—slow and fast—and its direction is described based on the fast phase. While difficult to tell at bedside, the slow phase and its change in velocity with subsequent "beats" can help localize the pathology [13]. For example, a decrease in velocity of the slow phase is almost always indicative of a central, specifically a cerebellar, vestibulopathy.

A *spontaneous* nystagmus associated with peripheral vestibular dysfunction is reliable and predictable. As mentioned earlier, VOR is mediated by tonic levels of afferent neuronal activity. Nystagmus results from imbalance in this tonicity due to peripheral vestibular dysfunction. Accordingly, a unilateral peripheral vestibular hypofunction would present with horizontal (or less commonly torsional) nystagmus, with the fast phase beating *toward* the *good* ear. This is present with the head still and is fatigable with visual fixation, which is an important distinction to be made with central dysfunction, which does not fatigue with fixation. Another important maneuver is to have the patient maintain *eccentric* (within approximately 30 ° of the target's central position) gaze in the horizontal and vertical orientation. Nystagmus should intensify when the gaze is directed away from the side of the peripheral lesion, while it slows down when looking toward the side of the lesion.

Finally, it is also important to note that normal physiologic nystagmus can be present when the eye is directed to two ends of the horizontal gaze, called end-gaze nystagmus. To distinguish this from a pathologic nystagmus, the clinician needs to evaluate nystagmus within the eccentric window of gaze.

Frenzel Lenses Augment Examination of Nystagmus

Frenzel lenses blur vision for the wearer and magnify the patient's eyes for the examiner, which aids twofold during examination: loss of ability to visually fixate may unmask nystagmus otherwise unnoticed and magnification of the wearer's eyes will augment the visibility of pathologic eye movements (Fig. 12.1). Frenzel lenses may not be routinely available on an inpatient service but are a useful adjunctive

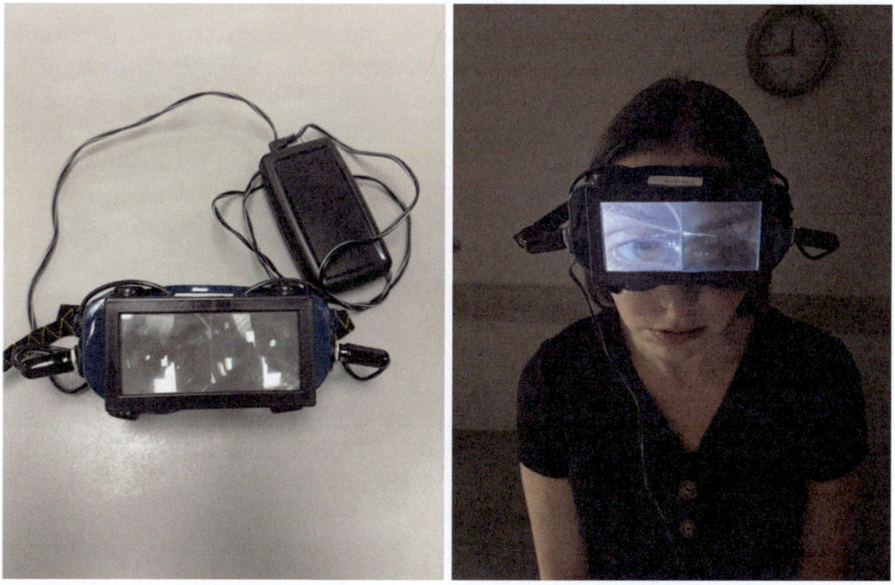

Fig. 12.1 Frenzel lenses illuminate and magnify the wearer's eyes to aid the examiner in identifying and characterizing pathologic eye movements. The eyes lose the ability to fixate, which helps to unmask nystagmus

tool for any clinician routinely evaluating dizziness in the hospital setting. For the dizzy-aware clinician, consider a modest investment in this tool [14].

Head Shake

The head-shake maneuver [15] is also helpful in identifying pathologic nystagmus. The patient's head is held with both hands and shaken vigorously (barring any pre-existing cervical pathology) for at least 30 seconds. Then the shaking is abruptly held, and the patient is asked to open their eyes and look straight ahead. This is best done with Frenzel lenses in place. A healthy patient should not display persistent nystagmus but could have 2–3 cycles of jerk nystagmus. If there is a unilateral peripheral hypofunction, the patient would display nystagmus with its quick phase away from the lesion. It is also possible for a reversal phase to occur where the quick phase occurs toward the lesion after several beats.

Bedside "Fistula" Testing

Pressure changes in the middle ear, and by extension the inner ear, can rarely elicit nystagmus, termed the *Hennebert sign* [16]. Pressure-induced nystagmus can be seen rarely, associated with a collection of pathologies that fall under the third-window syndromes, with the most common being superior semicircular canal dehiscence (SSCD). This can be elicited by having the patient perform a Valsalva maneuver or the nose pinch maneuver. A tragal pump maneuver can be performed by pressing the tragal cartilage into the ear canal in a plunging motion; this transmits pressure to the middle ear and will elicit a similar response to a patient-initiated Valsalva. The Tullio phenomenon [17] can be observed when application of a loud sound (a finger-snap or clap next to the ear) elicits nystagmus, or patient-reported vertigo or dizziness.

Saccades

This term refers to eye movement observed during rapid change in gaze from point A to point B. The most common test utilized is the finger–nose alternating test, with the patient alternatively fixating between the examiner's nose and then a finger held within the eccentric gaze range of 30 degrees. It is best described in accuracy, velocity, and stability [18]. Unfortunately, without more sophisticated testing capacity, it is difficult to quantify the degree of deviation from normal saccadic eye movements at the bedside. However, the patient will exhibit clear symptoms, such as rapid fatigue with repetitive tasks, inability to maintain visual fixation in between tasks, and grossly abnormal eye movements, which will indicate an abnormality.

Head Impulse Testing

The *head impulse maneuver* can also be helpful in identifying the laterality of a peripheral vestibular lesion. The clinician holds the patient's head with both hands over the ears and creates a brief and quick head movement in the horizontal plane while the patient maintains the gaze at the clinician's nose. Normally, the rapid head impulse movement to one side should elicit a compensatory eye movement to the opposite direction with minimal latency. However, if a peripheral dysfunction is present, then impulse toward that ear should display a delayed corrective saccade or a saccadic overshoot when the head is rapidly turned toward the side of the lesion [19] (Fig. 12.2).

Positional Testing

Given the high prevalence of benign positional vertigo, testing for positional triggers is of paramount importance. Again, it is recommended that the clinician use Frenzel lenses during maneuvers when available. A proper Dix–Hallpike maneuver is very useful for diagnosing posterior canal BPPV, the most common variant of BPPV. A positive test would typically show a torsional nystagmus that is geotropic, meaning the fast phase of the torsional movement pointing toward the floor. Rarely, the clinician may observe an ageotropic torsional nystagmus (fast phase to the ceiling), which may indicate a contralateral superior canal BPPV, a rare cause of positional vertigo.

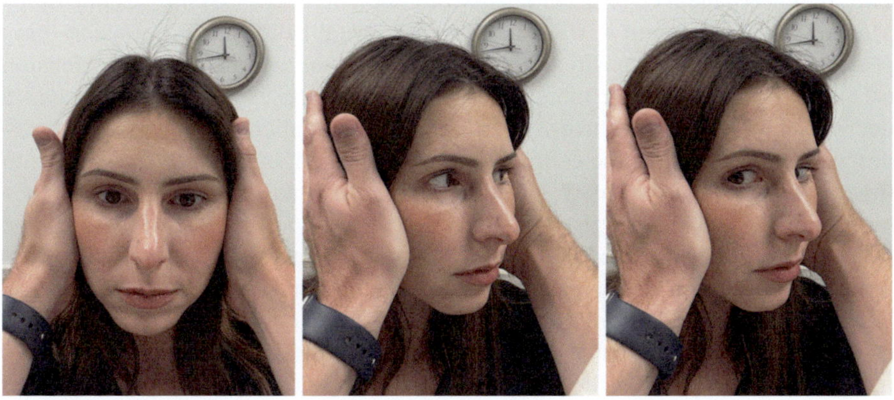

Fig. 12.2 Head impulse testing is performed in the plane of the horizontal semicircular canal. The patient is instructed to maintain gaze fixation on the examiner's nose. A quick thrust toward the pathologic side will cause an involuntary loss of fixation and a compensatory catch-up saccade if a peripheral lesion is present. This reflects dysfunction of the VOR due to a unilateral vestibular loss. The thrust can be *away from*, or *toward* the central position as per the examiner's preference

Horizontal canal BPPV may not be adequately elicited with the standard Dix–Hallpike maneuver. A supine roll test is more sensitive for this, and the authors recommend that this be performed together routinely for a more thorough evaluation. The supine roll test is also useful in patients who are physically limited to participate in the Dix–Hallpike, as it can elicit posterior canal pathology as well.

Adapting the Dix–Hallpike for Use in a Hospital Bed

The classic Dix–Hallpike test may be difficult to perform in a standard inpatient hospital bed, specifically due to headboards and rails that may prevent the ideal 30-degree head extension below the shoulder level. The mobility of a patient may be limited, traditional exam tables are not always available in every unit, and the time available to complete an inpatient examination may be short. Alternative positioning and maneuvers can adjust for these constraints, taking the mobility and frailty of the patient into account.

Additional Cervical Padding
One or more pillows or blankets can be stacked to accommodate the needed head extension during the maneuver. They are placed at the head of the bed under the expected position of the patient's shoulders when leaned back. When the patient leans back, the head is allowed to extend behind the stacked cushioning to mimic a Dix–Hallpike on a traditional exam table. The maneuver is then completed as in the classic setting.

Semont Maneuver
The Semont maneuver is an alternative to the classic Dix–Hallpike and Epley Maneuvers. The Semont is well suited to a hospital bed, as it utilizes side-lying positions with the head position naturally shifting without the need for extension off the back of the bed or table. The patient faces the examiner, turns head 45 degrees, and is forcefully thrown laterally so that the patient is laid onto the shoulder with the head facing the ceiling. Vertigo, if elicited, is allowed to resolve with time as the otoconia settle. With head position maintained, the patient is then rapidly brought back upright, then thrown to the opposite shoulder so that the head is facing down toward the bed or floor. If no vertigo is triggered during the first side-lying position, the patient is then brought upright, and the opposite side is tested. The first side-lying position, when positive, corresponds to the affected ear. For example, a patient with vertigo and nystagmus with the first side-lying position on the right shoulder with the head facing upward would be diagnosed with *right* benign positional vertigo (Fig. 12.3).

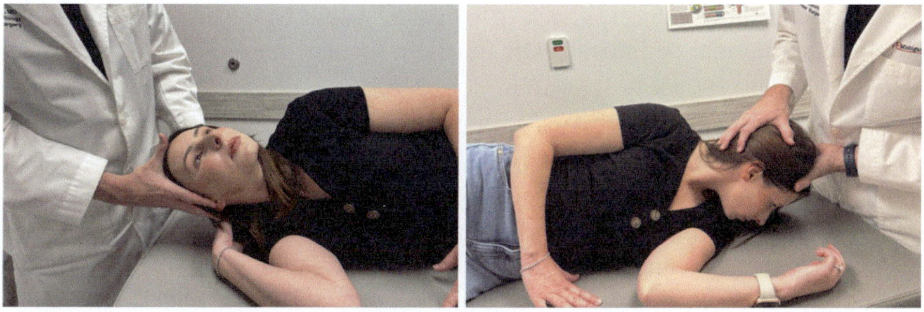

Fig. 12.3 The Semont maneuver is an alternative to the Epley and may be easier to perform in a hospital bed. From the upright position, the patient is quickly laid toward the test side (left image). If classic torsional nystagmus is elicited, position is maintained until the vertigo dissipates. The patient is then quickly brought upright and then toward the opposite side (Right Image) to complete the treatment. Note starting and ending head positions

Acute Vestibular Syndrome (AVS)

It is worth taking some time to be familiar with the acute presentation of AVS as well as the HINTS (Head Impulse, Nystagmus, Test of Skew) testing [20], which is a topic of interest in the emergency medicine literature. HINTS testing is a well-described and effective way to differentiate acute peripheral versus acute central pathology. It can also apply to the acutely dizzy admitted patient. The test is performed on a patient in the middle of an acute vestibular crisis—active spontaneous nystagmus at rest with or without associated imbalance, nausea, and vomiting. Diagnostic accuracy is very high for HINTS in identifying posterior circulation stroke clinically, with a sensitivity of over 95% and specificity above 90% when identifying all central causes of dizziness [21]. HINTS involves three testing domains.

Head Impulse

As a diagnostic tool to rule out stroke, head impulse testing should only be performed in a patient with active spontaneous nystagmus. Nystagmus not evident with visual fixation may be unmasked with the use of Frenzel lenses. The head impulse exam maneuver involves a sudden and unpredictable movement of the subject's head in either the left or right direction, while the subject attempts to visually fixate on a point immediately in front of them, such as the nose of the examiner. The examiner evaluates for "catch-up saccades" following the head movement (Fig. 12.2). If the patient's eye movement has increased latency relative to head movement, this implies VOR dysfunction and would be considered a finding supportive of a peripheral vestibular disturbance. On the other hand, compensatory eye movement without a catch-up saccade would suggest a central pathology. Note that in a normal healthy subject, a lack of saccades would be expected as well—this would imply normal peripheral VOR function; for this reason, only patients with active nystagmus should be tested.

Nystagmus

Evaluation of the nystagmus will point toward a peripheral or central source depending on noted characteristics. Horizontal nystagmus with or without a torsional component is suggestive of a peripheral vestibular lesion. The fast phase of the nystagmus in this case should remain unidirectional no matter the direction of gaze, and in some partially compensated lesions, the patient may be able to decrease the intensity of nystagmus with visual fixation.

In contrast, central lesions will exhibit horizontal, vertical, or purely torsional nystagmus [22]; in horizontal nystagmus, the fast phase may change directions depending on the direction of the patient's gaze. In most cases of central nystagmus, visual fixation is unable to overcome the pathologic eye movements.

Test of Skew

Dysconjugate vertical gaze is a central finding and can be elicited with alternate covering and uncovering of each individual eye. If the uncovered eye exhibits a vertical corrective saccade, this would be considered a positive finding (Fig. 12.4).

A positive finding on HINTS testing should lead to directed efforts at ruling out a posterior circulation stroke, including appropriate imaging.

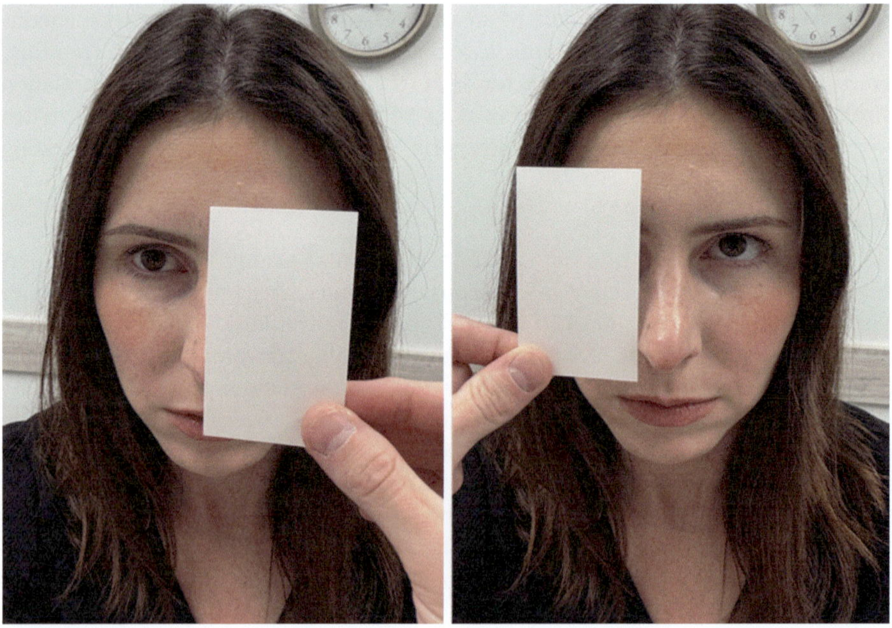

Fig. 12.4 In test of skew, the eyes are alternately covered, and vertical refixation saccades are identified. If eye position changes, the test is positive, suggesting a central lesion

Adjunctive Outpatient Testing

Finally, it is important for the clinician to recognize that a more exhaustive workup and testing are best done as an outpatient. Placing a referral for otolaryngology or neuro-otology practices prior to discharge to coordinate a battery of testing prior to specialist evaluation is beneficial for patient and clinician, and leads to improved patient outcomes. An audiometric evaluation characterizes associated hearing loss. Videonystagmography (VNG) is helpful for quantifying peripheral vestibular function as well as objectively documenting important vestibulo-ocular testing parameters. Rotary chair testing and video head impulse testing (vHIT) are also useful tools to further characterize the patient's vestibular function. Electrocochleography (ECochG) and vestibular-evoked myogenic potentials (VEMPs) are tests that are commonly performed but should only be recommended if there is sufficient clinical suspicion of cochlear and/or labyrinthine involvement, respectively. Finally, gait and movement disorders can be further investigated using posturography. The results are usually helpful in tailoring the patient's subsequent vestibular rehabilitation needs. See associated chapters for finer details on these testing modalities.

Diagnostic and Treatment Considerations for Peripheral Vertigo

This chapter is not meant to be a comprehensive guide for all causes of peripheral vestibular, central vestibular, and non-vestibular conditions and syndromes, although individual syndromes are discussed at length in other chapters of this book. Evaluation of the hospitalized dizzy patient should prioritize diagnosis of easily treatable conditions, ruling out central pathology, and facilitating appropriate referrals. Finally, empiric treatment of a presumed diagnosis and treatment of dizziness symptoms can allow for expedient discharge from the hospital as well as improved productivity of subsequent outpatient specialist evaluation(s) if needed.

Identification of Structural Lesions and Tumors

Typically, dizzy patients who require inpatient workup and management undergo a basic stroke workup that includes a CT of the head with or without contrast, despite the low diagnostic yield of CT [23, 24]. Contrasted MRI of the brain and internal auditory canals in appropriately selected patients will identify structural CNS lesions with associations to the patient's presentation. When considering MRI in a dizzy patient with high suspicion of CNS lesion, it is useful to obtain thin-slice (3 mm or less) imaging to improve sensitivity, which approaches 90% in the appropriate clinical context [25]. Appropriate specialty referrals can then be sought in the outpatient setting, unless the imaging findings show a time-sensitive pathology such as a stroke or other acute intracranial pathology.

Benign Paroxysmal Positional Vertigo.

BPPV is the most common cause of peripheral vertigo, encountered in the inpatient setting frequently. When identified during a patient's hospital stay, it can prevent unnecessary testing, imaging, specialty consultation, and reduce length of stay [26]. As such, BPPV should always be near the top of a diagnostic differential in a hospitalized dizzy patient. Perform an Epley maneuver, Semont maneuver, or Lempert (BBQ Roll) maneuver as indicated to attempt to reposition dislodged otoconia. This can be performed with the aid of a physical therapist, otolaryngologist, or neurologist.

Vestibular Neuritis and Labyrinthitis

Vestibular neuritis, when differentiated from central causes of vertigo, can be appropriately treated with a high-dose oral steroid burst and taper. A Cochrane review found a significant improvement in caloric function at 1 month, corroborated by a systematic review and metanalysis [27, 28], although benefit beyond 1 month in terms of caloric function and symptom improvement found no difference when compared to placebo. Despite this, corticosteroids remain the only available medical treatment in the acute setting. Our institutional dosing scheme is depicted in Box 12.1. Another aspect to keep in mind is that a significant portion of patients recovering from this pathology have residual vestibular dysfunction leading to imbalance requiring vestibular rehabilitation. Recognizing this early and placing outpatient referrals for therapy early in the hospitalization course allow for safe recovery from the inflammatory insult to the inner ear.

Meniere's Disease

An initial Meniere's disease flare may present similarly to vestibular neuritis, but symptoms are generally self-limited and resolve within minutes or hours. Commonly, there is associated fluctuation in hearing that helps with clinical diagnosis. A steroid burst (Box 12.1) can help to resolve the symptoms and allow for referral for outpatient management of this otologic condition. If the clinician is comfortable with outpatient follow-up, starting the patient on an empiric trial of diuretic therapy can be helpful in eventual diagnosis and treatment [29].

Box 12.1 Outpatient prednisone burst and taper

Days 1–7	60 mg once daily AM
Days 8–9	40 mg once daily AM
Days 10–11	20 mg once daily AM
Day 12	STOP medication

Symptom Control

Finally, management of symptoms, even without resolution of an underlying vestibular diagnosis, can nonetheless aid in improving patient symptoms, expediting discharge, and directing patients toward definitive management in the outpatient setting. Associated nausea can be treated with anti-emetic medication, such as ondansetron and prochlorperazine. Vestibular suppressant medications can be considered in the acute setting and include meclizine, an H1 antagonist with antihistaminergic and anticholinergic properties. Long-term use of meclizine is contraindicated, as it can prevent central and peripheral compensation for a vestibular insult [30]. However, it can be effective in symptomatic control of dizziness in acute vertigo attacks.

Vestibular Rehabilitation

A physical therapy assessment in the inpatient setting can triage patients at high risk for falls and allow for safe discharge with assistive devices such as walkers. As vestibular physical therapy is a mainstay first-line treatment for conditions such as BPPV and vestibular neuritis, an initial inpatient evaluation can help to start the process of vestibular rehabilitation and allow for an appropriate outpatient therapy referral. Vestibular physical therapy in patients with unilateral or bilateral vestibular hypofunction has been consistently shown to improve gaze and postural stability, functional status, and patient-reported symptoms of dizziness [31–33].

Surgical Management

Surgical or procedural intervention for peripheral dizziness should never be offered in the acute inpatient setting. All surgical interventions are performed electively after appropriate subspecialty referral and outpatient workup. However, a clinician with vestibular expertise may counsel on the possible role of surgical intervention for treatable disease processes, as surgery may be effective in appropriately selected patients. Meniere's disease patients with vertigo attacks refractory to maximal medical therapy may consider endolymphatic sac decompression surgery, which shows success rates as high as 80% [34]. A labyrinthectomy or vestibular nerve section is a more invasive option that can also bring dramatic improvement in symptoms in select patients [35]. Certain BPPV patients that are not able to achieve symptom resolution despite repetitive particle repositioning maneuvers may benefit from a surgical procedure to occlude the semicircular canal involved in their dizziness. Finally, cerebellopontine angle lesions associated with dizziness allow for a crucial point of discussion when deciding on a treatment strategy. During an inpatient consultation, it may be helpful to mention these interventions in the context of a balanced discussion of possible management options.

Final Thoughts and Conclusion

It is impossible to overstate the importance of a multidisciplinary approach to dizziness, which may include input from neurology, neurotology, otolaryngology, rehabilitative medicine, and even psychiatry. Unfortunately, patients and even clinicians can sometimes get frustrated at the lack of improvement among these challenging cases. As such, it is important to counsel patients on the importance of inpatient diagnosis where appropriate, symptom management where possible, and outpatient subspecialty evaluation. Assessment of functional concerns and patient safety can be completed with the aid of a physical therapy evaluation. In certain cases, recognizing the limits of an inpatient evaluation can help the clinician prioritize factors within their control and begin the process of outpatient management.

References

1. Kroenke K, Mangelsdorff AD. Common symptoms in ambulatory care: incidence, evaluation, therapy, and outcome. Am J Med. 1989;86(3):262–6. https://doi.org/10.1016/0002-9343(89)90293-3.
2. Kroenke K, Arrington ME, Mangelsdorff AD. The prevalence of symptoms in medical outpatients and the adequacy of therapy. Arch Intern Med. 1990;150(8):1685–9. https://doi.org/10.1001/archinte.150.8.1685.
3. Muncie HL, Sirmans SM, James E. Dizziness: approach to evaluation and management. Am Fam Physician. 2017;95(3):154–62.
4. Roy JE, Cullen KE. Vestibuloocular reflex signal modulation during voluntary and passive head movements. J Neurophysiol. 2002;87(5):2337–57. https://doi.org/10.1152/jn.2002.87.5.2337.
5. Peng GC, Hain TC, Peterson BW. A dynamical model for reflex activated head movements in the horizontal plane. Biol Cybern. 1996;75(4):309–19. https://doi.org/10.1007/s004220050297.
6. Goldberg JM. Afferent diversity and the organization of central vestibular pathways. Exp Brain Res. 2000;130(3):277–97. https://doi.org/10.1007/s002210050033.
7. Bronstein AM, Hood JD. The cervico-ocular reflex in normal subjects and patients with absent vestibular function. Brain Res. 1986;373(1–2):399–408. https://doi.org/10.1016/0006-8993(86)90355-0.
8. El Khiati R, Tighilet B, Besnard S, Chabbert C. Vestibular disorders and hormonal dysregulations: state of the art and clinical perspectives. Cells. 2023;12(4):656. https://doi.org/10.3390/cells12040656.
9. Saber Tehrani AS, Kattah JC, Kerber KA, et al. Diagnosing stroke in acute dizziness and vertigo: pitfalls and pearls. Stroke. 2018;49(3):788–95. https://doi.org/10.1161/STROKEAHA.117.016979.
10. Raisi-Estabragh Z, Kobo O, Elbadawi A, et al. Differential patterns and outcomes of 20.6 million cardiovascular emergency department encounters for men and women in the United States. J Am Heart Assoc. 2022;11(19):e026432. https://doi.org/10.1161/JAHA.122.026432.

11. Edlow JA, Carpenter C, Akhter M, et al. Guidelines for reasonable and appropriate care in the emergency department 3 (GRACE-3): acute dizziness and vertigo in the emergency department. Acad Emerg Med. 2023;30(5):442–86. https://doi.org/10.1111/acem.14728.
12. Edlow JA, Gurley KL, Newman-Toker DE. A new diagnostic approach to the adult patient with acute dizziness. J Emerg Med. 2018;54(4):469–83. https://doi.org/10.1016/j.jemermed.2017.12.024.
13. Yang A, Hullar TE. Relationship of semicircular canal size to vestibular-nerve afferent sensitivity in mammals. J Neurophysiol. 2007;98(6):3197–205. https://doi.org/10.1152/jn.00798.2007.
14. Dhonde P, Khadilkar S. Frenzel glasses: an affordable alternative. Pract Neurol. 2020;20(6):504. https://doi.org/10.1136/practneurol-2019-002495.
15. Cohen HS. A review on screening tests for vestibular disorders. J Neurophysiol. 2019;122(1):81–92. https://doi.org/10.1152/jn.00819.2018.
16. Pearlman RC. The fistula and Hennebert tests. J Am Audiol Soc. 1976;2(1):1–2.
17. Basura GJ, Cronin SJ, Heidenreich KD. Tullio phenomenon in superior semicircular canal dehiscence syndrome. Neurology. 2014;82(11):1010. https://doi.org/10.1212/WNL.0000000000000217.
18. Eggers SDZ, Bisdorff A, von Brevern M, et al. Classification of vestibular signs and examination techniques: nystagmus and nystagmus-like movements. J Vestib Res. 2019;29(2–3):57–87. https://doi.org/10.3233/VES-190658.
19. Shah VP, Silva LOJE, Farah W, et al. Diagnostic accuracy of the physical examination in emergency department patients with acute vertigo or dizziness: a systematic review and meta-analysis for GRACE-3. Acad Emerg Med. 2023;30(5):552–78. https://doi.org/10.1111/acem.14630.
20. Kattah JC, Talkad AV, Wang DZ, Hsieh YH, Newman-Toker DE. HINTS to diagnose stroke in the acute vestibular syndrome: three-step bedside oculomotor examination more sensitive than early MRI diffusion-weighted imaging. Stroke. 2009;40(11):3504–10. https://doi.org/10.1161/STROKEAHA.109.551234.
21. Newman-Toker DE, Kerber KA, Hsieh YH, et al. HINTS outperforms ABCD2 to screen for stroke in acute continuous vertigo and dizziness. Acad Emerg Med. 2013;20(10):986–96. https://doi.org/10.1111/acem.12223.
22. Cnyrim CD, Newman-Toker D, Karch C, Brandt T, Strupp M. Bedside differentiation of vestibular neuritis from central "vestibular pseudoneuritis". J Neurol Neurosurg Psychiatry. 2008;79(4):458–60. https://doi.org/10.1136/jnnp.2007.123596.
23. Guarnizo A, Farah K, Lelli DA, Tse D, Zakhari N. Limited usefulness of routine head and neck CT angiogram in the imaging assessment of dizziness in the emergency department. Neuroradiol J. 2021;34(4):335–40. https://doi.org/10.1177/1971400920988665.
24. Fakhran S, Alhilali L, Branstetter BF. Yield of CT angiography and contrast-enhanced MR imaging in patients with dizziness. AJNR Am J Neuroradiol. 2013;34(5):1077–81. https://doi.org/10.3174/ajnr.A3325.
25. Park MK, Kim KM, Lee N, Jung HH, Chae SW. The usefulness of magnetic resonance imaging for acute isolated vertigo patients in the emergency department. J Int Adv Otol. 2014;10(2):162.
26. Bhattacharyya N, Gubbels SP, Schwartz SR, et al. Clinical practice guideline: benign paroxysmal positional vertigo (Update). Otolaryngol–Head Neck Surg. 2017;156(3_suppl):S1–S47. https://doi.org/10.1177/0194599816689667.
27. Fishman JM, Burgess C, Waddell A. Corticosteroids for the treatment of idiopathic acute vestibular dysfunction (vestibular neuritis). Cochrane Database Syst Rev. 2011;11(5):CD008607. https://doi.org/10.1002/14651858.CD008607.pub2.
28. Leong KJ, Lau T, Stewart V, Canetti EFD. Systematic review and meta-analysis: effectiveness of corticosteroids in treating adults with acute vestibular neuritis. Otolaryngol–Head Neck Surg. 2021;165(2):255–66. https://doi.org/10.1177/0194599820982910.
29. Basura GJ, Adams ME, Monfared A, et al. Clinical practice guideline: Ménière's disease executive summary. Otolaryngol–Head Neck Surg. 2020;162(4):415–34. https://doi.org/10.1177/0194599820909439.

30. Roberts DS, Lin HW, Bhattacharyya N. Health care practice patterns for balance disorders in the elderly. Laryngoscope. 2013;123(10):2539–43. https://doi.org/10.1002/lary.24087.
31. McDonnell MN, Hillier SL. Vestibular rehabilitation for unilateral peripheral vestibular dysfunction. Cochrane Database Syst Rev. 2015;1(1):CD005397. https://doi.org/10.1002/14651858.CD005397.pub4.
32. Porciuncula F, Johnson CC, Glickman LB. The effect of vestibular rehabilitation on adults with bilateral vestibular hypofunction: a systematic review. J Vestib Res Equilib Orientat. 2012;22(5–6):283–98. https://doi.org/10.3233/VES-120464.
33. Hall CD, Herdman SJ, Whitney SL, et al. Vestibular rehabilitation for peripheral vestibular Hypofunction: an updated clinical practice guideline from the academy of neurologic physical therapy of the American Physical Therapy Association. J Neurol Phys Ther. 2022;46(2):118–77. https://doi.org/10.1097/NPT.0000000000000382.
34. Brinson GM, Chen DA, Arriaga MA. Endolymphatic mastoid shunt versus endolymphatic sac decompression for Ménière's disease. Otolaryngol–Head Neck Surg. 2007;136(3):415–21. https://doi.org/10.1016/j.otohns.2006.08.031.
35. Lucas JC, Hong RS. Recent surgical advances and continued controversies in medically refractory Meniere's disease. Curr Opin Otolaryngol Head Neck Surg. 2023;31(5):325–31. https://doi.org/10.1097/MOO.0000000000000907.

Part III
Common Vestibular Pathology

Chapter 13
Pathophysiology and Diagnosis of BPPV

Benjamin Campbell, Kyle Kimura, Robert Yawn, and Marc Bennett

Introduction

Benign paroxysmal positional vertigo (BPPV), a disorder of the inner ear characterized by sudden, repeated episodes of positional vertigo, is the most common of the peripheral vestibular disorders and is believed to be the leading cause of vertigo worldwide. It has a favorable prognosis for recovery, with approximately 50% of cases resolving spontaneously within 3 months, and is rarely associated with any serious underlying CNS disorder [1–3].

Epidemiology and Burden of Disease

BPPV is responsible for an estimated 5.6 million clinic visits annually, with a lifetime prevalence of 2.4% and an incidence that increases with age. [4–6] The average age of onset is approximately 50 years and the cumulative incidence by age 80 approaches 10% [5]. BPPV is more commonly seen in women, with a female-to-male ratio

B. Campbell
Altru Professional Center, Grand Forks, ND, USA
e-mail: ben.campbell@altru.org

K. Kimura · M. Bennett (✉)
Department of Otolaryngology Head and Neck Surgery, Vanderbilt University Medical Center, Nashville, TN, USA
e-mail: kyle.kumura@ascentist.com; marc.bennett@vanderbilt.edu

R. Yawn
College of Medicine – Memphis, Department of Otolaryngology Head-Neck Surgery, Memphis, TN, USA
e-mail: ryawn@uthsc.edu

J. C. Lucas et al. (eds.), *Diagnosis and Treatment of Vestibular Disorders*,
https://doi.org/10.1007/978-3-032-11740-3_13

approaching 2:1 [7]. In 2007, researchers from Germany and Switzerland created the REVERT registry in an attempt to quantify the disease burden of vertigo. In their study, they evaluated more than 4000 patients with diagnoses of vertigo and found that nearly one-third were subsequently diagnosed with BPPV [8].

In 2011, BPPV was associated with approximately $750 million in emergency department costs in the United States with total healthcare costs approaching $2 billion per year [9]. The estimated cost of diagnostic workup for a single patient has been reported at approximately $2000 [6, 10]. A major factor contributing to the high costs of diagnostic workup is the use of unnecessary testing in evaluating a patient with vertigo. According to a recent study, greater than 65% of patients with BPPV received some form of unnecessary testing, imaging, or therapy related to their diagnosis and treatment [10]. While not all imaging modalities are unnecessary, the vast majority of patients will receive a scan at some point during their evaluation. In fact, 70% of patients will have magnetic resonance imaging (MRI) and 45% will receive computed tomography (CT) [11]. Despite the prevalence and economic burden of BPPV, these reported costs may still underestimate the true disease burden by their inability to assess quality-of-life reduction in patients with BPPV as evidenced by increased levels of depression and anxiety [5].

Etiology and Risk Factors

While BPPV is most frequently idiopathic in nature, it has been linked to incidents of head trauma, vestibular neuritis, and other underlying vestibular disorders such as Meniere's disease [12]. Recent ear surgery, thought to be linked to utricular damage and release of otoconia, has been described as an independent risk factor and as mentioned previously, increasing age is also a risk factor [13]. Intubation has been proposed as another potential inciting incident, in that it allows for the entrance of detached otoconia into the posterior canal when the patient is supine with an extended neck [1]. Comorbidities associated with BPPV include hypertension, hyperlipidemia, and migraines [5]. Given that all of these comorbidities are vascular in nature, it is hypothesized that there could be underlying labyrinthine ischemia in BPPV patients that facilitates detachment of the otoconia [5]. Other studies have found that osteopenia and osteoporosis are associated with BPPV independent of patient age and gender [14]. More rarely, there have been case reports that cite certain types of swimming or diving as having an association with the development of BPPV [15].

Pathophysiology

There are currently two existing theories that attempt to explain the pathophysiology of BPPV, the canalithiasis theory and the cupulolithiasis theory (Fig. 13.1). The inciting event in both of these theories is the detachment of calcium carbonate otoconia from the macula of the utricle.[16] In the canalithiasis theory, the free-floating dislodged otoconia enter the endolymph of the semicircular canal and shift when the head moves relative to gravity. The inertial drag of the otoconia displaces the cupula and causes vertigo. This vertigo resolves when the otoconia settle. Alternatively, the cupulolithiasis theory suggests that the detached otoconia adhere to the cupula of the semicircular canal itself, which displaces the cupula during head position changes relative to gravity. While this theory would explain some of the more permanent forms of positional vertigo, it fails to explain the transient nature of BPPV or the torsional nystagmus that occurs during episodes [6].

Within the vestibular system, BPPV most commonly affects the posterior canal, which is seen in 85–95% of cases. The posterior canal is thought to be most commonly affected because of its most gravity-dependent position [16]. BPPV of the lateral canal is much less common and is responsible for 5–22% of cases [6, 16, 17]. When compared to posterior canal BPPV, the lateral canal variant tends to produce shorter, yet more severe episodes of vertigo; however, it also tends to spontaneously resolve more rapidly [18]. Lateral canal BPPV may even result from the treatment of posterior canal BPPV with canalith repositioning procedures in a process called canal conversion [6]. The final variant, superior (or anterior) canal BPPV, is quite rare, reported in about 1% of cases of BPPV [16, 17, 19].

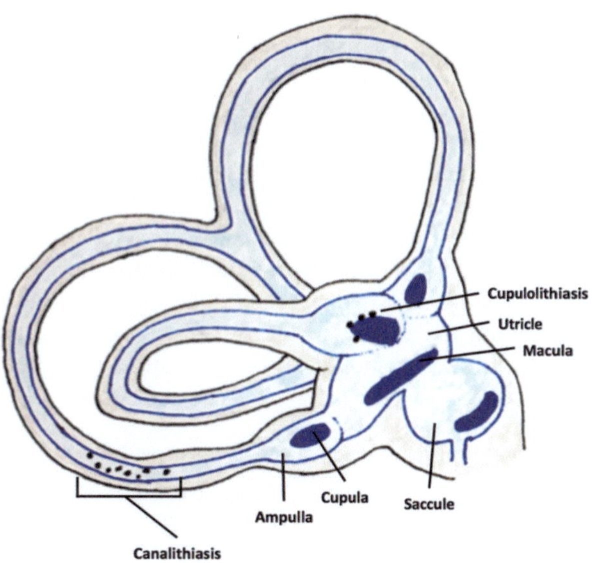

Fig. 13.1 Two pathophysiologic theories of BPPV—canalithiasis and cupulolithiasis

Presentation, Diagnosis, and Physical Exam

BPPV usually presents as episodes of brief positional vertigo, brought on by sudden head movements, which resolve in seconds to minutes. Patients usually notice that these episodes occur during specific daily activities, such as rolling over in bed, standing up, bending forward, or looking upwards. These vertiginous episodes may be associated with nausea and lightheadedness, but it is important to note that they are not associated with any hearing loss or tinnitus. Even though BPPV is characterized as an episodic disease, up to 50% of patients report feeling off-balance between episodes of vertigo, which can last hours to days [5].

The diagnosis of posterior canal BPPV can be made solely with an appropriate history and physical exam. The official diagnostic criteria of BPPV have two components: a history of repeated episodes of vertigo with head changes relative to gravity and a positive Dix–Hallpike maneuver (Table 13.1) [6]. A positive Dix–Hallpike maneuver is one that reproduces the patient's vertigo and causes a torsional, upbeating nystagmus that begins 2–20 seconds after the maneuver, increases in amplitude, and then resolves within 60 seconds of its onset [6]. Vestibular testing and imaging are not required if the two diagnostic criteria above are met; however, an atypical response to the Dix–Hallpike maneuver or persistent and continuous episodes of vertigo may merit additional workup.

Proper performance and interpretation of the Dix–Hallpike maneuver are of utmost importance, as the maneuver is currently the gold standard in diagnosis of posterior canal BPPV [6]. When performed by specialty clinicians, the Dix–Hallpike maneuver has an estimated 82% sensitivity and 71% specificity for posterior canal BPPV [20]. Testing by primary care physicians may have slightly lower sensitivity and specificity, necessitating repeat testing or referral to specialists if suspicion for BPPV is high [21].

To perform the Dix–Hallpike maneuver, the clinician must have the patient seated on an examination table (Fig. 13.2). The clinician will then assist the patient in moving from an upright position to a supine position while the patient's head is turned 45 degrees to one side. Ideally, the patient's neck should be extended 20 degrees after the patient reaches the supine position. This may be accomplished by hanging the patient's neck off of the examination table. The transition from upright to supine should be done relatively quickly and the patient should be

Table 13.1 Diagnostic criteria for posterior canal BPPV

History	Repeated episodes of vertigo with changes in head position relative to gravity
Dix–Hallpike maneuver *(requires all three)*	Provokes vertigo and torsional, upbeating nystagmus
	Latency period between completion of the maneuver and onset of vertigo and nystagmus
	Vertigo and nystagmus increase and then resolve within 60 seconds of their onset

Adapted from Bhattacharyya et al. [6]

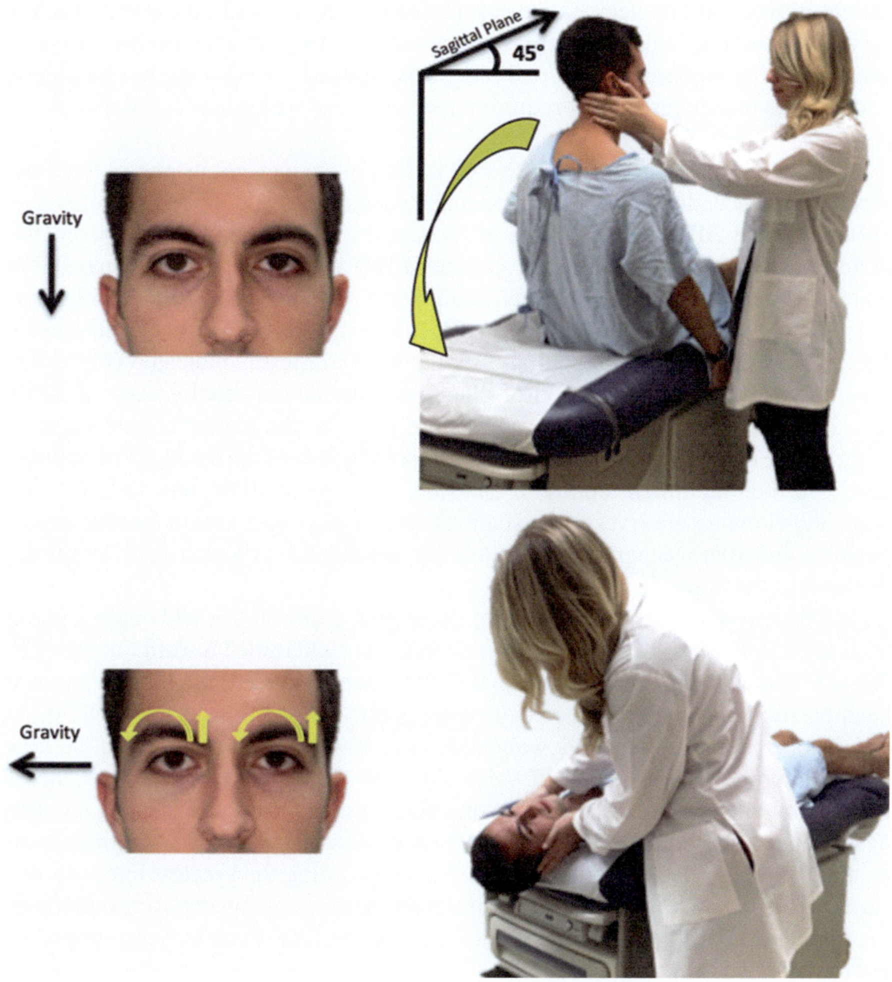

Fig. 13.2 Dix–Hallpike maneuver. (Adapted from Furman and Cass [22])

instructed to keep his or her eyes open. This should be repeated with the patient's head turned to the opposite side. In a positive test, the patient will experience symptoms of vertigo when the affected ear is downward and the clinician will observe upbeating, torsional nystagmus that begins 2–20 seconds after reaching the supine position. The torsional component of the nystagmus should be toward the downward ear [6]. The nystagmus will gradually increase before eventually decreasing and resolving altogether over approximately one minute's time [23]. The nystagmus and symptoms of vertigo associated with the Dix–Hallpike maneuver lessen with each subsequent maneuver; however, repeated maneuvers are not necessary in making the diagnosis, as the fatiguable nature of the nystagmus is not one of the diagnostic criteria for BPPV [6]. Because this maneuver requires quick patient movement and neck extension, patients with physical limitations, such as cervical spinal cord injury, severe rheumatoid arthritis with cervical involvement, vertebrobasilar ischemia, back pathology, or reduced fitness, may not be able to undergo the maneuver or may require the expertise of a physical or balance therapist [24].

Most commonly, the positive Dix–Hallpike maneuver elicits the classic crescendo–decrescendo, upbeating, torsional nystagmus, which is characteristic of posterior canal BPPV. Other forms of nystagmus seen during the maneuver may indicate the presence of a different variant of BPPV including lateral canal BPPV, which will cause pure horizontal nystagmus and superior canal BPPV, which will cause downbeating nystagmus [6, 25–27]. If either of these types of nystagmus is elicited, further examination with the supine head roll test is indicated (Fig. 13.3). This test is the preferred method of diagnosing the lateral canal variant of BPPV [16, 26, 29, 30]. To perform the supine head roll test, the patient should begin by lying supine on the examination table while looking toward the ceiling. The patient's head will then be turned rapidly to one side, stopping at 30 degrees to horizontal, while the clinician observes for nystagmus. The head is then returned to the neutral position, and after nystagmus has ceased, the maneuver is repeated again by turning the head to the opposite side [28].

In a patient with lateral canal BPPV, the supine head roll test will cause a purely horizontal nystagmus that is more intense with the head turned toward one side [26, 30–32]. The nystagmus of lateral canal BPPV changes direction with alterations in head position and can be one of two types: geotropic or apogeotropic [29, 30, 33, 34]. Geotropic nystagmus is downbeating (i.e., toward the ground). It is the most common form of lateral canal BPPV. For a patient with geotropic nystagmus, the ear affected by lateral canal BPPV is the one that is down during the greatest intensity nystagmus as determined by the patient. Conversely, apogeotropic nystagmus is upbeating, and the affected ear is the one that is up during the greatest intensity nystagmus [6]. It has been suggested that canalithiasis is the mechanism underlying geotropic nystagmus, while cupulolithiasis is the mechanism underlying apogeotropic nystagmus [35].

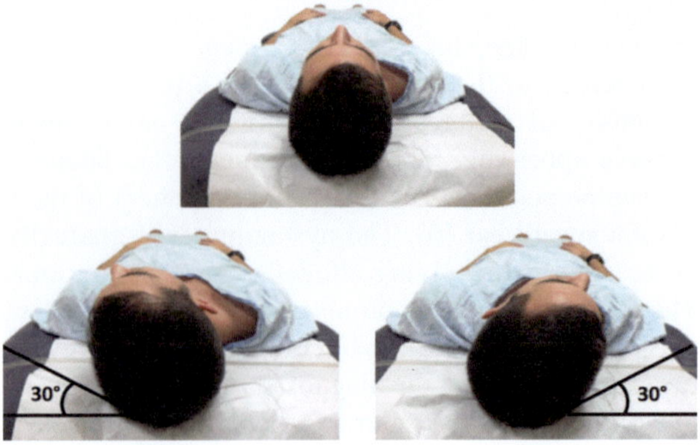

Fig. 13.3 Supine head roll test. (Adapted from Fife et al. [28])

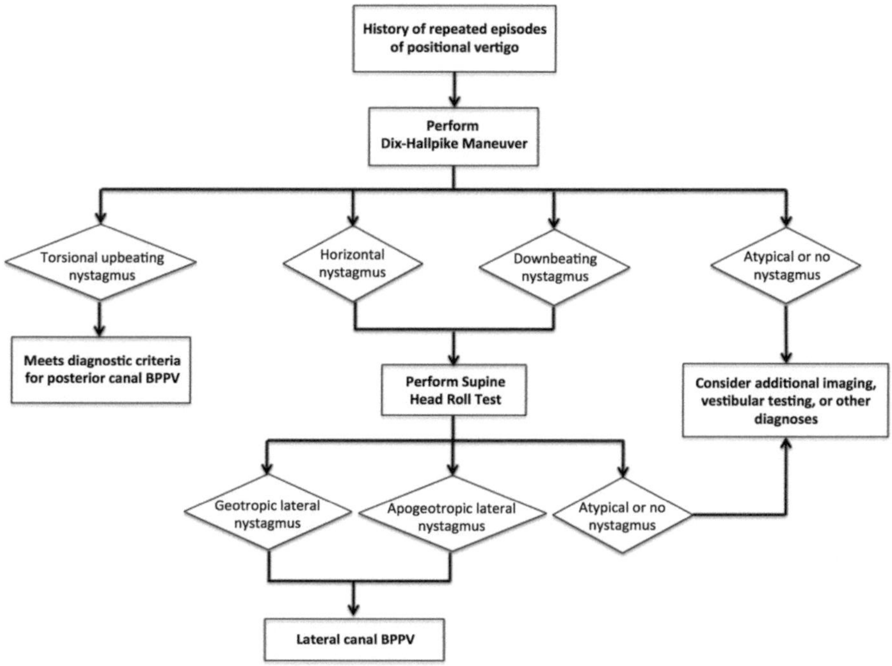

Fig. 13.4 Diagnostic flowchart for BPPV

Real-time interpretation of nystagmus in either the Dix–Hallpike maneuver or the supine head roll test may be difficult to observe due to its transient nature and potential inability of the patient to keep their eyes open. In these scenarios, video-oculographic recordings of the nystagmus, or videonystagmography (VNG), may be helpful, as it allows for the eye to be enlarged on screen, replayed at various speeds, and recorded to facilitate collaboration with other specialty physicians[6] (Fig. 13.4).

Differential Diagnosis and Additional Testing

In most cases, when a patient meets diagnostic criteria for BPPV, no further radiographic imaging or vestibular testing is necessary. However, if symptoms or testing is inconsistent with BPPV, radiology and vestibular testing may help with diagnosis. Radiographic imaging, in the form of a head CT with contrast or a brain MRI, should be obtained in patients who suffer from episodic vertigo with visual disturbances, severe headaches, or abnormal cranial nerve findings on physical examination to search for signs of ischemia, demyelination, or intracranial mass lesions [6]. Imaging can also be very helpful in patients who experience multiple recurrences. Vestibular testing should be considered for patients who have atypical nystagmus on either the Dix–Hallpike maneuver or the supine head roll test [6]. Patients who have failed treatment with canalith repositioning procedures or those who suffer from frequent recurrences of BPPV may also benefit from vestibular testing [6]. Finally, vestibular testing is also useful if the patient is suspected of having additional vestibular pathology aside from BPPV, which has been estimated to occur in 31–53% of patients with BPPV [1, 36, 37].

The differential diagnosis for BPPV contains many otologic and neurologic disorders. However, BPPV can often be distinguished by its self-resolving nature and inciting events prior to episodes of vertigo [6]. Other disorders may present with chronic symptoms of vertigo or symptoms that occur spontaneously without an identifiable trigger. While BPPV is not associated with hearing loss, Meniere's disease, which presents in a similar manner to BPPV with spontaneous, sustained episodes of vertigo, will often have associated aural fullness, tinnitus, or hearing loss[1]. Compared to BPPV, the episodes of vertigo in Meniere's disease are not brought on by positional changes, but rather occur spontaneously without an identifiable source [1]. Acute peripheral vestibular syndromes, such as vestibular neuritis and labyrinthitis, can also cause vertigo, but these episodes are often more insidious in nature, developing over the course of hours and lasting for days to weeks. In these syndromes, vertigo may also occur at rest [38]. Superior canal dehiscence syndrome and perilymph fistulas may also produce acute episodes of triggered vertigo; however, this vertigo is induced by inner ear pressure changes, such as loud sounds or Valsalva maneuvers rather than from changes in position [39]. Central nervous system (CNS) pathologies such as vestibular migraine, posterior circulation transient ischemic attacks (TIAs) or strokes, vertebrobasilar insufficiency, infratentorial lesions, and central positional vertigo can also present with episodes of vertigo [6]. Of these CNS pathologies, vestibular migraine is the most common, causing roughly 14% of vertigo cases, with a lifetime prevalence of 3.2%. [38, 40] Findings that suggest a neurologic cause of vertigo include down-beating nystagmus without a torsional component during the Dix–Hallpike maneuver, direction-changing nystagmus without change in head position, or nystagmus at rest [6]. Posterior circulation TIAs or strokes may be suspected when episodes of vertigo are accompanied by focal neurologic signs such as dysarthria or dysphagia [41]. Cervicogenic vertigo is triggered by head movements, but these head movements occur when the head is upright and are not positional changes relative to gravity. Other disorders on the differential for BPPV include anxiety attacks and panic disorder, medication side effects, and postural hypotension [6].

Summary

BPPV is a relatively common disorder of the inner ear that causes sudden episodes of positional vertigo and is one of the leading causes of vertigo worldwide. It is most frequently idiopathic and is believed to be caused by the presence of detached otoconia within the semicircular canals. While the differential diagnosis for vertigo is broad, BPPV can often be diagnosed solely through history and physical exam, consisting of the Dix–Hallpike maneuver or the supine head roll test. Treatment of BPPV will be discussed in a separate chapter of this book.

References

1. Baloh RW, Honrubia V, Jacobson K. Benign positional vertigo: clinical and oculographic features in 240 cases. Neurology. 1987;37:371–8.
2. Lynn S, Pool A, Rose D, Brey R, Suman V. Randomized trial of the canalith repositioning procedure. Otolaryngol Head Neck Surg. 1995;113:712–20.
3. Burton MJ, Eby TL, Rosenfeld RM. Extracts from the Cochrane library: modifications of the Epley (canalith repositioning) maneuver for posterior canal benign paroxysmal positional vertigo. Otolaryngol Head Neck Surg. 2012;147:407–11.
4. Schappert SM. National Ambulatory Medical Care Survey: 1989 summary. Vital Health Stat. 1992;13(110):1–80.
5. von Brevern M, Radtke A, Lezius F. Epidemiology of benign paroxysmal positional vertigo: a population based study. J Neurol Neurosurg Psychiatry. 2007;78:710–5.
6. Bhattacharyya N, Gubbels SP, Schwartz SR, Edlow JA, El-Kashlan H, Fife T, Holmberg JM, Mahoney K, Hollingsworth DB, Roberts R, Seidman MD, Steiner RWP, Do BT, Voelker CCJ, Waguespack RW, Corrigan MD. Clinical practice guideline: benign paroxysmal positional vertigo (update). Otolaryngol Head Neck Surg. 2017;156(3):S1–S47.
7. Neuhauser HK, Lempert T. Vertigo: epidemiologic aspects. Semin Neurol. 2009;29:473–81.
8. Benecke H, Agus S, Kuessner D, Goodall G, Strupp M. The burden and impact of vertigo: findings from the REVERT patient registry. Front Neurol. 2013;4:136.
9. Tehrani ASS, Coughlan D, Hsieh YH, Mantokoudis G, Korley FK, Kerber KA, Frick KD, Newman-Toker DE. Rising annual costs of dizziness presentations to U.S. emergency departments. Acad Emerg Med. 2013;20(7):689–96.
10. Wang H, Yu D, Song N, Yin S. Delayed diagnosis and treatment of benign paroxysmal positional vertigo associated with current practice. Eur Arch Otorrinolaringol. 2014;271:261–4.
11. Grill E, Strupp M, Müller M, Klaus J. Health services utilization of patients with vertigo in primary care: a retrospective cohort study. J Neurol. 2014;261:1492–8.
12. Karlberg M, Hall K, Quickert N, Hinson J, Halmagyi GM. What inner ear diseases cause benign paroxysmal positional vertigo? Acta Otolarygnol. 2000 Mar;120(3):380–5.
13. Atacan E, Sennaroglu L, Genc A, Kaya S. Benign paroxysmal positional vertigo after stapedectomy. Laryngoscope. 2001;111(7):1257–9.
14. Vibert D, Kompis M, Hausler R. Benign paroxysmal positional vertigo in older women may be related to osteoporosis and osteopenia. Ann Otol Rhinol Laryngol. 2003;112:885–9.
15. Aksoy S, Sennaroglu L. Benign paroxysmal vertigo in swimmers. Kulak Burun Bogaz Ihtis Derg. 2007;17(6):307–10.
16. Cakir BO, Ercan I, Cakir ZA. What is the true incidence of horizontal semicircular canal benign paroxysmal positional vertigo? Otolaryngol Head Neck Surg. 2006;134:451–4.
17. Parnes LS, Agrawal SK, Atlas J. Diagnosis and management of benign paroxysmal positional vertigo (BPPV). CMAJ. 2003;169:681–93.
18. Imai T, Ito M, Takeda N. Natural course of the remission of vertigo in patients with benign paroxysmal positional vertigo. Neurology. 2005;64:920–1.
19. Califano L, Vassallo A, Melillo MG, Mazzone S, Salaria F. Direction-fixed paroxysmal nystagmus lateral canal benign paroxysmal positional vertigo (BPPV): another form of lateral canalolithiasis. Acta Otorhinolaryngol Ital. 2013;33(4):254–60.
20. Lopez-Escamez JA, Lopez-Nevot A, Gamiz MJ. Diagnosis of common causes of vertigo using a structured clinical history. Acta Otorrinolaringol Esp. 2000;51:25–30.

21. Hanley K, O'Dowd T. Symptoms of vertigo in general practice: a prospective study of diagnosis. Br J Gen Pract. 2002;52:809–12.
22. Furman JM, Cass SP. Benign paroxysmal positional vertigo. N Engl J Med. 1999;341:1590–6.
23. von Brevern M, Bertholon P, Brandt T. Benign paroxysmal positional vertigo: diagnostic criteria. J Vestib Res. 2015;25:105–17.
24. Humphriss RL, Baguley DM, Sparkes V, Peerman SE, Moffat DA. Contraindications to the dix-Hallpike manoeuvre: a multidisciplinary review. Int J Audiol. 2003;42(3):166–73.
25. Heidenreich KD, Kerber KA, Carender WJ. Persistent positional nystagmus: a case of superior semicircular canal benign paroxysmal positional vertigo? Laryngoscope. 2011;121:1818–20.
26. Casani AP, Nacci A, Dallan I. Horizontal semicircular canal benign paroxysmal positional vertigo: effectiveness of two different methods of treatment. Audiol Neurootol. 2011;16:175–84.
27. Lopez-Escamez JA, Molina MI, Gamiz MJ. Anterior semicircular canal benign paroxysmal positional vertigo and positional downbeating nystagmus. Am J Otolaryngol. 2006;27:173–8.
28. Fife TD, Iverson DJ, Lempert T. Practice parameter: therapies for benign paroxysmal positional vertigo (an evidence-based review). Report of the quality standards Subcommittee of the American Academy of Neurology. Neurology. 2008;70:2067–74.
29. Fife TD. Positional dizziness. Continuum (Minneapolis, Minn). 2012;18(5, neuro-otology):1060–85.
30. Nuti D, Agus G, Barbieri MT. The management of horizontal-canal paroxysmal positional vertigo. Acta Otolaryngol. 1998;118:455–60.
31. Fife D, FitzGerald JE. Do patients with benign paroxysmal positional vertigo receive prompt treatment? Analysis of waiting times and human and financial costs associated with current practice. Int J Audiol. 2005;44:50–7.
32. Lee S-H, Choi K-D, Jeong S-H. Nystagmus during neck flexion in the pitch plane in benign paroxysmal positional vertigo involving the horizontal canal. J Neurol Sci. 2007;256:75–80.
33. White JA, Coale KD, Catalano PJ. Diagnosis and management of lateral semicircular canal benign paroxysmal positional vertigo. Otolaryngol Head Neck Surg. 2005;133:278–84.
34. Tirelli G, Russolo M. 360-degree canalith repositioning procedure for the horizontal canal. Otolaryngol Head Neck Surg. 2004;131:740–6.
35. Fife TD. Benign paroxysmal positional vertigo. Semin Neurol. 2009;29:500–8.
36. Roberts RA, Gans RE, Kastner AH. Prevalence of vestibulopathy in benign paroxysmal positional vertigo patients with and without prior otologic history. Int J Audiol. 2005;44:191–6.
37. Korres SG, Balatsouras DG. Diagnostic, pathophysiologic, and therapeutic aspects of benign paroxysmal positional vertigo. Otolaryngol Head Neck Surg. 2004;131:438–44.
38. Kentala E, Rauch SD. A practical assessment algorithm for diagnosis of dizziness. Otolaryngol Head Neck Surg. 2003;128:54–9.
39. Minor LB, Cremer PD, Carey JP. Symptoms and signs in superior canal dehiscence syndrome. Ann N Y Acad Sci. 2001;942:259–73.
40. Dunniway HM, Welling DB. Intracranial tumors mimicking benign paroxysmal positional vertigo. Otolaryngol Head Neck Surg. 1998;118:429–36.
41. Kerber KA. Acute continuous vertigo. Semin Neurol. 2013;33:173–8.

Chapter 14
Medical and Surgical Treatment of BPPV

Peng You, Sumit K. Agrawal, and Lorne S. Parnes

Introduction and Background

Benign paroxysmal positional vertigo (BPPV) is the most commonly encountered peripheral vestibular disorder. While Barany first described the presentation in 1921 [1], the term benign paroxysmal positional vertigo was not coined until 1952 by Dix and Hallpike [2]. The name of the disorder eloquently summarized its salient features that include sudden but brief episodes of vertigo elicited by certain head positioning.

In the context of BPPV, the symptoms of vertigo reflect inadvertent activation of the inner ear, which leads to an illusory sense of motion. Studies have found that 17–42% of patients with vertigo are eventually diagnosed with BPPV [3]. The majority of BPPV occurs without a known cause (primary BPPV). In comparison, secondary BPPV is thought to be related to closed head injury, otologic and non-otologic surgery, or inner ear diseases, such as sudden sensorineural hearing loss, Meniere's disease, vestibular neuritis, and even migraine [4]. The peak onset of primary BPPV is between the fifth decade and the sixth decade of life with a female-to-male ratio of 2–3 to 1 [5]. This gender difference is not observed in younger patients or those with an onset of BPPV following trauma [6].

The prevalence of the BPPV equates to a high healthcare burden, estimated to approach $2 billion per year [6]. However, delay in diagnosis and treatment is frequent, with cost and quality of life implications for patients and caregivers [6, 7]. For instance, in the elderly, it has been estimated that 9% of patients have unrecognized BPPV [8]. Furthermore, some authors have found that only 10–20% of patients with BPPV seen by physicians receive appropriate treatment [9]. Fortunately,

P. You · S. K. Agrawal · L. S. Parnes (✉)
Department of Otolaryngology-Head and Neck Surgery, Schulich School of Medicine and Dentistry, Western University, London, ON, Canada
e-mail: pyou2@uwo.ca; Sumit.Agrawal@lhsc.on.ca; Lorne.Parnes@lhsc.on.ca

J. C. Lucas et al. (eds.), *Diagnosis and Treatment of Vestibular Disorders*,
https://doi.org/10.1007/978-3-032-11740-3_14

BPPV is usually easily diagnosed through the history and physical exam. Moreover, the majority of patients can be treated using effective, non-invasive means.

Understanding of the pathophysiology and available treatment options is essential for clinicians tackling this common affliction. The pathophysiological mechanism of BPPV has been attributed to cupulolithiasis (particles adherent to the cupula) or canalithiasis (floating particles within a semicircular canal). The theory of canalithiasis is supported by in vivo discovery of endolymph particles by Parnes and McClure in 1992 [10]. A recent scanning electron microscopy study demonstrates that canaliths are displaced fragments from the utricular otolithic membrane [11]. On the other hand, the theory of cupulolithiasis describes particle or debris being adherent to the cupula and may represent the more chronic form of BPPV [4]. Details ofpathophysiology and diagnosis of BPPV will be elaborated in another chapter. Once the clinician arrives at an accurate diagnosis of BPPV, appropriate non-surgical and surgical management can be arranged.

Management

Non-surgical Management

BPPV is an eminently treatable inner ear disease. In the vast majority of cases, clinicians can offer non-invasive means to correct what is essentially a mechanical problem within one or more semicircular canals. Note that in BPPV associated with vestibular neuronitis, Meniere's disease, head trauma, and even the idiopathic type, there may be other concurrent vestibulo-pathologies in conjunction with the BPPV, most notably affecting the otolith organs. Clinicians should be mindful that treatment for the latter with vestibular rehabilitation therapy (VRT) can coincide with or follow the treatment for BPPV.

A crucial component of BPPV management is education and reassurance. BPPV is ultimately a benign condition, and patients should be made aware of its favorable prognosis. Left untreated, 25% of patients have spontaneous resolution by one month and up to 50% at three months [12]. While observation is an option, effective treatment can help avoid discomfort and possible injury associated with episodic vertigo [6]. Unfortunately, relapse and remissions can occur unpredictably in both treated and untreated patients [5]. Thus, education also helps patients anticipate and cope with recurrences.

The treatment of choice centers around appropriate repositioning maneuvers. The in-office techniques have been shown to be more efficacious than rigorous vestibular habituation therapy, such as that introduced by Brandt and Daroff [13]. Furthermore, studies have shown labyrinthine sedatives to be less efficacious than repositioning maneuvers or vestibular training [14]. Therefore, based on current evidence, clinicians should refrain from treating BPPV with vestibular suppressant medications [6, 14].

Posterior Canal BPPV

The Semont (aka Liberatory) maneuver was first described in 1988 and was based on the theory of cupulolithiasis [15]. Through rapid, stepwise changes in head position, the maneuver aimed to free stuck debris from the cupula. In time, the cupulolithiasis theory was supplanted by the canalithiasis theory, but as it turned out, the Semont maneuver still proved useful through its repositioning of the canaliths into the utricle. The patient is first seated upright with the head turned away from the affected ear (Fig. 14.1). Then, the patient quickly adopts a side-lying position to the affected side with the head angled up. After 5 minutes, the patient is moved to the

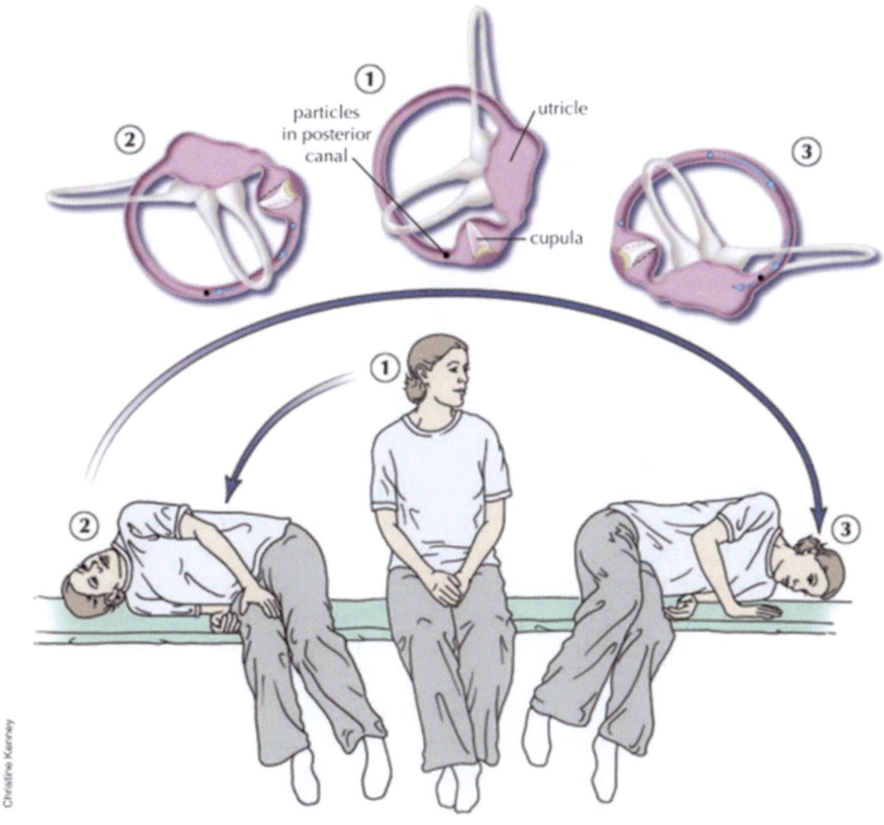

Fig. 14.1 Semont maneuver (right ear). The effect of the sequential movements on the labyrinth is depicted in the top panel. The transition from position 2 to 3 must be rapid. (Reprinted from Parnes, Agrawal and Atlas. Diagnosis and management of benign paroxysmal positional vertigo (BPPV) Fig. 7. Canadian Medical Association Journal September 30, 2003 169 (7) 681–693. © Canadian Medical Association 2003. This work is protected by copyright and the making of this copy was with the permission of the Canadian Medical Association Journal (www.cmaj.ca) and Access Copyright. Any alteration of its content or further copying in any form whatsoever is strictly prohibited unless otherwise permitted by law [4])

opposite side-lying position with the head angled down. The patient remains this way for 5–10 minutes before slowly being brought back to the sitting position. Most, if not all, clinicians now perform these steps much more quickly than originally described, perhaps 1 minute for each. Overall, the Semont maneuver has been shown to be efficacious, safe, and advantageous compared to a sham control [16]. The reported response rate ranges from 70% to 90% with a recurrence rate of approximately 29% [16, 17]. This maneuver may be considered for patients with cervical spine or vascular conditions, as it does not require hyperextension of the neck. Unfortunately, due to its rapid pace, the Semont maneuver can be difficult in elderly, obese, and infirm patients.

In the 1980s, based on the canalithiasis theory, Dr. John Epley devised a set of controlled head movements called the canalith repositioning procedure (CRP), now known colloquially as the Epley maneuver [4]. The premise was to return the canaliths, under the influence of gravity, from the posterior semicircular canal back into the utricle. Over time, the CRP has been simplified and has become the mainstay treatment for posterior canal BPPV. One modified form of CRP is the particle repositioning maneuver (PRM). First introduced by Parnes and Price-Jones, PRM offers a more simplistic 3-position maneuver and obviates the need for sedation and mastoid vibration described in the original CRP [4]. Currently, the terms CRP, PRM, and Epley manoeuver are used interchangeably. The procedure has been shown to be efficacious with 70–85% success rate after a single maneuver [18]. A Cochrane review of 11 relevant studies representing 745 participants concluded that the Epley manoeuver and its modifications are safe and effective [19].

The steps of the PRM are as follows [4] (Fig. 14.2):

1. Place the patient lengthwise on a table or stretcher in a sitting position.
2. Move the patient into the supine Dix–Hallpike position with head turned toward the side being treated. Place the neck in extension, hanging the head back over the edge of the stretcher. For those who cannot tolerate neck extension, tilt the stretcher back into Trendelenburg position.
3. Maintain this position for 1–2 minutes while observing for nystagmus.
4. While keeping the neck in full extension, turn the head 90° toward the opposite ear.
5. Continue to roll the patient another 90° until the head is diagonally opposite to the first Dix–Hallpike position. This step should be done in less than 3 seconds in order to generate a nystagmus response. The latter results from the gravitational pull on the canaliths, which induces an endolymph current and in turn induces cupular displacement and the resulting nystagmus.
6. Observe for "secondary-stage" nystagmus. Ideally, this secondary-stage nystagmus should beat in the same direction as the primary stage nystagmus.
7. After 30–60 seconds, the patient resumes a seated position. With a successful maneuver, there should be no nystagmus or vertigo when the patient returns to the sitting position.

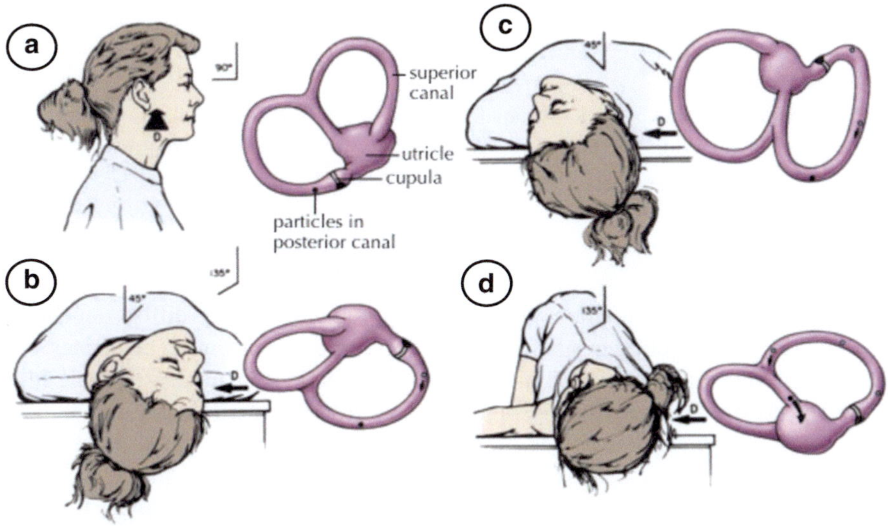

Fig. 14.2 Particle repositioning maneuver (right ear). Sequential movements and the corresponding position of the utricle and semicircular canals. (**a**) The patient is seated as viewed from the right side. (**b**) First step of particle repositioning maneuver and the same position assumed during normal Dix–Hallpike. This position is maintained for 1–2 minutes. (**c**) The patient's head is rotated toward the opposite side while neck remains extended. (**d**) In a steady motion, the patient is rolled onto the opposite side. Position D is maintained for another 1–2 minutes before the patient sits up to position A. D = direction of view of labyrinth, dark circle = position of particle conglomerate, open circle = previous position. (Reprinted from Parnes, Agrawal and Atlas. Diagnosis and management of benign paroxysmal positional vertigo (BPPV) Fig. 8. Canadian Medical Association Journal September 30, 2003 169 (7) 681–693. © Canadian Medical Association 2003. This work is protected by copyright and the making of this copy was with the permission of the Canadian Medical Association Journal (www.cmaj.ca) and Access Copyright. Any alteration of its content or further copying in any form whatsoever is strictly prohibited unless otherwise permitted by law [4])

Practitioners should pay careful attention to the patient's nystagmus during the PRM. Reversed/absent secondary stage nystagmus or a reversed nystagmus at the conclusion of PRM suggests that the canaliths have not returned to the utricle. The PRM should then be repeated after a short interval. While the original Epley maneuver described post-treatment activity limitations and mastoid vibration, neither has been shown to enhance the rate of success [20, 21]. However, on occasion, mastoid oscillation may be helpful in cases resistant to conventional repositioning.

Emerging evidence supports the utility of treating subjective BPPV. This is the term used for patients with convincing clinical histories but no nystagmus during Dix–Hallpike testing [4]. Proposed theories for this include subclinical nystagmus, a fatigued response, and less severe BPPV that activates the sensation of vertigo but not the vestibulo-ocular reflex. Studies have shown that repositioning maneuvers in those with subjective BPPV are nearly as effective as they are for patients with objective BPPV [22].

Table 14.1 Characteristic nystagmus associated with horizontal canal BPPV

	Direction of nystagmus	
Intensity of nystagmus	Ageotropic	Geotropic
Stronger on the left side	Right cupulolithiasis	Left canalithiasis
Stronger on the right side	Left cupulolithiasis	Right canalithiasis

Table reproduced from Parnes et al. [4]

Horizontal Canal BPPV

The choice of repositioning technique of horizontal canal BPPV differs depending on whether the presenting nystagmus is geotropic or apogeotropic. The former suggests canalithiasis and is more clinically responsive and well studied [6], Table 14.1.

When horizontal geotropic nystagmus is encountered with lateral supine head turns, barbecue roll or barrel roll can be used to rotate patients in the plane of the horizontal semicircular canal [23]. Starting in a supine position, the head is first turned toward the affected ear. The head and body are then turned away from the affected side in 90-degree increments. The patient holds each position for about 1 minute until a full 360-degree rotation is completed before they are returned to the seated position. An alternative strategy is the Gufoni maneuver [24]. The patient begins by lying sideways on the *unaffected* side for 1–2 minutes. The head is then rapidly turned 45 degrees toward the ground where the patient holds the position for two minutes before sitting up. A randomized control trial showed comparable success between Gufoni (response rate of 60.9%) and barbecue roll (69.1%) [25].

In the event of apogeotropic nystagmus, suggesting the likely mechanism to be cupulolithiasis, the Gufoni maneuver begins with the patient lying sideways on the *affected* side before turning the head rapidly toward the ground [6]. Similarly, the patient holds each position for 1–2 minutes before sitting up. Whereas the Gufoni maneuver depends on linear acceleration and positive inertia to move the canalith, Vannucchi and colleagues proposed forced prolonged positioning, which relies on gravitational sedimentation [26]. In forced prolonged position, the patient assumes a lateral decubitus position on the unaffected side for 12 hours (affected side if nystagmus is apogeotropic). A prospective observational study found the effectiveness of forced prolonged position to be similar to that of Gufoni's maneuver after a single application (with success rates of 76% and 89%, respectively) [27]. Practically, due to the time commitment, the forced prolonged positioning is not typically performed.

Superior Canal BPPV

In contrast to the posterior and superior canal variants, the data are sparse for effective therapeutic maneuvers for superior canal BPPV. Two commonly published maneuvers for the superior canal are the reverse Epley and Yacovino, with a mean success rate of 75.9% and 78.8%, respectively [28]. The reverse Epley is effectively a PRM of the unaffected side, thus isolating the contralateral and affected anterior canal. In comparison, the Yacovino maneuver is sequential head positioning where the patient starts in a supine 30-degree head hanging position, then a supine 30-degree head inclined position, and lastly a sitting head 30 degrees forward position.

Recurrences, Complications, and Failed Treatment

Spontaneous recurrence following the successful treatment of BPPV is high and should not be a deterrent for the clinician. Repositioning maneuvers are usually safe and can be repeated at the time of follow-up. While the follow-up after canal repositioning has not been standardized, a typical interval is one month [6]. Follow-up is also crucial in the event of bilateral BPPV. For bilateral BPPV, the more symptomatic side should be treated first with plans to address the other side in follow-up. The contralateral side is not repositioned during the initial visit given the theoretical risk of re-displacing the canaliths on the initially treated side.

Overall, repositioning maneuvers have very few associated side effects. The most frequent sequela is nausea, which is found in 16.7–32% of the cases [19]. In susceptible patients, prophylactic anti-emetics and or vestibular suppressants may be necessary. During repositioning for posterior canal BPPV, canaliths may be displaced from the posterior canal into the horizontal canal. This is termed canal conversion and occurs in less than 5% of the cases [29]. In the event of canal conversion, appropriate treatment of horizontal canal BPPV should ensue. Lastly, clinicians should be mindful of patients with vascular disease or C-spine disorders, as the diagnostic maneuvers and treatments have the potential, albeit very rarely, to cause injury to the vertebral arteries or C-spine structures, respectively [30].

In instances of multiple failed repositioning maneuvers, a tertiary center referral should be considered [6]. Recently developed repositioning chairs including the Epley Omniax rotator and the TRV hold great promise for refractory cases, multi-canal involvement, or patients with high-risk necks [31]. Because of high cost, they will be limited to tertiary care centers. In the event of refractory disease, surgical intervention may be considered.

Surgery

BPPV is highly amenable to repositioning maneuvers. As such, operative intervention is reserved for intractable cases or patients with severe and frequent recurrences that significantly impact the quality of life. Overall, less than 1% of BPPV patients require surgical intervention [32]. Aside from sporadic cases reports and small series of canal occlusion for horizontal or superior canal BPPV, virtually all surgical interventions have been for intractable posterior canal BPPV.

Given the associated operative risk for this "benign" disorder, preoperative planning is critical. Surgeons should precisely confirm the affected canal and its side. Preoperative testing should include audiometry, given the possible complication of hearing loss from inner ear surgery. Vestibular testing including videonystagmography (VNG), video head impulse testing (vHIT), and/or vestibular-evoked myogenic potentials (VEMP) is encouraged to establish baseline function in the operative ear and ensure normal vestibular function in the contralateral ear. Imaging with CT and or MRI should also be arranged for surgical planning and to rule out central lesions that may mimic BPPV.

Singular Neurectomy

The singular neurectomy for posterior canal BPPV was popularized by Gacek and involves transection of the posterior ampullary nerve within the singular canal [33]. To gain access to the singular canal, the surgeon begins with the exposure of the round window through a trans-canal approach. Some of the posterior canal wall and the bony overhang of the round window niche are drilled to expose the entire round window membrane. The singular canal lies 1–2 mm below the posterior–inferior margin of the round window membrane. After the singular nerve is exposed in its canal, it can be transected with a pick or small right-angled hook. The neurectomy removes the resting input from the affected posterior canal ampulla, creating both a dynamic and static vestibular asymmetry. Over time, compensation occurs by central adaptation that can be expedited by VRT.

Large case series of singular neurectomy showed favorable success in complete resolution of vertigo between 80% and 97% [34, 35]. However, with the necessary surgical exposure placing the vestibule at risk, singular neurectomy carries a significant risk of sensorineural hearing loss (SNHL). Smaller series reported complication rates of SNHL at 12%, 29%, and 41% of cases among 8, 7, and 12 neurectomies, respectively [36–38]. By comparison, Gacek's updated series of 252 neurectomies reported the rate of SNHL at 3.7% [34]. Therefore, surgeon's experience is crucial to the success of this technically challenging procedure.

Posterior Semicircular Canal Occlusion

Posterior semicircular canal occlusion was first introduced by Parnes and McClure in 1990 as a treatment for intractable BPPV [39]. They proposed that occluding the canal would render the cupula unresponsive to any kind of stimulation, be it from natural head movements or gravitational pull on the canaliths/cupuliths. While this creates a dynamic vestibular asymmetry, central adaption relieves the initial postoperative imbalance over time.

Exposure of the posterior semicircular canal is done through a standard postauricular incision and limited mastoidectomy [40] (Fig. 14.3). Following the identification of the posterior canal otic capsule, the bone is blue-lined. After that, a 1-mm

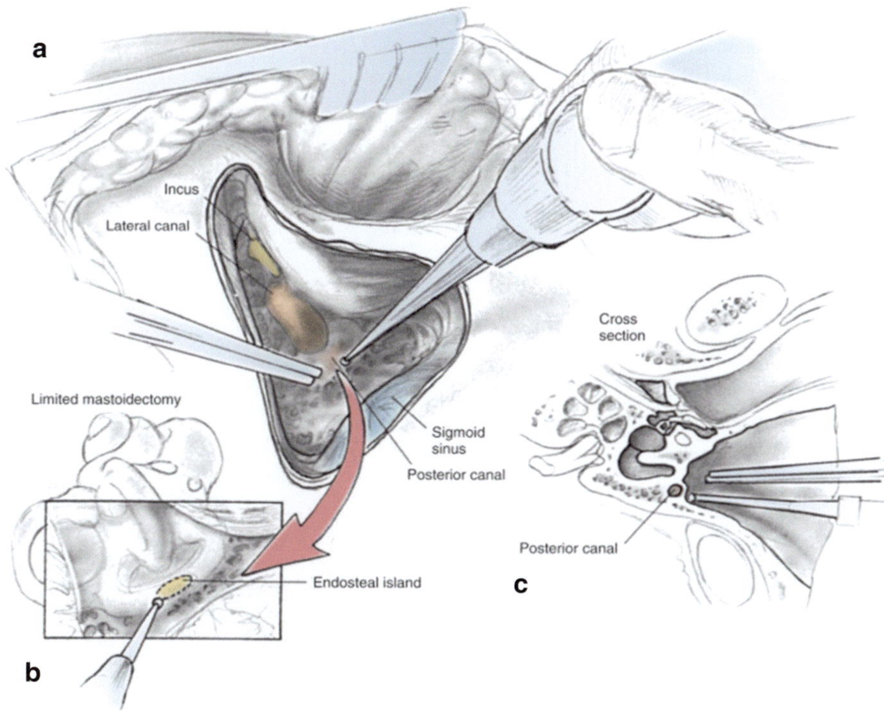

Fig. 14.3 Surgical exposure of posterior semicircular canal. (**a**) Exposure of posterior semicircular canal otic capsule using limited mastoidectomy. (**b**) Creating 1×3 mm endosteal island with a small diamond burr. C, cross-section view. (Reproduced with permission. This figure was published in Otologic Surgery 4th edition by Brackmann, Shelton, and Arriaga, in chapter: "Transmastoid semicircular canal occlusion for benign paroxysmal positional vertigo and other disorders," Page 408–416, Copyright Elsevier (2015) [40])

diamond burr is used to create a 1 by 3 mm endosteal island. The endosteal island is removed using a fine 90-degree pick, revealing the perilymph (Fig. 14.4). The perilymph can then be wicked away to expose the membranous labyrinth. A variety of material can be used for canal plugging including bone dust, or fascia. The option preferred by the originator of this technique is to fashion the plug from dry mastoid cortex bone chips mixed with fibrinogen sealant (Fig. 14.5). The plug is inserted through the fenestra with the intention of occluding the canal lumen and collapsing the membranous labyrinth (Fig. 14.6). A blunt 45-degree probe can then be used to pack the plug tightly in the canal. Afterwards, the fenestra and surrounding bone are covered with temporalis fascia and more fibrinogen glue to prevent postoperative a perilymph fistula (Fig. 14.7). With time, the bone chips within the canal ossify resulting in a permanent occlusion of the canal.

Initial experience of Parnes and McClure and subsequent case series found posterior semicircular canal occlusion to be effective in abolishing BPPV while preserving hearing [41]. Furthermore, canal occlusion is not limited to the

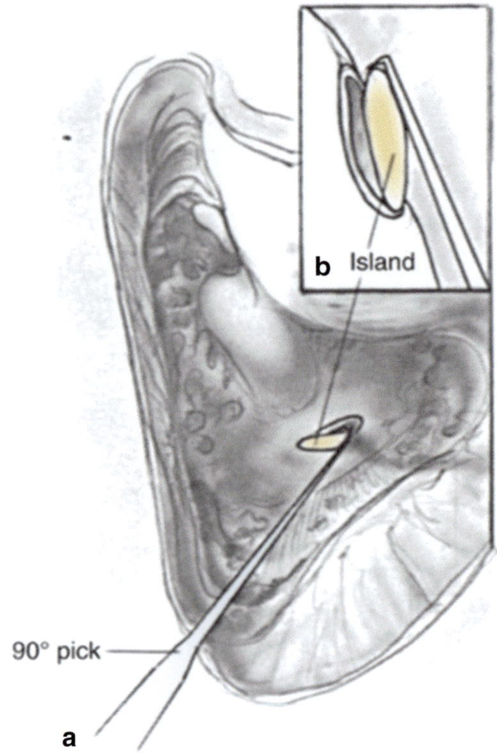

Fig. 14.4 (**a**) Lifting out the endosteal island with a fine 90-degree pick. (**b**) Magnified lateral view. (Reproduced with permission. This figure was published in Otologic Surgery 4th edition by Brackmann, Shelton, and Arriaga, in chapter: "Transmastoid semicircular canal occlusion for benign paroxysmal positional vertigo and other disorders," Page 408–416, Copyright Elsevier (2015) [40])

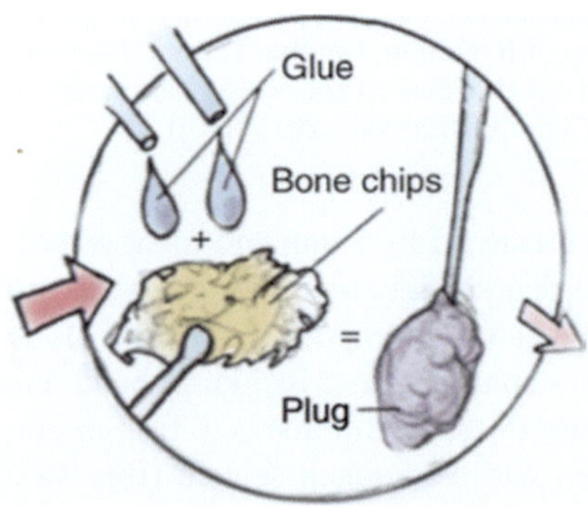

Fig. 14.5 Creating a plug with two-component fibrinogen glue and mastoid cortex bone chips. (Reproduced with permission. This figure was published in Otologic Surgery 4th edition by Brackmann, Shelton, and Arriaga, in chapter: "Transmastoid semicircular canal occlusion for benign paroxysmal positional vertigo and other disorders," Page 408–416, Copyright Elsevier (2015) [40])

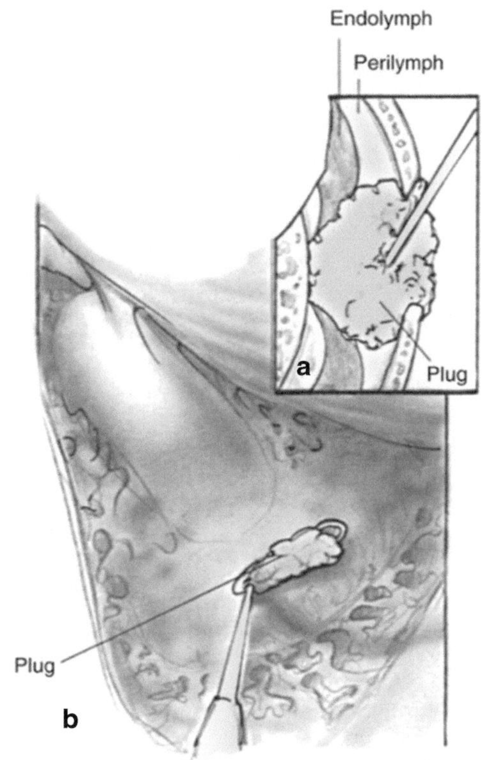

Fig. 14.6 (**a**) Tamping plug through the fenestra into the canal. (**b**) A cross section of the canal shows the intact but occluded membranous canal. (Reproduced with permission. This figure was published in Otologic Surgery 4th edition by Brackmann, Shelton, and Arriaga, in chapter: "Transmastoid semicircular canal occlusion for benign paroxysmal positional vertigo and other disorders," Page 408–416, Copyright Elsevier (2015) [40])

posterior semicircular canal as authors have reported cases of successful horizontal and anterior semicircular occlusion for treating the corresponding canal's intractable BPPV [42, 43]. Other variations include the use of argon laser for blue-lining the posterior canal or CO2 laser to produce canal fibrous occlusions [40]. Compared to singular neurectomy, this surgical approach carries fewer risks and less technical challenges. Of 74 posterior canal occlusions, Parnes and Agrawal showed only one case with a significant postoperative sensorineural hearing loss, which occurred three months postoperatively and was believed to be a result of labyrinthitis. This patient had also undergone two prior unsuccessful singular neurectomies in the same ear [40].

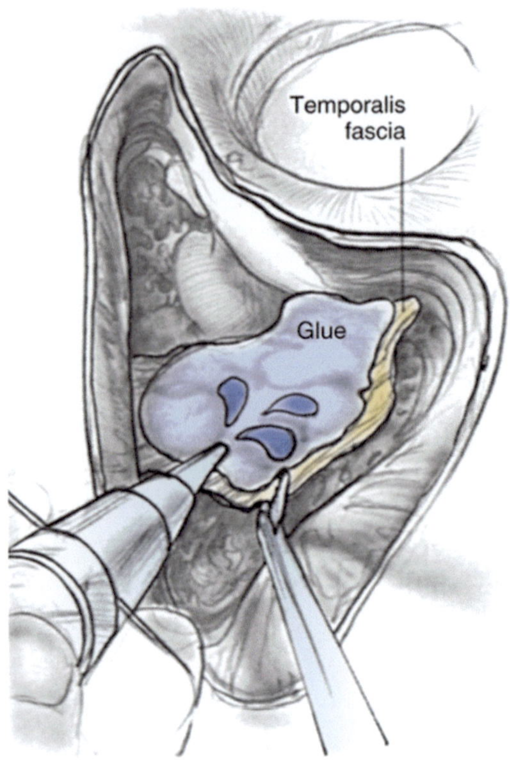

Fig. 14.7 Covering the fenestra and surrounding bone with fascia and glue. (Reproduced with permission. This figure was published in Otologic Surgery 4th edition by Brackmann, Shelton, and Arriaga, in chapter: "Transmastoid semicircular canal occlusion for benign paroxysmal positional vertigo and other disorders," Page 408–416, Copyright Elsevier (2015) [40])

References

1. Barany R. Diagnose von Krankheitserscheinungen im Bereiche des Otolithenapparatus. Acta Otolaryngol Stockh. 1921:434–7.
2. Dix MR, Hallpike CS. The pathology symptomatology and diagnosis of certain common disorders of the vestibular system. Proc R Soc Med. 1952;45:341–54.
3. Hanley K, O'Dowd T, Considine N. A systematic review of vertigo in primary care. Br J Gen Pract. 2001;51:666–71.
4. Parnes LS, Agrawal SK, Atlas J. Diagnosis and management of benign paroxysmal positional vertigo (BPPV). CMAJ. 2003;169:681–93.
5. Kim J-S, Zee DS. Clinical practice. Benign paroxysmal positional vertigo. N Engl J Med. 2014;370:1138–47.
6. Bhattacharyya N, Gubbels SP, Schwartz SR, et al. Clinical practice guideline: benign paroxysmal positional vertigo (update). Otolaryngol Head Neck Surg. 2017;156:S1–S47.
7. Fife D, FitzGerald JE. Do patients with benign paroxysmal positional vertigo receive prompt treatment? Analysis of waiting times and human and financial costs associated with current practice. Int J Audiol. 2005;44:50–7.
8. Oghalai JS, Manolidis S, Barth JL, Stewart MG, Jenkins HA. Unrecognized benign paroxysmal positional vertigo in elderly patients. Otolaryngol Head Neck Surg. 2000;122:630–4.
9. von Brevern M, Lezius F, Tiel-Wilck K, Radtke A, Lempert T. Benign paroxysmal positional vertigo: current status of medical management. Otolaryngol Head Neck Surg. 2004;130:381–2.
10. Parnes LS, McClure JA. Free-floating endolymph particles: a new operative finding during posterior semicircular canal occlusion. 1992. Laryngoscope. 2015;125:1033.

11. Kao WTK, Parnes LS, Chole RA. Otoconia and otolithic membrane fragments within the posterior semicircular canal in benign paroxysmal positional vertigo. Laryngoscope. 2016;90:709–14.
12. Lynn S, Pool A, Rose D, Brey R, Suman V. Randomized trial of the canalith repositioning procedure. Otolaryngol Head Neck Surg. 1995;113:712–20.
13. Soto Varela A, Bartual Magro J, Santos Pérez S, Vélez Regueiro M, Lechuga García R, Pérez-Carro Ríos A, Caballero L. Benign paroxysmal vertigo: a comparative prospective study of the efficacy of Brandt and Daroff exercises, Semont and Epley maneuver. Rev Laryngol Otol Rhinol (Bord). 2001;122:179–83.
14. Sundararajan I, Rangachari V, Sumathi V, Kumar K. Epley's manoeuvre versus Epley's manoeuvre plus labyrinthine sedative as management of benign paroxysmal positional vertigo: prospective , randomised study. J Laryngol Otol. 2011;125:572–5.
15. Semont A, Freyss G, Vitte E. Curing the BPPV with a liberatory maneuver. Adv Otorhinolaryngol. 1988;42:290–3.
16. Chen Y, Zhuang J, Zhang L, Li Y, Jin Z, Zhao Z, Zhao Y, Zhou H. Short-term efficacy of Semont maneuver for benign paroxysmal positional vertigo: a double-blind randomized trial. Otol Neurotol. 2012;33:1127–30.
17. Haynes DS, Resser JR, Labadie RF, Girasole CR, Kovach BT, Scheker LE, Walker DC. Treatment of benign positional vertigo using the semont maneuver: efficacy in patients presenting without nystagmus. Laryngoscope. 2002;112:796–801.
18. White J, Savvides P, Cherian N, Oas J. Canalith repositioning for benign paroxysmal positional vertigo. Otol Neurotol. 2005;26:704–10.
19. Hilton M, Pinder D. The Epley manoeuvre for benign paroxysmal positional vertigo. Cochrane Database Syst Rev. 2014:1–38.
20. Devaiah AK, Andreoli S. Postmaneuver restrictions in benign paroxysmal positional vertigo: an individual patient data meta-analysis. Otolaryngol Head Neck Surg. 2010;142:155–9.
21. Sargent EW, Bankaitis a E, Hollenbeak CS, Currens JW. Mastoid oscillation in canalith repositioning for paroxysmal positional vertigo. Otol Neurotol. 2001;22:205–9.
22. Tirelli G, D'Orlando E, Giacomarra V, Russolo M. Benign positional vertigo without detectable nystagmus. Laryngoscope. 2001;111:1053–6.
23. Lempert T, Tiel-Wilck K. A positional maneuver for treatment of horizontal-canal benign positional vertigo. Laryngoscope. 1996;106:476–8.
24. Ciniglio Appiani G, Catania G, Gagliardi M. A liberatory maneuver for the treatment of horizontal canal paroxysmal positional vertigo. Otol Neurotol. 2001;22:66–9.
25. Kim JS, Oh S-Y, Lee S-H, Kang JH, Kim DU, Jeong S-H, Choi K-D, Moon IS, Kim BK, Kim HJ. Randomized clinical trial for geotropic horizontal canal benign paroxysmal positional vertigo. Neurology. 2012;79:700–7.
26. Vannucchi P, Giannoni B, Pagnini P. Treatment of horizontal semicircular canal benign paroxysmal positional vertigo. J Vestib Res. 1997;7:1–6.
27. Korres S, Riga MG, Xenellis J, Korres GS, Danielides V. Treatment of the horizontal semicircular canal canalithiasis: pros and cons of the repositioning maneuvers in a clinical study and critical review of the literature. Otol Neurotol. 2011;32:1302–8.
28. Anagnostou E, Kouzi I, Spengos K. Diagnosis and treatment of Anterior-Canal benign paroxysmal positional vertigo: a systematic review. J Clin Neurol. 2015;11:262–7.
29. Herdman SJ, Tusa RJ. Complications of the canalith repositioning procedure. Arch Otolaryngol Head Neck Surg. 1996;122:281–6.
30. Bergin M, Bird P, Wright A. Internal carotid artery dissection following canalith repositioning procedure. J Laryngol Otol. 2010;124:575–6.
31. West N, Hansen S, Møller MN, Bloch SL, Klokker M. Repositioning chairs in benign paroxysmal positional vertigo: implications and clinical outcome. Eur Arch Otorrinolaringol. 2016;273:573–80.
32. Shaia WT, Zappia JJ, Bojrag DI, LaRouere ML, Sargent EW, Diaz RC. Success of posterior semicircular canal occlusion and application of the dizziness handicap inventory. Otolaryngol Head Neck Surg. 2006;134:424–30.

33. Gacek RR. Transection of the posterior ampullary nerve for the relief of benign paroxysmal positional vertigo. Ann Otol Rhinol Laryngol. 1974;83:596–605.
34. Gacek RR, Gacek MR. Results of singular neurectomy in the posterior ampullary recess. ORL J Otorhinolaryngol Relat Spec. 2002;64:397–402.
35. Silverstein H, White DW. Wide surgical exposure for singular Neurectomy in the treatment of benign positional vertigo. Laryngoscope. 1990;100:701–6.
36. Pournaras I, Kos I, Guyot J-P. Benign paroxysmal positional vertigo: a series of eight singular neurectomies. Acta Otolaryngol. 2008;128:5–8.
37. Fernandes CM. Singular neurectomy in South African practice. S Afr J Surg. 1993;31:79–80.
38. Epley JM. singular neurectomy: hypotympanotomy approach. Otolaryngol Head Neck Surg (1979). 1980;88:304–9.
39. Parnes LS, McClure JA. Posterior semicircular canal occlusion for intractable benign paroxysmal positional vertigo. Ann Otol Rhinol Laryngol. 1990;99:330–4.
40. Parnes LS, Agrawal SK. Transmastoid semicircular canal occlusion for benign paroxysmal positional vertigo and other disorders. In: Brackmann D, Clough S, Arriag M, editors. Otologic surgery. 4th ed. Elsevier Health Sciences; 2015. p. 408–16.
41. Agrawal SK, Parnes LS. Human experience with canal plugging. Ann N Y Acad Sci. 2001;942:300–5.
42. Zhu Q, Liu C, Lin C, Chen X, Liu T, Lin S, Fan J. Efficacy and safety of semicircular canal occlusion for intractable horizontal semicircular benign paroxysmal positional vertigo. Ann Otol Rhinol Laryngol. 2015;124:257–60.
43. Brantberg K, Bergenius J. Treatment of anterior benign paroxysmal positional vertigo by canal plugging: a case report. Acta Otolaryngol. 2002;122:28–30.

Chapter 15
Pathophysiology and Diagnosis of Meniere's Disease

Alexander L. Luryi, Elliot Morse, and Elias Michaelides

Introduction

In 1861, Prosper Meniere described a disease that consisted of episodic vertigo and fluctuating hearing loss. He hypothesized that the disease arose from the inner ear peripheral end organ. Over the following century, knowledge of the mechanics of the inner ear was refined, and consensus gradually built that endolymphatic hydrops was likely causative of Meniere's disease (MD) [1]. MD has been estimated to affect between 10 and 150 out of every 100,000 individuals, although the true prevalence is difficult to determine due to variable diagnostic criteria. It typically presents between ages 35 and 60 and occurs slightly more frequently in females [2]. This chapter discusses the underlying pathophysiology, clinical features, and diagnosis of MD.

[Alexander L. Luryi] has died before the publication of this book.

A. L. Luryi (Deceased)
Camden, NJ, USA

E. Morse
Department of Surgery, Yale University School of Medicine, New Haven, CT, USA
e-mail: elliot.morse@yale.edu

E. Michaelides (✉)
Department of Otolaryngology, Rush University College of Medicine, Chicago, IL, USA
e-mail: elias_michaelides@rush.edu

J. C. Lucas et al. (eds.), *Diagnosis and Treatment of Vestibular Disorders*,
https://doi.org/10.1007/978-3-032-11740-3_15

Clinical Features

Clinical Presentation

Classically, MD consists of a triad of recurrent vertigo, tinnitus, and sensorineural hearing loss, usually accompanied by aural fullness. As there is no definitive test for MD, the diagnosis is primarily clinical and requires a thorough history and physical examination. The American Academy of Otolaryngology-Head and Neck Surgery (AAO-HNS) diagnostic guidelines historically included categories of "certain," "definite," "probable," and "possible" Meniere's disease dependent on the presence of certain clinical features and test results. The 2015 update of the guidelines, shown in Table 15.1, simplified these into "definite" and "probable" MD based only on history, physical examination, and pure tone audiometry [3].

Although definite Meniere's disease is not diagnosed until both cochlear and vestibular symptoms manifest, patients often initially present with episodic hearing loss or vertigo alone [4, 5]. Most patients have unilateral disease, although approximately 25–35% develop contralateral symptoms during their disease course [6–9]. Longitudinal studies have shown that the incidence of bilateral disease is higher in patients with a family history of MD and earlier disease onset [7]. Simultaneous onset of bilateral disease is uncommon and occurs in approximately 1% of cases.

Even in patients with clinically unilateral disease, some degree of sensorineural hearing loss is frequently detected in the contralateral ear, suggestive of subclinical bilateral disease [4]. Additional testing, including auditory brain stem responses and electrocochleography, has revealed bilateral involvement in up to 50% of patients [10]. This becomes significant as bilateral disease can affect surgical treatment algorithms (see Chap. 15).

Vertigo

The frequency of vertigo attacks varies significantly between patients, ranging from 1–2 attacks per year to nearly continuous vertigo. These attacks are described as spinning or motion sensations and are usually not positional in nature. While

Table 15.1 2015 AAO-HNS guidelines for diagnosis of Meniere's disease

Definite	1. Two or more spontaneous episodes of vertigo, each lasting 20 min–12 hours 2. Audiometrically documented low- to mid-frequency sensorineural hearing loss in one ear, defining the affected ear, on at least one occasion before, during, or after one of the episodes of vertigo 3. Fluctuating aural symptoms (hearing, tinnitus, or fullness) in the affected ear 4. Not better accounted for by another vestibular diagnosis
Probable	1. Two or more spontaneous episodes of vertigo or dizziness, each lasting 20 min–24 hours 2. Fluctuating aural symptoms (hearing, tinnitus, or fullness) in the affected ear 3. Not better accounted for by another vestibular diagnosis

diagnostic guidelines allow a wide range of attack durations, attacks usually last between 1 and 4 hours, and most patients rate their attacks as moderate in severity. With follow-up over ten years, vertiginous symptoms resolve to some degree in the majority of patients, with approximately half reporting complete resolution [11, 12]. In patients in whom vertigo persists, there does not appear to be any association between disease duration and attack duration, frequency, or intensity, although findings vary [7].

Hearing Loss

MD typically causes a low-frequency sensorineural hearing loss. In the early stages of the disease, hearing may recover between attacks, but permanent deficits are seen with disease progression. Fourteen years after diagnosis, approximately 50% of patients have completely absent hearing in the affected ear [13]. Audiometric findings will be discussed later in this chapter (see section "Diagnosis").

Tinnitus

Most MD patients experience tinnitus. In the early stages of disease tinnitus occurs primarily with vertiginous episodes, becoming more intense immediately before attacks. Over time, tinnitus becomes persistent even between attacks, mirroring the development of hearing loss. Tinnitus in MD is typically low-frequency (125–250 Hz), matching hearing loss, and is described as "roaring" or "ringing" [14].

Other Symptoms

Most MD patients also report aural fullness in the affected side. Patients may describe a feeling of "pressure" or a "clogged sensation" in the ear. This sensation is typically rated as moderate to severe and usually peaks in intensity immediately prior to attacks [15]. Aural fullness usually does not resolve over time [11].

Many patients also report some degree of audiologic distortion during attacks. In particular, MD patients often report binaural pitch diplacusis, most commonly affecting lower frequency tones. This is attributed to asymmetric hearing loss in these patients [16–18].

Drop attacks (otolithic crises of Tumarkin) are infrequent but potentially dangerous events in MD, reported in approximately 5% of patients [19–21]. During attacks, patients experience a sudden loss of balance often likened to the sensation of being pushed, resulting in a fall without loss of consciousness [22]. These attacks usually occur later in the course of disease. The number of attacks experienced by patients ranges widely from 1 to greater than 10, and most often occur within one year of each other, with subsequent spontaneous remission [19, 20, 22, 23].

Variants

AAO-HNS guidelines previously defined variations of MD for patients presenting with isolated cochlear or vestibular symptoms. A significant proportion of these patients eventually progress to definite MD [24]. Some evidence exists that these isolated cochlear and vestibular symptoms are associated with EH isolated to the respective labyrinth organ [25]. Data on these atypical variants are sparse, and they are not included in current diagnostic guidelines [3].

Pathophysiology of Meniere's Disease

MD is associated with the overaccumulation of endolymph in the scala media, known as endolymphatic hydrops (EH) [26]. Evidence of this association is abundant, and most authors further believe that EH causes MD. However, many theories exist regarding the etiology of EH as well as the mechanisms through which EH causes the clinical features of MD.

Temporal Bone and Anatomic Studies

In the 1930s, Hallpike and Yamakawa independently reported EH in the temporal bones of MD patients [27, 28]. In addition to gross dilation of the endolymphatic system and obliteration of perilymph spaces, certain characteristic changes in temporal bone morphology and histology were found. These findings were confirmed by multiple groups in the following decades, and the gross and microscopic features of the temporal bone in MD are now well-known. Gross findings include abnormally small size of the endolymphatic duct and sac, decreased mastoid and petrous pneumatization, anteromedial displacement of the sigmoid sinus, and frequent jugular bulb abnormalities, including high-riding jugular bulbs and diverticula [29–33]. Three-dimensional modeling of the endolymphatic drainage system further reveals decreased volume and a reduced external aperture of the vestibular aqueduct. Approximately half of specimens exhibit an abnormal, constitutively open utriculo-endolymphatic valve [34].

Microscopic inner ear changes associated with MD are also well-characterized. These include dilation of the scala media of the cochlea with partial obliteration of the scala vestibuli by Reissner's membrane (Fig. 15.1), degeneration of the organ of

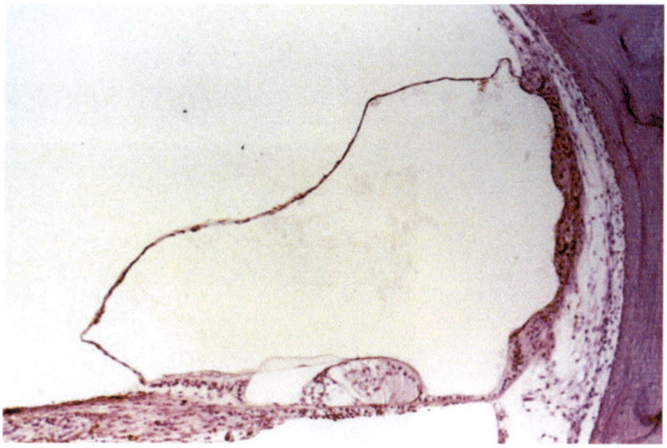

Fig. 15.1 Cochlear histopathology in a patient with MD. Reissner's membrane shows marked distension without significant changes in the organ of Corti. (Adapted with permission from Nomura, 2013 [178])

Corti, hypoplasia of the endolymphatic duct and sac, decreased afferent synapses and nerve endings to inner and outer hair cells, and decreased vascularity of the stria vascularis [35–38]. Dilation of the scala media affects the pars inferior more than the pars superior and the cochlear apex more than the base. Overall number of hair cells is usually conserved [39].

Imaging of MD was first accomplished in 2007 using trans-tympanic injection of gadolinium contrast, allowing visualization of obliterated perilymph spaces [40]. Further advances allowed for similar visualization using intravenous contrast (Fig. 15.2), although with lower intensity [41]. High-resolution magnetic resonance imaging (MRI) has revealed the nearly ubiquitous presence of EH in patients with MD with a strong correlation between degree of hydrops and severity of auditory and vestibular symptoms [42]. The integrity of the blood-labyrinth barrier was also found to deteriorate with increasing severity of EH, allowing higher concentrations of intravenous contrast in perilymph [43].

Temporal bone and imaging studies have shown that virtually all patients with MD exhibit EH [44–46]. However, the converse is not true, and EH is not uncommon in asymptomatic individuals. While this has led some authors to argue that EH is merely a marker of MD, data supporting a causative relationship is compelling. Most experts currently believe that EH is necessary but not sufficient for the development of MD.

Evidence that EH Causes MD

Animal models provide insight into the relationship between EH and MD. Surgical obliteration of the endolymphatic sac in guinea pigs (Fig. 15.3) yielded the first animal model for EH in the 1960s [47]. Similar models were created in the following decades with injected antigen-induced immune destruction of the endolymphatic sac or exogenous aldosterone-induced endolymph overproduction [48–50]. Following these interventions, guinea pigs developed a predominantly

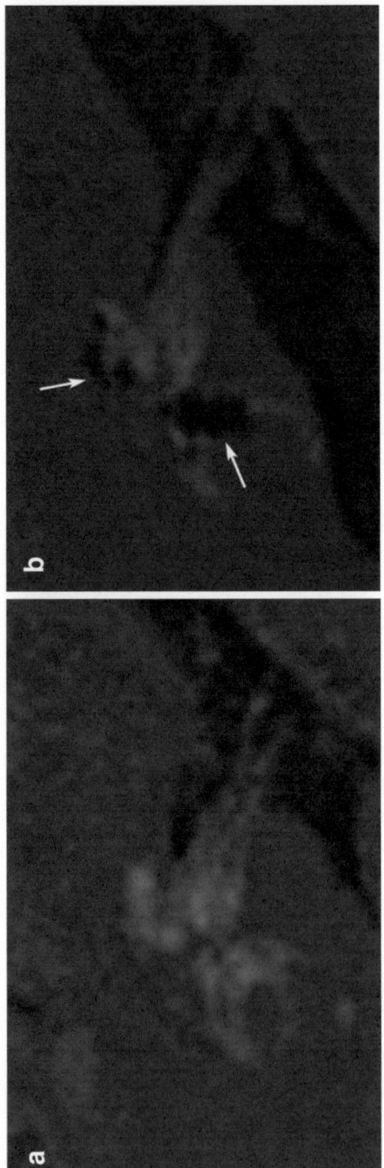

Fig. 15.2 T2-weighted 3D-FLAIR images with gadolinium with hybrid subtraction technique. (**a**) Normal inner ear with enhancement of perilymphatic space. (**b**) Meniere's disease with endolymphatic hydrops and partial obliteration of perilymph spaces (arrows). (Adapted with permission from Nomura, 2013 [178])

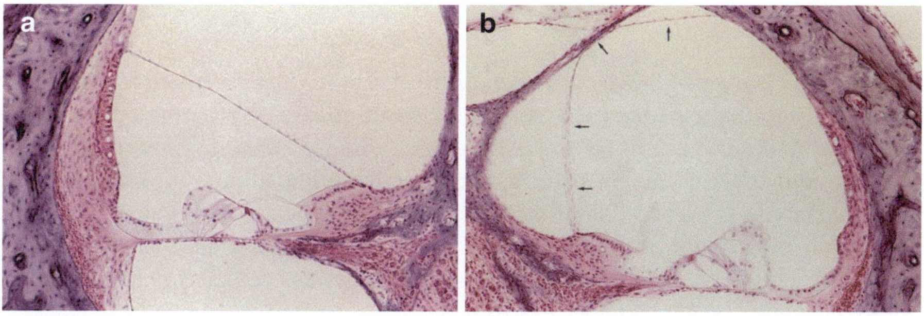

Fig. 15.3 Obliteration of the endolymphatic duct in the guinea pig. (**a**) Normal structure of guinea pig cochlea. (**b**) Marked distention of Reissner's membrane (arrows) into the perilymphatic space. (Adapted with permission from Nomura, 2013 [178])

low-frequency hearing loss and were found to have increased apoptosis and degeneration of the spiral ligament and stria vascularis [49, 51]. Interestingly, vertigo was absent in these animals. These early models demonstrated that the induction of EH alone resulted in inner ear dysfunction similar to what is seen in MD.

Recently developed mouse models resemble the pathologic state of MD more closely. Mice containing a germline mutation of the *Phex* gene causing X-linked hypophosphatemic rickets were found to develop EH in adulthood [52]. These mice also developed a predictable loss of hearing and vestibular function. Pathologic examination was consistent with MD, with spiral ganglion cell loss in the setting of preserved hair cells and a patent endolymphatic duct [53]. In addition, the *Phex* mouse validated the electrocochleography and vestibular-evoked myogenic potential findings in MD, which will be discussed later in this chapter [54].

The actions of diuretic medications also support a causative relationship between EH and MD. MD symptoms improve with acetazolamide, a diuretic and carbonic anhydrase inhibitor, which is thought to reduce endolymph volume by inhibiting the release of aqueous HCO_3^- into the endolymphatic space [55, 56]. Likewise, glycerol, an osmotic diuretic, temporarily improves hearing in early MD [57]. Thiazide diuretics, whose action is specific to the kidney, do not have as clear an effect on EH [58]. They are used to treat MD based on results from several small studies, and their benefit may be due to whole-body fluid shifts [59].

Etiology of Hydrops

The etiology of EH in MD is likely multifactorial. Many mechanisms have been proposed, including genetic, infectious, traumatic, mechanical, autoimmune, allergic, and vascular etiologies. None is capable of explaining all of the pathologic and clinical findings in MD, and findings in support of each have been conflicting.

Genetic

Familial MD is a well-known entity which affects approximately 5% of MD patients [60, 61]. These patients tend to have earlier onset of disease (fourth decade rather than fifth) and are more likely to have bilateral disease. Transmission usually follows an autosomal dominant pattern, and genetic anticipation is typical [60, 62]. However, some evidence suggests MD may have a genetic component beyond Mendelian inheritance in familial cases. For example, prevalence of MD varies widely by ethnicity, with significantly more Caucasians affected than people of Asian, Hispanic, or African ancestry [63].

A number of genes have been studied and may have a role in the pathogenesis of MD based on limited data. Examples include KCNE1 and KCNE3 [64–66], COCH [67, 68], FAM136A [69], certain major histocompatibility complex (MHC) genes [70, 71], and genes coding for aquaporin proteins [72–74]. However, no specific mutations have been conclusively identified to lead to MD, even in known familial cases [71].

Aquaporin proteins are of special interest due to their potential direct relationship with fluid shifts in the inner ear. The expression of aquaporin 2 is mediated by vasopressin, which has been associated with MD in multiple studies. Plasma vasopressin levels are elevated in MD and are even higher during MD attacks [75, 76]. High serum concentrations of vasopressin are known to worsen MD symptoms [72, 77], and lifestyle modifications to reduce vasopressin (increasing water intake, sleeping in total darkness, etc.) improve symptoms [78]. Furthermore, vasopressin has been shown to induce EH at concentrations similar to those observed during MD attacks [79]. These data, combined with the facts that MD symptoms respond to diuretic medications and that ion channel defects have been implicated in congenital deafness, suggest that a channelopathy may underlie the development of MD [55, 58, 80, 81].

Infectious

Multiple viral infections have been implicated in MD; however, conclusive evidence is lacking. In situ hybridization studies have revealed DNA from multiple herpesviruses in the endolymphatic sac, including varicella zoster virus (VZV), Epstein-Barr virus (EBV), and cytomegalovirus (CMV) [82]. While herpes simplex viruses 1 and 2 (HSV1 and HSV2) were not detected, one study revealed a higher rate of HSV1 and HSV2 DNA in singular nerve specimens from patients with MD compared with the general population, although this is an inconsistent finding [83, 84].

In prior decades, syphilis was thought to be the cause of MD in at least 5% of cases [85]. However, reported MD attributed to syphilis exhibited several distinct clinical features, including responsiveness to steroid therapy and early reduction of caloric responses [86]. Endolymphatic hydrops seen in otosyphilis was thought to be due to osteitic changes surrounding the endolymphatic duct, although recent temporal bone analyses do not support this theory [87]. While otosyphilis can produce a Meniere's-like syndrome, the vast majority of cases of MD are unrelated to syphilis, and the existence of a common pathogenic pathway is questionable.

Likewise, MD was historically theorized to occur as a consequence of severe acute or chronic otitis media [88]. The evidence for this was mostly anecdotal with several case series of patients who developed MD following middle ear infection. More recent data has not supported any relationship between otitis media and MD [89].

Autoimmune and Allergic

Autoimmunity is thought to account for between 5% and 30% of cases of MD [90, 91]. These patients are more likely to present with severe, bilateral disease. An autoimmune etiology for MD has been postulated since the 1980s, when a subset of MD patients was shown to have certain immunologic abnormalities [92]. A significantly increased prevalence of autoimmune [93] and allergic conditions [94, 95] has been documented in the MD population, and adequate medical control of allergies has been shown to improve symptoms of MD [96]. In conjunction with the possible association between MD and MHC genes, these trends have led some authors to believe in a significant if not dominant immunologic etiology for MD.

Immunologic evidence for an autoimmune etiology in MD is abundant but not conclusive. The endolymphatic sac is regarded as the site of immune function in the inner ear, and inflammatory cytokines have been reported in the endolymph [97, 98]. Patients with MD exhibit increased levels of autoantibodies and circulating antigen-antibody complexes [99, 100]. Their serum has been shown to react with unknown autoantigens, some of which are expressed in the inner ear [101, 102]. Small studies have revealed antibodies to type II collagen in patients with MD, and exogenous type II collagen administration has been shown to induce EH with spiral ganglion degeneration in animal models [103, 104]. Elevated antiphospholipid antibodies have also been described in MD [105].

Despite these data, no specific antigen or antibody has been detected in any significant sub-population of patients with MD [106]. Studies which have detected antibodies, HLA subtypes, or MHC polymorphisms associated with MD patients have been conflicting. While it does appear that the immune system may play a role in the pathogenesis of MD, further study, perhaps on a population level, is necessary to elucidate this.

Vasospastic/Vascular

MD is strongly associated with migraine, and the two conditions may share a common pathophysiology [107–111]. Since migraines are thought to be associated with cerebral vasospasm, vasospasm may play a role in MD as well [107, 112]. The stria vascularis is rapidly susceptible to ischemia, immediately resulting in loss of cochlear potential and eventually to strial atrophy [113]. One theory states that in patients with EH, the inner ear's venous outflow resistance is elevated, rendering cochlear structures, specifically the stria vascularis, additionally susceptible to vasospasm-mediated ischemia as well as to other vasculopathic processes, including atherosclerosis, vasculitis, or hyperviscosity [112]. In this model, MD attacks are caused by acute ischemia, and cumulative ischemic damage and reperfusion injury eventually lead to stromal atrophy and permanent cochlear and vestibular dysfunction.

Mechanical

Dislodged utricular otoconia have been established as the cause of vertigo in benign paroxysmal positional vertigo (BPPV). BPPV is common in patients with MD, and the same ear is usually affected, leading some authors to speculate about a relationship between the two conditions [114–116]. Dislodgement of saccular otoconia has been theorized to obstruct the endolymph drainage pathway, leading to EH. Three-dimensional CT imaging of patients with MD reveals loss of continuity and obliteration of the ductus reuniens, saccular duct, and endolymphatic sinus in the affected ear only, consistent with otoconial deposits [117]. Patients with MD also have increased otoconial deposits in the semicircular canals compared with age-matched controls [118]. The reported success of alternating middle ear pressure therapy in MD also supports this theory, as this may help move otoconia back to the vestibule [119]. However, otoconial obstruction of the endolymph drainage system has never been demonstrated in patients with MD, and this remains an area of active study. Trauma is thought to cause secondary EH via deposition of otoconial and other debris into the endolymph; however, evidence for a traumatic etiology for true MD is lacking [120, 121].

Pathophysiology of Symptoms in MD

Acute Symptoms

MD attacks were traditionally believed to be triggered by sudden increases in endolymphatic pressure, resulting in rupture of Reissner's membrane and endolymphatic potassium excitotoxicity [122]. This was thought to lead to loss of the endolymphatic ion gradient and cause global labyrinthine dysfunction [51]. However, in vivo studies have shown Reissner's membrane rupture to have only minor effects on endocochlear potential and to cause nystagmus inconsistent with that of MD attacks [123, 124]. While the membrane rupture theory is no longer believed, the true pathophysiology underlying symptoms in MD remains unknown. Vasospasm-mediated ischemia or otoconial obstruction of endolymph drainage may play a role (see section "Etiology of Hydrops").

One theory of MD attacks purports that excess endolymph which was stored in the apical cochlea forces open the utriculo-endolymphatic valve due to high pressures and an obstructed endolymphatic duct, resulting in fluid entry into the vestibule [125]. This causes severe vertigo, while hearing loss results from the accompanying cochlear fluid shifts. A similar mechanism has been proposed for drop attacks, which may occur when these sudden changes in endolymphatic fluid dynamics cause cochlear and vestibular end organ stimulation [126]. Alternatively, vestibular evoked myogenic potential (VEMP) testing suggests that drop attacks may be caused by damaged and unstable otolithic organs (see section "Diagnosis") [127].

Chronic Symptoms

Long-term damage to inner ear structures in MD appears to be mediated by oxidative stress. Nitric oxide (NO), generated by nitric oxide synthase (NOS), binds with hyperoxide to form peroxynitrite ($ONOO^-$), a highly reactive and unstable molecule which causes DNA degradation and disrupts mitochondrial and cell membranes [51]. NOS II, the inducible isoform of NOS, has been found to be overexpressed in the hydropic cochlea and vestibule in animal models [128–130], suggesting that damage to these organs is mediated by reactive oxygen species. Ultimately, this damage leads to atrophy of the stria vascularis and progressive denervation of the labyrinth.

Diagnosis

Diagnosis of MD relies chiefly on history, physical exam, and audiometry [3]. More advanced testing may be helpful to rule out other common inner ear, central nervous system, and systemic pathologies. A 2005 survey of the American Neurotology Society members showed that one-third of providers relied solely on history, physical exam, and audiometry for diagnosis of MD, while the remaining two-thirds pursued adjunct tests [131]. Exam findings and results of adjunct tests differ depending on if the patient is seen during or between attacks.

During Attacks

At attack onset, patients exhibit spontaneous nystagmus beating towards the affected ear ("irritative" nystagmus), followed by reversal away from the affected side in the following hours ("paralytic" nystagmus) [132–134]. A third phase of nystagmus has also been reported, termed "recovery" nystagmus, in which the nystagmus reverses direction for a second time as the patient's vertigo resolves [132, 135]. However, these reports are inconsistent, and doubt exists regarding the existence of this third phase [136–138]. Head-shake nystagmus (HSN) is observed in 60–70% of MD patients during attacks and also has irritative and paralytic phases [139]. The patterns of both spontaneous and head-shaking nystagmus are consistent with increased vestibular inputs from the affected ear early in an attack, causing nystagmus towards that ear, and diminished inputs later in the attack, reversing the direction of the nystagmus [140]. This may be due to rupture of the hydropic endolymphatic space leading to potassium excitotoxicity, although this theory has been challenged in recent years (see section "Pathophysiology of Meniere's Disease"). Patients rarely present during acute MD attacks, and therefore, clinicians cannot rely on findings during attacks for diagnosis.

Head impulse tests (HIT) can also be used to evaluate patients during attacks. Most reports show that HIT testing is abnormal during attacks in most patients, with some patients showing exaggerated, and others decreased, vestibulo-ocular reflexes [141].

Between Attacks

Abnormal findings are minimal between attacks. Spontaneous nystagmus is typically absent. HIT is often normal in early stages of MD but may remain abnormal between attacks in patients with advanced disease. HSN is observed in approximately 40% of patients between attacks and does not appear to have a directional predominance [142]. The presence of HSN between attacks is related to caloric function and increases in later stages of disease as caloric function declines [140].

Audiologic Testing

Audiometry typically reveals a sensorineural hearing loss, initially affecting low frequencies. Hearing loss in MD has been classified into stages based on the degree of hearing impairment between attacks, defined as stage 1 (four-tone threshold average ≤25 dB HL), stage 2 (26–40 dB HL), stage 3 (41–70 dB HL), and stage 4 (>71 dB HL). In one cross-sectional study of 115 patients, the average time from diagnosis in patients meeting criteria for stages 1–4 was 21, 27, 36, and 60 months, respectively [143]. With longitudinal follow-up, an evolution from an upsloping audiogram to an inverted "V," and finally to a down-sloping configuration may be seen (Fig. 15.4). However, the sensitivity and specificity of these findings are poor [144, 145].

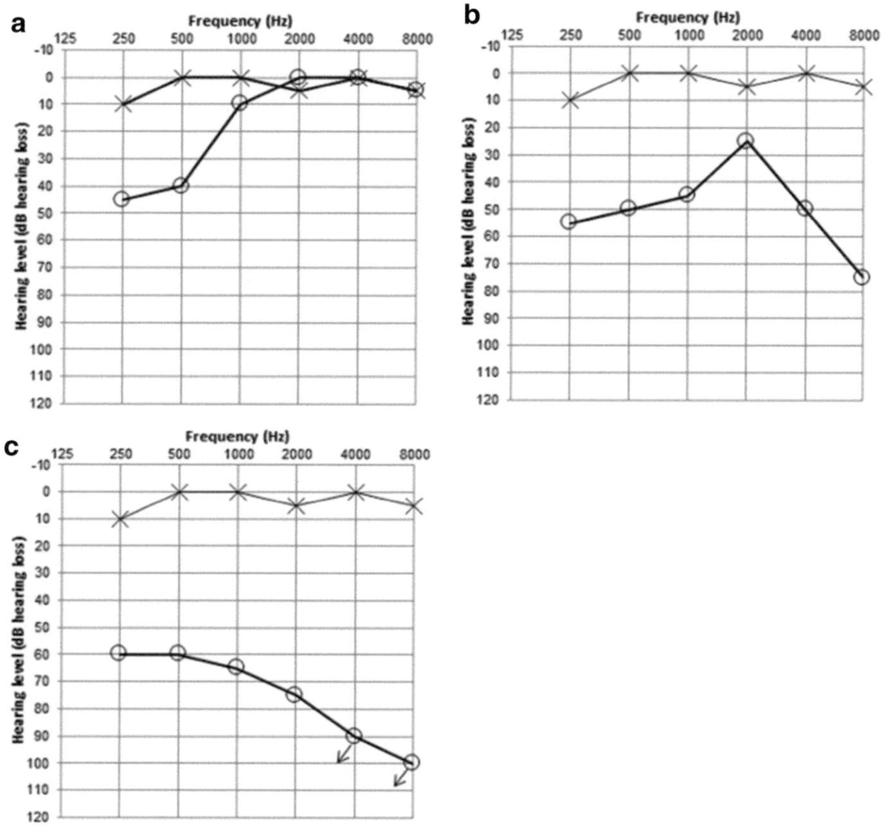

Fig. 15.4 Characteristic audiometry findings at various stages of right-sided MD. (**a**) Early MD; isolated low-frequency sensorineural hearing loss is seen. (**b**) Moderately advanced MD; "inverted V" audiogram. (**c**) Late MD; down-sloping severe to profound sensorineural hearing loss affecting all frequencies

Electrocochleography

Electrocochlography (ECoG) measures the electrical activity generated by the cochlea and vestibulocochlear nerve in response to stimuli. The main potentials recorded from ECoG are the summating potential (SP), which reflects hair cell activity, and the compound action potential (AP), which reflects activity of the cochlear nerve fibers. Thorough discussion of the physiology of ECoG in MD is found in Chap. 9; briefly, endolymphatic hydrops causes dilation of the scala media at the cochlear apex, which allows for greater displacement of the basilar membrane and greater electrical signals from outer hair cells without increased nerve firing.

This leads to an elevated SP/AP ratio; an SP/AP ratio greater than 0.5 is suggestive of MD, although cut-offs range from 0.35 to 0.50 in the literature [146, 147]. The SP/AP ratio is specific but not sensitive for MD, with reported specificities between 92% and100% and sensitivities generally under 70%. Efforts have been made to improve the sensitivity of ECoG using the SP/AP area, SP absolute value, or incorporating audiometric findings, and it remains a useful adjunct tool, particularly in cases where the diagnosis of MD is unclear [148–151].

Videonystagmography

Videonystagmography (VNG) is not necessary for diagnosis of MD but is often used to rule out central causes of vertigo. As described above, most MD patients do not have spontaneous nystagmus and have largely normal vestibular exams between attacks. Caloric testing, which is reliably abnormal during MD attacks, remains abnormal between attacks later in the disease course. This may be due to neuronal atrophy or thermal insulation related to the diameter of the hydropic endolymphatic system [152]. The remainder of VNG findings, including saccades, smooth pursuit, gaze, optokinetics, and positional maneuvers, are typically normal [141, 143, 152–154]. Abnormalities in these assessments of central function should prompt neurologic investigation.

Vestibular-Evoked Myogenic Potentials

Vestibular-evoked myogenic potentials (VEMPs) record otolith-mediated electromyographic reflexes from sternocleidomastoid (cVEMPs) or intraocular (oVEMP) muscles in response to high-intensity auditory or vibratory stimuli. cVEMPs principally evaluate saccular function, while oVEMPs evaluate the utricle (Chap. 8). VEMPs are often normal and occasionally increased in early-stage MD but become decreased or absent later in the course of disease. This is thought to be due to atrophy of the utricular and saccular maculae as disease progresses. VEMPs have low sensitivity for MD but may be useful to evaluate for certain other disease entities in questionable cases [155, 156].

Otoacoustic Emissions

Otoacoustic emission (OAE) testing refers to the detection of sounds produced by the inner ear by sensitive microphones placed within the ear canal. Transiently evoked OAE (TEOAEs) are OAEs produced in response to acoustic stimuli and have been shown to have attenuated frequency and amplitude in ears affected by

MD. This can occasionally be reversed with the administration of osmotic diuretics [157, 158]. Distortion-product OAEs (DPOAEs) are OAEs generated when pure tone stimuli at neighboring frequencies elicit combined outer hair cell motion. Multiple studies have shown that DPOAEs in patients with MD exhibit an exaggerated phase shift with changes in intracranial pressure induced by diuresis or tilt-table testing [159, 160].

Imaging

Imaging is not routinely indicated for MD diagnosis but may be used to rule out intracranial mass lesions and for research purposes. The perilymph spaces, which are obliterated in MD, are easily visualized on heavily T2-weighted fluid-attenuated inversion recovery imaging with gadolinium-based contrast [161]. Subtraction techniques can further improve the visibility of the endolymphatic space (Fig. 15.2) [162]. High-resolution MRI is sensitive but nonspecific for MD. Although cochlear hydrops is frequently seen in normal-hearing healthy patients, vestibular hydrops may be a more sensitive predictor of MD [163, 164].

Other Tests

Plasma antidiuretic hormone (ADH) levels have historically been used to aid in the diagnosis of MD. ADH levels are typically elevated between attacks and increase further during attacks, a phenomenon that has been linked to the presence of endolymphatic hydrops (see section "Pathophysiology of Meniere's Disease"). However, plasma ADH level is neither sensitive nor specific for MD [165–167].

Glycerol testing is the measurement of audiometry before and after administration of glycerol, an osmotic diuretic. Glycerol is thought to reduce the fluid burden of the cochlea through osmosis, leading to a partial and temporary improvement in hearing loss. However, this test is also neither sensitive nor specific. Furthermore, in the early stages of MD, this must be performed during attacks to capture patients with hearing loss, and in the later stages, hearing loss may be permanent regardless of the degree of hydrops. This limits the utility of this test, which is mentioned principally for historical purposes [165, 168].

Differential Diagnosis

The diagnosis of MD requires ruling out other common pathologies. Vestibular migraine (VM) is the most common cause of episodic vertigo and is diagnosed based on patient report of recurrent episodic vestibular symptoms with associated migrainous features and a personal history of migraines [169]. VM may be difficult to distinguish from MD, particularly in the early stages of MD when cochlear symptoms may be absent and hearing recovers fully in between attacks. Furthermore, concomitant aural symptoms (hearing disturbances, tinnitus, and aural pressure) are frequently seen in VM patients, and evidence exists that migraines are more prevalent in MD patients than in the general population [170].

Efforts have been made to establish accurate criteria to differentiate MD and VM. VM patients may have VEMPs and audiometric abnormalities that mimic those found in MD and may even exhibit EH [171]. There is debate whether the hydrops seen in VM patients is due to neurogenic inflammation in the inner ear, some patients suffer from both disorders simultaneously, or some MD patients are misdiagnosed with VM. Hearing loss is helpful in distinguishing MD and VM, as permanent unilateral hearing loss is relatively infrequent in VM patients compared to MD patients [170]. Multiple studies have worked to identify distinguishing features on VEMP testing and have suggested that differences in 500 Hz oVEMP responses may be useful [172–174]. In addition, caloric weakness is more common and more severe in MD than in VM patients [170, 175].

Some authors advocate for prophylactic anti-migraine medications in cases of diagnostic uncertainty. Medication response can help to differentiate between the disorders. However, a significant proportion of MD patients also respond to medications used for VM, and the two disorders may share a common pathogenesis (see section "Pathophysiology of Meniere's Disease") [176, 177].

Other diagnoses to consider include vestibular neuritis, labyrinthitis, perilymphatic fistula, otosclerosis, mass lesions, transient ischemic attacks, noise-induced hearing loss, and systemic disorders. These conditions tend to be easier to distinguish from MD based on history, audiometry, and imaging.

Conclusion

Meniere's disease is a complex disorder whose etiology continues to be elucidated. Diagnosis of MD requires a thorough history, physical exam, and audiometric evaluation, with additional audiologic testing in uncertain cases. As understanding of the pathophysiology of EH and MD advances in the coming decades, more reliable diagnostic tools and treatments will likely develop.

References

1. Sajjadi H, Paparella MM. Meniere's disease. The Lancet. 372(9636):406–14.
2. Tyrrell JS, Whinney DJ, Ukoumunne OC, Fleming LE, Osborne NJ. Prevalence, associated factors, and comorbid conditions for Meniere's disease. Ear Hear. 2014;35(4):e162–9.
3. Goebel JA. 2015 equilibrium committee amendment to the 1995 AAO-HNS guidelines for the definition of Mé niè re's disease. Otolaryngol Head Neck Surg. 2016;154:403–4.

4. Mancini F, Catalani M, Carru M, Monti B. History of Meniere's disease and its clinical presentation. Otolaryngol Clin N Am. 2002;35:565–80.
5. Paparella MM. Pathogenesis of Meniere's disease and Meniere's syndrome. Acta Otolaryngol Suppl. 1984;406:10–25.
6. Balkany TJ, Sires B, Arenberg IK. Bilateral aspects of Meniere's disease: an underestimated clinical entity. Otolaryngol Clin N Am. 1980;13:603–9.
7. Havia M, Kentala E. Progression of symptoms of dizziness in Ménière's disease. Arch Otolaryngol Head Neck Surg. 2004;130:431.
8. Mizukoshi K, Shojaku H, Aso S, Watanabe Y. Clinical study of elderly patients with Meniere's and related diseases. Auris Nasus Larynx. 2000;27:167–73.
9. Enander A, Stahle J. Hearing loss and caloric response in Menière's disease. A comparative study. Acta Otolaryngol (Stockh). 1969;67:57–68.
10. Stahle J, Friberg U, Svedberg A. Long-term progression of Menière's disease. Am J Otol. 1989;10:170–3.
11. Sumi T, Watanabe I, Tsunoda A, Nishio A, Komatsuzaki A, Kitamura K. Longitudinal study of 29 patients with Meniere's disease with follow-up of 10 years or more (in commemoration of Professor Emeritus Isamu Watanabe). Acta Otolaryngol (Stockh). 2012;132:10–5.
12. Green JD Jr, Blum DJ, Harner SG. Longitudinal followup of patients with Meniere's disease. Otolaryngol Head Neck Surg. 1991;104(6):783–8.
13. Green JD, Blum DJ, Harner SG. Longitudinal followup of patients with Meniere's disease. Otolaryngol Head Neck Surg. 1991;104:783–8.
14. Ueberfuhr MA, Wiegrebe L, Krause E, Gürkov R, Drexl M. Tinnitus in normal-hearing participants after exposure to intense low-frequency sound and in Ménière's disease patients. Front Neurol. 2017;7:239.
15. Levo H, Kentala E, Rasku J, PyykkF I. Aural fullness in M3ni2re's disease. Audiol Neurotol. 2014;19:395–9.
16. Albers GD, Wilson WH. Diplacusis: II. Etiology. Arch Otolaryngol Head Neck Surg. 1968;87:604–6.
17. Colin D, Micheyl C, Girod A, Truy E, Gallégo S. Binaural Diplacusis and its relationship with hearing-threshold asymmetry. PLoS One. 2016;11:e0159975.
18. Walsh TE. The diagnosis and treatment of Meniere's disease. Arch Otolaryngol Head Neck Surg. 1956;64:118–28.
19. Baloh RW, Jacobson K, Winder T. Drop attacks with Menière's syndrome. Ann Neurol. 1990;28:384–7.
20. Black FO, Effron MZ, Burns DS. Diagnosis and management of drop attacks of vestibular origin: Tumarkin's otolithic crisis. Otolaryngol Head Neck Surg. 1982;90:256–62.
21. Ozeki H, Iwasaki S, Murofushi T. Vestibular drop attack secondary to Meniere's disease results from unstable otolithic function. Acta Otolaryngol. 2008;128:887–91.
22. Kentala E, Havia M, Pyykkö I. Short-lasting drop attacks in Meniere's disease. Otolaryngol Head Neck Surg. 2001;124:526–30.
23. Janzen VD, Russell RD. Conservative management of Tumarkin's otolithic crisis. J Otolaryngol. 1988;17:359–61.
24. Kimura H, Aso S, Watanabe Y. Prediction of progression from atypical to definite Ménière's disease using electrocochleography and glycerol and furosemide tests. Acta Otolaryngol (Stockh). 2003;123:388–95.
25. Kato M, Sugiura M, Shimono M, Yoshida T, Otake H, Kato K, et al. Endolymphatic hydrops revealed by magnetic resonance imaging in patients with atypical Meniere's disease. Acta Otolaryngol. 2013;133:123–9.
26. Gurkov R, Pyyko I, Zou J, Kentala E. What is Meniere's disease? A contemporary reevaluation of endolymphatic hydrops. J Neurol. 2016;263(Suppl 1):S71–81.
27. Hallpike CS, Cairns H. Observations on the pathology of Ménière's syndrome: (section of otology). Proc R Soc Med. 1938;31(11):1317–36.
28. Paparella MM, Morizono T, Matsunaga T. Kyoshiro Yamakawa, MD, and temporal bone histopathology of Meniere's patient reported in 1938. Commemoration of the centennial of his birth. Arch Otolaryngol Head Neck Surg. 1992;118(6):660–2.

29. Hebbar GK, Rask-Andersen H, Linthicum FH Jr. Three-dimensional analysis of 61 human endolymphatic ducts and sacs in ears with and without Meniere's disease. Ann Otol Rhinol Laryngol. 1991;100(3):219–25.
30. Shambaugh GE Jr, Clemis JD, Arenberg IK. Endolymphatic duct and sac in Meniere's disease. Arch Otolaryngol. 1969;89(6):816–25.
31. Park JJ, Shen A, Keil S, Kuhl C, Westhofen M. Jugular bulb abnormalities in patients with Meniere's disease using high-resolution computed tomography. Eur Arch Otorrinolaringol. 2015;272(8):1879–84.
32. Sando I, Ikeda M. Pneumatization and thickness of the petrous bone in patients with Meniere's disease. A histopathological study. Ann Otol Rhinol Laryngol Suppl. 1985;118:2–5.
33. Paparella MM, Djalilian HR. Etiology, pathophysiology of symptoms, and pathogenesis of Meniere's disease. Otolaryngol Clin N Am. 2002;35(3):529–45. vi
34. Monsanto RD, Pauna HF, Kwon G, Schachern PA, Tsuprun V, Paparella MM, et al. A three-dimensional analysis of the endolymph drainage system in Meniere disease. Laryngoscope. 2017;127(5):E170–E5.
35. Lawrence M, McCabe BF. Inner-ear mechanics and deafness. Special consideration of Meniere's syndrome. JAMA J Am Med Assoc. 1959;171:1927–32.
36. Vasama JP, Linthicum FH Jr. Meniere's disease and endolymphatic hydrops without Meniere's symptoms: temporal bone histopathology. Acta Otolaryngol. 1999;119(3):297–301.
37. Kariya S, Cureoglu S, Fukushima H, Nomiya S, Nomiya R, Schachern PA, et al. Vascular findings in the stria vascularis of patients with unilateral or bilateral Meniere's disease: a histopathologic temporal bone study. Otol Neurotol. 2009;30(7):1006–12.
38. Okuno T, Sando I. Localization, frequency, and severity of endolymphatic hydrops and the pathology of the labyrinthine membrane in Meniere's disease. Ann Otol Rhinol Laryngol. 1987;96(4):438–45.
39. Nadol JB Jr, Thornton AR. Ultrastructural findings in a case of Meniere's disease. Ann Otol Rhinol Laryngol. 1987;96(4):449–54.
40. Nakashima T, Naganawa S, Sugiura M, Teranishi M, Sone M, Hayashi H, et al. Visualization of endolymphatic hydrops in patients with Meniere's disease. Laryngoscope. 2007;117(3):415–20.
41. Nakashima T, Naganawa S, Teranishi M, Tagaya M, Nakata S, Sone M, et al. Endolymphatic hydrops revealed by intravenous gadolinium injection in patients with Meniere's disease. Acta Otolaryngol. 2010;130(3):338–43.
42. Gurkov R, Flatz W, Louza J, Strupp M, Krause E. In vivo visualization of endolyphatic hydrops in patients with Meniere's disease: correlation with audiovestibular function. Eur Arch Otorrinolaringol. 2011;268(12):1743–8.
43. Tagaya M, Yamazaki M, Teranishi M, Naganawa S, Yoshida T, Otake H, et al. Endolymphatic hydrops and blood-labyrinth barrier in Meniere's disease. Acta Otolaryngol. 2011;131(5):474–9.
44. Merchant SN, Adams JC, Nadol JB Jr. Pathophysiology of Meniere's syndrome: are symptoms caused by endolymphatic hydrops? Otol Neurotol. 2005;26(1):74–81.
45. Rauch SD, Merchant SN, Thedinger BA. Meniere's syndrome and endolymphatic hydrops. Double-blind temporal bone study. Ann Otol Rhinol Laryngol. 1989;98(11):873–83.
46. Pyykko I, Zou J, Poe D, Nakashima T, Naganawa S. Magnetic resonance imaging of the inner ear in Meniere's disease. Otolaryngol Clin N Am. 2010;43(5):1059–80.
47. Kimura R, Schuknecht H. Membranous hydrops in the inner ear of the Guinea pig after obliteration of the endolymphatic sac. ORL. 1965;27(6):343–54.
48. Dunnebier EA, Segenhout JM, Wit HP, Albers FW. Two-phase endolymphatic hydrops: a new dynamic Guinea pig model. Acta Otolaryngol. 1997;117(1):13–9.
49. Watanabe K, Tomiyama S, Jinnouchi K, Yagi T. Apoptosis in the hydropic cochlea of Guinea pigs following immune reaction of the endolymphatic sac: immunohistochemical analysis. Eur Arch Otorrinolaringol. 2001;258(6):296–9.
50. Marshall AF, Jewells VL, Kranz P, Lee YZ, Lin W, Zdanski CJ. Magnetic resonance imaging of Guinea pig cochlea after vasopressin-induced or surgically induced endolymphatic hydrops. Otolaryngol Head Neck Surg. 2010;142(2):260–5.

51. Semaan MT, Alagramam KN, Megerian CA. The basic science of Meniere's disease and endolymphatic hydrops. Curr Opin Otolaryngol Head Neck Surg. 2005;13(5):301–7.
52. Megerian CA, Semaan MT, Aftab S, Kisley LB, Zheng QY, Pawlowski KS, et al. A mouse model with postnatal endolymphatic hydrops and hearing loss. Hear Res. 2008;237(1–2):90–105.
53. Semaan MT, Zheng QY, Han F, Zheng Y, Yu H, Heaphy JC, et al. Characterization of neuronal cell death in the spiral ganglia of a mouse model of endolymphatic hydrops. Otol Neurotol. 2013;34(3):559–69.
54. Wick CC, Semaan MT, Zheng QY, Megerian CA. A genetic murine model of endolymphatic hydrops: the Phex mouse. Curr Otorhinolaryngol Rep. 2014;2(3):144–51.
55. Sepahdari AR, Vorasubin N, Ishiyama G, Ishiyama A. Endolymphatic hydrops reversal following acetazolamide therapy: demonstration with delayed intravenous contrast-enhanced 3D-FLAIR MRI. AJNR Am J Neuroradiol. 2016;37(1):151–4.
56. Ikeda K, Kusakari J, Takasaka T, Saito Y. Early effects of acetazolamide on anionic activities of the Guinea pig endolymph: evidence for active function of carbonic anhydrase in the cochlea. Hear Res. 1987;31(3):211–6.
57. Klockhoff I, Lindblom U. Glycerol test in Meniere's disease. Acta Otolaryngol. 1966;Suppl 224:449+.
58. Shinkawa H, Kimura RS. Effect of diuretics on endolymphatic hydrops. Acta Otolaryngol. 1986;101(1–2):43–52.
59. Crowson MG, Patki A, Tucci DL. A systematic review of diuretics in the medical management of Meniere's disease. Otolaryngol Head Neck Surg. 2016;154(5):824–34.
60. Morrison AW, Bailey ME, Morrison GA. Familial Meniere's disease: clinical and genetic aspects. J Laryngol Otol. 2009;123(1):29–37.
61. Birgerson L, Gustavson KH, Stahle J. Familial Meniere's disease: a genetic investigation. Am J Otol. 1987;8(4):323–6.
62. Arweiler-Harbeck D, Horsthemke B, Jahnke K, Hennies HC. Genetic aspects of familial Meniere's disease. Otol Neurotol. 2011;32(4):695–700.
63. Ohmen JD, White CH, Li X, Wang J, Fisher LM, Zhang H, et al. Genetic evidence for an ethnic diversity in the susceptibility to Meniere's disease. Otol Neurotol. 2013;34(7):1336–41.
64. Hietikko E, Kotimaki J, Okuloff A, Sorri M, Mannikko M. A replication study on proposed candidate genes in Meniere's disease, and a review of the current status of genetic studies. Int J Audiol. 2012;51(11):841–5.
65. Campbell CA, Della Santina CC, Meyer NC, Smith NB, Myrie OA, Stone EM, et al. Polymorphisms in KCNE1 or KCNE3 are not associated with Meniere disease in the Caucasian population. Am J Med Genet A. 2010;152A(1):67–74.
66. Doi K, Sato T, Kuramasu T, Hibino H, Kitahara T, Horii A, et al. Meniere's disease is associated with single nucleotide polymorphisms in the human potassium channel genes, KCNE1 and KCNE3. ORL. 2005;67(5):289–93.
67. Fransen E, Verstreken M, Verhagen WI, Wuyts FL, Huygen PL, D'Haese P, et al. High prevalence of symptoms of Meniere's disease in three families with a mutation in the COCH gene. Hum Mol Genet. 1999;8(8):1425–9.
68. Sanchez E, Lopez-Escamez JA, Lopez-Nevot MA, Lopez-Nevot A, Cortes R, Martin J. Absence of COCH mutations in patients with Meniere disease. Eur J Hum Genet. 2004;12(1):75–8.
69. Requena T, Cabrera S, Martin-Sierra C, Price SD, Lysakowski A, Lopez-Escamez JA. Identification of two novel mutations in FAM136A and DTNA genes in autosomal-dominant familial Meniere's disease. Hum Mol Genet. 2015;24(4):1119–26.
70. Bernstein JM, Shanahan TC, Schaffer FM. Further observations on the role of the MHC genes and certain hearing disorders. Acta Otolaryngol. 1996;116(5):666–71.
71. Chiarella G, Petrolo C, Cassandro E. The genetics of Meniere's disease. Appl Clin Genet. 2015;8:9–17.
72. Mhatre AN, Jero J, Chiappini I, Bolasco G, Barbara M, Lalwani AK. Aquaporin-2 expression in the mammalian cochlea and investigation of its role in Meniere's disease. Hear Res. 2002;170(1–2):59–69.

73. Vrabec JT. Genetic investigations of Meniere's disease. Otolaryngol Clin N Am. 2010;43(5):1121–32.
74. Candreia C, Schmuziger N, Gurtler N. Molecular analysis of aquaporin genes 1 to 4 in patients with Meniere's disease. Cell Physiol Biochem. 2010;26(4–5):787–92.
75. Aoki M, Ando K, Kuze B, Mizuta K, Hayashi T, Ito Y. The association of antidiuretic hormone levels with an attack of Meniere's disease. Clin Otolaryngol. 2005;30(6):521–5.
76. Aoki M, Asai M, Nishihori T, Mizuta K, Ito Y, Ando K. The relevance of an elevation in the plasma vasopressin levels to the pathogenesis of Meniere's attack. J Neuroendocrinol. 2007;19(11):901–6.
77. Maekawa C, Kitahara T, Kizawa K, Okazaki S, Kamakura T, Horii A, et al. Expression and translocation of aquaporin-2 in the endolymphatic sac in patients with Meniere's disease. J Neuroendocrinol. 2010;22(11):1157–64.
78. Kitahara T, Okamoto H, Fukushima M, Sakagami M, Ito T, Yamashita A, et al. A two-year randomized trial of interventions to decrease stress hormone vasopressin production in patients with Meniere's disease-a pilot study. PLoS One. 2016;11(6):e0158309.
79. Takeda T, Takeda S, Kitano H, Okada T, Kakigi A. Endolymphatic hydrops induced by chronic administration of vasopressin. Hear Res. 2000;140(1–2):1–6.
80. Gates P. Hypothesis: could Meniere's disease be a channelopathy? Intern Med J. 2005;35(8):488–9.
81. Wangemann P. K+ cycling and the endocochlear potential. Hear Res. 2002;165(1–2):1–9.
82. Yazawa Y, Suzuki M, Hanamitsu M, Kimura H, Tooyama I. Detection of viral DNA in the endolymphatic sac in Meniere's disease by in situ hybridization. ORL J Otorhinolaryngol Relat Spec. 2003;65(3):162–8.
83. Vrabec JT. Herpes simplex virus and Meniere's disease. Laryngoscope. 2003;113(9):1431–8.
84. Gartner M, Bossart W, Linder T. Herpes virus and Meniere's disease. ORL J Otorhinolaryngol Relat Spec. 2008;70(1):28–31; discussion.
85. Pulec JL. Indications for surgery in mc Nicrc's discasc. Laryngoscope. 1977;87(4 Pt 1):542–56.
86. Pulec JL. Meniere's disease of syphilitic etiology. Ear Nose Throat J. 1997;76(8):508–510, 12 14, passim.
87. Miller ME, Makary C, Lopez IA, Ishiyama A. Endolymphatic hydrops in otologic syphilis: a temporal bone study. Otol Neurotol. 2010;31(4):681–6.
88. Paparella MM, de Sousa LC, Mancini F. Meniere's syndrome and otitis media. Laryngoscope. 1983;93(11 Pt 1):1408–15.
89. Lin YS, Lin LC, Lee FP, Lee KJ. The prevalence of chronic otitis media and its complication rates in teenagers and adult patients. Otolaryngol Head Neck Surg. 2009;140(2):165–70.
90. Dornhoffer JL, Arenberg IK. Immune mechanisms in Meniere's syndrome. Otolaryngol Clin N Am. 1997;30(6):1017–26.
91. Bovo R, Ciorba A, Martini A. Vertigo and autoimmunity. Eur Arch Otorrinolaringol. 2010;267(1):13–9.
92. Hughes GB, Kinney SE, Barna BP, Calabrese LH. Autoimmune reactivity in Meniere's disease: a preliminary report. Laryngoscope. 1983;93(4):410–7.
93. Gazquez I, Soto-Varela A, Aran I, Santos S, Batuecas A, Trinidad G, et al. High prevalence of systemic autoimmune diseases in patients with Meniere's disease. PLoS One. 2011;6(10):e26759.
94. Derebery MJ, Berliner KI. Prevalence of allergy in Meniere's disease. Otolaryngol Head Neck Surg. 2000;123(1 Pt 1):69–75.
95. Derebery MJ, Berliner KI. Allergy and its relation to Meniere's disease. Otolaryngol Clin N Am. 2010;43(5):1047–58.
96. Derebery MJ. Allergic management of Meniere's disease: an outcome study. Otolaryngol Head Neck Surg. 2000;122(2):174–82.

97. Wackym PA, Friberg U, Linthicum FH Jr, Bagger-Sjoback D, Bui HT, Hofman F, et al. Human endolymphatic sac: morphologic evidence of immunologic function. Ann Otol Rhinol Laryngol. 1987;96(3 Pt 1):276–81.
98. Adams JC. Clinical implications of inflammatory cytokines in the cochlea: a technical note. Otol Neurotol. 2002;23(3):316–22.
99. Yoo TJ, Shea J Jr, Ge X, Kwon SS, Yazawa Y, Sener O, et al. Presence of autoantibodies in the sera of Meniere's disease. Ann Otol Rhinol Laryngol. 2001;110(5 Pt 1):425–9.
100. Brookes GB. Circulating immune complexes in Meniere's disease. Arch Otolaryngol Head Neck Surg. 1986;112(5):536–40.
101. Kim SH, Kim JY, Lee HJ, Gi M, Kim BG, Choi JY. Autoimmunity as a candidate for the etiopathogenesis of Meniere's disease: detection of autoimmune reactions and diagnostic biomarker candidate. PLoS One. 2014;9(10):e111039.
102. Gottschlich S, Billings PB, Keithley EM, Weisman MH, Harris JP. Assessment of serum antibodies in patients with rapidly progressive sensorineural hearing loss and Meniere's disease. Laryngoscope. 1995;105(12 Pt 1):1347–52.
103. Yoo TJ, Yazawa Y, Tomoda K, Floyd R. Type II collagen-induced autoimmune endolymphatic hydrops in Guinea pig. Science. 1983;222(4619):65–7.
104. Yoo TJ, Stuart JM, Kang AH, Townes AS, Tomoda K, Dixit S. Type II collagen autoimmunity in otosclerosis and Meniere's disease. Science. 1982;217(4565):1153–5.
105. Mouadeb DA, Ruckenstein MJ. Antiphospholipid inner ear syndrome. Laryngoscope. 2005;115(5):879–83.
106. Kangasniemi E, Hietikko E. The theory of autoimmunity in Meniere's disease is lacking evidence. Auris Nasus Larynx. 2017.
107. Murofushi T, Ozeki H, Inoue A, Sakata A. Does migraine-associated vertigo share a common pathophysiology with Meniere's disease? Study with vestibular-evoked myogenic potential. Cephalalgia. 2009;29(12):1259–66.
108. Ibekwe TS, Fasunla JA, Ibekwe PU, Obasikene GC, Onakoya PA, Nwaorgu OG. Migraine and Meniere's disease: two different phenomena with frequently observed concomitant occurrences. J Natl Med Assoc. 2008;100(3):334–8.
109. Rassekh CH, Harker LA. The prevalence of migraine in Meniere's disease. Laryngoscope. 1992;102(2):135–8.
110. Gurkov R, Kantner C, Strupp M, Flatz W, Krause E, Ertl-Wagner B. Endolymphatic hydrops in patients with vestibular migraine and auditory symptoms. Eur Arch Otorrinolaringol. 2014;271(10):2661–7.
111. Cha YH, Kane MJ, Baloh RW. Familial clustering of migraine, episodic vertigo, and Meniere's disease. Otol Neurotol. 2008;29(1):93–6.
112. Foster CA, Breeze RE. The Meniere attack: an ischemia/reperfusion disorder of inner ear sensory tissues. Med Hypotheses. 2013;81(6):1108–15.
113. Mom T, Chazal J, Gabrillargues J, Gilain L, Avan P. Cochlear blood supply: an update on anatomy and function. Fr Orl. 2005;88:81–8.
114. Balatsouras DG, Ganelis P, Aspris A, Economou NC, Moukos A, Koukoutsis G. Benign paroxysmal positional vertigo associated with Meniere's disease: epidemiological, pathophysiologic, clinical, and therapeutic aspects. Ann Otol Rhinol Laryngol. 2012;121(10):682–8.
115. Gross EM, Ress BD, Viirre ES, Nelson JR, Harris JP. Intractable benign paroxysmal positional vertigo in patients with Meniere's disease. Laryngoscope. 2000;110(4):655–9.
116. Jahn AF. Benign positional vertigo and endolymphatic hydrops: what is the connection? J Laryngol Otol. 2017;131(8):658–60.
117. Yamane H, Sunami K, Iguchi H, Sakamoto H, Imoto T, Rask-Andersen H. Assessment of Meniere's disease from a radiological aspect – saccular otoconia as a cause of Meniere's disease? Acta Otolaryngol. 2012;132(10):1054–60.
118. Morita N, Cureoglu S, Nomiya S, Nomiya R, Joglekar SS, Harada T, et al. Potential cause of positional vertigo in Meniere's disease. Otol Neurotol. 2009;30(7):956–60.

119. Thomsen J, Sass K, Odkvist L, Arlinger S. Local overpressure treatment reduces vestibular symptoms in patients with Meniere's disease: a clinical, randomized, multicenter, double-blind, placebo-controlled study. Otol Neurotol. 2005;26(1):68–73.
120. Mirza S, Gokhale S. Pathophysiology of Meniere's disease. Up to date on Meniere's disease. InTech; 2017.
121. Ferster APO, Cureoglu S, Keskin N, Paparella MM, Isildak H. Secondary endolymphatic hydrops. Otol Neurotol. 2017;38(5):774–9.
122. Schuknecht H. Correlation of pathology with symptoms of Meniere's disease. Otolaryngol Clin N Am. 1968;1:433–40.
123. Valk WL, Wit HP, Albers FW. Rupture of Reissner's membrane during acute endolymphatic hydrops in the Guinea pig: a model for Meniere's disease? Acta Otolaryngol. 2006;126(10):1030–5.
124. Brown DH, McClure JA, Downar-Zapolski Z. The membrane rupture theory of Meniere's disease–is it valid? Laryngoscope. 1988;98(6 Pt 1):599–601.
125. Gibson WP. Hypothetical mechanism for vertigo in Meniere's disease. Otolaryngol Clin N Am. 2010;43(5):1019–27.
126. Brandt T. Vertigo: its multisensory syndromes. Springer Science & Business Media; 2013.
127. Ozeki H, Iwasaki S, Murofushi T. Vestibular drop attack secondary to Meniere's disease results from unstable otolithic function. Acta Otolaryngol. 2008;128(8):887–91.
128. Urushitani M, Nakamizo T, Inoue R, Sawada H, Kihara T, Honda K, et al. N-methyl-D-aspartate receptor-mediated mitochondrial Ca(2+) overload in acute excitotoxic motor neuron death: a mechanism distinct from chronic neurotoxicity after Ca(2+) influx. J Neurosci Res. 2001;63(5):377–87.
129. Michel O, Hess A, Su J, Bloch W, Stennert E, Addicks K. Expression of inducible nitric oxide synthase (iNOS/NOS II) in the hydropic cochlea of Guinea pigs. Hear Res. 2000;143(1–2):23–8.
130. Watanabe K, Tomiyama S, Jinnouchi K, Hess A, Michel O, Yagi T. Expression of inducible nitric oxide synthase (iNOS/NOS II) in the hydropic vestibule after injection of keyhole limpet hemocyanin into the endolymphatic sac of Guinea pigs. J Vestib Res. 2001;11(2):67–71.
131. Kim H, Wiet R, Battista R. Trends in the diagnosis and the management of Meniere's disease: results of a survey. Otolaryngol Head Neck Surg. 2005;132:722–6.
132. Bance M, Mai M, Tomlinson D, Rutka J. The changing direction of nystagmus in acute Menière's disease: pathophysiological implications. Laryngoscope. 1991;101:197–201.
133. Brown DH, McClure JA, Downar-Zapolski Z. The membrane rupture theory of Menière's disease–is it valid? Laryngoscope. 1988;98:599–601.
134. Hirai C, Yamamoto Y, Takeda T, Tasaki A, Inaba Y, Kiyokawa Y, et al. Nystagmus at the onset of vertiginous attack in Ménière's disease. Otol Neurotol. 2017;38:110–3.
135. Kuo S-W, Yang T-H, Young Y-H. Changes in vestibular evoked myogenic potentials after Meniere attacks. Ann Otol Rhinol Laryngol. 2005;114:717–21.
136. McClure JA, Copp JC, Lycett P. Recovery nystagmus in Ménière's disease. Laryngoscope. 1981;91:1727–37.
137. Aschan G, Stahle J. Nystagmus in Menière's disease during attacks; a nystagmographical study. Acta Otolaryngol (Stockh). 1957;47:189–201.
138. Nishikawa K, Nishikawa M. Nystagmus during attack in Menière's disease. Auris Nasus Larynx. 1986;13(Suppl 2):S147–51.
139. Kim C-H, Shin JE, Kim TS, Shim BS, Park HJ. Two-dimensional analysis of head-shaking nystagmus in patients with Meniere's disease. J Vestib Res Equilib Orient. 2013;23:95–100.
140. Lee S-U, Kee H-J, Sheen SS, Choi BY, Koo J-W, Kim K-S. Head-shaking and Vibration-induced Nystagmus During and Between the Attacks of Unilateral Ménière's Disease.
141. Lee S-U, Kim H-J, Koo J-W, Kim J-S. Comparison of caloric and head-impulse tests during the attacks of Meniere's disease. Laryngoscope. 2017;127:702–8.
142. Park HJ, Migliaccio AA, Della Santina CC, Minor LB, Carey JP. Search-coil head-thrust and caloric tests in Ménière's disease. Acta Otolaryngol (Stockh). 2005;125:852–7.

143. Zhang Y, Liu B, Wang R, Jia R, Gu X. Characteristics of the Cochlear symptoms and functions in Meniere's disease. Chin Med J. 2016;129:2445–50.
144. Paparella MM, McDermott JC, de Sousa LC. Meniere's disease and the peak audiogram. Arch Otolaryngol (Chicago, Ill : 1960). 1982;108:555–9.
145. Lee CS, Paparella MM, Margolis RH, Le C. Audiological profiles and Menière's disease. Ear Nose Throat J. 1995;74:527–32.
146. Mammarella F, Zelli M, Varakliotis T, Eibenstein A, Pianura CM, Bellocchi G. Is Electrocochleography still helpful in early diagnosis of Meniere disease? J Audiol Otol. 2017;21:72–6.
147. Hornibrook J. Tone burst electrocochleography for the diagnosis of clinically certain Meniere's disease. Front Neurosci. 2017;11:301.
148. Sass K. Sensitivity and specificity of transtympanic electrocochleography in Meniere's disease. Acta Otolaryngol. 1998;118:150–6.
149. Gibson WP. The use of electrocochleography in the diagnosis of Meniére's disease. Acta Otolaryngol Suppl. 1991;485:46–52.
150. Conlon BJ, Gibson WP. Electrocochleography in the diagnosis of Meniere's disease. Acta Otolaryngol. 2000;120:480–3.
151. Kim HH, Kumar A, Battista RA, Wiet RJ. Electrocochleography in patients with Meniere's disease. Am J Otolaryngol. 26:128–31.
152. McGarvie LA, Curthoys IS, MacDougall HG, Halmagyi GM. What does the dissociation between the results of video head impulse versus caloric testing reveal about the vestibular dysfunction in Ménière's disease? Acta Otolaryngol (Stockh). 2015;135:859–65.
153. Blödow A, Heinze M, Bloching MB, von Brevern M, Radtke A, Lempert T. Caloric stimulation and video-head impulse testing in Ménière's disease and vestibular migraine. Acta Otolaryngol (Stockh). 2014;134:1239–44.
154. Yacovino DA, Hain TC, Musazzi M. Fluctuating Vestibulo-ocular reflex in Ménière's disease. Otol Neurotol. 2017;38:244–7.
155. Katayama N, Yamamoto M, Teranishi M, Naganawa S, Nakata S, Sone M, et al. Relationship between endolymphatic hydrops and vestibular-evoked myogenic potential. Acta Otolaryngol. 2010;130:917–23.
156. Young Y-H, Huang T-W, Cheng P-W. Assessing the stage of Ménière's disease using vestibular evoked myogenic potentials. Arch Otolaryngol Head Neck Surg. 2003;129:815.
157. Kubo T, Sakashita T, Kusuki M, Nakai Y. Frequency analysis of evoked otoacoustic emissions in Meniére's disease. Acta Otolaryngol Suppl. 1995;519:275–81.
158. Harris FP, Probst R. Transiently evoked otoacoustic emissions in patients with Menière's disease. Acta Otolaryngol (Stockh). 1992;112:36–44.
159. Drexl M, Krause E, Gürkov R. A comparison of distortion product Otoacoustic emission properties in Ménière's disease patients and normal-hearing participants. Ear Hear. 2017:1.
160. Avan P, Giraudet F, Chauveau B, Gilain L, Mom T. Unstable distortion-product otoacoustic emission phase in MeniEre's disease. 2011.
161. Nakashima T, Naganawa S, Sugiura M, Teranishi M, Sone M, Hayashi H, et al. Visualization of endolymphatic hydrops in patients with Meniere's disease. Laryngoscope. 2007;117:415–20.
162. Naganawa S, Suzuki K, Nakamichi R, Bokura K, Yoshida T, Sone M, et al. Semi-quantification of endolymphatic size on MR imaging after intravenous injection of single-dose gadodiamide: comparison between two types of processing strategies. Magn Reson Med Sci. 2013;12:261–9.
163. Yoshida T, Sugimoto S, Teranishi M, Otake H, Yamazaki M, Naganawa S, et al. Imaging of the endolymphatic space in patients with Ménière's disease. Auris Nasus Larynx. 2017;45(1):33–8.
164. Baráth K, Schuknecht B, Naldi AM, Schrepfer T, Bockisch CJ, Hegemann SCA. Detection and grading of endolymphatic hydrops in Menière disease using MR imaging. AJNR Am J Neuroradiol. 2014;35:1387–92.

165. Taguchi D, Kakigi A, Takeda T, Sawada S, Nakatani H. Diagnostic value of plasma antidiuretic hormone, electrocochleography, and glycerol test in patients with endolymphatic hydrops. ORL J Otorhinolaryngol Relat Spec. 2010;71(Suppl 1):26–9.
166. Kakigi A, Takeda T. Antidiuretic hormone and osmolality in patients with Meniere's disease. ORL. 2009;71:11–3.
167. Takeda T, Kakigi A, Saito H. Antidiuretic hormone (ADH) and endolymphatic hydrops. Acta Otolaryngol Suppl. 1995;519:219–22.
168. Klockhoff I, Lindblom U. Endolymphatic hydrops revealed by glycerol test. Preliminary report. Acta Otolaryngol (Stockh). 1966;61:459–62.
169. Dieterich M, Obermann M, Celebisoy N. Vestibular migraine: the most frequent entity of episodic vertigo. J Neurol. 2016;263(Suppl 1):S82–9.
170. Neff BA, Staab JP, Eggers SD, Carlson ML, Schmitt WR, Van Abel KM, et al. Auditory and vestibular symptoms and chronic subjective dizziness in patients with Ménière's disease, vestibular migraine, and Ménière's disease with concomitant vestibular migraine. Otol Neurotol. 2012;33:1235–44.
171. Gürkov R, Kantner C, Strupp M, Flatz W, Krause E, Ertl-Wagner B. Endolymphatic hydrops in patients with vestibular migraine and auditory symptoms. Eur Arch Otorrinolaringol. 2014;271:2661–7.
172. Taylor RL, Zagami AS, Gibson WP, Black DA, Watson SR, Halmagyi MG, et al. Vestibular evoked myogenic potentials to sound and vibration: characteristics in vestibular migraine that enable separation from Meniere's disease. Cephalalgia. 2012;32:213–25.
173. Inoue A, Egami N, Fujimoto C, Kinoshita M, Yamasoba T, Iwasaki S. Vestibular evoked myogenic potentials in vestibular migraine. Ann Otol Rhinol Laryngol. 2016;125:931–7.
174. Zuniga MG, Janky KL, Schubert MC, Carey JP. Can vestibular-evoked myogenic potentials help differentiate Ménière disease from vestibular migraine? Otolaryngol Head Neck Surg. 2012;146:788–96.
175. Sharon JD, Hullar TE. Motion sensitivity and caloric responsiveness in vestibular migraine and Meniere's disease. Laryngoscope. 2014;124:969–73.
176. Soto E, Vega R. Neuropharmacology of vestibular system disorders. Curr Neuropharmacol. 2010;8:26–40.
177. Ghavami Y, Mahboubi H, Yau AY, Maducdoc M, Djalilian HR. Migraine features in patients with Meniere's disease. Laryngoscope. 2016;126:163–8.
178. Nomura Y. Morphological aspects of inner ear disease. Springer Science & Business Media; 2013.

Chapter 16
Medical Management of Meniere's Disease

Stephen P. Cass, Maria C. Machala, and Emily C. Ambrose

Introduction

Meniere's disease refers to the clinical syndrome of fluctuating sensorineural hearing loss, tinnitus, aural pressure, and episodic vertigo [1]. While the principle underlying pathological finding in Meniere's disease is endolymphatic hydrops, the cause of endolymphatic hydrops and the mechanisms of hearing loss and episodes of vertigo remain unknown. The acute vertiginous attacks characteristic of Meniere's disease are severe and incapacitating, lasting 20 minutes to several hours. Because no permanent changes initially occur in the function of the vestibular neuroepithelium and vestibular nerve, in-between the acute episodes of vertigo, most people feel their balance is normal. Recurrent episodes of vertigo occur with highly variable frequency. There may be days, weeks, or years between attacks. Over time, there is a tendency for the sensorineural hearing loss to become fixed and no longer fluctuate back to normal. Tinnitus and aural fullness often become permanent, and vestibular hypofunction ensues.

Meniere's disease most often presents as a unilateral disorder, but the contralateral ear can also become involved (bilateral Meniere's disease). The exact incidence of bilateral Meniere's disease is unknown, but a reasonable estimate is that about 20% of patients with unilateral Meniere's disease will eventually have bilateral involvement within 5 years.

As the exact cause of Meniere's disease has yet to be elucidated, there are no definitive curative therapies available. Medical treatment is available, however, and is aimed at [1] treating endolymphatic hydrops and managing possible Meniere's

S. P. Cass (✉) · M. C. Machala · E. C. Ambrose
Department of Otolaryngology, University of Colorado Anschutz Medical Campus, Aurora, CO, USA
e-mail: stephen.cass@ucdenver.edu; maria.machala@cuanschutz.edu; emily.ambrose@cuanschutz.edu

J. C. Lucas et al. (eds.), *Diagnosis and Treatment of Vestibular Disorders*,
https://doi.org/10.1007/978-3-032-11740-3_16

disease co-factors, [2] reducing symptoms associated with acute vertigo, and [3], in cases of persistent disabling vertigo, reducing vestibular function in the affected ear (vestibular function ablation).

Treating Endolymphatic Hydrops and Managing Meniere's Disease Co-factors

It is widely accepted that a structural inner ear abnormality, endolymphatic hydrops (excess endolymph within the scala media), is a necessary but not sufficient condition leading to the symptoms of Meniere's disease. Since it has been shown that endolymphatic hydrops can exist without ever-producing symptoms of Meniere's disease, it is believed that endolymphatic hydrops alone is not sufficient to cause Meniere's disease. There must be an additional factor(s) combining with endolymphatic hydrops to give rise to the symptomatic disease [3]. Therefore, medical treatment can be directed at both the formation of endolymphatic hydrops itself and possible co-factors that "activate" the disease.

Commonly accepted treatments for endolymphatic hydrops include a low salt diet and diuretic therapy (discussed further below). Potential Meniere disease co-factors include chronic cerebrovascular disease, episodes of reduced blood flow, and/or activation of the inflammatory processes within the inner ear. Possible contributors to these co-factors include migraine, sleep apnea, hypertension, atherosclerosis, autoimmune disease, immunologic dysfunction, and food and environmental intolerances and allergy. A primary goal of medical treatment should be identifying and treating these underlying conditions. This requires a team approach that includes primary care providers and medical specialists who can help to ensure optimal assessment and management of cardiovascular risk factors and any immunologic abnormalities.

Lifestyle Changes

Some triggers of Meniere attacks include caffeine, chocolate, stress, visual stimuli, and dropping barometric pressure. Trigger avoidance is recommended through dietary modifications with strong recommendation for low salt (daily sodium less than 1500 mg) diet, limiting stimulants including caffeine, and regular sleep cycle with adequate sleep [4]. Food intolerances should be considered, and a trial of elimination diets can be beneficial. Food and environmental allergies can be investigated and treated.

Diuretic Therapy

It is well accepted that excess endolymph within the scala media plays a major role in the development of Meniere's disease. Consequently, initial treatment is aimed at reducing excess fluid by means of a diuretic and a low sodium diet. Medical therapy directed at the underlying endolymphatic hydrops carries the potential advantage of affecting the level of sensorineural hearing, tinnitus, fullness, as well as recurrent vertigo. Furstenberg (1934) popularized the notion that endolymphatic hydrops could be modified by controlling sodium and water metabolism and recommended inducing a general dehydration of the extracellular fluid space using a regimen of a low salt diet and diuretic [5]. In 1941, Furstenberg and colleagues reported on the results of 35 patients with Meniere's disease treated with a low salt diet and diuretic [6]. Satisfactory control of vertigo was reported in 83% of patients, while hearing loss stabilized in 65%, but worsened in 26%. In a subsequent report of 125 patients treated with the Furstenberg regimen, good to excellent relief of vertigo was reported in 86% of severe, 94% of moderate, and 100% of mild cases of Meniere's disease. Hearing loss in these patients appeared to stabilize within the first 5 years of disease in the moderate to severe range of pure tone and speech audiometry [7].

Klockhoff and Lindblom (1967) also studied the effect of diuretic therapy in patients with Meniere's disease [8]. In the first 20 patients studied, patients with advanced disease (non-fluctuating sensorineural hearing loss) demonstrated no distinct improvement. But in all patients with fluctuating hearing loss, variable improvement of symptoms was noted. To answer the question whether the use of a diuretic truly had a positive effect or whether the improvements simply reflected the spontaneous course of the disease, Knockoff and Lindblom selected an additional 30 patients with Meniere's disease and fluctuating hearing loss and studied them in a double-blind fashion using a diuretic and a placebo. A significant positive effect during diuretic treatment was noted for hearing loss and vertigo, and no effect was found during use of a placebo. From this study, Klockhoff and Lindblom concluded that diuretics have a positive effect on vertigo and hearing loss, but that the effect was partial, in that worsening of symptoms can still occur during treatment, and longer follow-up of the study group suggested that hearing loss progressed in many patients while the severity of vertigo subsided.

In a study of 192 patients with Meniere's disease, Corvera and Corvera (1989) substantiated the clinical experience of Klockhoff and Lindbloom [9]. They found that while diuretics are useful in managing vertigo and fluctuating hearing loss in the early stages of Meniere's disease, they have no effect on preventing the long-term deterioration of hearing.

A recent meta-analysis published in 2016 concluded that multiple low-level evidence studies support potential benefit of diuretic therapy in the medical management of Meniere's disease [10]. Improvement in frequency of vertigo was most often reported, but improvement in hearing outcomes was less often reported. Overall, however, there are insufficient high-quality studies to clearly support the efficacy of diuretics in Meniere's disease [11]. It is our view that until a definitive study can be performed, diuretic therapy provides, at a minimum, a safe and inexpensive opportunity for patients to exert control over the disease, thereby enhancing non-specific treatment effects.

The thiazide diuretic hydrochlorothiazide, combined with the potassium-sparing diuretic triamterene, is the most widely used diuretic in Meniere's disease, given its low cost and relatively low side effect profile. It should be avoided in patients on lithium therapy or those with sulfonamide allergies. It should be avoided or used cautiously in patients with hypotension, renal disease, diabetes mellitus, and gout. Standard dosing is 25–37.5 mg. For acute flare-ups, the dose can be doubled temporarily until symptoms are under control.

Other commonly used alternatives to triamterene-hydrochlorothiazide include acetazolamide and spironolactone. We often use acetazolamide for patients with Meniere's disease who have underlying migraines and in patients with bilateral Meniere's disease. The rationale behind this is that acetazolamide is not only a diuretic, but it also causes cerebral vasodilation and carbonic anhydrase inhibition. Both of these mechanisms are thought to play an important role in migraine prophylaxis. It should also be avoided in patients with sulfonamide allergies. Typical side effects include paresthesia and increased risk of kidney stones. Spironolactone can be safely used in patients with a sulfonamide allergy. Loop diuretics such as furosemide can also be used but require close monitoring of serum sodium and potassium levels from the start of therapy and renal function if used long-term.

Betahistine

Betahistine is a vasodilator, a mild H1 histamine agonist, and a potent H3 histamine antagonist. The mechanism of action in Meniere's disease is unknown, but theories include reducing the endolymphatic pressure through improved circulation in the stria vascularis or inhibiting activity in the vestibular nuclei. It has been found to be a safe drug with a very low side effect profile. Betahistine was FDA-approved for Meniere's disease in the US market for a short period of time in the 1970s, but approval was then rescinded due to lack of evidence supporting its efficacy. However, based on clinical experience and several observational studies, it is still widely used elsewhere in the world.

A Cochran review of betahistine in Meniere's disease by James first published in 2001 and updated in 2011 included 7 trials involving 243 patients [12]. Most trials suggested a reduction of vertigo with betahistine, and some suggested a reduction in tinnitus, but none showed an effect on hearing. However, this Cochran review concluded that these trials were of low quality, and bias in the methods could have affected the results. In 2016, a carefully designed and executed trial of the medical treatment of Meniere's disease with betahistine (BEMED) was published [13]. This was a prospective, multicenter, double blind, randomized, placebo-controlled trial to assess the long-term effects of Betahistine dihydrochloride in two different doses and a placebo. The BEMED trial found a significant decline in vertigo attack rates in all 3 treatment arms over time and no difference in the number of vertigo attacks after.

nine months of treatment with betahistine at a daily dose of 48 mg or 144 mg, compared with a placebo.

Despite the uncertainty over efficacy, betahistine appears to remain frequently prescribed for Meniere's disease in Europe. In the USA, betahistine is not approved by the Food and Drug Administration but can be obtained through US compounding pharmacies with a prescription.

Episodic Treatment of Acute Symptoms

The severity of acute vertigo and vegetative symptoms (nausea, vomiting, etc.) associated with attacks of Meniere's disease can be blunted using vestibular suppressant and/or antiemetic medications. Effective vestibular suppressants include anticholinergics (i.e., scopolamine), antihistamines (i.e., meclizine), phenothiazine (i.e., promethazine), benzodiazepines (i.e., diazepam), and Zofran.

Thus, patients should be provided medications to be used to abort or lessen the severity of symptoms associated with episodes of acute vertigo in the form of fast-acting vestibular suppressants and an antiemetic medication. These medications not only reduce the intensity of the vertigo and reduce symptoms of nausea and vomiting, but they also give patients a form of control over their disease that is known to improve their well-being.

Vestibular suppressants include antihistamine and benzodiazepine medications. Given the sudden onset of vertigo with duration up to 24 hours, medications with short onset and short half-life should be used. Commonly used antihistamine agents include meclizine and dimenhydrinate due to their ability to cross the blood-brain barrier and likely due to their anticholinergic properties. The exact mechanism of vestibular suppression is unknown. The primary adverse effect is sedation, which can lead to falls and memory dysfunction. Use cautiously in elderly patients and in patients on concomitant sedating medications. Other side effects include dry mouth, dry eyes, blurry vision, constipation, and difficulty with urination due to anticholinergic properties. Commonly used benzodiazepines include diazepam, lorazepam, and clonazepam due to short onset of action. They cause central nervous system inhibition via GABA modulation. In addition to sedative effects, additional risks of benzodiazepines include tolerance and dependence. They should be avoided or used cautiously in patients with a history of drug or alcohol addiction (Table 16.1).

It is important to emphasize that vestibular suppressants should only be used to decrease the intensity of acute vertigo or nystagmus. They are not to be used for general imbalance or disequilibrium that can be associated with advanced

Table 16.1 Vestibular suppressants

Antihistamine	Dose	Onset of action (minutes)	Peak (hours)	Half-life (hours)
Meclizine	25–50 mg every 4–6 hours	60	Unknown	4–6
Dimenhydrinate	50 mg every 4–6 hours	15–60	1–2	Unknown
Benzodiazepines				
Lorazepam	0.5–1 mg BID	15–60	1–6	10–20
Clonazepam	0.5 mg BID	20–60	1–2	20–50
Diazepam	2–4 mg BID	30–60	1–2	20–50

Reference: Furman JM, Cass SP, Whitney S. Vestibular disorders: a case-study approach. 3rd ed. Oxford University Press, New York, 2010

Meniere's disease in older people, as suppressing the vestibular system will only magnify these symptoms. The chronic use of vestibular suppressants is not appropriate since these medications do not affect the formation of endolymphatic hydrops or reduce the frequency of vertiginous episodes in Meniere's disease. Furthermore, vestibular suppressants delay the adaptive mechanisms that function to reduce any residual vestibular imbalance following an acute episode of vertigo.

Nausea and vomiting are often associated with acute Meniere's attacks and can lead to dehydration and weakness. Antiemetics should be prescribed for the patient to have on hand in addition to vestibular suppressants. Common medications are rapidly dissolving ondansetron and rectal promethazine to mitigate the chance of vomiting the medication. Standard dose for rapidly dissolving ondansetron is 4 mg every 8 hours. Onset of action is within minutes and is typically well tolerated. There is a concern for prolonged QT syndrome and serotonin syndrome with high doses. The standard dose for a promethazine suppository is 12.5–25 mg every 6 hours, and side effects include sedation and anticholinergic effects.

Oral Corticosteroids

The mechanism of action of steroids on the inner ear is not well understood, but these medications decrease damage from an inflammatory response, regardless of the etiology. Oral corticosteroids are often used for symptom exacerbations, though this is done based primarily on expert opinion because evidence of benefit is limited. Short-term treatment protocols vary, using either oral decadron, methyprednisolone, or prednisone for several days up to 2 weeks. Longer-term treatment protocols are sometimes used when immune-related inner ear disease is suspected. Use of oral steroids is based on expert opinion, as no clinical trials have been performed.

Migraine

Migraine has been suggested as an associated factor in Meniere's disease since Prosper Meniere first described the condition in 1861. The pathophysiology of the relationship between the two has yet to be established; however, several studies have shown the higher incidence of migraine in patients with Meniere's disease compared to the normal population [14, 15]. We see this frequently at our institution and initiate migraine treatment early on.

The first line of treatment is conservative with avoidance of common migraine triggers, dietary changes, and dietary supplementation. These measures should be trialed for at least 4–6 weeks. Common triggers include hormonal changes, sleep deprivation, stress, visual motion, and barometric pressure changes. Common dietary triggers include monosodium glutamate (MSG), tyramine, and phenylethylamine. Supplements recommended by the American Academy of Neurology and the American Headache Society are magnesium (600 mg daily), riboflavin (400 mg daily), and feverfew (50–300 mg twice daily) with level B evidence and Coenzyme Q10 (100 mg three times daily) with level C evidence [16].

When conservative measures fail to reduce vertigo spells in patients with migraine and Meniere's disease, migraine prophylaxis should be considered. Common prophylactic medications include amitriptyline, verapamil, propranolol, and topiramate. We often see that patients with migraine experience medication side effects with higher intensity and frequency than in patients without migraine. For this reason, we will often start migraine prophylaxis at sub-therapeutic levels and gradually increase the medication based on the patient's tolerability. Patients should remain on each medication at optimal dose for at least 4–6 weeks before the trial is complete to accurately assess response. If no benefit is noted, medication should be gradually weaned off. For partial response, increased dosing or addition of another migraine prevention medication should be considered. If patients fail to show a response with a trial of each of these medications, we recommend a neurology referral.

Allergy Treatment

Allergy has been associated with symptoms of Meniere's disease beginning with the observations of Duke in 1923 [17]. Throughout the intervening decades, several observers noted in case reports the role that both inhalant and food allergy can play in patients with hearing loss, tinnitus, aural fullness, and dizziness. The observed role of allergy in Meniere's disease has been strikingly demonstrated by Viscomi, who demonstrated significant changes in ECOG SP/AP ratios in five patients given a food provocation allergen challenge [18]. The ECoG changes also correlated with skin wheal reaction and subjective symptoms.

Several outcome studies of allergy treatment of Meniere's disease are also available. Outcome studies by their nature are uncontrolled, non-placebo studies, but can provide insight into the question at hand. In the 1970s both Powers and Shaver reported that 32% of their patients with Meniere's disease responded to allergy treatment for vertigo or fluctuating hearing loss due to Meniere's disease [19, 20]. In 2000, Derebery reported favorable outcomes of allergy treatment with 82% feeling better subjectively, 48% with vertigo absent or substantially improved, and 61% with hearing stable or improved [21].

The prevalence of allergy in Meniere's disease may be greater than in comparison controls. Derebery reported that the prevalence of air-borne and food allergy in patients with Meniere's disease (42% reported known airborne allergy and 27% reported known food allergy) was greater than control patients [22]. Keles measured cytokine profiles, allergic parameters, and lymphocyte subgroups in Meniere's disease patients and a matched control group of healthy volunteers (N = 92) [23]. They found a history of allergy in 31/46 (67%) of Meniere patients and 16/46 (35%) in the control group. Elevated total IgE levels were found in 41% of Meniere patients and in 20% of the control group.

In summary, there is a long history of a suspected connection between Meniere's disease and allergy. Most evidence of a connection is clinical observations and uncontrolled case series, and scientifically robust evidence is not available. Basic science information regarding immunology of the inner ear is supportive, but pathophysiology remains unknown. Nevertheless, allergy evaluation and treatment should be considered whenever there is a suspected relationship between ingestion of a particular food and seasonal variation of symptoms in a patient with a known history of allergy.

Vestibular Physical Therapy

Vestibular physical therapy is a specialized exercise-based intervention for management of dizziness and imbalance. In patients with peripheral vestibular disorders such as Meniere's, vestibular physical therapy seeks to adapt to vestibular insult via vestibular ocular reflex (VOR) adaptation, habituation, and substitution. VOR adaptation exercise produces retinal slip through eye/head exercises, which involve moving the head while focusing on a stationary target. Habituation exercises focus on exposure by and desensitization to provoking stimuli. Substitution involves other eye movements (saccade modification or enhancing smooth pursuit) to effectively cancel the vestibular deficit and prevent the patient from perceiving smeared retinal images during head movements. Vestibular exercises have demonstrated efficacy in fall reduction, improved balance, decreased dizziness, and improved quality of life in patients with unilateral peripheral vestibular dysfunction [24]. However, this trend does not persist when isolated to Meniere's disease, which can be attributed to the fluctuating nature of the disease in its early stages [25]. Guidelines for use of vestibular physical therapy in patients with peripheral hypofunction (typically patients with advanced Meniere's disease) are available [26].

Hearing Loss and Tinnitus Management

As Meniere's disease progresses, functional hearing including pure tone thresholds and word recognition declines. End-stage Meniere's is associated with a flat, severe sensorineural hearing loss around 60–70 dB with fair to poor word recognition. Hearing aids can be difficult to fit a fluctuating loss, though patients who have preserved word recognition can adjust the hearing aid as needed. For a flat loss at end stage of Meniere's disease, a Contralateral Routing of Signals (CROS) aid may provide the best benefit, as poor word recognition typically prevents any benefit from a traditional hearing aid.

In addition to hearing loss, many patients experience tinnitus. Given the heterogeneous nature, varying emotional response, and the uncertainty of the neural basis for tinnitus, patient-specific treatment remains challenging; however, the goal of therapy is to reduce the tinnitus sound and emotional distress associated with it. Sound therapy options include hearing amplification, tinnitus maskers, and white noise generators. Other treatments include counseling, cognitive behavioral therapy, and mindfulness-based stress reduction [27].

References

1. Lopez-Escamez JA, Carey J, Chung WH, Goebel JA, Magnusson M, Mandalà M, Newman-Toker DE, Strupp M, Suzuki M, Trabalzini F, Bisdorff A. Diagnostic criteria for Menière's disease. J Vestib Res. 2015;25(1):1–7.
2. Palaskas C, Dobie R, Snyder J. Progression of hearing loss in bilateral Meniere's disease. Laryngoscope. 1988;98:287–90.
3. Foster CA, Breeze RE. Endolymphatic hydrops in Ménière's disease: cause, consequence, or epiphenomenon? Otol Neurotol. 2013;34(7):1210–4.
4. Nevoux J, Franco-Vidal V, Bouccara D, Parietti-Winkler C, Uziel A, Chays A, Dubernard X, Couloigner V, Darrouzet V, Mom T, Groupe de Travail de la SFORL. Diagnostic and therapeutic strategy in Menière's disease. Guidelines of the French Otorhinolaryngology-Head and Neck Surgery Society (SFORL). Eur Ann Otorhinolaryngol Head Neck Dis. 2017;134(6):441–4.
5. Furstenberg A, Lashmet F, Lathrop F. Meniere's symptom complex: medical treatment. Ann Otol Rhinol Laryngol. 1934;43:1035–46.
6. Fustenberg A, Richardson G, Lathrop F. Meniere's disease. Arch Otolaryngol Head Neck Surg. 1941;34:1083–92.
7. Boles R, Rice D, Hybels R, Work W. Conservative management of Meniere's disease: Furstenberg regimen revisited. Ann Otol Rhinol Laryngol. 1975;84:513–7.
8. Klockhoff I, Lindblom U. Meniere's disease and hydrocholorothiazide- a critical analysis of symptoms and therapeutic effects. Acta Otolaryngol. 1967;63:347–65.
9. Corvera J, Corvera G. Long-term Effect of acetazolamide and chlorthalidone on the hearing loss of Meniere's disease. Am J Otol. 1989;10:142–5.
10. Crowson MG, Patki A, Tucci DL. A systematic review of diuretics in the medical management of Meniere's disease. Otolaryngol Head Neck Surg. 2016;154(5):824–34.
11. Thirlwall AS, Kundu S. Diuretics for Ménière's disease or syndrome. Cochrane Database Syst Rev. 2006;3:CD003599.
12. James A, Burton MJ. Betahistine for Ménière's disease or syndrome. Cochrane Database Syst Rev. 2001;2001(1):CD001873.

13. Adrion C, Fischer CS, Wagner J, Gürkov R, Mansmann U, Strupp M, BEMED Study Group. Efficacy and safety of betahistine treatment in patients with Meniere's disease: primary results of a long term, multicentre, double blind, randomised, placebo controlled, dose defining trial (BEMED trial). BMJ. 2016;352
14. Neff BA, Staab JP, Eggers SD, Carlson ML, Schmitt WR, Van Abel KM, Worthington DK, Beatty CW, Driscoll CL, Shepard NT. Auditory and vestibular symptoms and chronic subjective dizziness in patients with Ménière's disease, vestibular migraine, and Ménière's disease with concomitant vestibular migraine. Otol Neurotol. 2012;33(7):1235–44.
15. Radtke A, Lempert T, Gresty MA, Brookes GB, Bronstein AM, Neuhauser H. Migraine and Ménière's disease: is there a link? Neurology. 2002;59(11):1700–4.
16. Loder E, Burch R, Rizzoli P. The 2012 AHS/AAN guidelines for prevention of episodic migraine: a summary and comparison with other recent clinical practice guidelines. Headache. 2012;52(6):930–45.
17. Duke WW. Meniere's syndrome caused by allergy. J AMA. 1923;
18. Viscomi GJ, Bojrab DI. Use of electrocochleography to monitor antigenic challenge in Meniere's disease. Otolaryngol Head Neck Surg. 1992;107(6):733–7.
19. Powers WH. Allergic factors in Meniere's disease. Trans Am Acad Opthalmol Otolaryngol. 1973;77:22–9.
20. Shaver EF Jr. Allergic management of Meniere's disease. Arch Oto. 1975;101(2):96–9.
21. Derebery MJ. Allergic management of Meniere's disease: an outcome study. Oto Head Neck Surg. 2000;122(2):174–82.
22. Derebery MJ, Berliner KI. Prevalence of allergy in Meniere's disease. Oto Head Neck Surg. 2000;123:69–75.
23. Keles E, Godekmerdan A, Kalidag T, Kaygusuz I, Yalcin S, Cengiz AH, Aral M. Meniere's disease and allergy: allergens and cytokines. J Laryngol Otol. 2004;118(9):688–93.
24. Hillier SL, McDonnell M. Vestibular rehabilitation for unilateral peripheral vestibular dysfunction. In: Cochrane Database Syst Rev, vol. 2; 2011.
25. van Esch BF, van der Scheer-Horst ES, van der Zaag-Loonen HJ, Bruintjes TD, van Benthem PP. The effect of vestibular rehabilitation in patients with Ménière's disease. Otolaryngol Head Neck Surg. 2017;156(3):426–34.
26. Hall CD, Herdman SJ, Whitney SL, Cass SP, Clendaniel RA, Fife T, Furman JM, Goebel J, Shepard NA, Woodhouse S. Vestibular rehabilitation for peripheral vestibular hypofunction: clinical practice guidelines. J Neurol Phys Ther. 2016;4:118–77.
27. Arif M, Sadlier M, Rajenderkumar D, James J, Tahir T. A randomised controlled study of mindfulness meditation versus relaxation therapy in the management of tinnitus. J Laryngol Otol. 2017;131(6):501–7.

Chapter 17
Surgical Treatment of Meniere's Disease

Neal M. Jackson and Michael J. LaRouere

Introduction

Meniere's disease was first described by Prosper Meniere in 1861 [1]. The classic disease description includes the tetrad of hearing loss, tinnitus, aural fullness, and vertigo spells. The disease tends to fluctuate and can be said to be predictably unpredictable. The spells can last from minutes to hours. Attacks can be associated with nausea, vomiting, headache, and fatigue. Medical management is sufficient for a majority of patients, but those who are recalcitrant may be a candidate for surgical intervention. Currently, a variety of surgical techniques are employed for patients with Meniere's disease who have failed medical treatment.

Historical Perspective/Evolution of Surgical Technique

The first surgery for Meniere's disease was vestibular nerve section which was popularized by neurosurgeon Walter Dandy [2, 3]. The transmastoid labyrinthectomy to remove the neuroepithelium of one side of the vestibular system was described in 1904 by Lake and came into fashion for otologists in the 1940s thanks to Cawthorne's influential endorsement of the procedure [4, 5]. Transmastoid endolymphatic sac decompression was described in the 1920s by Portmann and popularized in the 1960s [6, 7].

N. M. Jackson (✉)
Departments of Otolaryngology & Neurosurgery, Tulane University School of Medicine, New Orleans, LA, USA

M. J. LaRouere
Department of Otology and Neurotology, Michigan Ear Institute, Farmington Hills, MI, USA

St. John Providence Hospital, Novi, MI, USA

J. C. Lucas et al. (eds.), *Diagnosis and Treatment of Vestibular Disorders*,
https://doi.org/10.1007/978-3-032-11740-3_17

Approaches to the vestibular nerve in the internal auditory canal (IAC) and cerebellopontine angle (CPA) such as the translabyrinthine approach and the retrolabyrinthine approach became popular in the 1980s. The development of a retrosigmoid approach to the vestibular nerve became preferred due to lower cerebrospinal fluid (CSF) leak rates and better facial nerve outcomes.

The middle cranial fossa craniotomy approach for vestibular nerve section has been described but now is used much less due to a higher risk of facial nerve injury compared to other approaches. It does, however, offer the only approach that allows individual sectioning of either the inferior or superior vestibular nerve before they join to form the common vestibular nerve.

A cochleosacculotomy/labyrinthotomy has also been described as a transcanal technique which can be performed under local anesthesia. After lifting a tympanomeatal flap, the round window is entered with a pick with the goal of fracturing the osseous spiral lamina and cochlear duct. This results in complete loss of hearing in the ear [8]. This technique is not performed at our institution. We will focus this chapter on the techniques currently in use at our institution in the sections below.

Clinical Evaluation

The basic pathophysiology of Meniere's disease is postulated to be endolymphatic hydrops, causing high fluid pressure in the inner ear endolymph. Multiple etiologic theories have been proposed, and thus far, the exact pathophysiologic mechanism has remained elusive. Surgical techniques aimed at treating Meniere's disease work to either reduce pressure in the endolymphatic sac or to destroy the function of the vestibular apparatus completely.

Clinical evaluation includes pure tone audiometry which classically shows a low-frequency sensorineural hearing loss which may later involve the high frequencies. Repeated audiograms may show fluctuation and possibly even normalization of this low-frequency loss once the patient has been optimized. Videonystagmography (VNG) may show vestibular hypofunction or hyperfunction depending on when the test is obtained. Electrocochleography (ECOG) can be used to compare the summating potential (SP) to the action potential (AP), and if this SP/AP ratio exceeds 50%, then it is suggestive of Meniere's disease [9]. While ECOG does have good sensitivity, the specificity is poor, so the clinician must be wary of false negatives.

The differential diagnosis may include acoustic neuroma, benign positional vertigo, migraine-associated vertigo, endolymphatic sac tumor, autoimmune inner ear disease, and Lyme disease. It is important to rule out other diagnoses, especially when considering a surgical intervention for Meniere's disease.

As discussed in the previous chapter, the mainstay of treatment is medical. Preventive measures include avoiding dietary exacerbations (salt, caffeine), avoiding stress, and promoting adequate sleep. Pharmacologic interventions to lower the frequency and intensity of a Meniere's attack include diuretic therapy (triamterene-hydrochlorothiazide/Dyazide, furosemide/Lasix, etc.). Oral steroids have been shown to reduce the frequency of vertigo attacks and improve hearing in Meniere's disease patients; however, their effect is not long-lasting [10].

While a majority of patients do respond to lifestyle modifications and medical therapy, there are some patients who continue to face life-threatening or debilitating vertigo attacks as well as extremely bothersome ringing, fullness, and hearing loss. These patients who fail to respond to medical therapy are candidates for a more aggressive treatment such as surgical intervention.

Many factors go into the decision to pursue surgical treatment for Meniere's disease. Some are the frequency and severity of the Meniere's episodes, the patient's age and overall health, the hearing and vestibular status of both ears, and the patient's occupation. It is also essential to confirm the laterality of the problematic ear. The status of the contralateral ear must be taken into account, especially if a vestibular ablative technique is being considered, as up to 40% of patients with Meniere's disease develop it bilaterally [11].

Surgical intervention for Meniere's disease can be divided into two categories: vestibular preservation techniques (intratympanic steroid perfusion and endolymphatic sac decompression) and vestibular ablation techniques (intratympanic gentamicin perfusion, intramuscular streptomycin, labyrinthectomy, and vestibular nerve section via middle cranial fossa, translabyrinthine, retrolabyrinthine, or retrosigmoid approach). Of note, labyrinthectomy and translabyrinthine vestibular nerve section permanently destroy the hearing in the operated side.

Vestibular Preservation Techniques

Intratympanic Steroid Perfusion

One of the simplest invasive procedures is intratympanic/transtympanic injection of steroid. The goal is to place a steroid solution in the middle ear around the round window so that the medication may be absorbed into the inner ear and reduce inflammation within the inner ear [12]. There is evidence to show that intratympanic administration yields much higher concentrations of steroid in the labyrinth when compared to systemic administration [13, 14].

Intratympanic steroid perfusion has been shown to be effective in the treatment of symptoms in Meniere's disease [15]. In our institution, patients who are familiar with their disease will often know that their baseline for vertigo attacks has been recently lowered due to stress, environmental changes (e.g., aeroallergens), and medical metabolic issues. These patients may be effectively treated with oral steroids or intratympanic steroids. Patients with Meniere's disease who experience a sudden drop in hearing are also offered intratympanic steroids. We have found that the hearing drop associated with Meniere's disease appears to respond quite well to IT steroid therapy.

Patients who do not tolerate systemic steroids, including diabetic patients or others, may prefer a steroid injection as the risk of hyperglycemia and other side effects is much lower. All patients treated with intratympanic steroids must remain on continued medical management (salt avoidance, caffeine limitation, diuretic therapy, etc.). Injections may need to be repeated on an as-needed basis.

This procedure can easily be performed in the office with use of a microscope and 27 g needle. A typical agent is 10–24 mg/ml of dexamethasone.

Technique

With the patient in a reclined position in the examination chair, the microscope is used to visualize the tympanic membrane. A small area of the tympanic membrane is anesthetized with a minimal amount of topical phenol. The area of the drum should blanch white almost immediately, and this indicates that anesthesia has been achieved. A 27-gauge spinal needle is used due to its length to penetrate into the middle ear space and its small caliber size to minimize the chance of a long-term perforation. Approximately 0.2–0.5 cc of the steroid solution is infiltrated. The surgeon should see the fluid level rise within the middle ear space as the solution is injected. The patient is asked to lie in this turned position and not swallow or speak to minimize the Eustachian tube opening for 30 minutes.

The possible complications of the procedure are tympanic membrane perforation from insertion of the spinal needle, possible infection, and transient sensation of vertigo due to caloric stimulation of the room temperature steroid solution filling the middle ear space. It is not uncommon to repeat injections if symptoms of vertigo and hearing loss return.

Endolymphatic Sac Decompression Surgery

Surgery of the endolymphatic sac is done to reduce the endolymphatic pressure within the endolymphatic sac and the rest of the system. The objective of an endolymphatic sac decompression (ESD) is to remove the bony covering on the lateral aspect of the endolymphatic sac, which in theory allows the endolymphatic sac to expand more freely. Additionally, manipulation of the sac intraoperatively may, through hydraulic action, free sludge or loose otoconia from the endolymphatic duct. An alternative to simple sac decompression is to open the endolymphatic sac and insert a shunt into the endolymphatic sac and allow drainage of excess endolymph into the mastoid or subarachnoid space [7]. This procedure does not destroy the hearing in the operated ear. While the symptoms of hearing loss, tinnitus, and aural fullness may be improved, the main goal of patients who elect to have the procedure is to reduce the frequency and intensity of the vertigo attacks while not destroying the hearing. Patients will still be vulnerable to Meniere's attacks in the operated ear and need to continue lifestyle modifications and medical therapy.

Endolymphatic sac decompression surgery was first described in 1926 by Portmann and since then has been met with both endorsement and skepticism [6]. Part of the skepticism stems from a report in 1981 by Thomsen and colleagues who compared endolymphatic sac decompression with sham mastoidectomy surgery and concluded that the two procedures were equivalent [16]. In 1989, Glasscock and colleagues stopped using sac decompression due to a low rate of vertigo control [17]. However, at some other institutions, including ours, we have seen impressive results. Pillsbury et al. published in 1983 an alternative analysis of Thomsen's sham study in which 71% of the decompression patients improved and only 47% of the placebo group improved [18]. Welling and Nagaraja also re-evaluated the data of the Thomsen sham study and determined that endolymphatic sac surgery is effective [19]. A 1993 study by Telischi and Luxford found that 80% of patients who undergo endolymphatic sac decompression never required more aggressive procedures and 93% reported little to no dizziness subsequently [20].

Endolymphatic sac surgery can be either a simple decompression to remove the bony covering over the sac or it can include placement of a shunt from the sac either into the mastoid or into the subarachnoid space. Our preference is a simple decompression, as opening the sac has been associated with sensorineural hearing loss in up to 4% of our patients. In a study by Kato et al., 87% of patients reported significant improvement in QOL after decompression without shunting [21]. In a recent systematic review, sac decompression and mastoid shunt surgery were both effective in controlling vertigo in at least 75% of patients who failed medical management. It was noted that mastoid shunt with the use of silastic sheeting was associated with a greater risk of hearing loss than mastoid shunt without the use of silastic sheeting [22].

If patients improve after sac surgery and years later redevelop symptoms in the same ear, one option to consider is revision sac decompression surgery [23]. The most common finding at the time of revision surgery is a small but significant amount of bony regrowth over the sac, which can be removed using standard microsurgical techniques discussed below [24]. The surgeon must be meticulous to dissect scar tissue and bony regrowth over the endolymphatic sac while trying to leave surrounding dura intact. At our institute, we have found that if patients redevelop symptoms within two years of the original sac decompression, revision surgery has been unlikely to control symptoms. However, if symptoms recur greater than two years after the original operation, then revision surgery can be effective in controlling the vertigo spells.

Technique

An endolymphatic sac decompression is essentially a decompression of a portion of the pre-sigmoid posterior fossa dura. Facial nerve monitoring is universally employed at our institution. This decompression is accomplished by a standard postauricular incision and periosteal dissection down to mastoid cortex. No ear canal incisions or tympanomeatal flap needs to be raised as the dissection is completely postauricular. A standard cortical mastoidectomy using 6 and 4 cutting burrs is executed. Particular focus is made on identification of the sigmoid sinus, lateral and posterior semicircular canals, and posterior bony ear canal wall. The sigmoid sinus is decompressed inferiorly towards the jugular bulb. The bony ear canal does not need to be excessively thinned. Once the bony horizontal and posterior semicircular canals are identified, the surgeon's mental conceptualization of Donaldson's line (posterior from the horizontal canal and perpendicular to the posterior semicircular canal) is useful to approximate the likely location of the endolymphatic sac, which is always inferior to this imaginary line.

The retrofacial air cells are drilled away, and the presigmoid dura is decompressed with a diamond burr. It is our practice to remove bone over the sigmoid sinus and over the presigmoid dura. Using a high-speed drill with either a 5 or 3 diamond burr and "flicking" off bone with otologic instruments such as a Freer and a Gimmick, the last layer of bone is then removed. This dissection proceeds in a lateral to medial direction (from the sigmoid sinus towards the sac). It is important to identify the bony posterior semicircular canal as it can have an irregular position in the temporal bone. Entering into it with a drill could result in complete and permanent hearing loss in the ear. The endolymphatic sac is a duplication of the posterior fossa dura and thus appears and feels more dense than the surrounding posterior fossa dura. A crossed striped pattern due to increased vascularity is many times seen. Once the bone over and around the sac has been removed, the decompression is complete (see Fig. 17.1). The wound is irrigated with saline solution to remove

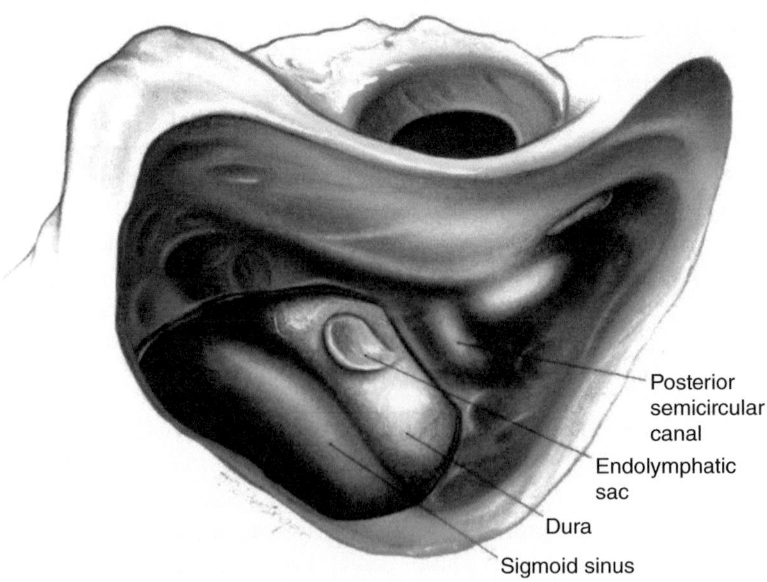

Fig. 17.1 Endolymphatic sac depicted in a left ear between the sigmoid sinus and posterior semicircular canal

bone dust, and the layers of soft tissue and skin are closed in the surgeon's standard fashion after mastoidectomy.

A variation of this procedure is to incise the sac with microinstruments and place a small permanent drainage tube into the sac to allow egress of excessive endolymph into either the subarachnoid space or the mastoid. Because of the increased risk of sensorineural hearing loss and possible fibroproliferative response, we do not open the endolymphatic sac at our institution.

Vestibular Ablative Techniques

Vestibular ablative techniques are indicated in patients who have failed medical management and vestibular preservation techniques. The goal of vestibular ablative techniques in Meniere's disease is to destroy all remaining vestibular function in the diseased ear. These procedures include vestibular nerve section and labyrinthectomy. In recent years, intratympanic injection of gentamicin has been used to either partially or totally destroy vestibular function in the diseased ear.

Although all vestibular ablation techniques destroy vestibular function, some (vestibular nerve section and intratympanic gentamicin) preserve hearing, while others (labyrinthectomy) destroy all remaining hearing in the operated ear. Thus, it is important to analyze both hearing status and vestibular status in both ears prior to proceeding with ablative techniques.

Intratympanic Gentamicin Perfusion

Intratympanic injection of an aminoglycoside can be performed to destroy vestibular function. Also known as a chemical labyrinthectomy, this technique generally uses clinically available gentamicin as it is the most vestibulotoxic aminoglycoside. The drug must reach the inner ear via intratympanic injection, tympanostomy tube, or microwick. At our institution, we prefer intratympanic injection.

Systemic administration of a related aminoglycoside, streptomycin, was first described in 1948 by Fowler [25]. Among the aminoglycosides, streptomycin and gentamicin have been the most studied for their ototoxicity. Gentamicin is preferred for clinical use for its preferential vestibulotoxicity and commercial availability. Several mechanisms explain the toxicity of aminoglycosides to the inner ear hair cells including (1) competitive inhibition of the calcium ion binding on calcium-receptor dependent plasma membrane transport channels, (2) accumulation in the hair cells by irreversibly entering through one-way channels in the cell membrane, (3) reducing the integrity of the hair cell plasma membrane, and (4) disruption of downstream intracellular messengers [26–28].

Use of ototoxic aminoglycoside therapy has evolved considerably since its introduction. In the 1950s, Schuknecht utilized high-dose streptomycin to treat Meniere's

[29]. In the 1980s, Graham and colleagues introduced titration of streptomycin therapy for bilateral Meniere's disease [30]. In 1991, Magnusson and Padoan described a rationale for low-dose intratympanic gentamicin [31]. Nedzelski et al. reported in 1993 that installation of gentamicin could lead to vertigo control in 83% of patients. In the study, in patients who had complete ablation of the vestibular system, there was over a 25% rate of sensorineural hearing loss, with 10% being profound in nature. Patients with normal hearing had a very low risk (5%) of hearing loss after treatment. However, about 30% patients with preexisting sensorineural hearing loss experienced a worsening loss after treatment [32].

There also seems to exist a small portion of patients who experience hearing loss after one treatment. This may be due to limited outer hair cell reserve as well as a mutation in a 12S ribosomal RNA [33]. It is therefore important to warn all patients of the potential risk of hearing loss with gentamicin injection.

There is no defined best protocol for administration of gentamicin. There are various successful methods that vary in treatment frequency, drug dosage, and clinical treatment endpoint criteria (e.g., total loss of caloric response on VNG, initiation of sensorineural hearing loss, or abatement of symptoms). A common practice today with gentamicin injection is serial low-dose injections every 2–4 weeks until vestibular symptoms abate or sensorineural hearing loss develops.

It is important to know that the vestibulotoxic effects of gentamicin are cumulative; thus, patients need to understand they may need multiple treatments. Also, the effects are not immediate but may take 3–5 days. Patients will report subjective dizziness as the vestibular injury occurs. Vestibular rehabilitation therapy can be effective in aiding in compensation.

Our technique for gentamicin injection is similar to the technique described above for steroid injection. With the patient in the supine position in the examination chair, the eardrum is visualized with the microscope, and a minimal amount of phenol is used to achieve anesthesia of the eardrum. Using a 27-gauge needle, 0.2–0.5 cc of a buffered 27.5 mg/mL gentamicin solution is injected into the middle ear space just superior to the round window. The patient is asked to stay in this position and not speak or swallow for the next 30 minutes to minimize drug loss into the Eustachian tube.

Intratympanic gentamicin administration can be repeated on a serial basis to gradually reduce vestibular function in the diseased ear. It is prudent to obtain pure tone audiometry to identify the occurrence of sensorineural hearing loss, as this may affect the decision to perform additional gentamicin treatments.

In Minor's protocol using transtympanic injection of gentamicin 40 mg/mL buffered with sodium bicarbonate to a final concentration of 26.7 mg/mL, over 90% of patients reported complete or substantial improvement in vertigo control. Hearing outcomes revealed 36% of patients saw improved hearing, 32% stayed the same, and 32% experienced a worsening of hearing. Three percent had profound sensorineural hearing loss (SNHL) [34].

Nedzelski et al. administered gentamicin 26.7 mg/mL via a tympanostomy tube with catheter three times per day over a four-day period. They reported over 90% complete or substantial improvement in vertigo. Hearing outcomes revealed that 26% improved, 51% were unchanged, and 25% worsened. Overall 16% experienced a profound SNHL [35].

Because of the risk of hearing loss, we prefer to offer endolymphatic sac decompression over gentamicin injection as our initial treatment of Meniere's disease in patients who have failed maximal medical treatment.

Vestibular Nerve Section/Vestibular Neurectomy

Vestibular nerve section has been the time-tested procedure that provides relief from vertigo attacks for Meniere's disease patients with good hearing. This technique requires a craniotomy, which offers the ability to access and transect the vestibular nerve between the labyrinth and the brainstem.

The evolution of vestibular nerve section has been fascinating. The first surgeon to perform regular transection of the cochleovestibular nerve and then selective vestibular nerve section was Walter Dandy, who performed over 600 procedures via a retrosigmoid approach in the 1930s–1940s [36, 37]. However, this was prior to the introduction of the surgical microscope, and the risk of facial nerve injury was 10%.

With the advent of the field of neurotology, a middle cranial fossa approach was developed [38]. Due to a higher risk of facial nerve injury and sensorineural hearing loss, the retrolabyrinthine approach was adopted [39]. Each approach had excellent vertigo control rates (over 90%). However, drawbacks to the retrolabyrinthine approach were found. These included a high rate of CSF leak and occasional difficulty with access due to a contracted mastoid. This led to the retrosigmoid approach being adopted as the most preferred method of vestibular nerve section in unilateral Meniere's disease. Vertigo control rates are excellent (96–97%) [40–43].

Complications of this procedure are low and include facial weakness (1%), hearing loss (1%), CSF leak (<5%), and headaches (10%). To minimize headaches, either fat or artificial bone is placed between the skin and the dura at closure [43–46].

Technique

Vestibular nerve section (VNS) is performed in conjunction with a neurosurgeon. The patient is positioned supine, and the head is turned away in the standard otologic position. Standard lateral skull base perioperative steps include facial nerve monitoring, lowering of $PaCO_2$, and administration of mannitol.

A standard curvilinear retrosigmoid incision is made behind the auricle and centered at the height of the root of the zygoma. Soft tissue dissection is performed down to the galea and attachments of the splenius capitus and sternocleidomastoid muscles. The root of the zygoma is an approximation for the level of the transverse sinus and take-off of the sigmoid sinus. The bone in this retrosigmoid area is exposed, and soft tissue is held by self-retainers. The bone around the sigmoid and lateral sinus is drilled away using a large cutting burr, followed by diamond burrs and ample irrigation. The surgeon may choose to perform a craniotomy with a retrosigmoid bone flap or a craniectomy with complete removal of the retrosigmoid bone.

Some otologic surgeons prefer to drill away some of the pre-sigmoid mastoid air cells to assist in identification of the sigmoid sinus before drilling retrosigmoid. If this is done, it is important to bone wax these air cells to prevent CSF leak. Others perform drilling only posterior to the sigmoid sinus with careful drilling techniques to avoid damage to the sinuses. Large diamond burrs are used around the sinuses to avoid injury.

The dura is incised about 1 cm posterior to the sigmoid sinus and about 1 cm inferior to the lateral sinus in a curvilinear fashion to allow egress of clear CSF and relaxation of the intracranial contents. The arachnoid is opened deeper and followed along the petrous dura to the suprameatal tubercle and then to the vestibulocochlear complex which lies between the brainstem and porous acousticus. Facial nerve stimulation is useful in confirmation of facial nerve position deep to the cochleovestibular complex. Gentle separation of the cochlear (inferior) and vestibular (superior) fibers is performed using a small probe in a motion parallel to the nerve. Many times there is a small blood vessel at the separation point. It is paramount to realize that vestibular nerve fibers are anatomically superior, the cochlear fibers are inferior, and the facial nerve fibers are "deep" out of the surgeon's view. Once the separation of cochlear and vestibular fibers is accomplished, the vestibular nerve is transected using microscissors (see Fig. 17.2).

Another technique of VNS is that of a translabyrinthine VNS. This involves a labyrinthectomy (described later) followed by opening of the internal auditory canal (IAC) and transecting the entire eighth nerve. In our experience, we have not found the results of the procedure to exceed those of a standard transmastoid labyrinthectomy. In addition, there is an added risk of CSF leak compared to a standard labyrinthectomy. However, some surgeons have found that tinnitus control rates may be better with a translabyrinthine VNS [47].

Labyrinthectomy

The most definitive procedure for the treatment of Meniere's disease is a labyrinthectomy, which destroys the inner ear and therefore prevents the patient from ever having Meniere's spells in that ear again. Patients with poor hearing who have

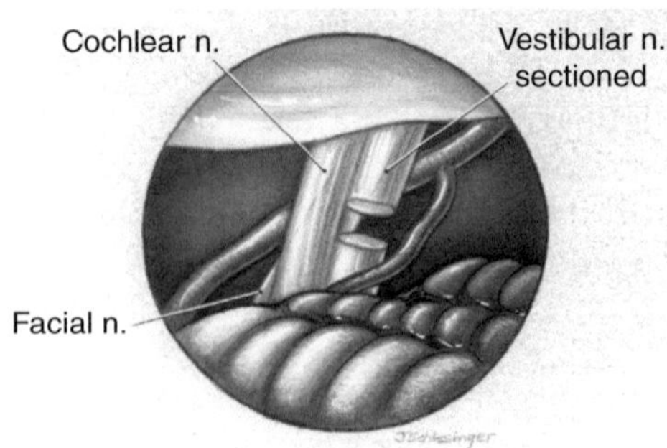

Fig. 17.2 Vestibular nerve section as seen through an endoscopic retrosigmoid approach. The facial nerve is seen deep to the cochlear and vestibular nerves

unilateral Meniere's disease with disabling symptoms are considered ideal candidates. The procedure is effective because it removes the neuroepithelium on one side of the vestibular system. Control of vertigo has been reported to be as high as 99% following transmastoid labyrinthectomy and over 90% following transcanal labyrinthectomy [48–50].

One of the downsides of labyrinthectomy is the loss of natural hearing in the operated ear. However, there are hearing rehabilitation options, including a contralateral routing of sound (CROS) hearing aid or a bone-anchored hearing aid (BAHA). Recently, some authors have been advocating for the role of concomitant labyrinthectomy and cochlear implantation (CI) in some patients with intractable Meniere's disease [51, 52].

Transcanal labyrinthectomy can be performed under local anesthesia. After the tympanomeatal flap is raised, the middle ear is evaluated, and landmarks such as horizontal segment of facial nerve, entire stapes footplate, and round window niche are identified. After cutting the stapedial tendon, the stapes and incus are removed. A drill is used to expose the vestibule by drilling between the oval and round windows. A right-angle hook can be used to remove the neuroepithelium from the ampullae of the semicircular canals. The contents of the utricle and saccule are removed. Gentamicin-soaked pledgets are placed in the labyrinth at the conclusion of the procedure because of the risk of retained neuroepithelium.

The major benefit of a transcanal labyrinthectomy (as opposed to the transmastoid labyrinthectomy) is that it can be performed swiftly and under local anesthesia with mild sedation. Thus, in the elderly or infirmed patient, the technique has appeal. Elimination of vertigo spells has been reported to be over 90% [48].

Transmastoid labyrinthectomy offers Meniere's disease patients the best control of vertigo symptoms (99%). As mentioned, there is complete loss of hearing in the operated ear, and thus the procedure is usually used for patients with poor hearing in the diseased ear. The advantage of a transmastoid labyrinthectomy is that all the vestibular neuroepithelium can be removed from all five areas of the labyrinth (three ampullated ends of the semicircular canals, saccule, and utricle) under direct vision. Vestibular compensation, which generally takes 1–2 months, is usually excellent.

Technique

Under general anesthesia, the ear is prepped in the standard fashion with facial nerve monitoring employed. A standard postauricular incision is made. Soft tissue dissection is performed to expose the temporalis fascia and periosteal tissue. Periosteal incisions are made in "T" or "7" configuration from the temporal line to the mastoid tip. Next, a standard mastoidectomy technique is employed, starting with a large cutting burr and large suction-irrigator. The goals of initial dissection are identification of tegmen tympani, posterior ear canal wall, and sigmoid sinus. The next areas to be identified are the antrum, horizontal semicircular canal, the incus in the epitympanum, and second genu of facial nerve (confirmed by using a facial nerve monitor with dissecting stimulator). Once the bony labyrinth has been exposed, there are different techniques for dissection. We prefer to initiate dissection of the superior half of the horizontal semicircular canal such that the lumen is encountered and the inferior portion of the canal is left to protect the facial nerve which is inferior. The arc of the superior canal is then exposed and can be followed to its ampullated end. The horizontal semicircular canal's ampullated end can then be opened inferior and lateral to the superior semicircular canal ampulla. The superior semicircular canal can then be followed posteriorly and then inferiorly until it connects with the posterior semicircular canal at the common crus. From the surgeon's perspective, the entire length of the SSC can be visualized during dissection, and it appears C-shaped. Surgeons in training can be instructed to "stay in the bowl" to find the superior canal. In contrast, the posterior canal lumen is seen on end and therefore appears as a dot. Surgeons in training are instructed to "follow the dot" of the posterior canal lumen from the common crus to the ampullated end and then to the vestibule. Of note, the two instances when the facial nerve is at risk of drill damage are when drilling the horizontal canal as the nerve lies just inferior to the horizontal canal and when the posterior canal proceeds posteriorly towards the facial nerve. The surgeon should shift the operating view more inferiorly and have the patient tilted away to facilitate following the canal while being mindful of the facial nerve. Once the vestibule is reached, the spherical recess of the saccule and the elliptical recess of the utricle are identified. The neuroepithelial contents of these two recesses, as well as the neuroepithelium of the ampulla of each semicircular canal, are removed with suction and a small weapon. Complete removal of the five sources of vestibular neuroepithelium (the ampulla of each semicircular canal, utricle, and saccule) is necessary to rid the inner ear of any remaining vestibular function (see Fig. 17.3).

Current Treatment Protocols

Patients who are diagnosed with Meniere's disease should be treated medically with low salt diet, low caffeine intake, and daily triamterene-hydrochlorothiazide (Dyazide). This is effectively applied in the majority of Meniere's disease patients. Patients who have occasional vertigo spells or drops in hearing can be treated with oral steroids or transtympanic steroid injection. Patients who persist with symptoms despite maximal medical therapy may be candidates for additional therapy. Patients with excellent hearing may be offered either gentamicin therapy as they are at low risk of sensorineural hearing loss or endolymphatic sac decompression. However, patients with preexisting hearing loss are offered endolymphatic sac decompression, as these patients would be at a higher risk of hearing loss if gentamicin were administered. If the sac surgery fails and if good hearing remains, then intratympanic gentamicin injection or vestibular nerve section are offered as these techniques may preserve hearing. In patients with poor hearing and unilateral Meniere's, transmastoid labyrinthectomy is offered.

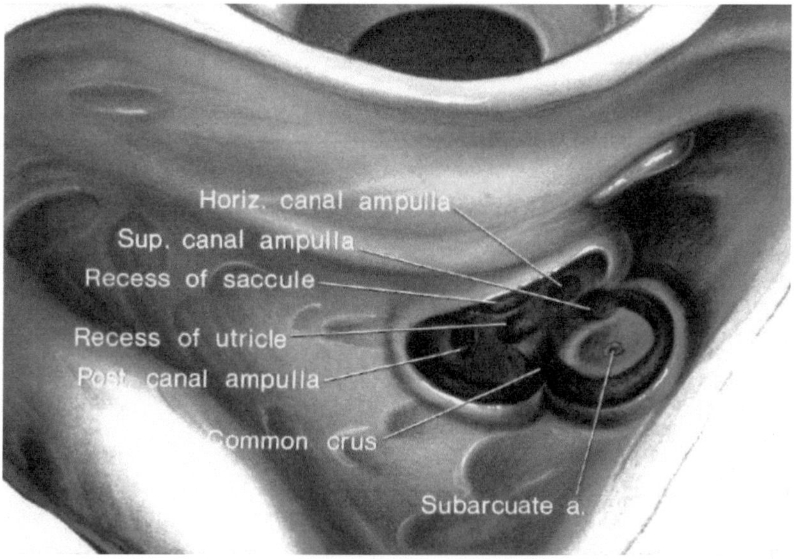

Fig. 17.3 Labyrinthectomy depicted in a right ear with delineation of each semicircular canal and the otolith organs

Challenging Clinical Scenarios

There are many situations which result in therapeutic dilemmas. For example, a patient may present with medically recalcitrant Meniere's in his or her only hearing ear. Thus, hearing preservation is strongly preferred. If this patient's Meniere's disease causes disabling symptoms, the sequential options of steroid therapy, endolymphatic sac decompression, and vestibular nerve section can be offered. Gentamicin must be carefully considered due to the risk of hearing loss, and labyrinthectomy would only be performed as a last resort of truly disabling vertigo.

Another difficult management decision occurs in patients with bilateral Meniere's disease and disabling vertigo spells. After testing (which includes an audiogram, VNG, and MRI), subjective symptoms seem to offer the most information concerning which ear is causing the symptoms. In general, if conservative treatment has failed, oral and/or intratympanic steroids are used. If the patient continues to have vertigo spells, then endolymphatic sac decompression surgery can be used, possibly in both ears (not simultaneously, however). Gentamicin can also be used but with caution as it is ablative. Rarely have we used VNS or labyrinthectomy in patients with bilateral MD. We have, however, used these techniques unilaterally upon clearly demonstrating that one ear is primarily the cause of the patient's severe vertiginous symptoms.

References

1. Meniere P. Sur une forme de surdite grave dependant d'une lesion de l'oreille interne. Gaz Med de Paris. 1861;16:29.
2. Dandy W. Effects on hearing after subtotal section of the cochlear branch of the auditory nerve. Bull Johns Hopkins Hosp. 1934;55:240–3.
3. Dandy W. The surgical treatment of Ménière's disease. Surg Gynecol Obstet. 1941;72
4. Lake R. Removal of semicircular canals in a case of unilateral aural vertigo. Lancet. 1904;1:421.
5. Cawthorne TE. The treatment of Ménière's disease. J LaryngolOtol. 1943;58:363–71.
6. Portmann G. Vertigo, surgical treatment of opening of the saccus endolymphaticus. Arch Otolaryngol Head Neck Surg 6:309, 192.
7. House WF. Subarachnoid shunt for drainage of endolymphatic hydrops. Laryngoscope. 1962;72:713–29.
8. Schuknecht HF. Cochlear endolymphatic shunt. Am J Otol. 1984;5:546–8.
9. Pou AM, Hirsch BE, Durrant JD, et al. The efficacy of tympanic electrocochleography in diagnosis of endolymphatic hydrops. Am K Otol. 1996;17(4):607–11.
10. Fischer LM, Derebery J. Oral steroid treatment for hearing improvement in Ménière's disease and endolymphatic hydrops. Otol Neurotol. 2012 Dec;33(9):1685–91.
11. Balkany. The Bilateral Aspects of Meniere' disease: an underestimated entity. Otolaryngol Clin North Am. 1980;12:603–9.
12. Shea JJ Jr. The role of dexamethasone or streptomycin perfusion in the treatment of Ménière's disease. Otolaryngol Clin N Am. 1997;30(6):1051.
13. Parnes LS, Sun AH, Freeman DJ. Corticosteroid pharmacokinetics in the inner ear fluids: an animal study followed by clinical application. Laryngoscope. 1999;109:1.
14. Chandrasekhar SS, Rubinstein RY, Kwartler JA. Dexamethasone pharmacokinetics in the inner ear: comparison and use of facilitation agents. Otolaryngol Head Neck Surg. 2000;122(4):521–8.
15. McRackan TR, Best J, Pearce EC, Bennett ML, Dietrich M, Wanna GB, Haynes DS, Labadie RF. Intratympanic dexamethasone as a symptomatic treatment for Meniere's disease. Otol Neurotol. 2014;35(9):1638–40.
16. Thomsen J, Bretlau P, Tos M, et al. Placebo effect in surgery for Ménière's disease. A double-blind, placebo-controlled study on endolymphatic sac shunt surgery. Arch Otolaryngol. 1981;107(5):271.
17. Glasscock, et al. What I think of sac surgery in 1989. Am J Otol 1989;10(3):230–233.
18. Pillsbury HC 3rd, Arenberg IK, Ferraro J, Ackley RS. Endolymphatic sac surgery. The Danish sham surgery study: an alternative analysis. Otolaryngol Clin N Am. 1983;16(1):123–7.
19. Welling DB, Nagaraja HN. Endolymphatic mastoid shunt: a reevaluation of efficacy. Otolaryngol Head Neck Surg. 2000;122(3):340.
20. Telischi FF, Luxford WM. Long-term efficacy of endolymphatic sac surgery for vertigo in Ménière's disease. Otolaryngol Head Neck Surg. 1993;109(1):83.
21. Kato BM, LaRouere MJ, Bojrab DI, et al. Evaluating quality of life after endolymphatic sac surgery: the Meniere's disease outcomes questionnaire. Otol Neurotol. 2004;25:339–44.
22. Sood A, Lambert P, et al. Endolymphatic sac surgery for Meniere's disease: a systematic review and meta-analysis. Otol Neurotol. 2014;35:1033Y1045.
23. Paparella MM. Revision of endolymphatic sac surgery for recurrent Meniere's disease. Otolaryngol Clin North Am. 2002;35(Issue 3):607–19.
24. Paparella MM1, Sajjadi H. Endolymphatic sac revision for recurrent Menière's disease. Am J Otol. 1988;9(6):441–7.
25. Fowler EP. Streptomycin treatment for vertigo. Trans Am Acad Ophthalmol Otolaryngol. 1948;52:293–301.
26. Ohmori WH. Mechano-electrical transduction currents in isolated vestibular hair cells of the chick. J Physiol. 1985;359:189–217.
27. Waguespack J, Ricci A. Aminoglycoside ototoxicity: permeant drugs cause permanent hair cell loss. J Physiol. 2005;567:359–60.

28. Williams S, Zenner H, Schacht J. Three molecular steps of aminoglycoside ototoxicity demonstrated in outer hair cells. Hear Res. 1987;30:11–8.
29. Schuknecht HP. Ablation therapy for the relief of Meniere's disease. Laryngoscope. 1956;66:859.
30. Graham MD, Sataloff RT, Kemink JL. Titration streptomycin therapy for bilateral Meniere's disease: a preliminary report. Otolaryngol Head Neck Surg. 1984;92(4):440–7.
31. Magnusson M, Padoan S. Delayed onset of ototoxic effects of gentamicin in treatment of Menière's disease. Rationale for extremely low dose therapy. Acta Otolaryngol. 1991;111(4):671–6.
32. Nedzelski J, Chiong C, Fradet G, et al. Intratympanic gentamicin instillation as treatment of unilateral Meniere's disease: update of an ongoing study. Am J Otol. 1993;13:278–82.
33. Prezant TR, Agapian JV, Bohlman MC, Bu X, Oztas S, Qiu WQ, Arnos KS, Cortopassi GA, Jaber L, Rotter JI. Mitochondrial ribosomal RNA mutation associated with both antibiotic-induced and non-syndromic deafness. Nat Genet. 1993;4(3):289–94.
34. Minor LB. Intratympanic gentamicin for control of vertigo in Meniere's disease: vestibular signs that specify completion of therapy. Am J Otol. 1999;20(2):209.
35. Kaplan DM, Nedzelski JM, Chen JM, et al. Intratympanic gentamicin for the treatment of unilateral Meniere's disease. Laryngoscope. 2000;110(8):1298.
36. Dandy WE. Ménière's disease: its diagnosis and method of treatment. Arch Surg. 1928;16:1127–52.
37. Dandy WE. Treatment of Ménière's disease by section of only the vestibular portion of the acoustic nerve. Bull Johns Hopkins Hosp. 1933;53:52–5.
38. House WF. Surgical exposure of the internal auditory canal and its contents through the middle cranial fossa. Laryngoscope. 1961;71:1363.
39. Silverstein H, Norrell H. Retrolabyrinthine surgery: a direct approach to the cerebellopontine angle. Otolaryngol Head Neck Surg. 1980;88:462–9.
40. Rosenberg S, Silverstein H, Hoffer M, et al. Hearing results after posterior fossa vestibular neurectomy. Otolaryngol Head Neck Surg. 1996;114:32–7.
41. Silverstein H, Norrell H, Smouha EE. Retrosigmoid-internal auditory canal approach vs. retrolabyrinthine approach for vestibular neurectomy. Otolaryngol Head Neck Surg. 1987 Sep;97(3):300–7.
42. Tewary AK, Riley N, Kerr AG. Long-term results of vestibular nerve section. J Laryngol Otol. 1998;112(12):1150–3.
43. Pappas DG Jr, Pappas DG Sr. Vestibular nerve section: long-term follow-up. Laryngoscope. 1997;107(9):1203–9.
44. Silverstein H, Norrell H, Rosenberg S. The resurrection of vestibular neurectomy: a 10-year experience with 115 cases. J Neurosurg. 1990;72(4):533–9.
45. Silverstein H, Jackson LE. Vestibular nerve section. Otolaryngol Clin North Am. 2002;35(3):655–73. ISSN 0030-6665
46. Setty BS, et al. Fully endoscopic Retrosigmoid vestibular nerve section for refractory Meniere disease. J Neurol Surg B Skull Base. 2016;77(04):341–9.
47. House JW, Brackmann DE. Tinnitus: surgical management. Ciba Found Symp. 1981;85:204–16.
48. Hammerschlag PE, Schuknecht HF. Transcanal labyrinthectomy for intractable vertigo. Arch Otolaryngol. 1981;107:152–6.
49. Graham MD. Transmastoid labyrinthectomy: further experiences with the indications, complications, and early postoperative results. J Laryngol Otol. 1981;95:1205–11.
50. Kemink JL, Telian SA, Graham MD, Joynt L. Transmastoid labyrinthectomy: reliable surgical management of vertigo. Otolaryngol Head Neck Surg. 1989;101(1):5–10.
51. Zwolan TA, Shepard NT, Niparko JK. Labyrinthectomy with cochlear implantation. Am J Otol. 1993;14(3):220–3.
52. MacKeith SA, Bottrill ID, Ramsden JD. Simultaneous labyrinthectomy with cochlear implantation in patients with bilateral Ménière's disease. Ann Otol Rhinol Laryngol. 2014;123(7):485–9.

Chapter 18
Pathophysiology and Diagnosis of Superior Canal Dehiscence

Gerard J. Gianoli

Introduction

Superior canal dehiscence (SCD) can be defined as both an anatomic anomaly found on CT scan and/or at surgical exploration (Figs. 18.1 and 18.2), or as a syndrome that frequently accompanies this anatomic deviation. It is now most recognized as part of the larger category of Third Mobile Window Disorders [1]. When SCD was first described in 1998 [2], it was felt to be a rare disorder. However, over the past 20 years, it has been recognized with increasing prevalence as varying clinical presentations have been elucidated. SCD has been called the great otologic mimicker due to the myriad of clinical presentations that may be identical to other major otologic disorders, such as patulous eustachian tube, otosclerosis, Meniere's disease, perilymph fistula, acute vestibular neuritis, and vestibular migraine [3]. This variety of presentations may lead to a delay in diagnosis, misdiagnosis, and in some cases inappropriate treatment. The correct diagnosis is important since relief of symptoms can be attained among the majority of SCD patients with appropriate treatment.

Included in the spectrum of SCD is the asymptomatic patient, which presumably includes most SCD patients prior to the onset of their symptoms. There are many patients with anatomic dehiscence of the superior canal that have no symptoms. Due to this, simply noting the anatomic presence of SCD does not signify causation for the patient's symptomatology. It has been recognized since the initial description of the problem in 1998 that a "second event" is suspected to be the root cause of the onset of the symptoms of SCD. The leading suspected "second events" are head

G. J. Gianoli (✉)
The Ear and Balance Institute, Covington, LA, USA

Department of Otolaryngology, Tulane University, New Orleans, LA, USA

J. C. Lucas et al. (eds.), *Diagnosis and Treatment of Vestibular Disorders*,
https://doi.org/10.1007/978-3-032-11740-3_18

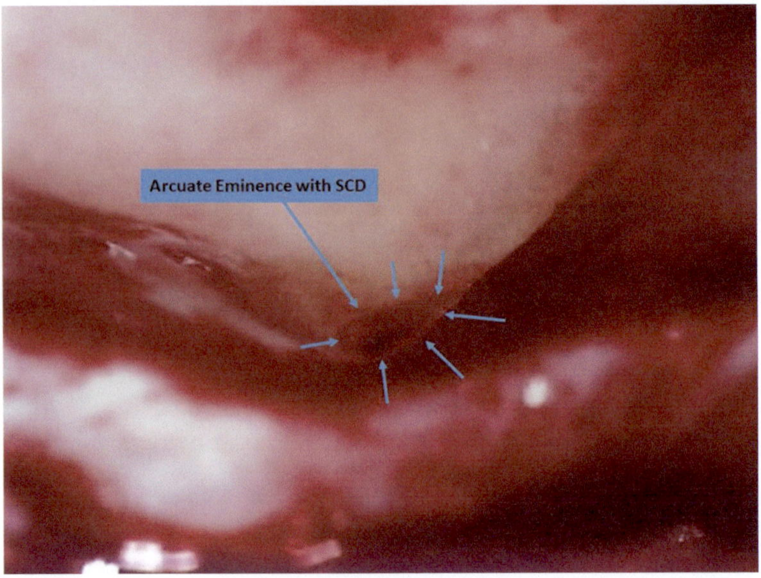

Fig. 18.1 Intraoperative view of the middle fossa floor exploration demonstrating SCD at the arcuate eminence

Fig. 18.2 CT scan demonstrating SCD

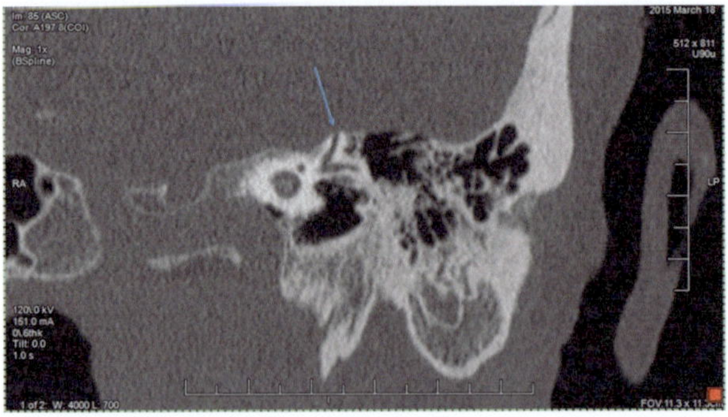

trauma and major pressure-altering events—affecting middle ear or intracranial pressure. This is the presumed reason why SCD syndrome is rarely seen in the pediatric population.

The diagnostic criteria for SSCD published by the Barany Society are as follows [4]:

Barany Society Criteria for Diagnosis of SCD

1. At least one of the following symptoms consistent with the presence of a "third mobile window" in the inner ear:
   Bone conduction hyperacusis
   Sound-induced vertigo and/or oscillopsia time-locked to the stimulus

Pressure-induced vertigo and/or oscillopsia time-locked to the stimulus
Pulsatile tinnitus

2. At least one of the following signs or diagnostic tests indicating a "third mobile window" in the inner ear:
   Nystagmus characteristic of excitation or inhibition of the affected superior semicircular canal evoked by sound, or by changes in middle ear pressure or intracranial pressure
   Low-frequency negative bone conduction thresholds on pure tone audiometry
   Enhanced VEMP responses (low cervical VEMP thresholds or high ocular VEMP amplitudes)
3. High-resolution temporal bone CT imaging with multiplanar reconstruction demonstrating dehiscence of the superior semicircular canal
4. Not better accounted for by another vestibular disease or disorder

Incidence and Etiology

An anatomic dehiscence of bone overlying the superior semicircular canal at its interface with middle cranial fossa dura has been proposed to be a developmental abnormality [2]. In utero between 32 and 40 weeks' gestation, which is beyond the time of the labyrinth reaching adult size, the incidence of SCD approaches 89% [5]. Bone overlying the middle fossa floor (or conversely, covering the tegmen mastoideum and tegmen tympani) thickens progressively in utero and throughout early childhood, such that a one-year-old with CT findings of SCD may see it "disappear" by the time they are 3 or 4 years old [6]. Sugihara and colleagues [7] in a review of 1006 temporal bone CT scans demonstrated progressive thickening of superior semicircular canal (SSC) bone throughout the first 8 years of life with a concomitant progressive lower incidence of SCD during that time period. At this age, the incidence of the anatomic finding of SCD is believed to be relatively stable, rendering 0.5% with frank dehiscence and 1–2% of the general population with exceedingly thin bone ($\leq$0.1 mm thickness) in this area [8]. Either frank dehiscence or thin bone of the superior semicircular canal (SSC) theoretically places these individuals at risk for developing SCD syndrome later in life.

The thickness of the calvarium and the area of the middle fossa floor overlying the SSC slowly thins throughout the course of life [9]. This has been submitted as evidence pointing toward an acquired etiology for SCD as opposed to the "congenital or developmental etiology" [9]. Additionally, a small number of patients have been identified who acquire SCD from erosive processes such as arachnoid granulations, cholesteatomas, other tumors, and fractures. The authors have also identified a few cases of iatrogenic SCD acquired due to skull base approaches for tumor resections. More recently, the CDH23 gene (associated with Usher syndrome and non-syndromic hearing loss) [10] and the EYA4 gene (otosclerosis and SCD) [11] have been found to be a genetic risk factor for development of SCD.

The prevalence of SCD has been found to be higher in analyzed CT scans compared to temporal bone histology. Carey et al. identified complete absence of bone over the superior canal histologically in 0.5% of 1000 vertically sectioned adult temporal bones [8]. There was an additional 1.4% with very thin (≤0.1 mm) bone covering the superior canal. Added together, the prevalence of thin or dehiscent superior canals approached 2%. This study also reported that 50% of the SCD cases had bilateral involvement. Carey and colleagues [8] also analyzed 36 infant temporal bones and concluded that the thickness of the bone overlying the superior canal was consistently thin. The thickness of the bone covering the superior canal gradually thickened with age, reaching adult levels by age 3. Further supporting the theory of a congenital/developmental origin for the anatomic defect of SCD is a study by DeJong and colleagues [12] demonstrating significantly less temporal bone volume among SCD patients compared to controls.

Roberto et al. [13] used tetracycline staining to investigate the deposition of bone in the dog model at 10, 25, and 50 days of age. This study demonstrated progressive deposition of endochondral and endosteal bone at the superior semicircular canal postnatally. The bone deposition decreased with age. These findings are in agreement with the observations in the study by Carey et al. In a related study, Hirvonen and colleagues [14] reported a CT study of the thickness of the superior canal in a group of patients with SCD and those without SCD. Among those with SCD, the contralateral superior canal bone was thinner (or dehiscent), compared to those patients without SCD. This finding supports the notion of SCD as a developmental anomaly related to bony deposition in early life. Alternatively, thin bone present early in life could also be a predisposing cause for eventual regression of bone and acquisition of SCD later in life.

Several observations point to an SCD as a developmental anomaly with a "second event" required to produce symptoms. Among these observations are:

1. The above studies demonstrate the development of bone over the superior semicircular canal occurring later (postnatally) than other parts of the inner ear.
2. The clinical observation of the presence of asymptomatic SCD noted during intraoperative exploration of the middle cranial fossa for encephalocele repair (Fig. 18.3).
3. Symptoms from SCD are rarely present in the pediatric population, in spite of a higher incidence of the anatomic dehiscence in children than among adult patients.

These observations support the notion that a second event is required in addition to the congenital anomaly of thin or absent superior canal bone in order to produce clinical symptoms. Roughly 25–45% of patients report an event they attribute to symptom onset for SCD [15, 16]. This "second event" is typically noted to be either head trauma, a Valsalva-type episode, or some other type of pressure-altering event that affects either middle ear or intracranial pressure.

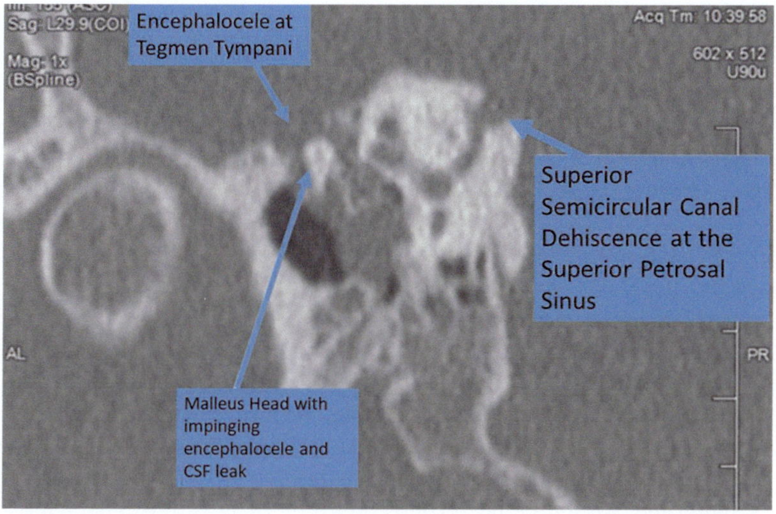

Fig. 18.3 CT scan demonstrating an encephalocele in a patient with an asymptomatic SCD

Case 1

In 1998 (shortly after the authors started treating SCD), an 8-year-old female was referred for tympanomastoidectomy for LEFT chronic suppurative otitis media and suspicion of cholesteatoma. A preoperative CT scan demonstrated RIGHT SCD. She had no complaints of vertigo/dizziness, autophony, or Tullio's phenomenon. No vestibular evaluation was performed because she was asymptomatic, and no surgical treatment was directed toward the RIGHT SCD at that time. She underwent successful LEFT tympanomastoidectomy and was lost to follow-up.

In 2010, she returned because of the new onset of RIGHT pulsatile tinnitus, episodic vertigo, dizziness, and near-constant unsteadiness. The vertigo spells were provoked by straining. Work-up revealed an abnormal RIGHT cVEMP and an abnormal RIGHT fistula (Hennebert) test. MRI scan was normal, and a CT scan performed at that time re-confirmed the RIGHT SCD.

Comment: This case illustrates three important points: (1) SCD can be asymptomatic, and the author would argue that most symptomatic SCD patients are asymptomatic initially. (2) Most pediatric SCD patients are asymptomatic. (3) This case supports the notion that SCD is congenital/developmental with symptoms acquired later in life.

Clinical Presentation

SCD was first reported by Minor et al. [2] in eight patients who exhibited the symptoms of short-lived vertigo spells in response to certain sounds or activities that would cause transient increases in intracranial or middle ear pressure (Valsalva, coughing, sneezing, nose-blowing, autoinsufflations). These activities would produce a torsional nystagmus, which directly implicates stimulation of the superior semicircular canal. Activities causing increased middle ear pressure (sound, positive pressure in the ear canal, autoinsufflations) induce nystagmus with the slow phase upward and the superior pole of the eye directed *away* from the affected ear. Activities causing a transient elevation in intracranial pressure (Valsalva against a closed glottis, jugular venous compression) or negative pressure in the ear canal resulted in the slow phase of nystagmus directed downward and the superior pole of the eye torquing *toward* the affected ear. The clinical findings of Tullio's phenomenon and pressure-inducing nystagmus associated with SCD have been termed Minor's syndrome. Although the vertigo caused by SCD is most characteristically reported as short-lived, other characterizations of vestibular symptoms have been reported as well, including more prolonged vertigo spells, chronic disequilibrium, and drop attacks [17].

In a publication [18] on SCD in 1999, Smullen et al. reported three SCD patients who had very disparate symptoms. One patient was asymptomatic and had middle fossa exploration to repair an encephalocele. Another patient had "symptoms that mimicked" Meniere's syndrome that resolved with SCD capping repair. The last patient had symptoms of straining-induced and positional vertigo which were also resolved with capping repair. Since these first reports of SCD, other variations on clinical presentations have been identified. In a review of their experience with SCD, Zhou et al. [3] described SCD as the "great otologic mimicker" because of the variety of presentations and the variety of other diagnoses with which SCD can be confused.

Case 2

A 74-year-old male was referred after a fall from a ladder 2 years prior. The head injury resulted in an intracranial bleed and a prolonged hospital stay. After regaining consciousness, he began to note left hearing loss, Tullio's phenomenon, autophony, chronic imbalance, and strain-induced vertigo spells. None of these symptoms had been present prior to the head trauma. Audiometry demonstrated left low-frequency mixed hearing loss with a large conductive component and intact acoustic reflexes. Fistula (Hennebert) test, Valsalva test, and cVEMP were abnormal on the left side. MRI scan demonstrated no CP angle, IAC, or brainstem pathology. CT scan demonstrated a very large left SCD and a much smaller right SCD. Left SCD repair alleviated his symptoms.

Comment: This case illustrates a "classic" presentation of SCD with an obvious second event (the head injury) as the provocateur of the onset of symptoms. The very large left SCD noted on CT scan was almost certainly present prior to the head injury but was asymptomatic before then.

Although the clinical presentation for SCD can vary, the most recognizable presentation includes Tullio's phenomenon, pressure-induced vertigo (transient increases in intracranial or middle ear pressure), pulsatile tinnitus, conductive hyperacusis, and autophony. While these are the most characteristic presentations of SCD, they are certainly not present in all SCD patients, and their absence cannot be used as a means to exclude the diagnosis of SCD. The more nonspecific symptoms of vestibulopathy such as head-movement-induced disequilibrium are much more common, but not particularly helpful in making the diagnosis of SCD. Pressure and aural fullness are common. Complaints of hearing loss, distorted hearing, and hyperacusis are also common. SCD patients may have been given a variety of other diagnoses prior to presenting in the office.

Vague cognitive and neurobehavioral symptoms are also frequently reported by SCD patients. While these have been reported in SCD patients, they are not specific to SCD patients and can be seen in other chronic vestibular syndromes. These include depression, "brain fog," short-term memory problems, and difficulty with concentration. These symptoms have been documented as present and improved after surgical repair of SCD by Wackym et al. [19].

Physical Exam

Routine head and neck exam is typically normal in SCD patients. Microscopic otoscopy, unless there has been prior surgical intervention, is normal as well. The vestibular component of the physical exam should include evaluation with infrared video goggles. This may be unremarkable, but if there has been any vestibular loss, it may reveal spontaneous nystagmus and head thrust or head shake abnormalities. In some extreme cases, one can identify a spontaneous torsional eye movement that is synchronous with the pulse. Tuning fork testing in locations (such as the malleolus) not normally used to stimulate the ear can sometimes show positive results in SCD patients.

Testing

Much of the literature discusses Vestibular Evoked Myogenic Potentials (VEMP) and high-resolution CT scan as the extent of testing for SCD. While the CT scan is imperative and the VEMP is often helpful, the authors feel this limited testing is inadequate for patients presenting with SCD. Since SCD is a disorder that can mimic many other otologic disorders, can cause many secondary pathologies, and may require invasive surgery to resolve, a full audiovestibular test battery is warranted.

CT scan slices should be performed at the submillimeter level, preferably ≤0.24 mm thickness but no thicker than 0.6 mm. The thinner slice scan gives a more accurate portrayal of the defect. Thicker scans are prone to high levels of inaccuracy [20]. MRI should be performed to evaluate concomitant intracranial abnormalities, but not for confirmation of SCD. One of the more frequent findings in SCD patients is Chiari malformation [21]. Additionally, MRI findings suggestive of elevated intracranial pressure should be sought (i.e., empty sella, vertical tortuosity of the optic nerves, prominent arachnoid spaces around the optic nerves, flattening of the globe, slit-like ventricles, venous sinus abnormalities, Chiari/cerebellar ectopia). MRI, however, may be useful postoperatively to determine whether surgical occlusion of the SSC has been successful via the lack of superior semicircular canal signal at the occlusion site.

Audiometric testing may be normal, show some degree of sensorineural hearing loss in the affected ear, or more characteristically, demonstrate a low-frequency conductive loss (some with bone scores at supra-threshold levels). To distinguish the low-frequency conductive loss patient who has SCD from an otosclerotic patient or other patient with middle ear pathology, impedance testing is warranted. The SCD patient should typically have a normal tympanogram and intact acoustic reflexes, whereas patients with otosclerosis will show absent acoustic reflexes [22].

Case 3

A 45-year-old female was diagnosed with otosclerosis and underwent middle ear exploration. No stapes fixation was noted at the time of surgery. She was referred for further evaluation. The patient reported a progressive hearing loss and no significant vestibular symptoms. The patient, however, did report autophony, pulsatile tinnitus, and could hear her eye movement. The audiogram demonstrated a low-frequency conductive loss with elevated bone scores, but acoustic reflexes were normal. Further testing demonstrated that cVEMP was abnormal, as was the fistula (Hennebert) test. MRI scan was unremarkable, and CT scan demonstrated a large SCD.

Comment: This case illustrates another variation for SCD presentation, principally hearing loss mimicking otosclerosis and lacking vestibular symptoms. Clinicians should maintain a high index of suspicion and evaluate prospective stapedectomy patients with acoustic reflex testing. An otosclerotic patient should have absent reflexes, while an SCD patient usually has intact acoustic reflexes.

VEMP (Vestibular Evoked Myogenic Potentials), both cervical and ocular, may show abnormal responses compared to lab norms, may show an asymmetric result in unilateral cases, or may be completely normal. cVEMP responses may be present at lowered threshold levels. Elevated amplitude of response has also been suggested as an indication of SSCD in oVEMP. The oVEMP response at 4 kHz has been proposed as particularly specific to SSCD [23]. In cases with vestibular loss, the VEMP response may be absent. Electrocochleography is frequently abnormal in SCD patients, which will often normalize after successful surgery [24].

The authors feel a full vestibular evaluation should be performed on anyone who is to undergo SCD surgery. Abnormalities identified are helpful in the consultation of (1) whether to proceed with surgery, (2) outcome expectations, and (3) documentation of vestibular status akin to preoperative audiometry. Patients with SCD have varied vestibular test profiles, including the possibilities of severe unilateral vestibular hypofunction and occasionally severe bilateral vestibular hypofunction. In this setting, successful surgical treatment of SCD will result in continued vestibular symptoms from these deficits. Additionally, BPPV is a frequent secondary pathology that may need treatment along with SCD.

Case 4

A 31-year-old male was referred for evaluation of suspected bilateral SCD. His chief complaint was constant imbalance/oscillopsia punctuated by short-lived spells of rotary vertigo induced by certain sounds and straining. He particularly had trouble with balance in the dark. Prior workup included an audiogram demonstrating a symmetric high-frequency sensorineural loss beyond 6 kHz, CT scan demonstrating SCD bilaterally and cVEMP within normal threshold stimulation and normal amplitudes on the left side with an absent response on the right side. No other vestibular evaluation had been performed.

Vestibular evaluation at our office demonstrated electrocochleography, Valsalva testing, fistula (Hennebert) testing, and Tullio's testing that were all abnormal and strongly suggestive of SCD. However, there was also significant bilateral caloric weakness, severely reduced gains on rotary chair, and high-frequency VOR testing indicating significant loss of vestibular function bilaterally. Further, on posturography, the patient would free fall on SOT 5 and 6.

Comment: The limited test battery of CT scan, audiometry, and VEMP did not completely describe this patient's pathology and missed important information—bilateral vestibular loss. The more extensive testing clearly explains why VEMP testing was not typical of SCD patients (i.e., reduced threshold response or large amplitude response). When there is global vestibular loss, one should expect a reduced or absent VEMP response as in this case. Knowing the severe bilateral loss allows the clinician to better counsel the patient on expectations if surgery is performed. In this case, surgery could resolve the Tullio's phenomenon and the strain-induced vertigo spells but is unlikely to improve his chronic disequilibrium to any measurable degree since his bilateral vestibular loss will persist. Without preoperative testing, postoperative vestibular weakness will likely be attributed to the surgical intervention, exposing the surgeon to the possibility of litigation.

Video Head Impulse Testing (VHIT) has been introduced to several labs recently. However, because clinical experience with this testing technology has not yet been widespread and has only been available for a limited time, the authors recommend caution when using this as a means to determine "normal" semicircular canal function. Recent studies have shown poor correlation of VHIT with caloric irrigation studies [25, 26]. Due to this, we cannot recommend using this in place of caloric irrigation. However, in the context of SCD, VHIT may prove to be invaluable in determining superior canal function preoperatively and postoperatively. In patients who have undergone SCD occlusion, VHIT may be helpful in determining whether the posterior semicircular canal has also been occluded.

Pathophysiology

The most commonly espoused theory for the pathophysiology of SCD is the "third mobile window theory." This theory posits that the flexible nature of the SCD allows for egress of endolymph in and out of the superior semicircular canal, resulting in abnormal stimulation of the superior canal cupula. Additionally, low-frequency sound energy transmitted through the inner ear is allowed to dissipate through this bony defect, resulting in the conductive air-bone gap noted in some SCD patients. Merchant and Rosowski [27] proposed that SCD could be classified among a number of lesions that produce a third mobile window on the scala vestibuli side of the cochlea. Included among these are lateral or posterior canal dehiscence, enlarged vestibular aqueduct, dehiscence of the internal auditory canal, carotid dehiscence (into the cochlea), diffuse dehiscence (such as in Paget's disease), and other congenital anomalies of the inner ear. The hearing loss in these pathologic third mobile window cases exhibits poor air conduction thresholds and good bone conduction thresholds.

However, the Third Mobile Window theory does not completely explain all of the clinical findings of SCD. Among these are

1. The presence of asymptomatic SCD patients who have been verified both radiographically and surgically during repair of encephalocele [18].
2. The presentation of SCD patients with only auditory and no vestibular findings or vice versa.
3. Ménière's-type vertigo spells (prolonged vertigo lasting several hours) and the findings of endolymphatic hydrops on MRI in 23–80% of SCD patients [18, 28–31].
4. The absence of symptoms until later in life, typically beyond 30 years of age.
5. Higher incidence of SCD among pediatric patients but lower incidence of symptomatology in the pediatric population.
6. SCD symptoms in patients who have "Near Dehiscence" (i.e., thin bone without dehiscence).

7. SCD patients with sensorineural hearing loss and/or vestibular loss.
8. Successful resolution of Tullio's phenomenon with round window reinforcement. (Theoretically, according to third mobile window theory, round window reinforcement should worsen Tullio's phenomenon by shunting more sound pressure to the vestibular end organ.)

It has been proposed that a second event such as trauma or a major pressure-altering event (Valsalva-type maneuver) causes a disruption of very thin bone over the superior canal, thus creating an SCD. However, this only explains adult onset of symptoms and not the other findings, nor does it explain a true dehiscence in an asymptomatic patient [18].

Gianoli and Soileau [32] proposed the theory that alteration of intracranial pressure may result in increased compliance at the round and oval windows and, if pressure changes were extreme, potential disruption of the windows resulting in a frank middle ear perilymph fistula. This theory could explain the above exceptions to the Third Mobile Window theory and why a second event of head trauma or pressure-altering event frequently brings on symptoms. It also explains why round window reinforcement has been noted to resolve SCD symptoms in many patients. Gianoli and Soileau further proposed a staging system for SCD (Fig. 18.4):

Stage 1: Asymptomatic SCD—anatomic dehiscence with no symptoms
Stage 2: Minor's syndrome—Tullio's phenomenon and Valsalva-induced vertigo, correlating with increased compliance of the inner ear windows and temporal lobe dura due to oscillating intracranial pressure transmission
Stage 3: Meniere's syndrome—Vertigo and hearing loss mimicking Meniere's disease, correlating with suspected intermittent oval or round window perilymphatic fistula and subsequent healing
Stage 4: End stage—Profound hearing loss and/or vestibular areflexia, because of repeated damage from stage 3 (see illustrative case above)

Case 5

A 44-year-old female diagnosed with left Meniere's disease was referred for further evaluation. She complained of a 3-year history of left-sided fluctuating hearing loss, fullness/pressure, tinnitus, and episodic vertigo lasting several hours per spell. She had failed medical management. At her initial office visit with us, she reported Tullio's phenomenon and possible strain-induced vertigo spells. She also noted autophony to voice, heartbeat, eye movements, and heel strike. Evaluation demonstrated an abnormal left ECOG but also an abnormal left cVEMP, Tullio's test, Valsalva test, and fistula (pressure) test. Audiometry demonstrated an asymmetric hearing loss with a left low-frequency mixed hearing loss pattern. The MRI scan was negative, and CT scan demonstrated a left SCD. The patient's vestibular symptoms resolved with SCD repair.

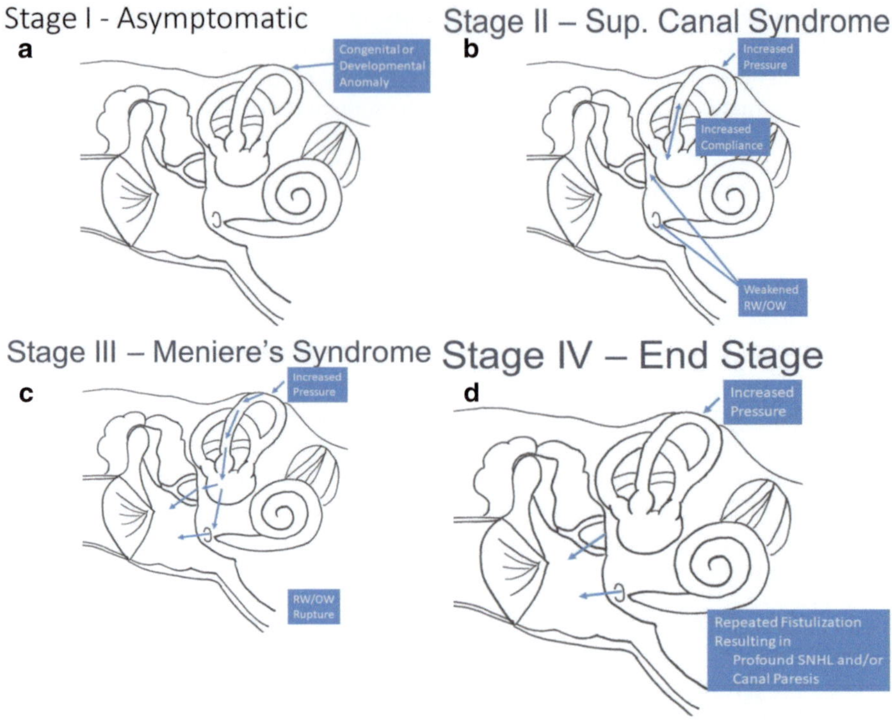

Fig. 18.4 SCD staging proposed by Gianoli and Soileau. (**a**) Stage 1 is the initial developmental/congenital defect in an asymptomatic patient. (**b**) Stage 2 develops after repeated fluctuation of intracranial pressure. This causes increased compliance of the round and/or oval windows and dura, resulting in Minor's syndrome. (**c**) Stage 3 is defined as the pressure increase resulting in intermittent perilymph fistulas. These cause Meniere's-type spells of hours-long vertigo. (**d**) Stage 4 is the terminal stage when repeated PLF have damaged the inner ear, resulting in profound hearing loss and/or vestibular areflexia

Comment: This patient illustrates a classic Meniere's syndrome presentation of SCD. It should be kept in mind that Meniere's syndrome is one of the myriad presentations for SCD and, in particular, should be assessed in those who do not respond to medical management for Meniere's.

Other Dehiscences

Among patients who present with symptoms and testing consistent with SCD, there are some who do not have SCD. These patients may be found to have dehiscence of labyrinthine bone in other areas. Among these are posterior semicircular canal dehiscence at the posterior fossa dura or at the jugular bulb, horizontal canal dehiscence (usually due to erosive processes such as cholesteatoma), cochlear dehiscence

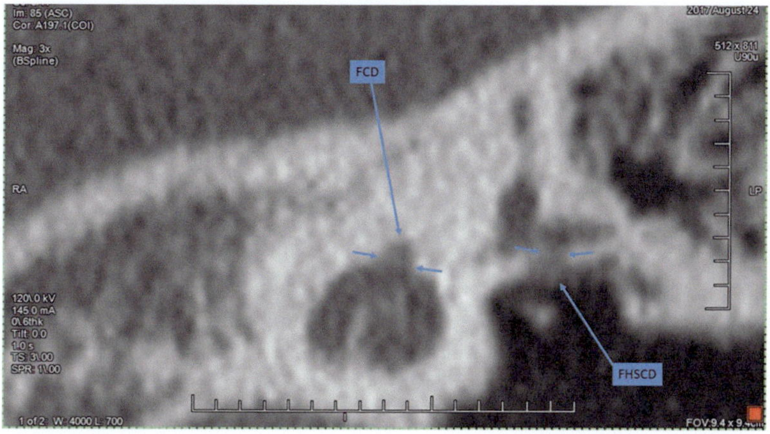

Fig. 18.5 CT scan demonstrating dehiscence of the cochlea at the region of the labyrinthine segment of the facial canal (FCD) and suspicious for dehiscence of the horizontal semicircular canal at the tympanic segment of the facial canal (FHSCD)

at the labyrinthine segment of the facial nerve (Fig. 18.5), cochlear dehiscence at the carotid artery, and horizontal canal dehiscence near the second genu of the facial nerve (Fig. 18.5). Each of these has minor variations from the typical presentation of SCD, but the most common uniting symptom seems to be pressure-induced dizziness/vertigo from either internal or external sources, although some may have autophony and Tullio's phenomenon. These dehiscences may be clinically identical in their presentation to SCD patients. Finally, patients may present with a syndrome identical to SCD but have no radiographically visible dehiscence. The collection of patients presenting with this syndrome has been named "CT-Negative otic capsule dehiscence syndrome" by Wackym et al. [33]

Case 6

A 23-year-old male was referred for vertigo, dizziness, and unilateral hearing loss after being struck by an industrial cable the previous year. The patient also had concomitant facial fractures and closed head injury. The patient reported that the vertigo was provoked by straining and possibly sound. He also noted autophony to heartbeat and voice. Evaluation demonstrated an abnormal cVEMP, fistula (Hennebert) test, and Valsalva test. MRI scan demonstrated no CPA, IAC, or brainstem pathology. CT scan demonstrated a posterior semicircular canal dehiscence at the junction of a high-riding jugular bulb. Surgical decompression of the jugular bulb with repair of the dehiscence resolved the patient's symptoms.

Comment: Many patients will present with SCD symptoms that do not have SCD. The clinician should look for other defects of the labyrinth which could possibly explain the symptomatology.

Near Dehiscence and Multiple Dehiscences

Many clinicians have noted patients with SCD symptoms and no bony defect of the SSC or any other place in the labyrinthine bone. Some of these patients will have extreme thinning of the SSC bone to the point where the bone itself is flexible enough to transmit pressure to the inner ear. These so-called near dehiscences share many features but typically do not have reduced thresholds on cVEMP testing. They also have a generally favorable outcome with SCD surgery [34]. A recent review examined 48 patients with thin bone overlying the superior semicircular canal demonstrating successful surgical repair with significant improvement in SCD symptoms. The measurement considered critical to include in the near dehiscent group was ≤0.5 mm thickness at the thinnest location [35].

Among SSCD patients, concomitant dehiscences in other locations have been identified [36]. In a review of 157 patients by Ionescu et al. [37], as many as 18.5% of SSCD patients had an additional otic capsule dehiscence in another area. However, a review by Shankar et al. compared 50 SCD patients with 50 non-SCD control patients finding no significant difference in the additional otic capsule defects [38]. The SCD group and the non-SCD group had 4% additional dehiscences.

Tegmen Dehiscence and Ossicular Head Impingement

Among the anomalies frequently seen with SCD are multiple dehiscences of the tegmen tympani and tegmen mastoideum as well as dehiscence of the geniculate ganglion [39]. Usually these are of no significance unless there has been dural herniation through the dehiscence resulting in an encephalocele and possible CSF leak. An encephalocele with prolapse onto the ossicular heads can cause a conductive hearing loss and autophony, which can accompany SCD. Similarly, a large tegmen tympani dehiscence may allow impingement of the ossicular heads without a prolapsing encephalocele (Fig. 18.6). If SCD repair does not include repair of this type of defect, some residual symptoms of autophony and conductive loss may persist.

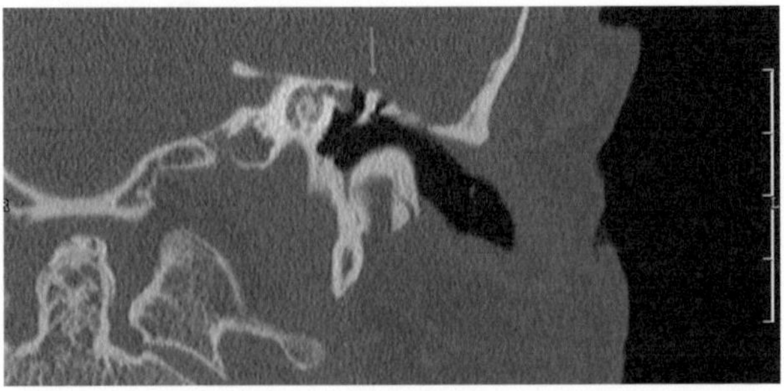

Fig. 18.6 CT scan of an SCD patient with concomitant dehiscence of the tegmen tympani with temporal lobe dura impinging on the ossicular heads (arrow)

Conclusions

We continue to learn about SCD and its implications since its first description in the literature 27 years ago. The pathophysiology is likely due to a combination of a third mobile window, increased round/oval window compliance, and concomitant intermittent PLF likely due to fluctuations in middle ear and/or intracranial pressure. The diagnosis of SCD requires a high degree of suspicion due to its varying presentation but must include (1) symptoms consistent with SCD, (2) physiologic testing consistent with SCD, and (3) high-resolution CT scan demonstrating SCD. None of these three elements is sufficient alone. Lastly, a comprehensive audiovestibular test battery is warranted for appropriate management of these complex patients.

References

1. Gianoli GJ, Thomson P, editors. Third mobile window syndrome of the inner ear: superior semicircular canal dehiscence and associated disorders. Cham: Springer; 2022.
2. Minor LB, Solomon D, Zinreich JS, Zee DS. Sound- and/or pressure-induced vertigo due to bone dehiscence of the superior semicircular canal. Arch Otolaryngol Head Neck Surg. 1998;124:249–58.
3. Zhou G, Gopen Q, Poe DS. Clinical and diagnostic characterization of canal dehiscence syndrome: a great otologic mimicker. Otol Neurotol. 2007;28(7):920–6.
4. Ward BK, van de Berg R, van Rompaey V, Bisdorff A, Hullar TE, Welgampola MS, Carey JP. Superior semicircular canal dehiscence syndrome: diagnostic criteria consensus document of the committee for the classification of vestibular disorders of the Bárány Society. J Vestib Res. 2021;31(3):131–41. https://doi.org/10.3233/VES-200004. PMID: 33522990; PMCID: PMC9249274.
5. Bom Braga GP, Noble JH, Gebrim EMMS, Labadie RF, Bento RF. The influence of the subarcuate artery in the superior semicircular canal dehiscence and its frequency on stillbirths: illustrative cases and systematic review. Acta Otolaryngol. 2017;22:1–6.
6. Meiklejohn DA, Corrales CE, Boldt BM, Sharon JD, Yeom KW, Carey JP, Blevins NH. Pediatric semicircular canal dehiscence: radiographic and histologic prevalence, with clinical correlation. Otol Neurotol. 2015;36(8):1383–9.
7. Sugihara EM, Babu SC, Kitsko DJ, Haupert HS, Thottam PJ. Incidence of pediatric superior semicircular canal dehiscence and inner ear anomalies: a large multicenter review. Otol Neurotol. 2016;37:1370–5.
8. Carey JP, Minor LB, Nager GT. Dehiscence or thinning of the bone overlying the superior semicircular canal in a temporal bone survey. Arch Otolaryngol Head Neck Surg. 2000;126(2):137–47.
9. Davey S, Kelly-Morland C, Phillips JS, Nunney I, Pawaroo D. Assessment of superior semicircular canal thickness with advancing age. Laryngoscope. 2015;125(8):1940–5.
10. Noonan KY, Russo J, Shen J, Rehm H, Halbach S, Hopp E, Noon S, Hoover J, Eskey C, Sunders J. CDH23 related hearing loss: a new genetic risk factor for semicircular canal dehiscence? Otol Neurotol. 2016;37(10):1583–8.
11. Ocal FCA, Kavus H, Satar B, Pehli van D. One genetic defect and two related entities in monozygotic twins: otosclerosis and superior semicircular canal near dehiscence syndrome. J Audiol Otol. 2022;26(2):97–102. https://doi.org/10.7874/jao.2021.00381. Epub 2021 Nov 9. PMID: 34748697; PMCID: PMC8996085.

12. de Jong MA, Carpenter DJ, Kaylie DM, Piker EG, Frank-Ito DO. Temporal bone anatomy characteristics in superior semicircular canal dehiscence. J Otol. 2017;12(4):185–91.
13. Roberto M, Favia A, Lozupone E. Postnatal bone growth in the semicircular canals of the dog. Ital J Anat Embryol. 1998;103:27–34.
14. Hirvonen TP, Weg N, Zinreich SJ, Minor LB. High-resolution CT findings suggest a developmental abnormality underlying superior canal dehiscence syndrome. Acta Otolaryngol. 2003;123(4):477–81.
15. Minor LB. Clinical manifestations of superior semicircular canal dehiscence. Laryngoscope. 2005;115:1717–27.
16. Formeister EJ, Krishnan PS, Schoo DP, Andresen N, Sayyid Z, Wei O, Carey JP. Traumatic events preceding the development of superior canal dehiscence syndrome. Otolaryngol Head Neck Surg. 2024;171(1):212–7. https://doi.org/10.1002/ohn.697. Epub 2024 Mar 5. PMID: 38440913; PMCID: PMC11211056.
17. Brantberg K, Ishiyama A, Baloh RW. Drop attacks secondary to superior canal dehiscence syndrome. Neurology. 2005;64(12):2126–8. https://doi.org/10.1212/01.WNL.0000165953.48914.B0. PMID: 15985585.
18. Smullen JL, Andrist EC, Gianoli GJ. Superior semicircular canal dehiscence: a new cause of vertigo. J LA State Med Soc. 1999;151:397–400.
19. Wackym PA, Balaban CD, Mackay HT, Wood SJ, Lundell CJ, Carter DM, Siker DA. Longitudinal cognitive and neurobehavioral functional outcomes before and after repairing otic capsule dehiscence. Otol Neurotol. 2016;37(1):70–82.
20. Tavassolie TS, Penninger RT, Zuñiga MG, Minor LB, Carey JP. Multislice computed tomography in the diagnosis of superior canal dehiscence: how much error, and how to minimize it? Otol Neurotol. 2012;33(2):215–22.
21. Kuhn JJ, Clenney T. The association between semicircular canal dehiscence and Chiari type I malformation. Arch Otolaryngol Head Neck Surg. 2010;136(10):1009–14.
22. Picavet V, Govaere E, Forton G. Superior semicircular canal dehiscence: prevalence in a population with clinical suspected otosclerosis-type hearing loss. B-ENT. 2009;5(2):83–8.
23. Manzari L, Burgess AM, McGarvie LA, Curthoys IS. An indicator of probable semicircular canal dehiscence: ocular vestibular evoked myogenic potentials to high frequencies. Otolaryngol Head Neck Surg. 2013;149(1):142–5. https://doi.org/10.1177/0194599813489494. Epub 2013 May 14. PMID: 23674567.
24. Arts HA1, Adams ME, Telian SA, El-Kashlan H, Kileny PR. Reversible electrocochleographic abnormalities in superior canal dehiscence. Otol Neurotol. 2009;30(1):79–86.
25. Jung J, Suh MJ, Kim SH. Discrepancies between video head impulse and caloric test in patients with enlarged vestibular aqueduct. Laryngoscope. 2017;127(4):921–6.
26. Rubin F, Simon F, Verillaud B, Herman P, Kania R, Hautefort C. Comparison of video head impulse test and caloric reflex test in advanced unilateral definite Menière's disease. Eur Ann Otorhinolaryngol Head Neck Dis. 2018;135(3):167–9. https://doi.org/10.1016/j.anorl.2017.08.008. Epub 2017 Dec 20. PMID: 29274769.
27. Merchant SN, Rosowski JJ. Conductive hearing loss caused by third window lesions of the inner ear. Otol Neurotol. 2008;29:282–9.
28. Ray A, Hautefort C, Guichard JP, Horion J, Herman P, Kania R, Houdart E, Verillaud B, Vitaux H, Attyé A, Eliezer M. MRI contribution for the detection of endolymphatic hydrops in patients with superior canal dehiscence syndrome. Eur Arch Otorhinolaryngol. 2021;278(7):2229–38. https://doi.org/10.1007/s00405-020-06282-3. Epub 2020 Aug 14. PMID: 32797276.
29. Lorente-Piera J, Prieto-Matos C, Manrique-Huarte R, Garaycochea O, Domínguez P, Manrique M. Otic capsule dehiscences simulating other inner ear diseases: characterization, clinical profile, and follow-up-is Ménière's disease the sole cause of vertigo and fluctuating hearing loss? Audiol Res. 2024;14(2):372–85. https://doi.org/10.3390/audiolres14020032. PMID: 38666903; PMCID: PMC11047452.
30. Sone M, Yoshida T, Morimoto K, Teranishi M, Nakashima T, Naganawa S. Endolymphatic hydrops in superior canal dehiscence and large vestibular aqueduct syndromes. Laryngoscope.

2016;126(6):1446–50. https://doi.org/10.1002/lary.25747. Epub 2015 Nov 3. PMID: 26525170.
31. Johanis M, De Jong R, Miao T, Hwang L, Lum M, Kaur T, Willis S, Arsenault JJ, Duong C, Yang I, Gopen Q. Concurrent superior semicircular canal dehiscence and endolymphatic hydrops: a novel case series. Int J Surg Case Rep. 2021;78:382–6. https://doi.org/10.1016/j.ijscr.2020.12.074. Epub 2020 Dec 26. PMID: 33421957; PMCID: PMC7804363.
32. Gianoli G. Superior semicircular canal dehiscence repair. In: Babu S, editor. Practical otology for the otolaryngologist. San Diego: Plural Publishing; 2013. p. 287–96.
33. Wackym PA, Wood SJ, Siker DA, Carter DM. Otic capsule dehiscence syndrome: Superior semicircular canal dehiscence syndrome with no radiographically visible dehiscence. Ear Nose Throat J. 2015;94(8):E8–E24.
34. Ward BK, Wenzel A, Ritzl EK, Gutierrez-Hernandez S, Della Santina CC, Minor LB, Carey JP. Near-dehiscence: clinical findings in patients with thin bone over the superior semicircular canal. Otol Neurotol. 2013;34(8):1421–8.
35. Hong M, Mozaffari K, Uy B, Kim WJ, Umesh A, Chandla A, Unterberger A, Yang I, Gopen Q. Postoperative outcomes of patients with thin bone overlying the superior semicircular canal: a single institution's experience. World Neurosurg. 2022;166:e93–8. https://doi.org/10.1016/j.wneu.2022.06.118. Epub 2022 Jun 30. PMID: 35779752.
36. Manzari L. Multiple dehiscences of bony labyrinthine capsule. A rare case report and review of the literature. Acta Otorhinolaryngol Ital. 2010;30(6):317–20. PMID: 21808455; PMCID: PMC3146321.
37. Ionescu EC, Reynard P, Damien M, Ltaief-Boudrigua A, Hermann R, Gianoli GJ, Thai-Van H. Why should multiple dehiscences of the otic capsule be considered before surgically treating patients with superior semicircular canal dehiscence? A radiological monocentric review and a case series. Front Neurol. 2023;14:1209567. https://doi.org/10.3389/fneur.2023.1209567. PMID: 37614976; PMCID: PMC10442812.
38. Shankar A, Nagururu NV, Pearl MS, Shankar A, Carey JP, Ward BK. Superior canal dehiscence and the risk of additional dehiscences: a retrospective CT cohort study. Otol Neurotol. 2024;45(7):e525–31. https://doi.org/10.1097/MAO.0000000000004228. PMID: 38995721.
39. Gianoli GJ. Deficiency of the superior semicircular canal. Curr Opin Otolaryngol Head Neck Surg. 2001;9:336–41.

Chapter 19
Surgical Treatment of Superior Semicircular Canal Dehiscence Syndrome

Francis X. Creighton and John P. Carey

Background

Superior canal dehiscence syndrome (SCDS) was first described by Minor in 1998 [1]. It is a disease characterized by the clinical findings of sound-induced vertigo and eye movements, chronic disequilibrium, conductive hearing loss (CHL), and decreased hearing thresholds for bone-conducted sounds. Conductive hyperacusis may lead to autophony (hearing their own voice), pulsatile tinnitus, or hearing their eye movements. The presence of a dehiscence creates a mobile third window within the labyrinth, leading to physiologic stimuli causing excitatory ampullofugal or inhibitory ampullopetal deflection of the cupula [1].

Symptoms caused by abnormal openings into the labyrinth have been known for decades. Fenestration of the semicircular canals was known to produce eye movements in response to sound in animals as early as 18 years ago [2]. The Tullio phenomenon, or eye movements in response to loud sound, was initially identified in humans suffering from advanced syphilis secondary to gummatous osteomyelitis and labyrinthine fistulae [3]. Subsequent reports have identified the Tullio phenomenon in perilymphatic fistula [4], head trauma [5], and cholesteatoma with semicircular canal erosion and fenestration [6]. The Hennebert sign (eye movement induced by pressure in the external auditory canal) is also often present in cases of abnormal openings into the labyrinth. These symptoms can be present in SCDS and help to lead to the understanding of the constellation of symptoms encompassing this syndrome.

F. X. Creighton · J. P. Carey (✉)
Johns Hopkins Outpatient Center, Baltimore, MD, USA
e-mail: Francis.creighton@jhmi.edu; jcarey@jhmi.edu

J. C. Lucas et al. (eds.), *Diagnosis and Treatment of Vestibular Disorders*,
https://doi.org/10.1007/978-3-032-11740-3_19

The exact mechanism by which SCDS causes its audiological and vestibular symptoms is still under investigation, but it is generally accepted that the dehiscence of the superior semicircular canal functions as a mobile "third window" in the bony labyrinth. This third window allows a low impedance outlet for fluid waves in the labyrinth to shunt flow from the cochlea to the labyrinth, which both activates the vestibular system and decreases pressure driving the traveling fluid wave in the cochlea. Cadaveric and animal models have supported this, showing measurable fluid velocities across the dehiscence, a decrease in intracochlear pressures in the scala typmani and scala vestibuli, a decrease in cochlear differential pressure, and a decrease in round window velocity, most notably in lower frequencies [7–9].

Epidemiology

The anatomic prevalence of superior canal dehiscence within a temporal bone library consisting of 1000 specimens revealed a 0.5% prevalence of complete dehiscence of the superior canal into the middle fossa or superior petrosal sinus [10]. In 1.4% of specimens, the bone was 0.1 mm or thinner. The prevalence of SCDS is not known with certainty, but it is likely that only a subset of patients with SCD actually experience symptoms. Re et al. found a SCD prevalence rate of 5.8% on temporal bone CT in a series of 191 consecutive patients scanned for all causes. Individuals identified with SCD then underwent otoneurological examinations. Of those identified with SCD on CT imaging, only 0.5% had symptoms or signs consistent with SCDS [11].

The effect of dehiscence size on the clinical manifestation of SCDS is currently debated in the literature. Small case series have found dehiscences greater than or equal to 2.5 mm often present with both vestibular and cochlear symptoms, whereas those less than 2.5 mm often present with either vestibular or cochlear symptoms, but not both [12]. However, in multivariate analysis, the length of the dehiscence was only shown to correlate with the size of the air-bone gap [13]. Assessments of the surface area of SSCDs have shown that larger dehiscences are associated with larger cVEMP and oVEMP amplitudes [14] Cadaveric models of SSCD have shown that larger dehiscences decrease intracochlear pressure and decrease the cochlear drive at low frequencies. This effect seems to saturate around 3 mm in length. Paradoxically, at higher frequencies, pinpoint dehiscences appear to cause a decrease in the cochlear drive, while larger dehiscences do not appear to effect at these frequencies [7, 15]. Cadaveric studies have also shown that the location of the SSCD along the arc of the canal does not have a major effect on intracochlear pressures. This is consistent with clinical studies showing that the location of the SCD did not correlate with the amount of hearing loss, although dehiscences located closer to the ampulla were found to be commonly seen in patients with auditory symptoms [16].

Diagnostic Evaluation

Patients with SCDS generally present with a primary complaint of dizziness, and when evaluating a patient with this complaint, a thorough history is the most effective diagnostic tool. Vertigo symptoms related to SCDS are usually induced by loud sounds or pressure changes and are brief in duration. Dizziness or oscillopsia induced by loud sounds is present in 90% of SCDS patients [17]. Vestibular symptoms induced by pressure changes, such as coughing or straining, are present in 73% of patients, with 67% exhibiting both pressure and sound-related symptoms [17]. Chronic disequilibrium and cognitive impairment ("brain fog") may also be attributed to SCDS.

In addition to dizziness, auditory symptoms are also a common feature of SCDS. Autophony, defined as the hyperperception of one's own voice, breathing, or other internal sounds, is present to varying degrees in up to 60% of patients [17]. Hyperacusis for bone-conducted sound [18] is present in 52% of SCDS patients [17]. Hyperacusis symptoms include patients hearing their own pulse, eye movements, or the impact of their feet during walking. Patients with SCDS can occasionally hear in the affected ear a 512 Hz tuning fork placed against the foot or ankle [19]. Pulsatile tinnitus is present in about one-third of patients seen at our institution.

Evoked eye movements in the plane of the superior canal are the hallmark of SCDS [20]. The eyes should be examined under Frenzel lenses, infrared video goggles, or by some other means to eliminate the effect of visual fixation. Using an audiometer, pure tones at levels up to 110 dB nHL should be delivered in one ear at a time, covering the frequency range of 125–4000 Hz. Sound-evoked eye movements at one or more frequencies were noted in 82% of SCDS patients using such stimuli [17]. Among our patient population, eye movements can also be induced with Valsalva maneuvers (34%) or pressure in the external auditory canal (23%).

Depending on the type of stimulus, either excitation or inhibition of the superior canal may occur, as shown in Fig. 19.1. Valsalva against pinched nostrils, pressure in the external auditory canal (e.g., tragal compression), or sound will produce excitatory effects (ampullofugal deflection of cupula). Valsalva against a closed glottis, jugular venous compression, or negative external canal pressure will produce inhibitory secondary to ampullopetal cupula deflection. Pressure or sound-evoked eye movements almost always occur in the plane of the superior canal, as shown in Fig. 19.2. In the case of larger dehiscences, eye movements may be shifted out of the superior canal plane [21]. However, if eye movements are not in this direction, the diagnosis of SCDS should be questioned, and alternative diagnoses of posterior canal dehiscence [22] or horizontal canal fistula [23] must be considered.

The audiogram (Fig. 19.3) is an important part of the SCDS evaluation. A minority of patients have auditory symptoms in the absence of any vestibular signs or symptoms [17, 19, 24, 25]. Conductive hearing loss, and bone conduction thresholds less than 0 dB nHL (conductive hyperacusis) are often greatest at lower frequencies [24, 25]. It is important to consider SCDS in patients with CHL and normal otologic exam, as case reports exist of SCDS being misdiagnosed as otosclerosis

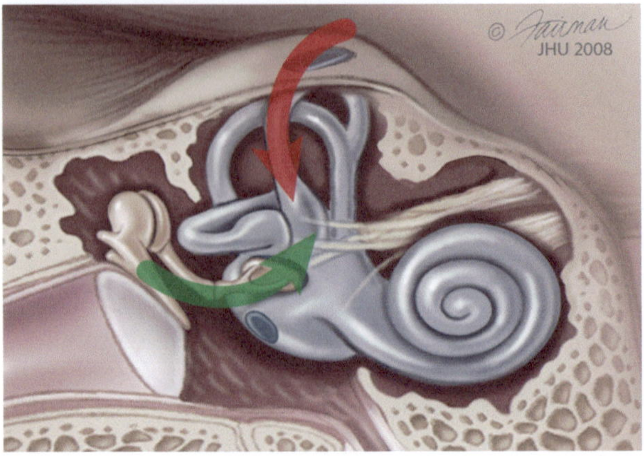

Fig. 19.1 Route of excitatory and inhibitory pressure changes causing stimulation of the superior canal ampulla in SCDS. Superior canal excitation is caused by ampullofugal displacement of the cupula (green arrow), typically by positive external auditory canal pressure, nasal Valsalva, or sound. Superior canal inhibition is caused by ampullopetal displacement of the cupula (red arrow) from negative external auditory canal pressure or glottic Valsalva maneuver, which transiently increases intracranial pressure

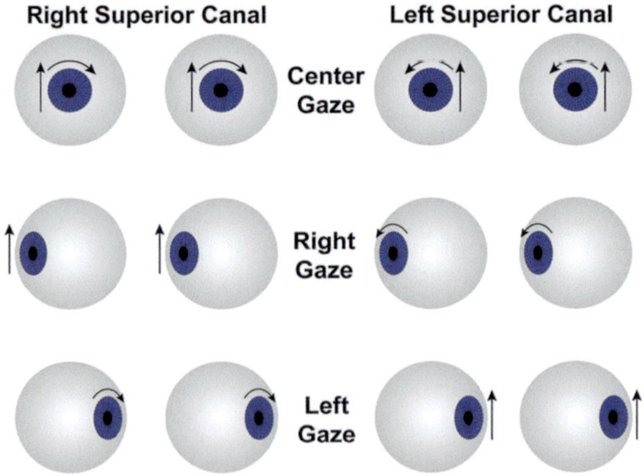

Fig. 19.2 Direction of the slow phase of eye movements with superior canal excitation. Eye movement occurs in the plane of the superior canal regardless of the direction of gaze. There are both vertical and torsional components when the patient is looking directly ahead (center gaze). The torsional and vertical components can be separated by having the patient look to the right or left during stimulation

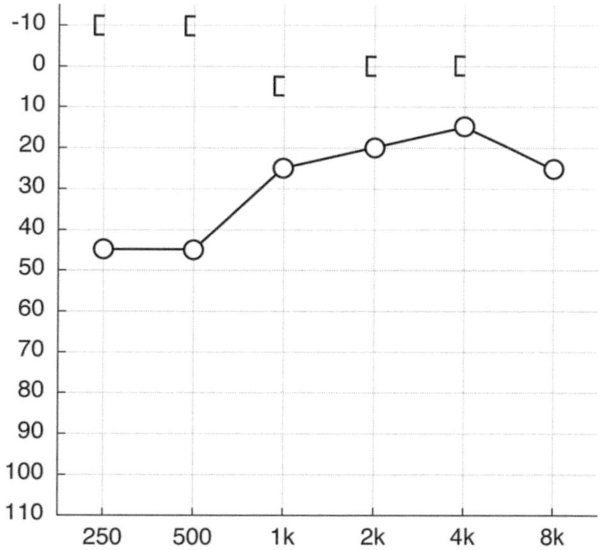

Fig. 19.3 Typical audiogram in a patient with right-sided SCDS. Circles represent air conduction and brackets represent bone conduction. Note that there is a negative bone conduction threshold at 250 and 500 Hz, and the air-bone gap is largest at low frequencies. X-axis: kilohertz (k). Y-axis: decibel (dB)

[19]. The key differences between SCDS and otosclerosis are (1) that conductive hyperacusis does not occur in otosclerosis, and (2) that the acoustic stapedial reflex, which is often normal in superior canal dehiscence, should be absent in an ear affected with otosclerosis.

Electrocochleography (ECochG) has been used in the past for diagnosing SCDS. Initial studies of ECochG showed elevated summating potential (SP) to action potential (AP) ratios >0.4 were reported in all (n = 21) patients with unilateral SCDS, with normalization of the SP/AP ratio postoperatively [26]. More recent studies, though, have failed to reproduce the post-operative results [27].

Cervical vestibular evoked myogenic potentials, or cVEMPs, are inhibitory electromyographic (EMG) signals measured over the contracted sternocleidomastoid (SCM) muscle ipsilateral to the ear being stimulated by multiple loud clicks or tone bursts (Fig. 19.4). It is thought that cVEMPs are activated through the stapes footplate to the saccule and vestibular nerve [28]. In SCDS, abnormally low thresholds and enlarged peak-to-peak amplitudes are demonstrated [4, 17]. The theory is that a dehiscent semicircular canal lowers the impedance of the vestibular system, resulting in a lower resistance for pressure and sound transmission [18, 19]. Thus, cVEMP signals are enhanced with lower thresholds in patients with SCDS. For air-conducted 500 Hz tone bursts, for example, we have found that cVEMP thresholds were 80–95 dB SPL for 13 patients with SCDS (83.85 ± 1.40 dB SPL, mean ± SD), 20–30 dB lower than in normal control subjects (110.25 ± 1.28 dB SPL) [29]. It has been argued that cVEMP is better than 90% sensitive and specific for SCD [30], while other series have found the sensitivity and specificity closer to 80% [31]. The cVEMP is not measurable in all patients and is especially likely to be absent in patients who have had previous middle ear surgery. The cVEMP threshold may also be decreased in other conditions, such as enlarged vestibular aqueduct syndrome [32].

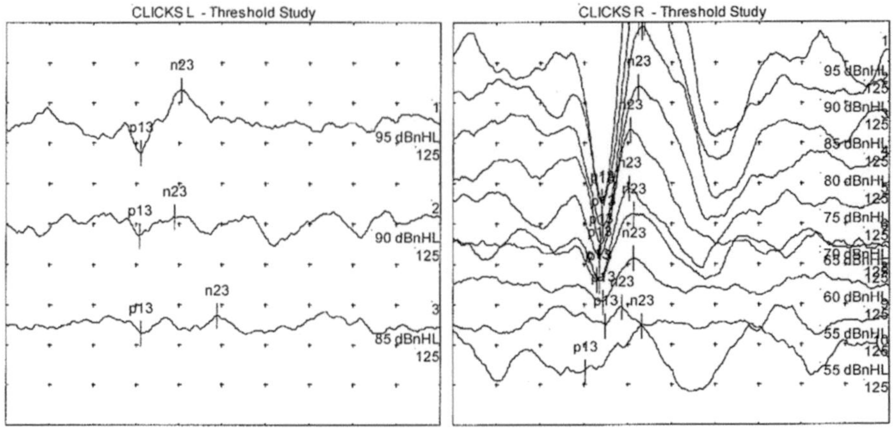

Fig. 19.4 Typical cervical vestibular evoked myogenic potential (cVEMP) results in a patient with right-sided SCDS and an intact left side. The cVEMP is initially measured with clicks at 95 dB nHL, and the stimulus amplitude is decreased until the response is no longer measurable. In the left ear, the patient has a cVEMP response at 95 dB but not with lower amplitude stimuli. In the right ear, the amplitude of the cVEMP is much larger at 95 dB, and the response continues to be detectable at amplitudes as small as 60 dB. Thus, in this example, the cVEMP threshold is 95 dB nHL on the left and 60 dB nHL on the right

Ocular VEMP (oVEMP) is also used for the diagnostic evaluation of suspected SCDS. An excitatory EMG response is obtained from the contralateral inferior oblique muscle, with the pathway thought to be a result of utricular activation. We have demonstrated that oVEMP results in response to air-conducted sound provide greater sensitivity and specificity than cVEMP for diagnosing SCDS [33]. In 29 patients with surgically confirmed SCDS, a peak-to-peak amplitude greater than 17.1 μV corresponded to 100% sensitivity and 98% specificity. The performance of oVEMP is also less time-consuming compared to cVEMP. oVEMPs may also be a good screening test for SCDS. In a prospective study, SCDS patients were more likely to have abnormal oVEMPs when compared to healthy controls [34].

For the diagnosis of SCD to be considered, imaging of the temporal bone using computed tomography (CT) must show the absence of bone over the superior canal. If the superior canal appears surrounded with bone on CT, the diagnosis of SCDS is effectively excluded; however, the appearance of a dehiscence on CT does not rule out thin bone covering the SC below the resolution of the scanner. Thus, CT is a highly sensitive test for SCD, but it is not specific [31].

Optimal imaging uses high-resolution CT (HRCT) formatted in the plane of the superior canal [31, 35]. Unfortunately, the term "high-resolution" has been applied to a wide variety of CT scanning parameters, which continue to change as technology is updated. In a review of temporal bone CT scans done in the general population, 9% of scans had apparent SCD, with one observer calling as many as 12% [36]. Many of these are likely false dehiscences caused by the limits of resolving thin bone. In scans with greater than 1 mm thickness, thin structures are subjected to partial volume artifacts. Furthermore, with bone structures less than 0.1 mm in thickness, volume artifacts can give the impression that bone is absent, thus leading to a higher rate of dehiscence [11].

A properly done scan should have a resolution near 0.2 mm. This requires attention to a number of parameters. The most important of these is slice thickness. Collimation of the x-ray beam to 0.5 mm allows the data to be represented by nearly isotropic voxels, so that the images can be reformatted in any plane without distortion.

Helical CT scanning, in which the table moves along the z-axis while the gantry rotates and scans, may lead to some loss of resolution. The "step, scan, and repeat" mode is preferred. The field of view used to reconstruct the images of the inner ear should be of the smallest size possible, so that the labyrinth is displayed to maximal resolution over the fixed size of the image matrix (usually 512 × 512 pixels). Image filters should be set for bone edge detection, as those filters that produce less "noisy" images are likely to filter out a thin layer of bone that might remain over the canal. Images should be reconstructed in the plane of the superior canal as well as orthogonal to it so that any dehiscence can be definitively demonstrated (Fig. 19.5). Parallel (Pöschl position) and perpendicular (Stenver) reformatted planes can allow for more accurate assessment. In one study of 850 patients (1700 temporal bones), the prevalence of any semicircular canal dehiscence decreased from 7% to 2.5% when use of HRCT was combined with a semicircular canal evaluation whereby dehiscence was confirmed in two perpendicular planes [19]. However, even optimized scans are not without the risks of false positive findings, so the diagnosis of SCD must never be based on a CT scan alone. The authors cannot stress enough that a finding of SCD on CT should be considered in the context of findings on physical exam, cVEMP or oVEMP, audiogram, and the patient's symptoms before concluding that the patient has SCDS.

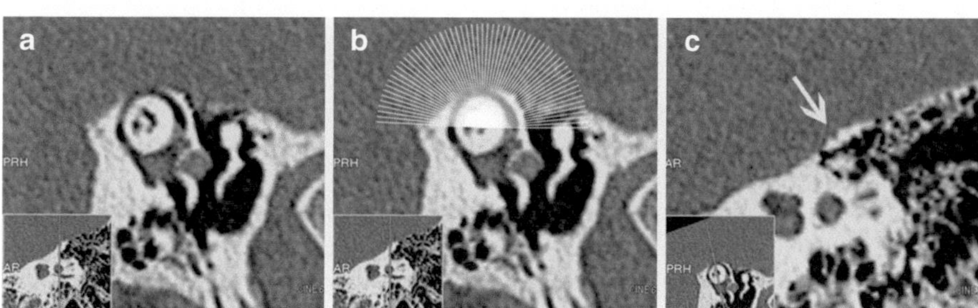

Fig. 19.5 CT scan demonstrating SCD. Panel (**a**) CT image is reformatted in the plane of the superior canal. An area of dehiscence between the superior canal and the middle fossa is present. Panel (**b**) Orthogonal reconstructions are performed at 3° intervals for 180° around the superior canal. These planes of reconstruction are shown as white lines. Panel (**c**) An orthogonal reconstruction demonstrating SCD. The region of the reconstruction is shown in small view in the lower left

Differential Diagnosis

In assessing a patient with possible SCDS, it is important to consider other possible diagnoses, such as otosclerosis, Meniere's disease, patulous Eustachian tube, perilymphatic fistula, and vertiginous migraine.

The CHL component of SCDS can appear similar to otosclerosis because both occur in adulthood in ears that appear normal on physical exam [19]. The audiograms differ in that SCDS patients often have conductive hyperacusis, and if there is no previous history of middle ear surgery, the acoustic reflex is often intact. Otosclerosis is also not associated with decreased cVEMP or oVEMP thresholds, vertigo symptoms, or CT findings of SCD.

Menière's disease is characterized by the triad of low-frequency hearing loss, vertigo, aural fullness, and tinnitus [37]. Although the hearing loss in Menière's disease is classically sensorineural hearing loss, CHL has also been described [38]. The attacks of vertigo associated with Menière's disease are usually severe and last hours with normal periods between attacks. The dizziness associated with SCDS can be chronic, but distinct vertigo attacks are often shorter and associated with exposure to noise or pressure changes.

Autophony is often the predominant symptom in patients with a patulous eustachian tube [39], but it can also be the most disturbing symptom in SCDS. One distinguishing feature between the two conditions is that patients with patulous Eustachian tube typically have autophony for their own breath sounds, whereas patients with SCDS usually do not [39]. A history of vertigo symptoms and hyperacusis of bone-conducted sound is not typical of a patulous eustachian tube. The audiogram, VEMP testing, and CT will typically differentiate a patulous eustachian tube from SCDS.

A perilymphatic fistula, along with fenestrations of other semicircular canals, is often considered in the differential diagnosis of SCDS [40]. A perilymphatic fistula is a leak of perilymph within the vestibular labyrinth and generally is used to describe a fistula involving the round or oval window. The leak creates an abnormal compliance that allows fluid to move and stimulate the vestibular end organs in response to sound or pressure changes. The diagnosis of a perilymphatic fistula should be considered in the context of a recent stapes surgery, temporal bone fracture, or barotrauma injury. In these cases, acute vertigo is usually accompanied by a sensorineural hearing loss. A fistula in the horizontal canal can be acquired in cases of cholesteatoma or prior mastoidectomy [41]. Spontaneous perilymphatic fistula is a controversial diagnosis and should be considered as a diagnosis of exclusion [42].

One of the most common causes of spontaneous (non-positional) vertigo is migraine-associated vertigo, and it should be considered in the differential with SCDS [43]. The incidence of migraine is 17.6% of females and 5.7% of males [44], and approximately 25% of migraine patients report some vertigo [45]. Thus, migraine is much more common than SCDS, and inevitably, we have found some patients with radiographically apparent SCD whose symptoms were non-specific and better explained by migraine. Particularly challenging are those patients who have specific symptoms of both SCDS and migraine. For example, it may be difficult to determine if their sound sensitivity is due to one more than the other. Their chronic disequilibrium may be related to migraine, or it may be due to the constant transmission of intracranial pressure pulsations through the dehiscence to the labyrinth. Moreover, the physiological disturbances of the labyrinth caused by SCDS could serve as triggers to exacerbate migraine in susceptible individuals. However, the neurotologist must also consider that failure to recognize and treat coexistent migraine can lead to disappointing results in SCDS surgery.

Pre-operative Decision-Making

The decision to undergo surgery for SCD plugging is often more difficult than settling on the diagnosis. The physician must help the patient weigh the severity of symptoms against the risks and benefits of surgery. In the authors' institution, approximately 72% with SCDS opt to have surgical SC plugging, with the remaining patients opting to live with their symptoms or make lifestyle changes to avoid situations that exacerbate the symptoms, like loud noise. This number may be a reflection of the referral pattern of patients seeking care at our institution.

The dizziness handicap inventory (DHI) [46] is an instrument that may be helpful in gauging vestibular symptom severity. This questionnaire grades dizziness symptoms on a scale from 0 to 100. It has previously been validated for surgical treatment of benign paroxysmal positional vertigo (BPPV) [47], acoustic neuroma surgery [48, 49], and ablative procedures for Menière's disease [50]. We measured the DHI in 19 patients with SCDS before they underwent SCD repair via a middle fossa approach. The average pre-op DHI score was 44 ± 24 (mean ± SD) [51]. This compares with the handicap caused by untreated primary benign paroxysmal positioning vertigo, in which the DHI score averaged 38.5 in one series [52], and with the handicap caused by active Menière's disease, in which the DHI score averaged 39.6 ± 21.1 in another series [53]. The comparisons indicate a high degree of dizziness handicap for SCDS patients who seek surgical treatment.

Auditory symptoms are the primary complaint in a significant number of SCDS patients [25]. Autophony or conductive hyperacusis can often be quite disabling, especially in patients for whom singing or speaking is important. There is no medical treatment for autophony symptoms due to SCDS, as the sound transmission is via bone, not the eustachian tube. Thus, for SCDS patients who are significantly disturbed by autophony or conductive hyperacusis, surgery is the only option for relief.

CHL is a common symptom in SCDS [54]. It is often limited to low frequencies and usually only affects one ear, so many patients do not have a significant disability. In most patients, the CHL improves with surgery [54], and resolution of a large sensorineural hearing loss has even been reported [55]. However, plugging of SCD does carry a risk of hearing loss, and this risk is greater in patients who have had previous inner ear surgery, including stapes surgery [54]. In a retrospective review of 43 cases of SCDS who underwent repair via middle fossa approach with plugging, 25% developed a mild high-frequency hearing loss [56]. Long-term follow-up of 242 patients who have undergone repair at our institution shows 2.5% of patients ultimately developing a profound sensorineural hearing loss [57]. Patients should be carefully counseled on these risks, and those with hearing loss as their primary symptom of SCDS should strongly consider non-surgical options such as a hearing aid.

As part of the pre-operative decision-making process, it is important to provide patients with counseling on their likely post-operative course and possible complications of SCD. Although dizziness symptoms are often the motivation for surgery, it is common for imbalance symptoms to be worse during the immediate post-operative period. At the author's institution, all patients are evaluated by inpatient physical therapy post-operatively to determine if continued inpatient or outpatient therapy is required.

In the initial post-operative period, there are often decreased VOR gains in all ipsilateral canals. Whether this is due to labyrinthine inflammation or loss of perilymph is not clear [58]. This is typically transient in the horizontal and posterior canal, but plugging of the superior canal will cause a permanent vestibular sensory deficit due to the hydrodynamic insufficiency of the canal. This can be seen as decreased VOR in the superior canal plane (rotating the head to align the superior canal in the vertical orientation and quickly thrusting the patient's head down in that vertical plane) [3]. However, patients can adapt very well to this single-canal insufficiency. Low-frequency, low-acceleration head movements will generate useful inhibitory signals from the contralateral posterior canal, and recent studies of video head impulse testing post-operatively have shown evidence of central compensation within one week [58]. Vestibular physical therapy can take advantage of the contralateral posterior canal's function and of other gaze-stabilizing mechanisms in promoting compensation for the loss caused by SCD plugging. In our experience, the compensated state after SCD plugging allows the patient to lead a much more active lifestyle than did the SCDS condition.

Complications of SCD plugging are rare, but can be serious. The most common complication is post-operative BPPV, which occurs in 4–24% of all patients [57, 59]. It is important to monitor for this in the early post-operative period, as it is easy to dismiss as normal vestibular hypofunction. A Dix-Hallpike maneuver, looking at the posterior and horizontal canal, should be performed in patients with abnormal bouts of vertigo with head positioning. As mentioned above, hearing loss is a real risk of SCD repair. As noted above, one fourth of patients undergoing MFC repair at our institution developed mild high-frequency SNHL [56]. While fortunately, this hearing loss is mild, profound SNHL does occur in 2–3% of patients at our institution [57]. Surgery for SCD via a middle fossa approach shares the risk of perioperative complications common to any craniotomy [60]. Cerebrospinal fluid (CSF) leak may occur if the dura is violated, especially if air cells into the mastoid are exposed during surgery or if there is a tegmen dehiscence. Intracranial hematoma is a rare post-operative complication that can occur after any middle fossa surgery. In 220 primary middle fossa approaches at our institution, epidural hematoma occurred in

1.4% of the time [57]. The patient's mental status should be closely monitored during the acute post-operative period, and the onset of unusually severe pain should also be a warning sign. If this complication occurs, the patient must be quickly returned to the operating room for hematoma evacuation to prevent more serious sequela.

The age and general state of health of the patient should also be considered in the decision to undergo surgery. In older patients, it is more difficult to elevate the middle fossa dura without tearing the dura and causing CSF leak [61]. Language impairment due to damage to the dominant temporal lobe must be considered. Post-operative vestibular adaptation and recovery can be a longer and more difficult process in older patients.

Outcomes

In the properly selected patient, the vast majority of patients have improvement of symptoms following surgical repair. In a study of 93 post-operative patients, 95% of patients reported that their symptoms had improved postoperatively. Importantly, this reported benefit did not seem to decrease the further out patients were from surgery, implying that patients can expect longevity of their surgical repair. It was also noted in this study that auditory symptoms, such as tinnitus, autophony, and sensitivity to sound, were noted to have the greatest improvement in patient-reported outcomes. Symptoms such as headaches, imbalance, dizziness, and cognitive impairment were noted to have a lower reported improvement by patients. This is important to consider when managing patient expectations preoperatively. For patients with headache or cognitive impairment as a major symptom, we routinely treat patients for migraine-related imbalance prior to consideration of any surgical intervention [62].

Bilateral Dehiscences

At our institution, 38% of individuals diagnosed with SCDS have the appearance of bilateral SCD on high-resolution CT scan. Fortunately, one side is usually responsible for most of the symptoms and can be readily identified by the patient. In some cases, symptoms and signs can be elicited from both ears, including decreased VEMP thresholds, conductive hyperacusis, and sound- or pressure-induced eye movements. In such patients who have bilateral SCDS, every effort should be made to identify the more symptomatic ear and operate on that side first. In most cases, symptoms will either resolve after operating on the more symptomatic side or abate to the point that contralateral surgery is not required. While exceedingly rare, some patients do ultimately require bilateral surgery. We recommend that the second side should only be considered for plugging surgery after at least 6 months have passed since the initial operation. Plugging of both superior canals significantly impairs the ability to sense downward head rotation in the vertical plane, so these patients are at risk of developing vertical oscillopsia during ambulation, particularly while walking down stairs.

Revision Surgery

While the majority of patients have improvement post-operatively, some patients will ultimately need revision surgery. This can be due to a variety of reasons. In a review of 23 patients undergoing revision surgery, the majority of patients were found to have a canal plug in the correct location, but that was not entirely covering the dehiscence. Results of these revision surgeries did not show a significant increase in complication rates or hearing loss, but did show a decreased rate of resolution of symptoms compared with patients undergoing initial surgery [63]. We have found success in both revision middle fossa approaches, as well as transmastoid approaches, and decide the best approach on a case-by-case basis.

Operative Technique

Since the initial description of SCDS, much has been learned about the pathophysiology and treatment outcomes. Multiple surgical approaches have been described and recently reviewed by Shaia and Diaz [64]. The middle cranial fossa approach was described first [1], and the technique is detailed in the following paragraphs. Since the initial description of surgical treatment of SCDS, several alternative approaches have been described. Most notable are transmastoid SCD plugging, transmastoid resurfacing, or endoscopic-assisted middle cranial fossa resurfacing [65–67].

Advocates of the transmastoid approach have noted that it avoids a craniotomy, involves no temporal lobe retraction, and may lead to better stability of the canal plug. Moreover, most otolaryngologists are more familiar with the transmastoid anatomy [68, 69]. Case series using transmastoid plugging have reported success rates of 94% [65]. A modification of the original middle fossa approach has been made with the introduction of intraoperative endoscopy. The technique allows for a smaller, 2 cm diameter craniotomy. This method permits resurfacing, but exposure adequate for canal plugging is not attained. Others have described the use of a mini-craniotomy (2 × 3 cm) and angled rigid endoscopes for enhanced visualization of more medial defects [67].

We favor the middle fossa approach over the transmastoid approach for the vast majority of patients. There are several reasons for this. First, the transmastoid approach does not allow direct visual confirmation of the dehiscence. This presents several problems, and transmastoid plugging of a superior canal that was later found to be intact has been described [68]. Furthermore, without direct access to the dehiscence, the transmastoid approach requires drilling, irrigation, and suctioning on the bony canal. Once the canal is opened, these manipulations could contaminate or remove perilymph and cause collapse of the membranous labyrinth or serous labyrinthitis. Anatomically, the transmastoid approach is not always possible in patients with a low-hanging dura or extensive tegmen dehiscences [68]. In the transmastoid approach, the plug is also placed closer to the sensory epithelia of the ampulla and the utricle. This may be more traumatic to these structures, risking disturbance of their baseline firing rates. Furthermore, opening the superior canal distal to the dehiscence may place the plug into the common crus, causing loss of sensory function of the posterior canal as well [70].

Transmastoid Repair

Despite these drawbacks, we do perform transmastoid repairs in select cases. Patients with multiple medical comorbidities requiring anticoagulation, and those who have undergone prior MFC repair, are often best approached via the mastoid. We have also found that patients whose dehiscences are located medially along the canal are often difficult to access via the MFC [71].

The transmastoid approach is set up with electrophysiological monitoring and image navigation in a similar fashion to the middle fossa craniotomy approach described below. A cortical mastoidectomy is performed, with care taken to thin the tegmen to allow for maximum exposure of the canal. Once the canal is clearly identified, image navigation is used to determine the location of the dehiscence along the arc of the canal. Once the location of the dehiscence has been confirmed with navigation, two small labyrinthotomies are made with a 1 mm diamond burr on low speed. One is made on the ampullopetal side of the dehiscence, and the other is made on the ampullofugal side of the dehiscence.

Plugging is performed in a manner similar to the middle fossa craniotomy approach described below. Care must be taken when plugging the canal via a transmastoid approach to not place an excessive amount of material into the labyrinth. Due to the need to isolate the dehiscence, which cannot be directly visualized via this approach, the labyrinthotomies are placed closer towards the cupula (ampullopetally) and closer to the common crus (ampullofugally). Excessive plugging could lead to deflection of the cupula, which can cause long-term vestibular dysfunction, or accidental plugging of the posterior canal, which can cause a reduction in the function of that canal as well.

When performing the transmastoid repair, we switch to basic salt solution irrigation when opening the bony labyrinth. Basic salt solution's electrolyte composition is the most similar to perilymph of all commercially available solutions. The goal of switching the basic salt solution is to limit changes in the electrolyte composition of the exposed perilymph, with the goal of reducing injury to the inner ear. After completion of plugging, a titanium plate is placed over the mastoid bowl at the end of the case to limit patient sensitivity to mastoid pressure, inducing vertigo or auditory distortions.

Middle Fossa Craniotomy

Our preferred technique for SCD repair is to plug the canal via a middle cranial fossa approach. The approach has evolved to involve a smaller craniotomy and the use of CT-guided image navigation to aid in both craniotomy planning and localization of the dehiscence. We routinely utilize image-guidance to minimize the risk of applying suction to the dehiscence when attempting to identify the dehiscence, in what is often a field of tegmen dehiscences. On the day of or prior to surgery, the patient undergoes a CT scan. We use the LandmarX® image guidance system (Medtronic Corporation, Minneapolis, MN), which allows us to fuse the low-resolution, whole-head dataset with a high-resolution scan of the temporal bone. The latter is invaluable for the precise localization of the dehiscence.

The navigation system allows placement of the craniotomy for optimum exposure to the superior canal while avoiding mastoid air cells. The precise placement of the craniotomy centered over the trajectory of the dehiscence also allows for a smaller craniotomy. Craniotomy size less than 3 × 3 cm has been performed with excellent access to the dehiscence for plugging and resurfacing (Fig. 19.6).

On the day of surgery, after the anesthesiologist has intubated the patient and placed any necessary lines and monitors, the table is rotated 180° so that the head faces the surgeon. The head is placed on a horseshoe headrest. Positioning of the head should ensure no strain is placed on the neck and minimize significant rotation of the neck. Additionally, the contralateral ear should be centered within the headrest to avoid bending of the neuromonitoring equipment.

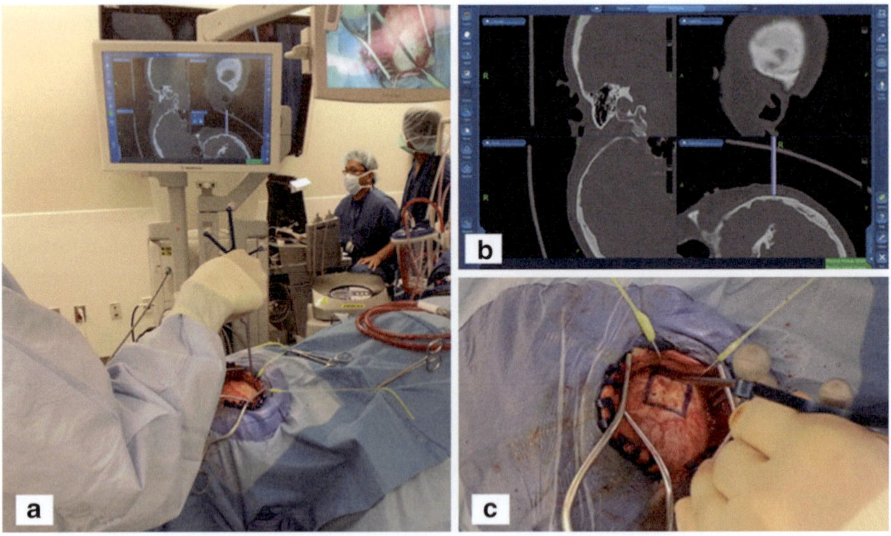

Fig. 19.6 Navigation and placement of craniotomy. Panel (**a**) Surgeon positioned at head of bed with navigation on the left side. Panel (**b**) Trajectory view mode is used to "sight" a line from the surface of the skull to the dehiscence. Panel (**c**) The lower border of craniotomy (marked in purple) is centered here on the skull

The surgeon is positioned at the head of the bed, and thus it serves the scrub technologists to be located on the right side of the patient while the CT navigation system is on the left (Fig. 19.6a). Given this design, both arms of the patient should be tucked and secured. Care should be made to ensure pressure points are protected and no undo traction is placed on the shoulder that could lead to brachial plexus injury.

Dexamethasone 0.1 mg/kg and appropriate prophylactic antibiotics are given intravenously. Mannitol dosed at 0.5 g/kg should be prepared to be administered just prior to making the craniotomy.

An area of the scalp away from the area of the middle fossa approach incision is prepped and sterilely draped for placement of the reference frame. In positioning of the reference frame, the surgeon should anticipate the position of the eventual incision, the location of the surgeon's hands during surgery, the location of microscope, the location of the navigation system, as well as the patient's anatomy, including the thickness of the bone and the location of the superior sagittal sinus (for the right) or mastoid emissary vein (for the left). For right-sided surgery, we position the reference frame in a parasagittal orientation. For left-sided approaches, the reference frame is placed in the post-auricular. When the site is chosen, a 1-cm incision is made, and a small patch of periosteum is cleared from the bone. The reference frame is anchored (Fig. 19.7a). The reference frame is then registered with surface point mapping to allow navigation during surgery. Typically, the precision of the navigation registration is ≤1 mm. The surgeon should be cognizant of any tape used to secure the endotracheal tube and its potential for distorting the skin during point mapping, leading to inaccuracy during navigation system registration.

a b

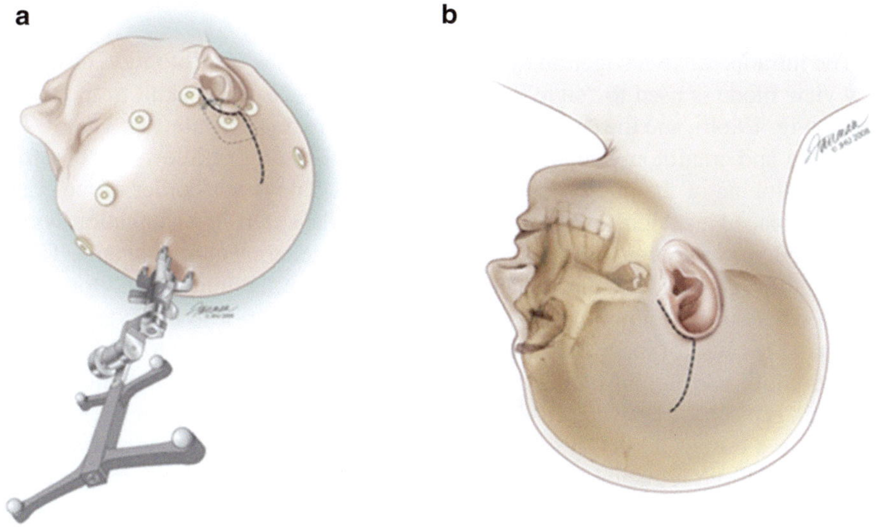

Fig. 19.7 (**a**) Placement of the reference frame. Fiducial markers are shown on the scalp. Planned area of the incision and craniotomy is shown as dashed lines. (**b**) Incision planning

After registration is complete, the neuromonitoring team places the necessary sound probes and electrodes for facial nerve monitoring, somatosensory evoked potential monitoring, ECochG, and auditory brainstem response (ABR). ECochG is performed using gold foil tip electrodes (Etymotic Research Inc., Elk Grove, IL, USA), which are placed adjacent to the tympanic membrane in the external auditory canal. The electrodes are placed under otomicroscopic visualization by the surgeon, with conductive gel placed in the EAC leading onto the tympanic membrane. Bone wax is placed at the external auditory meatus to prevent surgical prep solution from entering the external canal. The ECochG compression fittings, output cables, and ground electrode are secured to the pinna with water-tight Tegaderm™ adhesive dressing and tape.

The incision is then marked on the scalp extending from the helical root around the helix to a location over the external auditory canal, and then superiorly (Fig. 19.7b). The exact orientation of the incision is determined with the aid of the image guidance system to allow for the optimal trajectory and position of the craniotomy to access the dehiscence. Hair around the area of the planned incision is shaved, and the area is infiltrated with 1% lidocaine with 1:100,000 epinephrine. The skin is sterilized widely enough to include the previously placed reference frame in the field and to be prepared for the rare case in which a craniotomy may need to be enlarged in order to control bleeding or evacuate a hematoma. After the skin incision is completed, bleeding is controlled using Raney clips along the skin edges. A large piece of true temporalis fascia is harvested for later use in plugging the superior canal, repair of any tegmen defects, or cerebrospinal fluid leak that may occur (Fig. 19.8). Afterward, the temporalis muscle is divided, and the area of the craniotomy is exposed. Fishhook and cerebellar retractors are used to improve visualization of the proposed craniotomy site.

The intraoperative navigation system is used to plan the craniotomy. The trajectory view mode is used to "sight" a line from the surface of the skull to the dehiscence (Fig. 19.6b), and the craniotomy is centered here on the skull (Fig. 19.6c). The trajectory and craniotomy should be oriented in a position that allows for comfortable positioning of the microscope and the surgeon. The lower border of the craniotomy is placed just high enough to avoid the mastoid air cells. If a navigation system is not used, the craniotomy should be centered on the external auditory canal. This is slightly different from the placement used for drilling of the internal auditory canal (IAC), where the craniotomy is placed with its center anterior to the external auditory canal because of the more anterior location of the IAC relative to the labyrinth.

The width and height of the craniotomy are enough to accommodate a Fisch retractor, typically 3 cm wide by 4 cm high (Fig. 19.6c). Care is taken to ensure the anterior and posterior cuts of the craniotomy are parallel to facilitate stable placement of the Fisch retractor. Once the craniotomy is marked, the bone is opened by drilling troughs around the borders beginning with a 4-mm cutting burr. As the bone is thinned, a 4-mm diamond burr is used to drill until an eggshell layer of bone remains over the dura. This is fractured with a blunt instrument. During the drilling of the cortex, bone dust is collected and placed in sterile saline for later use during plugging of the dehiscence.

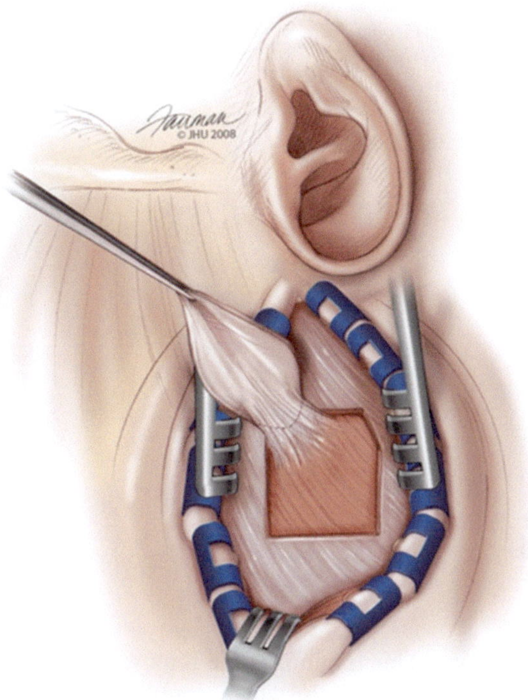

Fig. 19.8 Harvest of temporalis fascia after incision is opened and Raney clips are applied

Penfield instruments are used to elevate the bone flap away from the dura. The bone flap is placed in saline for later cranioplasty. Bleeding from branches of the middle meningeal artery, which traverses the field, often must be controlled with bipolar cautery. The dura is slightly further elevated from the edges of the craniotomy to accommodate the retractor. The sharp edges of the craniotomy are removed using 2- and 1-mm Kerrison rongeurs, and the bone chips created in this process are saved for later use as plugs for the superior canal.

The initial dural dissection is accomplished with the use of large, saline-soaked cotton balls with strings. We find that the large cotton balls soaked in saline are the least traumatic means for the dural elevation. A hemostatic agent, such as (Floseal®) or gelatin powder (Gelfoam®) mixed as a paste with thrombin, is generously applied in advance of the cotton balls. The Fisch middle cranial fossa retractor is then placed and used to gently elevate the dura off of the floor of the middle fossa (Fig. 19.9). Retraction of the temporal lobe is minimized, and the distal end of the retractor is most often in contact with the petrous bone. Extradural retraction is felt to distribute the pressure to the dura as opposed to the underlying brain parenchyma [72]. Dura mater of the middle fossa can be very thin, especially if tegmen dehiscences are also present. The image navigation system is frequently useful during exploration to identify the precise location of the superior canal and its dehiscence. The surgeon is careful to only suction on the cotton balls and not to directly suction the area of the

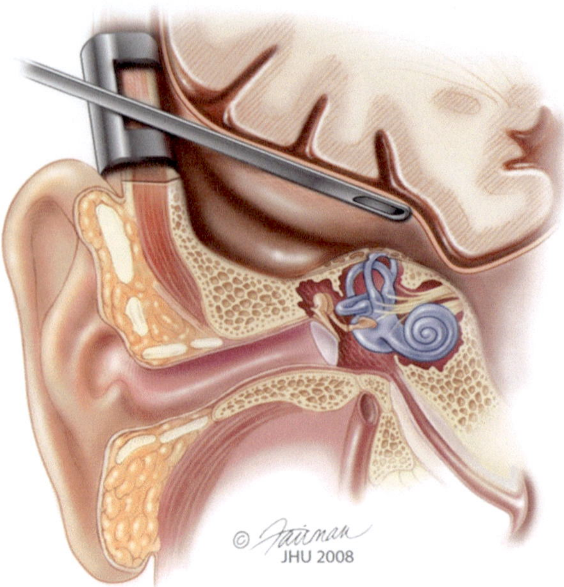

Fig. 19.9 Elevation of the dura using the Fisch retractor to expose the superior canal

dehiscence. This minimizes the removal of excessive perilymph or tearing of the membranous labyrinth, which could cause sensorineural hearing and vestibular loss. More recently, irrigation fluid has been changed from saline to warm basic salt solution to more closely represent the electrolyte composition of perilymph.

Once the superior canal dehiscence has been identified, attention is immediately shifted towards plugging the dehiscence (Figs. 19.10 and 19.11). The uncovering of the dehiscence and the subsequent plugging of the anterior and posterior limbs of the canal are communicated with the intraoperative monitoring technician to facilitate close monitoring of the ECochG. Copious amounts of irrigation are used once the dehiscence has been uncovered (Fig. 19.11a, b) to limit the risk of perilymph aspiration. From the harvested temporalis fascia, small moist pieces of fascia are slid into the two open lumens of the bony superior canal with gentle pressure from a curved pick (Figs. 19.10 and 19.11c). Several pieces are placed at each end so as to push the plugs several millimeters beyond the dehiscence. Bone dust is also used to reinforce the fascia and aid in plugging. This is done so as to prevent a recurrence should further bone erosion occur from the ends of the present dehiscence. Note that hydraulic pressure tends to push previously placed pieces of fascia out of one end of the dehiscence while the other is being packed. In fact, we look for this as the final confirmation that the correct holes are being plugged. To prevent fascia from becoming displaced, bone chips matching the diameter of the canal are firmly lodged so as to "cork" each end of the dehiscence (Figs. 19.10 and 19.11d). Any degradation of the ECochG response serves as a warning that too much pressure may be built up within the inner ear.

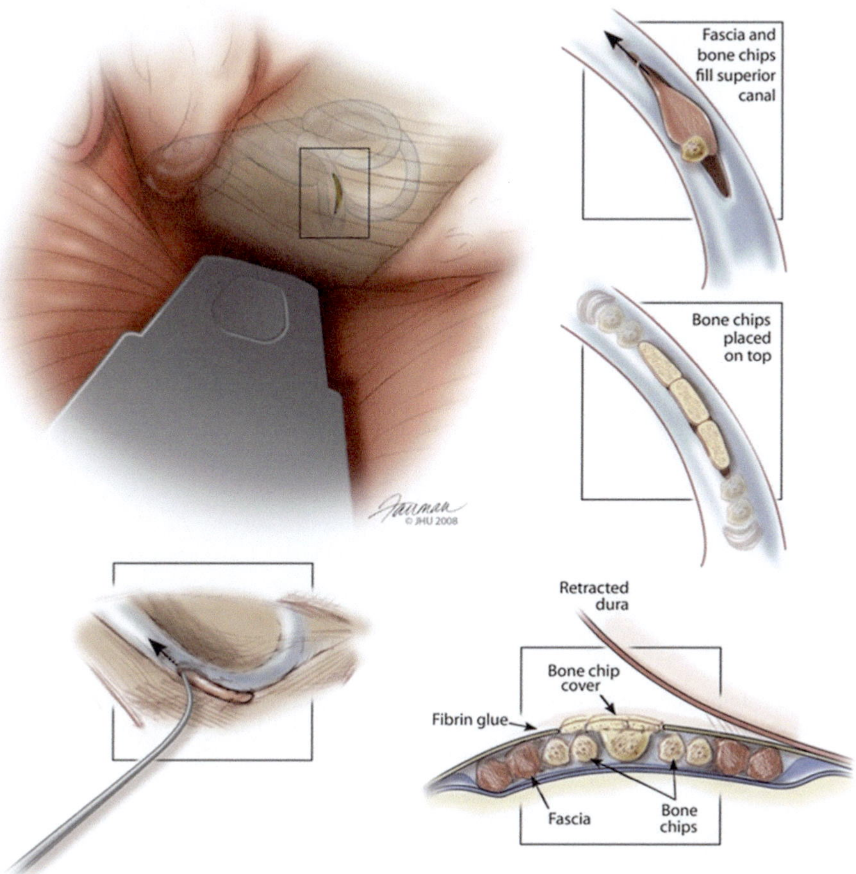

Fig. 19.10 Schematic drawing of plugging of the superior canal dehiscence. Area of the superior canal is identified while the dura is retracted. Fascia followed by bone chips is used to plug both ends of the superior canal

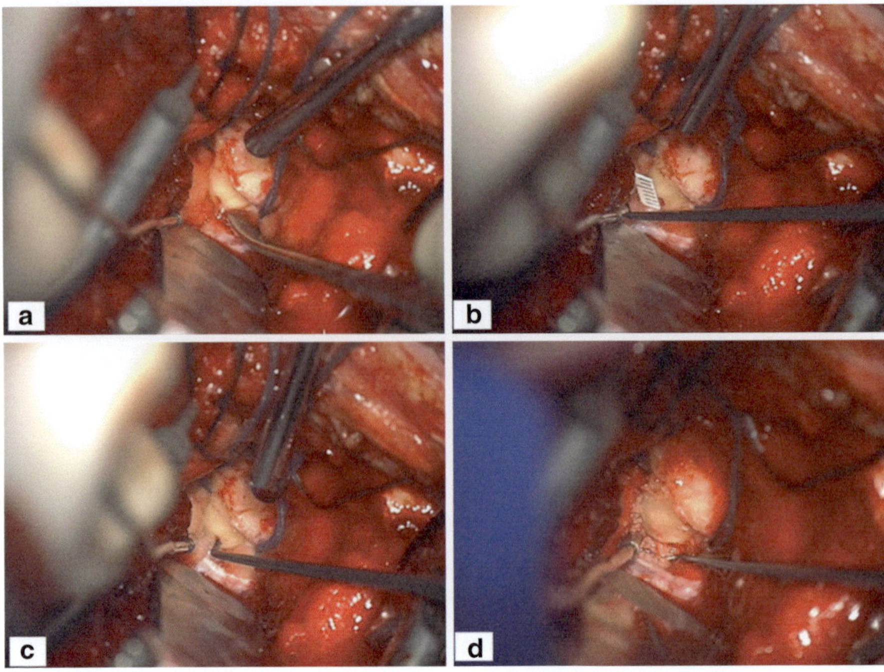

Fig. 19.11 Intraoperative view. Panel (**a**) Uncovering the dehiscence. Panel (**b**) Measuring the ~2 mm dehiscence. Panel (**c**) Packing the dehiscence with fascia and bone dust. Panel (**d**) Final appearance of dehiscence after bone chips have been placed

Following plugging of both sides of the dehiscence, the middle fossa floor is resurfaced using hydroxyapatite bone cement (HydroSet, Stryker®). All cotton balls used during the dissection are removed prior to placement. The bone cement is allowed to set for 2 minutes in warm lactated Ringer's solution. The remaining harvested temporalis fascia is placed over the bone cement, followed by fibrin glue.

Closure is achieved by anchoring the previously harvested bone flap in place using titanium plates (Fig. 19.12). A burr may be used to recess the plates into the bone so that they are not palpable post-operatively, or the plates and screws may be covered with hydroxyapatite bone cement. The temporalis muscle is approximated with absorbable sutures, and the skin is closed with staples and/or nylon suture. A drain is not typically used. The wound is cleaned, and a formal mastoid dressing is applied.

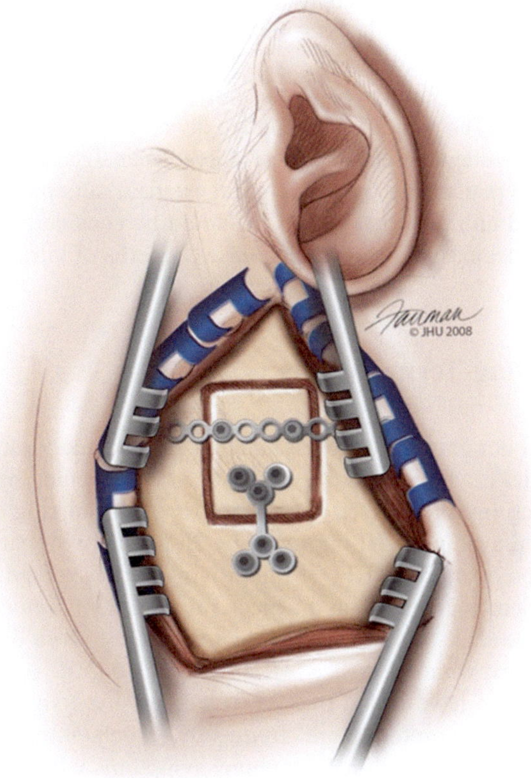

Fig. 19.12 Closure of the craniotomy. The bone flap is replaced using titanium plates

Post-operative Care

Patients are closely monitored in the post-anesthesia care unit for 4 hours prior to transfer to the surgical ward, with frequent neurological checks overnight due to the risk of epidural hematoma. Post-operative patients are treated with intravenous dexamethasone, generally dosed 6 mg IV every 6 hours with a taper beginning on the second post-operative day. Longer courses may be considered for patients who experience post-operative sensorineural hearing loss or loss of sensory function in the horizontal or posterior canals as manifested on head thrust testing. Patients are encouraged to be out of bed in a chair and ambulating starting on the first post-operative day. An oral diet can be started the day after surgery. The typical hospitalization lasts a total of 2 or 3 days.

Patients frequently experience nausea during the initial hours after surgery. This is best controlled using intravenous promethazine. Due to the risk of sedation, low doses should be given initially, starting at 6.25 mg and increasing up to 25 mg dosing every 4–6 hours. There are also many other medications available to control nausea, some of which may be traditionally preferred in neurosurgical patients due to the risk of sedation associated with promethazine. However, for nausea related to simulation of the vestibular end organs, we have found superior results with promethazine.

Post-operative pain is usually not severe and is localized to the area of the incision. The pain is mostly due to division of the temporalis muscle and is often worse with chewing. Routine post-operative analgesics are sufficient to control the pain. If the patient is experiencing intense pain, an epidural hematoma may be the cause, and an immediate head CT should be considered. Any change in mental status or consciousness should also raise concerns of intracranial bleeding.

Long-Term Results

In our experience, most patients are extremely satisfied with the surgery. Relief of dizzy symptoms has recently been documented by measuring the dizziness handicap inventory (DHI) [46] prior to SCD plugging surgery and 3 months afterward. On average, DHI improved by 26 points, with patients with more severe dizziness (preoperative DHI ≥30) improving by an average of 39 points [51]. This improvement is greater than the mean improvement seen after surgical labyrinthectomy for Menière's disease, which decreased DHI score by 17, and after vestibular neurectomy, which decreased DHI score by 16 [50].

We have found that when patients have significant autophony or hyperacusis, these symptoms are frequently much improved immediately after surgery. Occasionally, some autophony symptoms will take time to resolve, which is likely due to fluid collecting in the middle ear during the immediate post-operative period and causing conductive hearing loss. Utilizing a created autophony index, Crane et al. found a statistically lower mean score with 94% of patients reporting plugging improved their autophony symptoms [73].

The results for improving hearing with SCD surgery are less clear. Dramatic results have been observed in individual patients [55], but are not common. In a series of 6 patients with an air-bone gap prior to SCD plugging who had no previous history of ear surgery, 4 (66%) had at least partial closure of the air-bone gap after surgery [54]. However, in patients with previous middle cranial fossa or stapes surgery, the risk of hearing loss was high in this series. In a study from our institution, the average patient experienced a 10 dB improvement in air conduction hearing, although individual results varied from a 45 dB gain to a 45 dB hearing loss [31]. There has even been a report of improvement in sensorineural hearing loss after SCD surgery [55]. However, as discussed earlier, there is a risk of mild high-frequency sensorineural hearing loss with 25% of patients suffering permanent loss [56].

Balance can be significantly impaired in the immediate post-operative setting. Hypofunction of the canals can be assessed with head thrust testing in the plane of the canal. Agrawal et al. [73] noted that 1 mm increases in dehiscence length increased the odds of immediate postoperative hypofunction 2.6-fold (95%

confidence interval, 1.3–5.1). The prevalence of vestibular hypofunction was significantly higher in the early compared with the late postoperative period. Despite this, even patients with large dehiscences have recovery of dynamic and static measures of balance [74]. Patients should undergo fall risk assessment, and involvement of vestibular physical therapy in the inpatient post-operative period is beneficial.

Summary

The diagnosis of SCDS is based on an appropriate patient history, physical exam findings, including eye movements in response to sound or pressure, and other supporting studies, including the audiogram, VEMPs, and CT scanning. The spectrum and severity of SCDS symptoms vary significantly between individuals, and one must carefully weigh the potential benefit of surgery against the risks and probability of success in each patient.

Superior canal dehiscence plugging may be performed via a transmastoid or middle fossa approach, with the authors preferring the middle fossa for the majority of patients. Overall, patients experience an improvement in dizziness, autophony, and hyperacusis symptoms. Although there is often an improvement in hearing after surgery, this must be carefully weighed against the risk of hearing loss, which is significant in patients who have had previous middle fossa or stapes surgery.

Bibliography

1. Minor LB, Solomon D, Zinreich JS, Zee DS. Sound- and/or pressure-induced vertigo due to bone dehiscence of the superior semicircular canal. Arch Otolaryngol Head Neck Surg. 1998;124:249–58.
2. Tullio P. Das ohr und die entstehung de sprache und schrift. Berlin: Urban Scharzenberg; 1929.
3. Mayer O, Fraser JS. Pathological changes in the ear in late congenital syphilis. J Laryngol Otol. 1936;51:683–714.
4. Fox EJ, Balkany TJ, Arenberg IK. The Tullio phenomenon and perilymph fistula. Otolaryngol Head Neck Surg. 1988;98:88–9.
5. Kacker SK, Hinchcliffe R. Unusual Tullio phenomena. J Laryngol Otol. 1970;84:155–66.
6. Ishizaki H, Pyykko I, Aalto H, Starck J. Tullio phenomenon and postural stability: experimental study in normal subjects and patients with vertigo. Ann Otol Rhinol Laryngol. 1991;100:976–83.
7. Pisano DV, Niesten MEF, Merchant SN, Nakajima HH. The effect of superior semicircular canal dehiscence on intracochlear sound pressures. Audiol Neurootol. 2012;17(5):338–48. https://doi.org/10.1159/000339653.
8. Rosowski JJ, Songer JE, Nakajima HH, Brinsko KM, Merchant SN. Clinical, experimental, and theoretical investigations of the effect of superior semicircular canal dehiscence on hearing mechanisms. Otol Neurotol. 2004;25(3):323–32.
9. Chien W, Ravicz ME, Rosowski JJ, Merchant SN. Measurements of human middle- and inner-ear mechanics with dehiscence of the superior semicircular canal. Otol Neurotol. 2007;28(2):250–7. https://doi.org/10.1097/01.mao.0000244370.47320.9a.

10. Carey JP, Minor LB, Nager GT. Dehiscence or thinning of bone overlying the superior semicircular canal in a temporal bone survey. Arch Otolaryngol Head Neck Surg. 2000;126:137–47.
11. Re M, Gioacchini FM, Salvolini U, et al. Multislice computed tomography overestimates superior semicircular canal dehiscence syndrome. Ann Otol Rhinol Laryngol. 2013;122:625–31.
12. Pfammatter A, Darrouzet V, Gartner M, et al. A superior semicircular canal dehiscence syndrome multicenter study: is there an association between size and symptoms? Otol Neurotol. 2010;31:447–54.
13. Chien WW, Janky K, Minor LB, Carey JP. Superior canal dehiscence size: multivariate assessment of clinical impact. Otol Neurotol. 2012;33:810–5.
14. Hunter JB, O'Connell BP, Wang J, et al. Correlation of superior canal dehiscence surface area with vestibular evoked myogenic potentials, audiometric thresholds, and dizziness handicap. Otol Neurotol. 2016;37(8):1104–10. https://doi.org/10.1097/MAO.0000000000001126.
15. Niesten MEF, Stieger C, Lee DJ, et al. Assessment of the effects of superior canal dehiscence location and size on intracochlear sound pressures. Audiol Neurootol. 2015;20(1):62–71. https://doi.org/10.1159/000366512.
16. Niesten MEF, Hamberg LM, Silverman JB, et al. Superior canal dehiscence length and location influences clinical presentation and audiometric and cervical vestibular-evoked myogenic potential testing. Audiol Neurootol. 2014;19(2):97–105. https://doi.org/10.1159/000353920.
17. Minor LB. Clinical manifestations of superior semicircular canal dehiscence. Laryngoscope. 2005;115:1717–27.
18. Watson SR, Halmagyi GM, Colebatch JG. Vestibular hypersensitivity to sound (Tullio phenomenon): structural and functional assessment. Neurology. 2000;54:722–8.
19. Halmagyi GM, Aw ST, McGarvie LA, et al. Superior semicircular canal dehiscence simulating otosclerosis. J Laryngol Otol. 2003;117:553–7.
20. Cremer PD, Minor LB, Carey JP, Della Santina CC. Eye movements in patients with superior canal dehiscence syndrome align with the abnormal canal. Neurology. 2000;55:1833–41.
21. Minor LB, Cremer PD, Carey JP, Della Santina CC, Streubel SO, Weg N. Symptoms and signs in superior canal dehiscence syndrome. Ann N Y Acad Sci. 2001;942:259–73.
22. Krombach GA, DiMartino E, Schmitz-Rode T, et al. Posterior semicircular canal dehiscence: a morphologic cause of vertigo similar to superior semicircular canal dehiscence. Eur Radiol. 2003;13:1444–50.
23. Sheehy JL, Brackmann DE. Cholesteatoma surgery: management of the labyrinthine fistula–a report of 97 cases. Laryngoscope. 1979;89:78–87.
24. Merchant SN, Rosowski JJ. Conductive hearing loss caused by third-window lesions of the inner ear. Otol Neurotol. 2008;29:282–9.
25. Mikulec AA, McKenna MJ, Ramsey MJ, et al. Superior semicircular canal dehiscence presenting as conductive hearing loss without vertigo. Otol Neurotol. 2004;25:121–9.
26. Adams ME, Kileny PR, Telian SA, et al. Electrocochleography as a diagnostic and intraoperative adjunct in superior semicircular canal dehiscence syndrome. Otol Neurotol. 2011;32:1506–12.
27. Wenzel A, Ward BK, Ritzl EK, et al. Intraoperative neuromonitoring for superior semicircular canal dehiscence and hearing outcomes. Otol Neurotol. 2015;36(1):139–45. https://doi.org/10.1097/MAO.0000000000000642.
28. Welgampola MS, Colebatch JG. Characteristics and clinical applications of vestibular-evoked myogenic potentials. Neurology. 2005;64:1682–8.
29. Welgampola MS, Myrie OA, Minor LB, Carey JP. Vestibular-evoked myogenic potential thresholds normalize on plugging superior canal dehiscence. Neurology. 2008;70:464–72.
30. Zhou G, Gopen Q, Poe DS. Clinical and diagnostic characterization of canal dehiscence syndrome: a great otologic mimicker. Otol Neurotol. 2007;28:920–6.
31. Crane BT, Minor LB, Carey JP. Three-dimensional computed tomography of superior canal dehiscence syndrome. Otol Neurotol. 2008;29:699–705.
32. Sheykholeslami K, Schmerber S, Habiby Kermany M, Kaga K. Vestibular-evoked myogenic potentials in three patients with large vestibular aqueduct. Hear Res. 2004;190:161–8.

33. Zuniga MG, Janky KL, Nguyen KD, Welgampola MS, Carey JP. Ocular versus cervical VEMPs in the diagnosis of superior semicircular canal dehiscence syndrome. Otol Neurotol. 2013;34:121–6.
34. Janky KL, Nguyen KD, Welgampola M, Zuniga MG, Carey JP. Air-conducted oVEMPs provide the best separation between intact and superior canal dehiscent labyrinths. Otol Neurotol. 2013;34:127–34.
35. Belden CJ, Weg N, Minor LB, Zinreich SJ. CT evaluation of bone dehiscence of the superior semicircular canal as a cause of sound- and/or pressure-induced vertigo. Radiology. 2003;226:337–43.
36. Williamson RA, Vrabec JT, Coker NJ, Sandlin M. Coronal computed tomography prevalence of superior semicircular canal dehiscence. Otolaryngol Head Neck Surg. 2003;129:481–9.
37. Minor LB. Meniere's disease and migraine. Arch Otolaryngol Head Neck Surg. 2005;131:460.
38. Muchnik C, Hildesheimer M, Rubinstein M, Arenberg IK. Low frequency air-bone gap in Meniere's disease without middle ear pathology. A preliminary report. Am J Otol. 1989;10:1–4.
39. Poe DS. Diagnosis and management of the patulous eustachian tube. Otol Neurotol. 2007;28:668–77.
40. Minor LB. Labyrinthine fistulae: pathobiology and management. Curr Opin Otolaryngol Head Neck Surg. 2003;11:340–6.
41. Hakuba N, Hato N, Shinomori Y, Sato H, Gyo K. Labyrinthine fistula as a late complication of middle ear surgery using the canal wall down technique. Otol Neurotol. 2002;23:832–5.
42. Friedland DR, Wackym PA. A critical appraisal of spontaneous perilymphatic fistulas of the inner ear. Am J Otol. 1999;20:261–76; discussion 276-269.
43. Eggers SD. Migraine-related vertigo: diagnosis and treatment. Curr Pain Headache Rep. 2007;11:217–26.
44. Tepper SJ. A pivotal moment in 50 years of headache history: the first American Migraine Study. Headache. 2008;48:730–1; discussion 732.
45. Kayan A, Hood JD. Neuro-otological manifestations of migraine. Brain J Neurol. 1984;107(Pt 4):1123–42.
46. Jacobson GP, Newman CW. The development of the dizziness handicap inventory. Arch Otolaryngol Head Neck Surg. 1990;116:424–7.
47. Shaia WT, Zappia JJ, Bojrab DI, LaRouere ML, Sargent EW, Diaz RC. Success of posterior semicircular canal occlusion and application of the dizziness handicap inventory. Otolaryngol Head Neck Surg. 2006;134:424–30.
48. Tufarelli D, Meli A, Labini FS, et al. Balance impairment after acoustic neuroma surgery. Otol Neurotol. 2007;28:814–21.
49. Humphriss RL, Baguley DM, Moffat DA. Change in dizziness handicap after vestibular schwannoma excision. Otol Neurotol. 2003;24:661–5.
50. Badke MB, Pyle GM, Shea T, Miedaner J. Outcomes in vestibular ablative procedures. Otol Neurotol. 2002;23:504–9.
51. Crane BT, Minor LB, Carey JP. Superior canal dehiscence plugging reduces dizziness handicap. Laryngoscope. 2008;118:1809–13.
52. O'Reilly RC, Elford B, Slater R. Effectiveness of the particle repositioning maneuver in subtypes of benign paroxysmal positional vertigo. Laryngoscope. 2000;110:1385–8.
53. Perez N, Martin E, Garcia-Tapia R. Dizziness: relating the severity of vertigo to the degree of handicap by measuring vestibular impairment. Otolaryngol Head Neck Surg. 2003;128:372–81.
54. Limb CJ, Carey JP, Srireddy S, Minor LB. Auditory function in patients with surgically treated superior semicircular canal dehiscence. Otol Neurotol. 2006;27:969–80.
55. Wilkinson EP, Liu GC, Friedman RA. Correction of progressive hearing loss in superior canal dehiscence syndrome. Laryngoscope. 2008;118:10–3.
56. Ward BK, Agrawal Y, Nguyen E, et al. Hearing outcomes after surgical plugging of the superior semicircular canal by a middle cranial fossa approach. Otol Neurotol. 2012;33:1386–91.

57. Xie Y, Sharon JD, Pross SE, et al. Surgical complications from superior canal dehiscence syndrome repair: two decades of experience. Otolaryngol Head Neck Surg. 2017;157(2):273–80. https://doi.org/10.1177/0194599817706491.
58. Mantokoudis G, Saber Tehrani AS, Wong AL, Agrawal Y, Wenzel A, Carey JP. Adaptation and compensation of vestibular responses following superior canal dehiscence surgery. Otol Neurotol. 2016;37(9):1399–405. https://doi.org/10.1097/MAO.0000000000001196.
59. Barber SR, Cheng YS, Owoc M, et al. Benign paroxysmal positional vertigo commonly occurs following repair of superior canal dehiscence. Laryngoscope. 2016;126(9):2092–7. https://doi.org/10.1002/lary.25797.
60. Sanna M, Taibah A, Russo A, Falcioni M, Agarwal M. Perioperative complications in acoustic neuroma (vestibular schwannoma) surgery. Otol Neurotol. 2004;25:379–86.
61. Oghalai JS, Buxbaum JL, Pitts LH, Jackler RK. The effect of age on acoustic neuroma surgery outcomes. Otol Neurotol. 2003;24:473–7.
62. Alkhafaji MS, Varma S, Pross SE, et al. Long-term patient-reported outcomes after surgery for superior canal dehiscence syndrome. Otol Neurotol. 2017;38(9):1319–26. https://doi.org/10.1097/MAO.0000000000001550.
63. Sharon JD, Pross SE, Ward BK, Carey JP. Revision surgery for superior canal dehiscence syndrome. Otol Neurotol. 2016;37(8):1096–103. https://doi.org/10.1097/MAO.0000000000001113.
64. Shaia WT, Diaz RC. Evolution in surgical management of superior canal dehiscence syndrome. Curr Opin Otolaryngol Head Neck Surg. 2013;21:497–502.
65. Beyea JA, Agrawal SK, Parnes LS. Transmastoid semicircular canal occlusion: a safe and highly effective treatment for benign paroxysmal positional vertigo and superior canal dehiscence. Laryngoscope. 2012;122:1862–6.
66. Deschenes GR, Hsu DP, Megerian CA. Outpatient repair of superior semicircular canal dehiscence via the transmastoid approach. Laryngoscope. 2009;119:1765–9.
67. Carter MS, Lookabaugh S, Lee DJ. Endoscopic-assisted repair of superior canal dehiscence syndrome. Laryngoscope. 2014;124:1464–8.
68. Agrawal SK, Parnes LS. Transmastoid superior semicircular canal occlusion. Otol Neurotol. 2008;29:363–7.
69. Crovetto M, Areitio E, Elexpuru J, Aguayo F. Transmastoid approach for resurfacing of superior semicircular canal dehiscence. Auris Nasus Larynx. 2008;35:247–9.
70. Carey JP, Migliaccio AA, Minor LB. Semicircular canal function before and after surgery for superior canal dehiscence. Otol Neurotol. 2007;28:356–64.
71. Cheng YS, Kozin ED, Lee DJ. Endoscopic-assisted repair of superior canal dehiscence. Otolaryngol Clin N Am. 2016;49(5):1189–204. https://doi.org/10.1016/j.otc.2016.05.010. Review. PubMed PMID: 27565386.
72. Driscoll CL, Jackler RK, Pitts LH, Banthia V. Extradural temporal lobe retraction in the middle fossa approach to the internal auditory canal: biomechanical analysis. Am J Otol. 1999;20:373–80.
73. Agrawal Y, Migliaccio AA, Minor LB, Carey JP. Vestibular hypofunction in the initial postoperative period after surgical treatment of superior semicircular canal dehiscence. Otol Neurotol. 2009;30:502–6.
74. Janky KL, Zuniga MG, Carey JP, Schubert M. Balance dysfunction and recovery after surgery for superior canal dehiscence syndrome. Arch Otolaryngol Head Neck Surg. 2012;138:723–30.

Chapter 20
Miscellaneous Third Window Syndromes

Robert M. Conway, Gerard J. Gianoli, and Jacob C. Lucas

Introduction

Third window syndromes are a general classification of different disorders that involve an abnormal opening, "window," into the bone of the inner ear. The inner ear is almost entirely encased by otic capsule bone, with the exception being the oval and round windows. Under normal physiologic conditions, the inner ear functions as a closed hydraulic system with two compliant windows—the oval and round windows—that allow for the transmission and dissipation of acoustic energy, where the round window dissipates with an opposite phase to the acoustic energy entering via the oval window. Third window disorders can cause changes to these normal fluid mechanics by creating an alternative pressure outlet, which may result in auditory and vestibular symptoms [1]. While there are other "windows" in the inner ear, including the vestibular and cochlear aqueducts, these have not been shown to affect fluid dynamics in their normal physiologic state [2].

The most described third window syndrome is Superior Semicircular Canal Dehiscence (SSCD). While not covered in depth in this chapter, SSCD has a wide array of clinical presentations that overlap with other third window disorders. These include enlarged vestibular aqueduct syndrome (EVAS), posterior and lateral semicircular canal dehiscence, X-linked gusher syndrome (incomplete partition

R. M. Conway
Department of Otology and Neurotology, Michigan Ear Institute, Farmington Hills, MI, USA

Department of Otology and Neurotology, Michigan Ear Institute, Farmington Hills, MI, USA

G. J. Gianoli
The Ear and Balance Institute, Covington, LA, USA

Department of Otolaryngology, Tulane University, New Orleans, LA, USA

J. C. Lucas (✉)
Michigan Ear Institute, Farmington Hills, MI, USA

J. C. Lucas et al. (eds.), *Diagnosis and Treatment of Vestibular Disorders*,
https://doi.org/10.1007/978-3-032-11740-3_20

type III), and cochlear fistula. Although each condition involves a distinct anatomic site and mechanism, they share the common pathophysiologic principle of abnormal pressure transmission and fluid displacement within the inner ear. Dehiscence can occur throughout the otic capsule at any subsite; one recent effort to describe a uniform classification system led to "otic capsule dehiscence" (OCD) as a global term encompassing all subtypes of anatomic third window.

Pathophysiology and Clinical Presentation

When acoustic energy is transmitted to the inner ear, there is propagation of a pressure wave in the cochlea through the scala vestibuli, displacing the basilar membrane and exiting the round window. When a third window is present, energy is shunted away from the basilar membrane due to decreased impedance toward the window, sometimes leading to an air-bone gap on audiometry with intact acoustic reflexes. Similarly, this third window can affect bone conduction as well, causing a suprathreshold bone conduction and contributing to vestibular activation. This activation of the vestibular system is the basis of the "Tullio Phenomenon," first described by Pietro Tullio during the early twentieth century, when pigeons would get sound-induced nystagmus after fenestration of a third window in their semicircular canals [3]. Similarly, Camille Hennebert noted pressure-induced nystagmus (PIN) or vertigo elicited by pressure changes in the EAC in patients with third window disorder related to congenital syphilis [4]. Both Tullio phenomenon and Hennebert's sign provide the underpinnings for a related condition—perilymphatic fistula.

Patients with a third window typically present with hearing loss, autophony, aural fullness, and vestibular symptoms. Third window syndromes may present with a conductive component of hearing loss, and include EVA, posterior canal dehiscence, cochlear-facial dehiscence, and carotid canal dehiscence [5–7]. Air-bone gaps (ABG) in third window syndromes are related to a mix of increased air conduction thresholds due to acoustic energy being shunted away from the basilar membrane toward the pathologic window, as well as a decrease in bone conduction threshold related to vibration of the perilymph leading to enhanced cochlear stimulation [8]. Vestibular symptoms occur in a similar manner, with acoustic stimulus being transmitted toward the dehiscence, passing and activating sensory epithelia of the labyrinth [9]. In general, the presence of a conductive gap on audiometry is loosely correlated with the size of the dehiscence among SSCD patients, with 3 mm being a critical size—i.e., less than 3 mm typically do not have a conductive gap, and the bigger the dehiscence beyond 3 mm, the greater the air bone gap [10]. Interestingly, the size of the dehiscence in SSCD also correlates with cVEMP results, but it does not correlate very well with vestibular symptomatology. The size of EVAs is weakly correlated with the size of the air-bone gap, but for the other non-SSCD TMWS disorders, this has not yet been studied.

Diagnostic Evaluation

While a thorough history and physical examination are the cornerstone of evaluation in patients with a third window syndrome, a high degree of suspicion is required, given the significant overlap with other middle and inner ear disorders. Emphasis on triggers such as sound- and pressure-induced vertigo are important factors to elicit further evaluation into third window syndromes. Physical exam findings may be normal. A fistula test can be performed by performing pneumatic otoscopy with observance of phase-locked eye movements, which may be present in cases of perilymphatic fistula and other third window syndromes. The direction of the eye movements seen on fistula testing may give a hint as to the source of the dehiscence. For example, upward clockwise torsional movement with positive pressure in the right ear suggests a right-sided SSCD, whereas horizontal movement would suggest a horizontal canal dehiscence.

Audiometry may demonstrate a conductive hearing loss with intact acoustic reflexes, as previously discussed; some diseases, such as an EVA, can present with other audiologic patterns, such as progressive sensorineural hearing loss (SNHL) [11, 12]. Vestibular testing, particularly vestibular evoked myogenic potentials (VEMPs), can help aid in the diagnosis as well. VEMPs evaluate otolithic function by presenting an intense acoustic or vibratory stimulus to the ear, which is detected by the saccule or utricle. A reflex arc is then activated through the vestibular nuclei, which triggers a muscle response, which is noted on the recording surface electromyography. The cervical VEMP (cVEMP) assesses the saccule and inferior vestibular nerve by an electrode placed on the ipsilateral sternocleidomastoid muscle, while the ocular VEMP (oVEMP) assesses the utricle and superior vestibular nerve via the contralateral inferior oblique muscle. In third window syndromes, the dehiscent bone allows an abnormally large stimulus to be transmitted to the vestibular system. This leads to the typical results of a decreased threshold and increased amplitude for both cVEMP and oVEMP in third window syndromes [13]. Additional testing to help corroborate a TMWS diagnosis includes nasal and glottic Valsalva testing and Tullio testing. Recording the eye movements and patient symptoms with Valsalva maneuvers during VNG testing is most helpful. Regarding Tullio testing, a 500 Hz pulse tone is utilized and recorded before and after stimulation, as well as documenting patient symptomatology. While neither the Valsalva nor Tullio testing is standardized, they both offer a means to objectively document the patients' presenting symptoms of sound or strain-induced dizziness.

Imaging is another important aspect of the diagnostic evaluation, with computed tomography (CT) scans being the mainstay modality. CT imaging can reliably locate the pathologic window in most cases [14]. Certain diseases, such as perilymphatic fistula, will often have a negative CT, with the diagnosis being largely clinical/surgical. Even in cases where a third window is definitively present, careful clinical consideration is required, as radiologic presence of a third window is significantly more prevalent than clinical third window syndromes, along with confounding diseases, such as vestibular migraine, which may be causing symptoms as well [15–17]. Lastly, identification of one otic capsule dehiscence should elicit a search for concomitant dehiscences in the same ear. Ionescu et al. recently reported an 18% incidence of concomitant dehiscences among a cohort of 157 SSCD patients [18]. Knowing in advance the presence of multiple dehiscences could significantly alter treatment recommendations.

Specific Syndromes

Enlarged Vestibular Aqueduct

Enlarged vestibular aqueduct syndrome (EVAS) is a congenital inner ear malformation in which the vestibular aqueduct, which connects the endolymphatic sac to the inner ear, is dilated. When enlarged, the vestibular aqueduct may act as a third window, allowing dissipation of acoustic energy toward the aqueduct rather than the cochlea.

The prevalence of EVA among children with SNHL is between 5% and 15%, with 60–70% of cases being bilateral [19–21]. EVAS is strongly associated, if not obligatory, in patients with Pendred syndrome, a mutation in the SLC26A4 gene. Normally, the vestibular aqueduct is <1 mm in size at its midpoint, with a mean value of around 0.5 mm [22]. Valvassori and Clemis initially described criteria for EVA as a diameter greater than 1.5 mm at the midpoint. However, this was a study of 50 patients suspected of inner ear congenital malformations using planar tomography in the 1970s. More recently, the Cincinnati criteria (using a database of 1600 children and High-resolution CT scanning) described EVA as greater than or equal to 1 mm at the midpoint or 2 mm at the operculum, improving specificity for patients with sensorineural hearing loss without another known cause [21, 23, 24].

Patients with EVAS typically present with a progressive or fluctuating sensorineural hearing loss that can be pre- or post-lingual in nature and may be preceded by head trauma. Jackler et al. presented a series of patients in which follow-up over 7 years demonstrated a worsening of 25 dB and a 29% drop in speech discrimination [25]. This same study demonstrated a heterogeneous presentation of these patients, ranging from normal hearing to profound deafness [25]. Vestibular symptoms, including vertigo, imbalance, and nausea, can also affect patients with EVA. These symptoms have a higher incidence in bilateral EVA, and while vestibular testing may have some benefit, there can be a discordance of vestibular signs and symptoms present [26]. As a third window syndrome, these patients can also present with conductive hearing component, typically worse in the low frequencies [6, 27]. Likewise, these patients have been found to have similar findings on VEMP testing as other third window syndromes, with decreased thresholds and increased amplitudes [28].

Treatment of EVAS is largely limited and, at least initially, is typically conservative in nature. It is generally recommended to limit lifestyle activities that are associated with an increased risk of head trauma, primarily contact sports, as this may precipitate a drop in hearing [29]. Endolymphatic sac surgery, both occlusion and shunts, has been performed in an attempt to prevent further hearing decline in patients without significant improvement, negating the need for surgical intervention in these patients [25, 30]. Hearing aids are a useful treatment option for patients with EVAS while they have serviceable hearing. As hearing loss progresses, frequent programming may be needed. Once hearing loss has progressed beyond aidable conditions, cochlear implantation is often considered. Cochlear implantation in patients with EVAS provides excellent results, similar to those with normal progressive SNHL [31, 32]. These patients do have an increased risk of intraoperative gusher; despite this, it is a safe and effective procedure for these patients [33].

Lateral Semicircular Canal and Posterior Canal Semicircular Canal Dehiscence

Lateral semicircular canal dehiscence (LSCD) and posterior semicircular canal dehiscence (PSCD) are less common but clinically significant causes of third window syndrome. Similar to SSCD, they consist of a bony defect of a semicircular canal resulting in an abnormal connection in the bone of the inner ear. The underlying etiology between SSCD and LSCD differs, with the latter often being associated with chronic ear disease, iatrogenic trauma, or other erosive pathology [34]. In contrast, PSCD may arise de novo in the absence of antecedent pathology and is uniquely associated with a high-riding jugular bulb and fibrous dysplasia (Fig. 20.1) [35, 36]. The dehiscence may occur at the level of the posterior fossa dura, at the jugular bulb, or within the vestibular aqueduct.

The incidence is not entirely known; however, radiologic studies of asymptomatic patients demonstrated a prevalence of 1.2% [37]. PSCD tends to be more common in the right ear, which can be potentially explained by patients more likely to have right-dominant jugular venous drainage [38].

The lateral semicircular canal lies more superficially than the posterior semicircular canal, in close proximity to the middle ear and mastoid cavities. This makes it vulnerable to chronic middle ear problems, such as cholesteatoma and chronic otitis media. Incidence of labyrinthine fistula in chronic otitis media and cholesteatoma is around 7% [39]. Chronic otitis media is hypothesized to lead to resorption osteitis from osteoclastic activation secondary to chronic inflammation and granulation tissue, while cholesteatoma is thought to cause erosion from osteolytic compounds produced by cholesteatoma or direct pressure [40].

Symptoms of PSCD and LSCD mirror SSCD and may include autophony, aural fullness, conductive hearing loss, and pressure/sound-induced vertigo. However, symptoms tend to be more variable as the underlying process may lead to erosion of the membranous labyrinth as well, leading to a frank fistula. Due to this variability, PCSD symptoms can range from mild conductive hearing loss, as expected in typical third window syndromes, to extensive sensorineural hearing loss more typical of a complete labyrinth defect [38]. Typical LSCD patients are described as

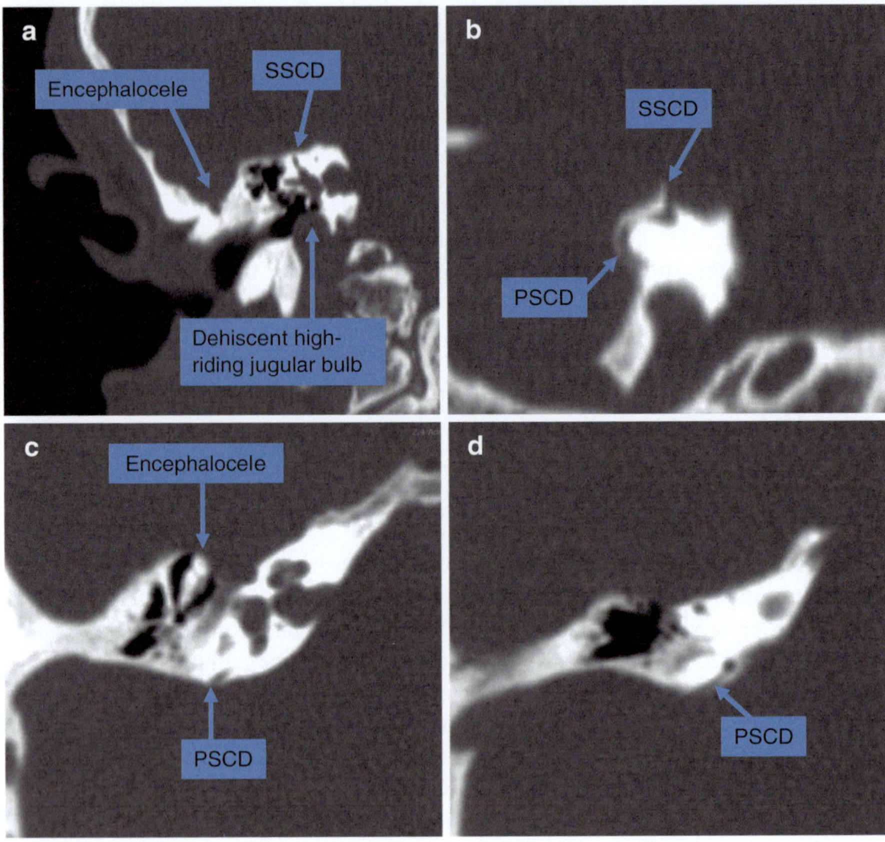

Fig. 20.1 Multiple right-sided otic capsule dehiscence sites are demonstrated in one temporal bone. (**a**) CT coronal view showing dehiscence of the superior semicircular canal (*SSCD*) and the jugular bulb, alongside a temporal encephalocele. (**b**) CT "Stenver" oblique sagittal view shows both superior and posterior canal dehiscence (*SSCD* and *PSCD*, respectively). Sequential sagittal views highlight the PSCD in (**c**, **d**)

vertiginous with a positive fistula test, in the setting of chronic ear disease. However, LSCD symptoms are not always predictive of the disease, as many of these patients present solely with chronic otorrhea and hearing loss related to the underlying disease process [39, 41].

Due to the limited prevalence of the disease, there is no standard treatment for PSCD. If symptoms are limited, observation is typically appropriate and the preferred treatment option. If severe or bothersome symptoms exist, surgical repair may be warranted. Mikulec and Poe presented a patient who underwent transmastoid plugging of the posterior canal with conductive hearing loss and vestibular symptoms that had significant improvement postoperatively [7]. The benefit of plugging is increased surgical efficacy, as the dehiscence does not need to be completely exposed. Surgical plugging does increase the risk of sensorineural hearing loss and disrupts normal canal mechanics [42]. Gubbels et al. performed a resurfacing of the posterior semicircular canal after decompression of a high-riding jugular bulb with successful resolution of vestibular symptoms [35]. Resurfacing has the benefit of preserving canal fluid dynamics in SSCD patients, which may help long-term vestibular function; however, there is concern for residual symptoms in some cases. It is presumed that a similar dynamic would apply to PSCD cases [43].

Management of LSCD differs significantly from PSCD and can be controversial in nature. Historically, standard management of LSCD in the setting of cholesteatoma involves performing a canal wall down mastoidectomy while leaving cholesteatoma matrix on the dehiscent aspect of the lateral semicircular canal [44]. This approach allows exteriorization of disease while avoiding opening the labyrinth and the associated risk of sensorineural hearing loss associated with this, although literature does not demonstrate a difference in audiologic outcomes [39]. The disadvantage of this approach is in symptomatic patients, in whom there is no improvement in their third window symptoms. Removal of cholesteatoma matrix from the fistula site is advocated for by some surgeons, with data supporting similar audiologic outcomes with improvement in vertigo and other third window symptoms [45]. Special considerations are needed when considering repair of lateral canal fistula, including quick repair with previously harvested graft (fascia, cartilage, bone wax) as well as constant irrigation and avoidance of any suction over the fistula site. This can be done as an intact canal wall or canal wall down mastoidectomy, with some authors advocating that other aspects of the cholesteatoma disease should be the guiding factor, not the mere presence of a fistula [41].

In 2022, Gianoli and colleagues reported a different type of LSCD located at the ampullated end of the LSC where the tympanic segment of the facial nerve crosses [46]. This is likely a congenital or developmental anomaly. Sixteen cases were reported, and 10 had resolution of symptoms with medical management, whereas 4 had surgery. The surgery included reinforcement of the round window and the oval window, inclusive of the tympanic segment of the facial nerve. Garvis and colleagues more recently reported on a series of 34 patients with LSCD in this area with similar clinical and test findings [15].

Lateral Skull Base Surgery and Third Window

Third window phenomena may complicate approaches to the pathology of the lateral skull base. Especially in "hearing preservation" approaches for temporal bone neoplasms, all inner structures including the cochlea and labyrinth are at risk of violation. Injury or breach of the otic capsule may occur during exposure of the internal auditory canal (IAC) as part of a middle fossa or retrosigmoid craniotomy for vestibular schwannoma surgery. During the retrosigmoid approach, the endolymphatic sac, vestibule, and posterior semicircular canal can be opened during tumor exposure and lead to third window symptoms. Similarly, during a middle fossa exposure of the internal auditory canal, the superior semicircular canal and cochlea may be inadvertently unroofed; the superior semicircular canal may even be intentionally "blue-lined" to augment exposure to orient the surgeon to the axis of the IAC. Up to 20% of hearing preservation approaches to the internal auditory canal may manifest third window symptoms postoperatively [47].

Two other iatrogenic etiologies have been found to cause auditory TMWS but lack vestibular symptoms. These include endolymphatic sac surgery and posterior fossa surgery resulting in pneumocephalus [48]. Meniere's patients undergoing endolymphatic sac decompression surgery have also been shown to produce a postoperative low-frequency air-bone gap, like what we see in TMWS [49]. Pneumocephalus in the posterior fossa has been reported to cause aural fullness, autophony, and pulsatile tinnitus, mimicking TMWS [48].

Cochlear Dehiscence

Cochlear dehiscences are a rare cause of third window syndrome (with the exception of the cochlear-facial dehiscence) but can cause significant symptoms. These dehiscences involve a bony communication between the cochlea and another structure. They can involve the carotid canal (carotid-cochlear fistula), the facial nerve (cochlear-facial nerve fistula), or the internal auditory canal (Incomplete Partition Type III). While all involve the cochlea and are technically a third window, symptoms can differ between the different locations.

Cochlear-Facial Dehiscence (CFD)

A dehiscence between the basal turn of the cochlea and labyrinthine segment of the facial nerve is another potential form of cochlear dehiscence (Fig. 20.2). This dehiscence can be secondary to an event such as trauma, cholesteatoma, or facial nerve tumor, but may be idiopathic in nature. Fang et al. performed a histological study of over 1000 temporal bones and noted an incidence of complete dehiscence in 0.59% of patients [50]. The mean bony partition width in this study was 0.23 mm, with increased age, female gender, and non-Caucasian individuals having thinner bony partition [50]. Of important note, almost 35% of patients had a <1 mm bony partition, which could appear dehiscent on CT scan [50]. These patients can present with typical third window symptoms; however, some have been identified after cochlear implantation due to postoperative facial nerve stimulation [51, 52]. While direct repair of this area is difficult due to anatomical constraints, Wackym et al. performed round window reinforcement for CFD patients with significant improvements in many domains, including third window symptoms and dizziness handicap inventory [53].

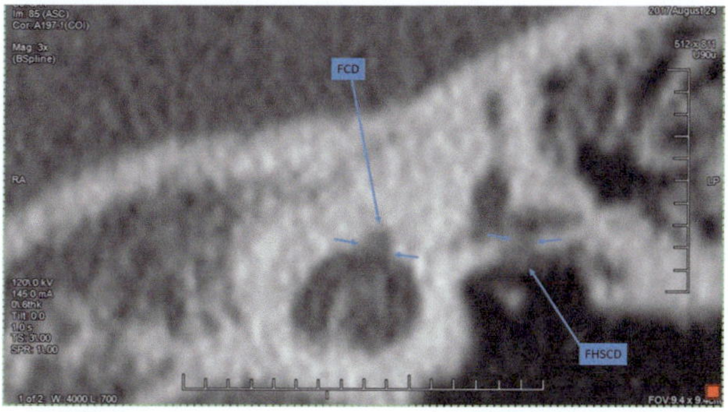

Fig. 20.2 CT scan demonstrating dehiscence of the cochlea at the region of the labyrinthine segment of the facial canal (FCD) and suspicious for dehiscence of the horizontal semicircular canal at the tympanic segment of the facial canal (FHSCD). (Source: See Chap. 18)

Carotid-Cochlear Dehiscence (CCD)

Carotid-Cochlear dehiscence involves a dehiscence of bone between the basal turn of the cochlea and the petrous carotid artery. This area can be evaluated on imaging, which is referred to as the carotid-cochlear interval (CCI), and thickness typically ranges between 0 and 7 mm [54, 55]. This type of dehiscence is extremely rare with no known cause. Patients can present with typical third window symptoms, but pulsatile tinnitus tends to be more prominent given the proximity to arterial flow. Observation is the preferred treatment method given the high risk of surgical intervention in this area. Special consideration must be taken in these patients if performing cochlear implantation as there is a theoretical risk of implant extrusion through the dehiscence, although this has not been previously reported.

Incomplete Partition Type III

Incomplete partition type III (IP-III) is a type of cochlear malformation present in X-linked deafness type 2 (DFNX2), which is secondary to a loss of POU3F4 protein function. This protein is expressed in early development and signals development of the inner ear, leading to abnormal development in the otic capsule [56]. While this is the most common cause of X-linked deafness, overall it is a very rare entity, accounting for 1–2% of nonsyndromic genetic deafness [57].

The primary cochlear abnormalities that can be seen on CT scan include absent interscalar septa, absent modiolus, and absent cribriform plate between the basal turn of the cochlea and IAC. Other primary characteristics outside of the cochlea include thin otic capsule bone, dilated IAC, cystic vestibule, and dysplastic oval and round windows [58]. The third window aspect of this involves the absent cribriform plate, which causes a cochlear-IAC fistula.

Males with IP-III will present typically with a severe-profound sensorineural or mixed hearing loss that is progressive in the first years of life. Female carriers of this disease are typically normal but may have mild hearing loss [59]. Conductive hearing loss resulting from IP-III demonstrates intact acoustic reflexes on immittance testing, contrasting with the *absent* reflexes seen in ossicular fixation and otosclerosis. The presence of intact reflexes suggests that the conductive loss relates to third window phenomena, similar to SSCD [60].

Management of IP-III depends on the degree of hearing loss. The minority of patients, those with mild-severe hearing loss, can often benefit from using a conventional hearing aid [61]. As most patients typically present or have early progression to severe-profound hearing loss, a cochlear implant is often the only option available. Cochlear implantation in this patient population needs to be done with extreme caution. The biggest concern is that these patients are almost guaranteed to have a cerebrospinal fluid (CSF) gusher during cochleostomy, making placement more difficult as well as a concern for misplacement of the electrode into the IAC [62].

"Otic Capsule Dehiscence": A Unifying Classification Scheme

An all-encompassing classification system for the family of third mobile window syndromes has been proposed and expanded upon by Ionescu et al. (Fig. 20.3). Classification of the otic capsule dehiscence (OCD) is dictated by the location of the third window and its interface with meningeal (Type I), vascular (Type II), or petrous bone (Type III) structures. The unifying classification includes SSCD alongside all other third window phenomena. A pictorial overview of the OCD-type classification schema is depicted in Fig. 20.3.

Type I: OCD-Meningeal

OCD-Meningeal type dehiscences encompass classic SSCD (Type Ia) and include PSCD (Type Ib). In the case of SSCD, the dehiscence of the superior canal lies in contact with the middle fossa dura, while PSCD interfaces with the posterior fossa dura.

Type II: OCD-Vascular

OCD-Vascular dehiscence syndromes include otic capsule defects, which interface with local temporal bone vasculature. Otic capsule defects may involve the cochlea or vestibular apparatus structures. Possible dehiscence sites include the superior semicircular canal at the superior petrosal sinus (Type IIa) (Fig. 20.4). Dehiscence into the internal jugular vein may involve the vestibular aqueduct, cochlear aqueduct, or PSC (Type IIb). Type IIb dehiscence syndromes feature exercise-induced vertigo and pulsatile tinnitus as prominent symptoms. Type IIc OCD corresponds to cochlear dehiscence into the carotid artery.

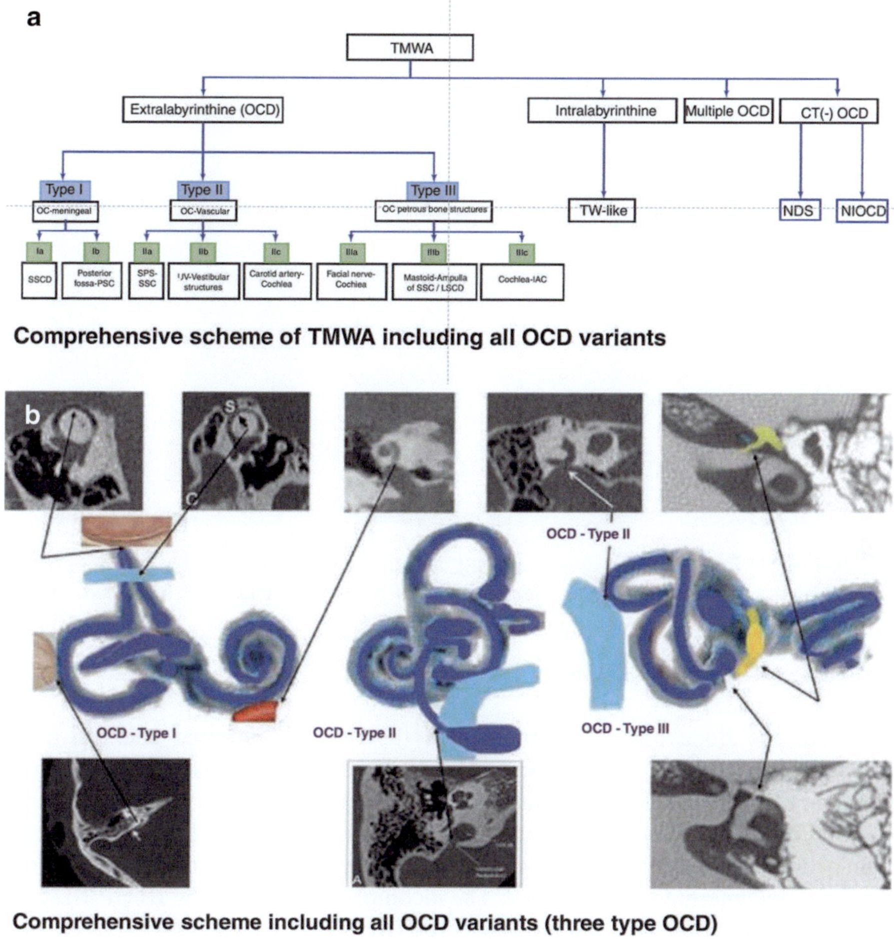

Fig. 20.3 (**a**) The OCD classification scheme is laid out in images with correlating anatomy. (**b**) Proposed classification scheme of third window syndromes as described by Ionescu et al. IAC internal auditory canal, IJV internal jugular vein, LSCD lateral semicircular canal, OC otic capsule, OCD otic capsule dehiscence, SSCD superior semicircular canal dehiscence, NDS near dehiscence syndrome, NIOCD non-identified otic capsule dehiscence, SPS superior petrosal sinus, PSC posterior semicircular canal, SSC superior semicircular canal, TW third window. (Source: Gianoli and Thomson [63])

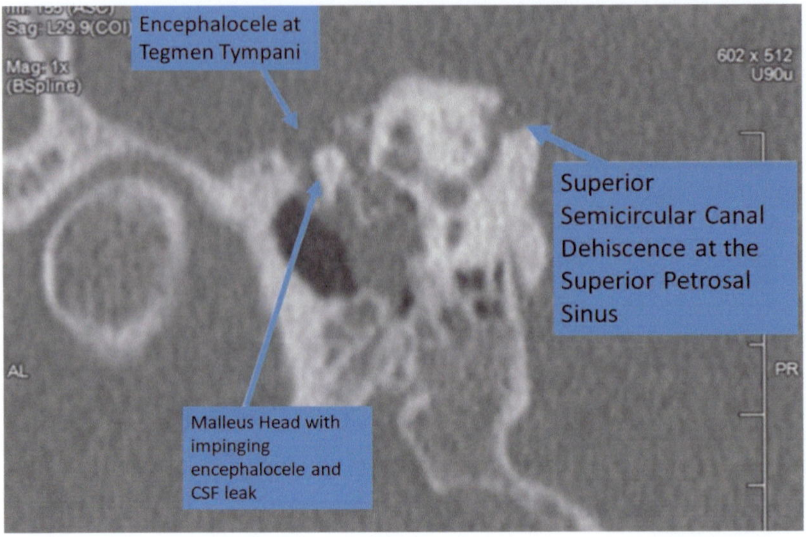

Fig. 20.4 OCD Type IIa demonstrated with SSC dehiscence interfacing with the superior petrosal sinus. Note the coexisting encephalocele impacting the malleus head. (Source: See Chap. 18)

Type III: OCD-Petrosal Bone

OCD-Petrous Bone anomalies encompass the recently reported cochlear-facial dehiscence (Type IIIa) as described earlier. Superior canal dehiscence into a mastoid air cell is a particularly rare cause of OCD; this underpins Type IIIb anomalies, which are described as hyperpneumatized portions of the temporal bone in communication with the membranous inner ear. Type IIIc OCD includes dehiscence involving the internal auditory canal. The incomplete partition type-III (IP-III) congenital malformation may qualify as a "Type IIIc" OCD variant.

Intralabyrinthine, Multiple OCD, and CT-Negative OCD

Additional variants may not perfectly qualify for the OCD schema. These include intralabyrinthine dehiscences, hypermobile stapes, and membranous stapes cases. Intralabyrinthine dehiscence includes a dehiscent interface between multiple inner ear structures, such as might be seen with an enlarged vestibular aqueduct (EVA), causing a secondary dehiscence of the PSC. Patients may have multiple dehiscence sites, such as a superior canal and posterior canal combined dehiscence (Fig. 20.1). Finally, patients may present with classic third window symptoms and positive electrophysiologic testing (reduced threshold on VEMP), but have negative imaging; CT-negative OCD allows for classification of this minority of patients, which may include occult perilymphatic fistula as an example.

Conclusion

Third window syndromes share an aspect of similar physiology and pathologic changes; however, each disorder has unique presentation and treatment. When patients present with third window-like symptoms and a negative CT scan, high clinical suspicion is required to evaluate for these other causes. Vestibular testing, specifically VEMP testing, Fistula testing, Valsalva testing, and Tullio testing, can be beneficial in many cases given the present third window pathology. Treatment is targeted toward the underlying cause of the third window syndrome and severity of patient symptoms. Classification of these syndromes involves ongoing and active research efforts, and improved diagnostic testing to characterize unique dehiscence locations will continue to evolve as they are more commonly identified and reported in the contemporary literature.

References

1. Merchant SN, Rosowski JJ. Conductive hearing loss caused by third-window lesions of the inner ear. Otol Neurotol. 2008;29(3):282–9. https://doi.org/10.1097/mao.0b013e318161ab24.
2. Gopen Q, Rosowski JJ, Merchant SN. Anatomy of the normal human cochlear aqueduct with functional implications. Hear Res. 1997;107(1–2):9–22. https://doi.org/10.1016/s0378-5955(97)00017-8.
3. Tullio P. Some experiments and considerations on experimental otology and phonetics. Presented at: 1929, Bologna, Italy.
4. Hennebert C. Reflexe oto-oculo-moteur. Int Zentralbl Ohrenheilkd Rhino Laryngol. 1905;3:405.
5. Kim HHS, Wilson DF. A third mobile window at the cochlear apex. Otolaryngol Head Neck Surg. 2006;135(6):965–6. https://doi.org/10.1016/j.otohns.2005.04.006.
6. Merchant SN, Nakajima HH, Halpin C, et al. Clinical investigation and mechanism of air-bone gaps in large vestibular aqueduct syndrome. Ann Otol Rhinol Laryngol. 2007;116(7):532–41. https://doi.org/10.1177/000348940711600709.
7. Mikulec AA, Poe DS. Operative management of a posterior semicircular canal dehiscence. Laryngoscope. 2006;116(3):375–8. https://doi.org/10.1097/01.mlg.0000200358.93385.5c.
8. Rosowski JJ, Songer JE, Nakajima HH, Brinsko KM, Merchant SN. Clinical, experimental, and theoretical investigations of the effect of superior semicircular canal dehiscence on hearing mechanisms. Otol Neurotol. 2004;25(3):323–32. https://doi.org/10.1097/00129492-200405000-00021.
9. Minor LB, Solomon D, Zinreich JS, Zee DS. Sound- and/or pressure-induced vertigo due to bone dehiscence of the superior semicircular canal. Arch Otolaryngol Head Neck Surg. 1998;124(3):249–58. https://doi.org/10.1001/archotol.124.3.249.
10. Yuen HW, Boeddinghaus R, Eikelboom RH, Atlas MD. The relationship between the air-bone gap and the size of superior semicircular canal dehiscence. Otolaryngol Head Neck Surg. 2009;141(6):689–94. https://doi.org/10.1016/j.otohns.2009.08.029.
11. Nakashima T, Ueda H, Furuhashi A, et al. Air-bone gap and resonant frequency in large vestibular aqueduct syndrome. Am J Otol. 2000;21(5):671–4.
12. Govaerts PJ, Casselman J, Daemers K, De Ceulaer G, Somers T, Offeciers FE. Audiological findings in large vestibular aqueduct syndrome. Int J Pediatr Otorhinolaryngol. 1999;51(3):157–64. https://doi.org/10.1016/s0165-5876(99)00268-2.

13. Welgampola MS, Myrie OA, Minor LB, Carey JP. Vestibular-evoked myogenic potential thresholds normalize on plugging superior canal dehiscence. Neurology. 2008;70(6):464–72. https://doi.org/10.1212/01.wnl.0000299084.76250.4a.
14. Ho ML, Moonis G, Halpin CF, Curtin HD. Spectrum of third window abnormalities: semicircular canal dehiscence and beyond. AJNR Am J Neuroradiol. 2017;38(1):2–9. https://doi.org/10.3174/ajnr.A4922.
15. Garvis WJ, Johnson BA, Kluesner KE, Garvis SM. Characteristics of the facial canal-lateral canal dehiscence: the under-recognized third window. OTO Open. 2025;9(1):e70085. https://doi.org/10.1002/oto2.70085.
16. Razskazovskiy V, McCall AA, Branstetter BF. Prevalence of cochlear-facial and other non-superior semicircular canal third window dehiscence on high-resolution temporal bone CT. AJNR Am J Neuroradiol. 2023;44(11):1309–13. https://doi.org/10.3174/ajnr.A8032.
17. Smetak MR, Cass ND, Manzoor NF, et al. Vestibular migraine confounds management of superior canal dehiscence syndrome. Otol Neurotol. 2022;43(7):835–9. https://doi.org/10.1097/MAO.0000000000003584.
18. Ionescu EC, Reynard P, Damien M, et al. Why should multiple dehiscences of the otic capsule be considered before surgically treating patients with superior semicircular canal dehiscence? A radiological monocentric review and a case series. Front Neurol. 2023;14:1209567. https://doi.org/10.3389/fneur.2023.1209567.
19. Madden C, Halsted M, Benton C, Greinwald J, Choo D. Enlarged vestibular aqueduct syndrome in the pediatric population. Otol Neurotol. 2003;24(4):625–32. https://doi.org/10.1097/00129492-200307000-00016.
20. Elmoursy MM. The incidence of enlarged vestibular aqueduct among hearing-impaired children: hospital-based tertiary care referral center. Egypt J Otolaryngol. 2022;38(1):145. https://doi.org/10.1186/s43163-022-00333-8.
21. Valvassori GE, Clemis JD. The large vestibular aqueduct syndrome. Laryngoscope. 1978;88(5):723–8. https://doi.org/10.1002/lary.1978.88.5.723.
22. Juliano AF, Ting EY, Mingkwansook V, Hamberg LM, Curtin HD. Vestibular aqueduct measurements in the 45° oblique (Pöschl) plane. AJNR Am J Neuroradiol. 2016;37(7):1331–7. https://doi.org/10.3174/ajnr.A4735.
23. Boston M, Halsted M, Meinzen-Derr J, et al. The large vestibular aqueduct: a new definition based on audiologic and computed tomography correlation. Otolaryngol Head Neck Surg. 2007;136(6):972–7. https://doi.org/10.1016/j.otohns.2006.12.011.
24. Dewan K, Wippold FJ, Lieu JEC. Enlarged vestibular aqueduct in pediatric sensorineural hearing loss. Otolaryngol Head Neck Surg. 2009;140(4):552–8. https://doi.org/10.1016/j.otohns.2008.12.035.
25. Jackler RK, De La Cruz A. The large vestibular aqueduct syndrome. Laryngoscope. 1989;99(12):1238–42. https://doi.org/10.1288/00005537-198912000-00006; discussion 1242–1243.
26. Zalewski CK, Chien WW, King KA, et al. Vestibular dysfunction in patients with enlarged vestibular aqueduct. Otolaryngol Head Neck Surg. 2015;153(2):257–62. https://doi.org/10.1177/0194599815585098.
27. Pang J, Wang Y, Cheng Y, et al. Conductive hearing loss in large vestibular aqueduct syndrome—clinical observations and proof-of-concept predictive modeling by a biomechanical approach. Int J Pediatr Otorhinolaryngol. 2021;146:110752. https://doi.org/10.1016/j.ijporl.2021.110752.
28. Zhou G, Gopen Q. Characteristics of vestibular evoked myogenic potentials in children with enlarged vestibular aqueduct. Laryngoscope. 2011;121(1):220–5. https://doi.org/10.1002/lary.21184.
29. Noordman BJ, van Beeck CE, Witte B, Goverts T, Hensen E, Merkus P. Prognostic factors for sudden drops in hearing level after minor head injury in patients with an enlarged vestibular aqueduct: a meta-analysis. Otol Neurotol. 2015;36(1):4–11. https://doi.org/10.1097/MAO.0000000000000659.

30. Welling DB, Martyn MD, Miles BA, Oehler M, Schmalbrock P. Endolymphatic sac occlusion for the enlarged vestibular aqueduct syndrome. Am J Otol. 1998;19(2):145–51.
31. Claró́s P, Fokouo JVF, Clarós A. Cochlear implantation in patients with enlarged vestibular aqueduct. A case series with literature review. Cochlear Implants Int. 2017;18(3):125–9. https://doi.org/10.1080/14670100.2016.1268754.
32. Au G, Gibson W. Cochlear implantation in children with large vestibular aqueduct syndrome. Am J Otol. 1999;20(2):183–6.
33. Aschendorff A, Marangos N, Laszig R. Large vestibular aqueduct syndrome and its implication for cochlear implant surgery. Am J Otol. 1997;18(6 Suppl):S57.
34. Meyer A, Bouchetemblé P, Costentin B, Dehesdin D, Lerosey Y, Marie JP. Lateral semicircular canal fistula in cholesteatoma: diagnosis and management. Eur Arch Otorrinolaringol. 2016;273(8):2055–63. https://doi.org/10.1007/s00405-015-3775-6.
35. Gubbels SP, Zhang Q, Lenkowski PW, Hansen MR. Repair of posterior semicircular canal dehiscence from a high jugular bulb. Ann Otol Rhinol Laryngol. 2013;122(4):269–72. https://doi.org/10.1177/000348941312200409.
36. McCall AA, Curtin HD, McKenna MJ. Posterior semicircular canal dehiscence arising from temporal bone fibrous dysplasia. Otol Neurotol. 2010;31(9):1516–7. https://doi.org/10.1097/MAO.0b013e3181be6b12.
37. Erdogan N, Songu M, Akay E, et al. Posterior semicircular canal dehiscence in asymptomatic ears. Acta Otolaryngol. 2011;131(1):4–8. https://doi.org/10.3109/00016489.2010.502184.
38. Gopen Q, Zhou G, Poe D, Kenna M, Jones D. Posterior semicircular canal dehiscence: first reported case series. Otol Neurotol. 2010;31(2):339–44. https://doi.org/10.1097/MAO.0b013e3181be65a4.
39. Copeland BJ, Buchman CA. Management of labyrinthine fistulae in chronic ear surgery. Am J Otolaryngol. 2003;24(1):51–60. https://doi.org/10.1053/ajot.2003.10.
40. Jang CH, Merchant SN. Histopathology of labyrinthine fistulae in chronic otitis media with clinical implications. Am J Otol. 1997;18(1):15–25.
41. Portier F, Lescanne E, Racy E, Nowak C, Lamblin B, Bobin S. Studies of labyrinthine cholesteatoma-related fistulas: report of 22 cases. J Otolaryngol. 2005;34(1):1–6. https://doi.org/10.2310/7070.2005.00001.
42. Ward BK, Agrawal Y, Nguyen E, et al. Hearing outcomes after surgical plugging of the superior semicircular canal by a middle cranial fossa approach. Otol Neurotol. 2012;33(8):1386–91. https://doi.org/10.1097/MAO.0b013e318268d20d.
43. Rodgers B, Lin J, Staecker H. Transmastoid resurfacing versus middle fossa plugging for repair of superior canal dehiscence: comparison of techniques from a retrospective cohort. World J Otorhinolaryngol Head Neck Surg. 2016;2(3):161–7. https://doi.org/10.1016/j.wjorl.2016.11.001.
44. Freeman P. Fistula of the lateral semicircular canal. Clin Otolaryngol Allied Sci. 1978;3(3):315–21. https://doi.org/10.1111/j.1365-2273.1978.tb00706.x.
45. Chen R, Delsing CPA, Saxby A, Kong JHK, Jufas N, Patel NP. Underwater endoscopic ear surgery for repair of lateral semicircular canal fistulae secondary to cholesteatoma—a pilot safety analysis. Aust J Otolaryngol. 2024;7:40. https://doi.org/10.21037/ajo-24-3.
46. Gianoli G, Soileau J, Shore B. Description of a new labyrinthine dehiscence: horizontal semicircular canal dehiscence at the tympanic segment of the facial nerve. Front Neurol. 2022;13:879149. https://doi.org/10.3389/fneur.2022.879149.
47. Ben-Shlomo N, Rahimi A, Abunimer AM, et al. Incidence of iatrogenic inner ear breaches from vestibular schwannoma surgery: a review of 1,153 hearing preservation approaches. J Neurol Surg Part B Skull Base. 2020:s-0040-1702361. https://doi.org/10.1055/s-0040-1702361.
48. Ikeda R, Kikuchi T, Sato S, et al. Pulsatile tinnitus caused by pneumocephalus after Janneta surgery. Auris Nasus Larynx. 2021;48(4):793–6. https://doi.org/10.1016/j.anl.2020.05.024.
49. Kim SH, Ko SH, Ahn SH, Hong JM, Lee WS. Significance of the development of the inner ear third window effect after endolymphatic sac surgery in Ménière disease patients. Laryngoscope. 2012;122(8):1838–43. https://doi.org/10.1002/lary.23332.

50. Fang CH, Chung SY, Blake DM, et al. Prevalence of cochlear-facial dehiscence in a study of 1,020 temporal bone specimens. Otol Neurotol. 2016;37(7):967–72. https://doi.org/10.1097/MAO.0000000000001057.
51. Blake DM, Tomovic S, Vazquez A, Lee HJ, Jyung RW. Cochlear-facial dehiscence--a newly described entity. Laryngoscope. 2014;124(1):283–9. https://doi.org/10.1002/lary.24223.
52. Chen J, Chen B, Zhang L, Li Y. Severe and persistent facial nerve stimulation after cochlear implantation in a patient with cochlear-facial dehiscence: a case report. J Int Med Res. 2021;49(11):3000605211057823. https://doi.org/10.1177/03000605211057823.
53. Wackym PA, Balaban CD, Zhang P, Siker DA, Hundal JS. Third window syndrome: surgical management of cochlea-facial nerve dehiscence. Front Neurol. 2019;10:1281. https://doi.org/10.3389/fneur.2019.01281.
54. Shoman NM, Samy RN, Pensak ML. Contemporary neuroradiographic assessment of the cochleo-carotid partition. ORL J Otorhinolaryngol Relat Spec. 2016;78(4):193–8. https://doi.org/10.1159/000369622.
55. Gunbey HP, Aydın H, Cetin H, et al. MDCT assessment of the cochlear-carotid interval. Neuroradiol J. 2011;24(3):439–43. https://doi.org/10.1177/197140091102400315.
56. Phippard D, Lu L, Lee D, Saunders JC, Crenshaw EB. Targeted mutagenesis of the POU-domain gene *Brn4/Pou3f4* causes developmental defects in the inner ear. J Neurosci. 1999;19(14):5980–9. https://doi.org/10.1523/JNEUROSCI.19-14-05980.1999.
57. Corvino V, Apisa P, Malesci R, Laria C, Auletta G, Franzé A. X-linked sensorineural hearing loss: a literature review. Curr Genomics. 2018;19(5):327–38. https://doi.org/10.2174/1389202919666171218163046.
58. Hong R, Du Q, Pan Y. New imaging findings of incomplete partition type III inner ear malformation and literature review. AJNR Am J Neuroradiol. 2020;41(6):1076–80. https://doi.org/10.3174/ajnr.A6576.
59. Saylisoy S, Incesulu A, Gurbuz MK, Adapinar B. Computed tomographic findings of X-linked deafness: a spectrum from child to mother, from young to old, from boy to girl, from mixed to sudden hearing loss. J Comput Assist Tomogr. 2014;38(1):20–4. https://doi.org/10.1097/RCT.0b013e3182a0d05f.
60. Snik AF, Hombergen GC, Mylanus EA, Cremers CW. Air-bone gap in patients with X-linked stapes gusher syndrome. Am J Otol. 1995;16(2):241–6.
61. Dasgupta S, Hong J, Morris R, Iqbal J, Lennox-Bowley A, Saniasiaya J. X-linked gusher disease DFNX2 in children, a rare inner ear dysplasia with mixed hearing and vestibular loss. Audiol Res. 2023;13(4):600–14. https://doi.org/10.3390/audiolres13040052.
62. Sennaroğlu L, Bajin MD. Incomplete partition type III: a rare and difficult cochlear implant surgical indication. Auris Nasus Larynx. 2018;45(1):26–32. https://doi.org/10.1016/j.anl.2017.02.006.
63. Gianoli GJ, Thomson P, editors. Chapter 4, figure 4.7. Third mobile window syndrome of the inner ear: superior semicircular canal dehiscence and associated disorders. Springer; 2022.

Chapter 21
Vestibular Migraine

Amy Schettino and Dhasakumar Navaratnam

Introduction

Vestibular migraine is a clinical syndrome of the central nervous system that is characterized by episodic vestibular symptoms and a history of migraines. It affects approximately 1% of the population [1] and is one of the most common diagnoses in children presenting with vertigo [2].

One of the earliest case reports consistent with vestibular migraine was recorded in the second century AD by a Greek physician [3] who made a clear distinction between chronic, brief, and vertiginous type headaches. He labeled this latter type ἑτεροκρανίη, meaning "heterocrania," which evolved into "hemicrania," and eventually became the familiar term "migraine." Beginning in the late 1800s, the relationship between migraine headaches and vertigo was again anecdotally noted in countries throughout Europe [4–6], but the first studies directly targeting the association between migraine and vertigo were not published until the late 1970s [7, 8]. Hundreds of articles have since investigated this syndrome, and although the term "vestibular migraine" was coined in 1917 [6], then reintroduced in 1999 [9], many other names have been used interchangeably, including benign recurrent vertigo, episodic vertigo, migraine-associated vertigo or dizziness, migraine-related vestibulopathy, migrainous vertigo, and benign paroxysmal vertigo of childhood.

A. Schettino (✉)
Department of Surgery, Yale University, School of Medicine, New Haven, CT, USA
e-mail: amy.schettino@yale.edu

D. Navaratnam
Departments of Neurology (OL,DN) Neuroscience (DN) and Surgery (DN), Yale University, School of Medicine, New Haven, CT, USA
e-mail: dhasakumar.navaratnam@yale.edu

J. C. Lucas et al. (eds.), *Diagnosis and Treatment of Vestibular Disorders*,
https://doi.org/10.1007/978-3-032-11740-3_21

Such varied terminology reflects much of the uncertainty that surrounded vestibular migraine in the past, and over the last few decades, this lack of standardization has hampered the advancement of research. In 2012, the Bárány Society and International Headache Society jointly released the first criteria for the diagnosis of vestibular migraine as a distinct clinical entity [10], which has sparked several large-scale clinical trials and will hopefully propel investigations to improve the quality of life for these patients.

Diagnostic Criteria (Table 21.1)

Table 21.1 Diagnostic criteria for vestibular migraine

1. Vestibular migraine
A. At least five episodes with vestibular symptoms[a] of moderate or severe intensity,[b] lasting 5 min to 72 h
B. Current or previous history of migraine with or without aura according to the *International Classification of Headache Disorders* (1CHD)[d]
C. One or more migraine features with at least 50% of the vestibular episodes:[e]
Headache with at least two of the following characteristics: one-sided location, pulsating quality, moderate or severe pam intensity, aggravation by routine physical activity
Photophobia and phonophobia[f]
Visual aura[g]
D. Not better accounted for by another vestibular or ICHD diagnosis[h]
2. Probable vestibular migraine
A. At least five episodes with vestibular symptoms[a] of moderate or severe intensity,[b] lasting 5 min to 72 h[c]
B. Only one of the criteria B and C for vestibular migraine is fulfilled (migraine history or migraine features during the episode)
C. Not better accounted for by another vestibular or ICHD diagnosis[h]

Reprinted from Lempert et al. [10] with permission from IOS Press. Available at IOS Press through https://doi.org/10.1007/S00115-013-3768-x

[a]Vestibular symptoms, as defined by the Bàràny Society's Classification of Vestibular Symptoms and qualifying for a diagnosis of vestibular migraine, include the following:

Spontaneous vertigo including the following:

Internal vertigo, a false sensation of self-motion

External vertigo, a false sensation that the visual surround is pinning or flowing

Positional vertigo, occurring after a change of head position

Visually induced vertigo, triggered by a complex or large moving visual stimulus

Head motion-induced vertigo, occurring during head motion

Head motion-induced dizziness with nausea. Dizziness is characterized by a sensation of disturbed spatial orientation. Other forms of dizziness are currently not included in the classification of vestibular migraine

[b]Vestibular symptoms are rated "moderate" when they interfere with, but do not prohibit, daily activities and "severe" if daily activities cannot be continued

[c]Duration of episodes is highly variable: about 30% of patients have episodes lasting minutes, 30% have attacks for hours, and another 30% have attacks over several days. The remaining 10% have attacks lasting seconds only, which tend to occur repeatedly during head motion, visual stimulation, or after changes of head position. In these patients, episode duration is defined as the total

(continued)

Table 21.1 (continued)

period during which short attacks recur. At the other end of the spectrum, there are patients who may take 4 weeks to fully recover from an episode. However, the core episode rarely exceeds 72 h

[d]Migraine categories 1.1 and 1.2 of the ICDH-2

[e]One symptom is sufficient during a single episode. Different symptoms may occur during different episodes. Associated symptoms may occur before, during, or after the vestibular symptoms

[f]Phonophobia is defined as sound-induced discomfort. It is a transient and bilateral phenomenon that must be differentiated from recruitment, which is often unilateral and persistent. Recruitment leads to an enhanced perception and often distortion of loud sounds in an ear with decreased hearing

[g]Visual auras are characterized by bright scintillating lights or zigzag lines, often with a scotoma that interferes with reading. Visual auras typically expand over 5–20 min and last for less than 60 min. They are often, but not always, restricted to one hemifield. Other types of migraine aura, e g., somatosensory or dysphasic aura, are not included as diagnostic criteria because their phenomenology is less specific and most patients also have visual auras

[h]History and physical examinations do not suggest another vestibular disorder or such a disorder is considered but ruled out by appropriate investigations or such disorder is present as a comorbid or independent condition, but episodes can be clearly differentiated. Migraine attacks may be induced by vestibular stimulation. Therefore, the differential diagnosis should include other vestibular disorders complicated by superimposed migraine attacks

Epidemiology

The lifetime prevalence of vestibular migraine has been reported to be around 1% [1], and the diagnosis is fairly common in specialized neurology or otolaryngology clinics. Among patients seen in a dizziness clinic, it accounts for 7% of the diagnoses [11], while it affects between 9% and 21% of patients seen in a migraine clinic [12, 13]. It is considered the most common cause of episodic spontaneous vertigo in adults, as well as the most common cause of vertigo and dizziness in children and adolescents [2, 14, 15]. However, as official acceptance of this disorder has been relatively recent, it is unsurprising that it has been historically overlooked, with one study of an interdisciplinary vertigo center finding that vestibular migraine was diagnosed at over 10 times the rate at which it was initially suspected by the referring provider [16].

Vestibular migraine disproportionately affects women, with studies reporting that females are affected between 1.5 and 5.6 times more often than males [9, 11, 17–19]. However, Neuhauser et al. [1] noted that there was no significant difference in the odds ratio for female sex in vestibular migraine compared with migraine alone, so the predominance of women affected by vestibular migraine simply reflects the demographics of the migraine population. Vestibular migraine may present at any age; however, the first episode of vertigo is often around 40 years old [9, 18], and the majority present between 20 and 60 years old [9]. Park and Viire [20] have suggested that the hormonal fluctuations of menopause play a role in triggering the initial episode of vestibular migraine. Migraine often precedes the onset of vestibular migraine [9, 11, 18], with a recent multicenter database analysis reporting over a decade between the onset of headaches and the initial episode of vertigo [18]. In some cases, vestibular migraine may present years after the resolution of migraine attacks [9]. A family history is common as well, with between 35% and 78% of these patients reporting headaches or vertigo in a first or second-degree relative [9, 18, 21–23].

Vestibular migraine exists at the intersection of migraine and vertigo. Migraine affects nearly 12% of the adult population of Western countries [24], while symptoms of vertigo are reported by 3–10% of the population [25–28], and dizziness affects up to 30% of the population [28, 29]. These are two very common neurological disorders, and the overlap between them is considerable, as 50% of patients with migraine also report at least occasional dizziness or vertigo [18], and up to 15% of patients with migraine are concurrently affected by vestibular migraine [11]. Many studies have found that the concurrence of these two symptoms is 1.6–3 times higher than expected based on chance alone [1, 11, 30, 31], suggesting a link beyond that of coincidence.

Many vestibular migraine patients are not affected by a separate vestibular disorder [32]; in fact, it was this substantial population of patients with unexplained vestibular symptoms that led to the discovery and classification of vestibular migraine as an independent diagnosis. However, several neurotologic disorders, such as benign paroxysmal positional vertigo (BPPV), Ménière's disease, and motion sickness, do affect migraine patients more often than controls, and as much as 57% of vestibular migraine patients have an additional comorbid vestibular condition [33]. Among those patients with dual vestibular diagnoses, the most common combination is vestibular migraine and BPPV, followed by vestibular migraine and Ménière's disease [34]. One study found that 12.5% of patients with vestibular migraine also met criteria for BPPV, and this subset made up 4.2% of the patients referred to a single center's neurotology clinic over a 1-year period [35]. Ménière's disease has been reported to affect between 17% and 23% of vestibular migraine patients [36–38].

Pathophysiology

While the pathophysiology of functional vestibular symptoms in healthy individuals is fairly well-understood [39], the underlying mechanisms of vestibular migraine are still unclear. It is accepted that migraine interacts with the vestibular system at both the central and peripheral levels [40, 41] to produce the wide range of vestibular symptoms experienced by patients, but the overarching hypotheses of the disease process come from our limited understanding of migraine alone [42].

It is now generally accepted that headache is caused by activation of the trigemino-vascular system, which innervates the pia mater, dura mater, and cranial blood vessels. Second and third-order neurons of this system project throughout the cortex, brainstem, and hypothalamus [43]. When this system is sensitized, vasoactive neuropeptides, including substance P, calcitonin gene-related protein, and neurokinin A, are released and lead to vasodilation, mast cell degranulation, and neurogenic inflammation [44]. Approaching migraine from an electrophysiological standpoint, many feel the key lies in understanding cortical spreading depression, a transient, widespread wave of neural depolarization, followed by suppression of electrical activity and delayed restoration of transmembrane concentration gradients [9]. This phenomenon is thought to play a role in migraine aura as well as migraine initiation, but cortical spreading depression has not been definitively linked to aura in humans, and it is unclear if or how it might then activate the trigemino-vascular system [45].

Though the vestibular symptoms of vestibular migraine are not equivalent to a migraine sensory aura, some suggest that they may be triggered by cortical spreading depression that reaches the vestibular brainstem nuclei [9]. However, it has been pointed out that the duration of depolarization does not fit with the length of clinical episodes that last seconds to days. Older theories on vestibular migraine have suggested the involvement of vasospasm of the internal auditory artery or infarct of the anterior inferior cerebellar artery, as the symptom onset is rather sudden, and migraine with aura is independently associated with cerebrovascular risk [46–48]. These proposed mechanisms similarly fail to account for the wide range of clinical manifestations seen with vestibular migraine [42].

Several studies have suggested an autosomal dominant inheritance pattern [49–51], with a decreased penetrance in males as evidenced by the high female-to-male ratio. Genetic predisposition to vestibular migraine appears to be heterogeneous [52], and several chromosomal foci, notably 6q, 22q12, 11q, and 5q35, have been identified in association with families reporting migraine and vestibulopathy [52–55]. Other investigations, targeting a gene linked with several ataxia and hemiplegic migraine syndromes, have suggested that a mutation in the voltage-gated calcium channel CaV2.1 (P/Q type; CACNA1A) may promote cortical spreading depression, and thus migraine and vestibular migraine [32, 56–58]. The rare form of familial hemiplegic migraine itself has been linked to two other ion channel/transporter genes ATP1A2 and SCN1A [59, 60]. A more recent extensive meta-genetic analysis with GWAS of 59,624 individuals identified 38 genomic loci that were associated with migraine, including one on the X chromosome (migraine, including vestibular migraine, is more common in women) [61, 62]. The data from this study also replicated prior work that had identified 13 genomic loci implicated in migraine, since 10 of the 13 loci were also found in this study [61, 62]. Somewhat unexpectedly, only a few of these genes were associated with neuronal function and ion channels, and corroborated by absent eQTL signal in brain. A significant number of the genes that were identified were associated with vascular disease or smooth muscle function. Two of the genes (Jag1 and Hey2) implicated in the study are involved in the Notch pathway, important for hair cell development [61, 62].

More recent research has focused on the neuroanatomical foci of vestibular processing and the structural changes accompanying vestibular migraine. The ventral posterior lateral and ventral posterior medial nuclei, known primarily as thalamic relay nuclei for somatosensory information, have been shown to process vestibular inputs as well [63]. Increased thalamic activation has been demonstrated in vestibular migraine patients [64, 65], and temporary sensitization of these nuclei may underlie migraine attacks [42]. The posterior insular-opercular region is also under study as a site of potential interaction between nociceptive and vestibular pathways [66–68]. Though thalamocortical pathways seem to be more active in patients with vestibular migraine [64, 65, 69], there appear to be no microstructrual changes in white matter in patients with vestibular migraine or migraine with or without aura compared to controls [70]. Conversely, the volume of gray matter in patients with vestibular migraine differs significantly from that of healthy controls [71, 72] in areas involved with multisensory vestibular and nociceptive processing.

Clinical Manifestations

The presentation of vestibular migraine varies widely between patients, as well as between episodes for a single patient. However, according to the Bárány Society and International Headache Society criteria, all patients with vestibular migraine will have at least five distinct episodes of vestibular symptoms, a prior history of migraine, and at least one migraine feature with 50% or more of the vestibular episodes [73].

Vestibular Symptoms

The clinical course and presentation of vestibular migraine are extremely variable. The most commonly reported vestibular symptom is episodic spontaneous vertigo, which one study found affects 67% of patients. Some 24% of patients report positional vertigo [1], and the initial type of vertigo may transform into another form of vertigo or dizziness, such as positional dizziness or disequilibrium with gait disturbance, over the course of a single attack [7, 74, 75]. Additionally, patients may experience different combinations of vestibular symptoms with each attack, which helps differentiate vestibular migraine from other neurotologic diseases such as BPPV or Ménière's disease that rarely present with more than one type of vertigo [76]. Other vestibular manifestations include postural imbalance, head motion-induced dizziness (where head movements trigger imbalance, illusory motion, and nausea) [77, 78], and visually induced vertigo (which is provoked by moving visual imagery such as traffic and movies) [78–80].

Episodes of vestibular symptoms range in duration from seconds to days, even for an individual patient [8, 9, 11, 81]. While 10% of patients report attacks lasting a few seconds, 30% report several minutes, 30% report several hours, and 30% report several days. Most attacks last between 5 min to 72 h, though patients may need longer to recover even after the cessation of symptoms [75]. Around 30% of patients experience vertigo without headache [11, 22, 81], but at least 50% of these episodes must be accompanied by other typical features of migraine, such as visual aura, photophobia, phonophobia, osmophobia, or exacerbation by movement [82]. Without accompanying headache, these symptoms are vital for accurate diagnosis and often must be directly elicited through thorough history taking or a dizziness diary [76]. Nausea and vomiting commonly accompany acute attacks but are not specific to vestibular migraine [40, 41]. Around 25% of patients have headache along with vertigo, and in these cases, the vertigo may occur before, with, or during the migraine attack, which is identified by the presence of unilaterality, pulsating quality, moderate to severe intensity, and worsening with physical activity [1, 10].

Signs of central vestibular dysfunction may also occur during attacks, including gaze-induced nystagmus, saccadic pursuit, central positional nystagmus, and horizontal or vertical spontaneous nystagmus [75]. Of these, central positional nystagmus is the most frequently reported and is typically low-velocity, sustained, and without latency [40, 41]. Central vestibular findings are reported to manifest in 8.6–66% of patients [8, 9, 40, 78, 80, 81] and become more frequent and severe over the course of the condition [80].

Migraine Symptoms

Some patients do not report migraine headaches ever occurring with vestibular episodes, but most patients have episodes both with and without headache [9, 11, 22, 81]. In many cases, patients experience a blunted version of their migraine headache with vestibular migraine attacks [22, 83]. Patients may still experience full migraine attacks in between vestibular episodes, or the intensity of their migraine headaches may have decreased over several years.

Triggers and Other Symptoms

Triggers of vestibular migraine attacks have been reported and appear similar to those for migraine attacks. Provocation has been noted due to stress, physical exertion, sleep irregularities, specific foods, dehydration, hormonal changes, and intense sensory stimulation, but requires further study before being included in the diagnostic criteria [10, 32, 84].

Up to 52% of patients may experience auditory symptoms, such as hearing loss, tinnitus, and aural pressure [8, 22, 38, 78, 85, 86]. Hearing loss in vestibular migraine is typically mild and transient, but does increase suspicion for Ménière's disease. To differentiate the two conditions, one study found that around 18% of patients with vestibular migraine progress to bilateral sensorineural hearing loss with a downsloping pattern. While some patients may still meet the criteria for Ménière's disease, the bilateral high-frequency hearing loss of vestibular migraine does not fit the typical findings of unilateral low-frequency hearing loss in Ménière's [80].

The onset of a vestibular syndrome has not been shown to influence the development of a new psychiatric disorder; however, a positive psychiatric history does increase the risk of a reactive psychiatric disorder in response to a vestibular vertigo syndrome [87]. Patients with vestibular migraine report higher levels of psychological strain than those with other types of vestibular vertigo [88], and around 50% of vestibular migraine patients present with comorbid psychiatric disorders, most commonly affective disorders and anxiety [87]. As the psychological impact of vestibular migraine can severely affect patients' quality of life, some investigators have drawn attention to the necessity of identifying functional dizziness in combination with a vestibular syndrome [33, 39, 89]. Functional dizziness, formerly psychogenic or somatoform dizziness, includes chronic subjective dizziness, phobic postural vertigo, space motion discomfort, and visual vertigo [39]. One study estimated that 35% of patients with vestibular migraine had concomitant chronic subjective dizziness [33]. Although diagnosis may be difficult because of the overlapping symptoms of functional dizziness and the Bárány Society/IHS criteria for vestibular migraine [33], it is important to recognize that patients' experiences of their illness are heavily influenced by their behavioral responses to it, and treatment strategies should address the physiological, functional, and psychiatric manifestations of the disorder [39].

Differential Diagnosis

The differential diagnosis of vestibular migraine is long [90, 91]. More frequent conditions that need to be considered include orthostatic hypotension, Ménière's disease, BPPV, head trauma and TBI, and peripheral neuropathy. Less common conditions include multiple sclerosis, vestibular neuronitis, stroke, tumors in the subtentorial space, and seizures. It is important to recognize that while the positive features of migraine (e.g., associated unilateral throbbing headache made worse with exercise) are often useful in helping distinguish it from other conditions, it can also lead to false attribution since migraine is present in up to 15% of the population [92].

Orthostatic hypotension is an often-troubling complaint in patients [93]. In distinguishing migraine-associated vertigo, patients may not complain of syncope, making the differentiation difficult. Patients will, however, state their symptoms to be worse when standing from a seated or lying down position. Other common associations include the use of blood pressure medications (frequently beta blockers and calcium channel blockers) and alpha adrenergic blockers used for the treatment of prostate disorders. A tilt table test is a useful adjuvant to test for orthostasis. The list of medications related to orthostasis is long, including diverse agents that reduce blood pressure as a therapeutic intent or as an inadvertent side effect (amitriptyline, trazodone, nitroglycerin, chlorpromazine, clozapine, levodopa/carbidopa, cyclobenzaprine, tizanidine, baclofen, sildenafil) [94]. Although carotid occlusions and arrhythmias can cause orthostasis, these conditions are self-evident and usually do not present to the dizzy clinic.

Ménière's disease is a common condition and typically presents with the characteristic triad of fullness, hearing loss, and tinnitus, usually in a unilateral distribution [95]. On occasion, the distinction can be difficult as many patients with Ménière's disease often have associated features of migraine-associated vertigo, and may have bilateral disease. Our practice in this case is to treat both conditions simultaneously.

BPPV is an easier condition to distinguish owing to its peculiar positional symptoms, usually when looking up, and often when lying or turning in bed [96], and classic eye findings. Other helpful features in separating it from migraine are the brief duration and absence of symptoms between episodes (e.g., patients with migraine complain of symptoms that are constant with exacerbations by movement).

Dizziness after head trauma is a common presentation [97]. It has been debated how much of the dizziness is due to central or peripheral causes [98]. The latter is often present in the immediate aftermath, and a variety of conditions, including BPPV, perilymphatic fistulas, and superior canal dehiscence, have been identified. These conditions have their own distinguishing features and are discussed separately in this book. More commonly, patients will present several months to years after TBI with symptoms of dizziness. Objective findings are elusive, and these patients are often labeled as malingering. A recent school of thought places these patients in the migraine overlap group and reports some benefit from treating them as migraine sufferers [99, 100].

Peripheral neuropathy can be a mimic and can be distinguished by symptoms made worse in the dark, associated history of diabetes or other conditions (B12 deficiency, medications, etc.) that give rise to a neuropathy. Physical exam findings will demonstrate a loss of light touch, position, and vibration sense in a distal to proximal gradient in a glove and stocking fashion. Deep tendon reflexes are usually absent or diminished. However, a recent paper identified peripheral vestibular disorders in 60% of patients with diabetic neuropathy, complicating the suggested simple dichotomy [101].

Patients with multiple sclerosis (MS) often present with dizziness. These patients will have a history suggestive of MS, including optic neuritis, internuclear ophthalmoplegias, and other transient focal neurological dysfunction. These patients will also have associated MRI abnormalities demonstrating a classical FLAIR and T2 signal in the subcortical white matter with enhanced signal on the T1 sequence after gadolinium administration. A confounding mimic in patients with MS is BPPV, which is present in increased frequency in these patients [102].

Vestibular neuronitis is distinguished by a monophasic, sudden, severe dizziness that worsens over a day or two and recovers over weeks to months with clear evidence of unilateral vestibular dysfunction (unilateral gaze evoked nystagmus in the opposite direction, ipsilateral corrective saccades with head thrusts, and ipsilateral turning with Fukuda stepping) [103].

Stroke, particularly involving the posterior inferior cerebellar artery, can present as a sudden onset of dizziness with associated nausea and vomiting. Cerebellar and brainstem findings (gaze-evoked nystagmus and skew deviation) are variably present [104]. Since these patients present with a single episode, confusion with migraine is not the norm. However, since migraine sufferers have an increased incidence of stroke, separating a stroke from a more severe episode of migraine-associated vertigo can be difficult and may need recourse to MRI to confirm a stroke.

Though possible, tumors of the cerebellopontine angle do not typically present with acute vertigo, likely since they are slow growing and allow the brainstem to adapt to the reduced vestibular input [105]. With eighth nerve tumors, there is associated loss of hearing. An MRI will enable separation of the more benign migraine-associated vertigo.

Seizures, particularly of the temporal cortex and less commonly the parietal cortex, have been associated with dizziness [106]. Typically, these patients have other features of epilepsy, including frank seizures. Less commonly, patients can have isolated dizziness associated with a cortical epileptic focus. These patients are often vexing since EEG can fail to detect seizure activity in the deep cortex, and may require prolonged recordings and recourse to indirect evidence of seizures (asymmetric slowing in the period leading to, during and after the clinical symptoms).

Treatment

Unfortunately, research in this field has not yet identified a definitive therapy for vestibular migraine. Furthermore, a recent Cochrane review [107] concluded that there were insufficient randomized controlled trials to point to any medications effective in preventing vestibular migraine. Therefore, most of the proposed medications are currently supported by data showing their efficacy in treating migraine or studies of vestibular migraine with small sample sizes. However, vestibular migraine may be managed with a wide range of therapies, including pharmacotherapy, lifestyle modification, dietary adaptations, vestibular physical therapy, and cognitive therapy. These treatment options allow for effective management of symptoms in most patients, with a 50% or greater decrease in attack frequency as a feasible target [108] (Table 21.2).

When approaching the variety of available management options, it is important to adapt each treatment regimen to the individual experience of each patient. A patient who does not feel significantly disturbed by their attacks may simply opt for reassurance that no larger medical problem exists. However, patients who feel significantly impaired by each episode are likely to benefit from intervention or a combination of strategies.

Lifestyle and dietary modification are the simplest and safest forms of intervention and are often used as an initial step before supplementing other therapies. Similar to patients with migraine and Ménière's disease, patients with vestibular migraine are encouraged to keep a diary of episodes in order to identify and avoid triggers. Adaptations often include stress reduction, more regular sleeping patterns, regular aerobic exercise, and avoidance of specific foods. In a few cases, patients have initiated hormonal management with their gynecologist [22]. A structured plan of dietary manipulation has also been shown to reduce attacks and involves avoiding aged cheeses, processed meats, red wine, artificial sweeteners, chocolate, caffeine, and alcohol [22, 109, 110].

Table 21.2 Patient factors

Patient factors that may influence medication selection	
Patient factor	Suggested initial therapy
Hypertension Angina Essential tremor Panic attacks Anxiety	Beta blockers
Depression Sleep disturbance Chronic tension headaches Chronic pain	TCAs
Hypertension Asthma	Flunarizine
Obesity Headaches	Topiramate
Vertigo predominates Vertigo is part of aura	Lamotrigine
Depression	Venlafaxine
Headaches predominate	Valproate Beta blockers

Vestibular rehabilitation therapy has been shown to benefit patients with vestibular migraine, either alone or in combination with pharmacotherapy [111–113]. The optimal duration of vestibular therapy is unknown, but studies have demonstrated a significant reduction in symptoms with four to five visits spread over 2–3 months [112, 113]. The therapist should have experience in treating vestibular disorders and teaching vestibular exercises, as exercises too advanced or inappropriate for the condition may temporarily worsen dizziness, and the patient will be unlikely to return for future sessions [114].

In patients with a known or suspected psychiatric component to their dizziness, it may be helpful to incorporate cognitive behavioral therapy or select a medication with antidepressant activity, such as a selective serotonin reuptake inhibitor (SSRI) [115]. Psychiatric comorbidities, as discussed previously, affect approximately 50% of patients with vestibular migraine.

If pharmacotherapy is indicated, it should be selected based on the side effect profile and patient comorbidities, then titrated in a step-wise fashion. In several cases, patients have required a combination of two or more drugs before noticing an improvement [22]. Patients with infrequent but long episodes are best suited for abortive therapy, while those with short, frequent attacks may benefit most from prophylactic medication.

Though there have been several studies of abortive medications for acute episodes of vestibular migraine, the evidence is weak. Oral zolmitriptan (2.5 mg) was an effective, but statistically nonsignificant, abortive agent in a study of ten patients [116], and intramuscular and oral sumitriptan was found to significantly improve vertigo and migraine, based on 20 patients in a study of 129 patients with migraine-associated dizziness [117]. Oral almotriptan (12.5 mg) as a single dose within 1 h of the onset of a vertigo attack was also found to be significantly beneficial in a retrospective study of 26 patients with vestibular migraine [118]. Conversely, a case series of three patients noted that while triptans alleviated vertigo, they appeared to exacerbate or trigger headache [119]. Interestingly, a randomized controlled trial of ten patients found that oral rizatriptan (10 mg) was effective in decreasing motion sickness in individuals with migrainous vertigo, but not in patients with migraine alone [120]. Intravenous methylprednisolone (1000 g/day for 1–3 days) has also been used to abort prolonged attacks and was noted to effectively reduce symptoms in four patients [121]. Symptomatic treatment may be necessary during acute episodes, such as fluid replacement for vomiting, dimenhydrinate (50 mg q4–6h, max 400 mg/day) [122] as an antivertigo, antiemetics such as prochlorperazide, promethazine, metoclopramide, or cyclizine [123], and ibuprofen or paracetamol for headache.

The majority of the proposed pharmacotherapy for vestibular migraine consists of prophylactic medications, borrowed from their proven application in migraine or related vestibular disorders. These medications typically fall under the classification of antihypertensive, antidepressant, or neuroleptic medications. While no large randomized controlled trial yet exists to confirm the efficacy of any specific medication in treating vestibular migraine, multiple studies have found that prophylactic treatment significantly reduces vestibular migraine symptoms compared with placebo or no treatment.

Beta-adrenergic inhibitors, such as metoprolol and propranolol, have been established as effective prophylactic treatment for migraine, but their neurological mechanism of action and role in vestibular migraine are not yet clear [109, 124, 125]. Their prophylactic use in vestibular migraine is currently supported by multiple case series advocating for the use of propranolol, atenolol, and metoprolol in episodic vertigo and migraine-associated dizziness, as well as a recent retrospective study and randomized controlled trial which both noted significant improvement in vestibular symptoms using propranolol in patients with vestibular migraine [9, 19, 109, 126–128]. The efficacy of metoprolol in vestibular migraine is currently under investigation in a large randomized controlled trial (PROVEMIG). While there is no evidence to suggest they are superior to any other prophylactic pharmacologic therapy, beta-blockers may be particularly beneficial in patients with comorbid hypertension and angina, and they are typically well-tolerated [109, 129, 130]. Occasional side effects include syncope and bronchospasm. However, there are several contraindications to their use, including a history of bronchospasm, brittle diabetes, congestive heart failure, cardiac arrhythmia, or depression (Table 21.3).

Calcium channel blockers have been shown to exhibit antimigraine activity, and flunarizine, verapamil, and cinnarizine have been studied in relation to vestibular migraine in several smaller clinical trials. A randomized controlled trial of 100 patients with migrainous vertigo demonstrated a decrease in the frequency and severity of vertigo in the group treated nightly with 10 mg flunarizine for 3 months, and no effect on headache [131]. Both groups in this study were treated for acute attacks with betahistine and paracetamol. Other retrospective studies have found

Table 21.3 Medication doses and contraindications

Medication	Daily dosage range	Contraindications
Metoprolol	100–200 mg oral	History of bronchospasm Congestive heart failure Cardiac arrhythmia Brittle diabetes Reynaud's disease Depression
Propranolol	40–160 mg oral	
Flunarizine	5–10 mg oral	Cardiac conduction abnormalities
Cinnarizine	37.5–75 mg oral	
Verapamil	80–240 mg oral	
Amitriptyline	10–100 mg oral	Epilepsy Long QT syndrome
Nortriptyline	10–75 mg oral	
Venlafaxine	37.5–150 mg oral	Concurrent use of MAOI
Sertraline	50–200 mg oral	
Acetazolamide	250–500 mg oral	
Topiramate	50–100 mg oral	
Valproate	600 mg oral	History of pancreatitis Liver disease Pregnancy
Lamotrigine	75–100 mg oral	

Prescribed medication doses and contraindications as found in the literature
MAOI monoamine oxidase inhibitor

similar efficacy of flunarizine, but have not demonstrated superiority to other prophylactic medications [19, 127, 132]. Side effects of flunarizine have included weight gain, sedation, depression, and reversible parkinsonism, with some studies reporting discontinuation rates between 7% and 18% [9, 133, 134]. Cinnarizine is effective in the prevention of motion sickness [135] and has been shown to be safe and efficacious in reducing headache and vertigo in a retrospective study of 24 patients with vestibular migraine or migraine-associated vertigo [136]. Another study noted that cinnarizine and dimenhydrinate significantly reduced vertigo and headache crises in the following 6 months compared to only lifestyle modifications [137]. Verapamil showed promise in two patients from a case series on chronic migrainous vertigo [79], and it is frequently listed as a possible migraine prophylaxis. However, a meta-analysis found it was no better than a placebo for migraine alone [124], and it has not been systematically evaluated in the treatment of vestibular migraine [22, 138]. One randomized controlled trial attempted to differentiate vestibular migraine from persistent postural-perceptual dizziness on the basis of vestibular migraine's potential response to verapamil, and instead found that sertraline was more effective in reducing both headache and dizziness [139].

Tricyclic antidepressants (TCAs) have a broad range of activity, including inhibition of sodium channels, elevation of GABA levels, and inhibition of central norepinephrine and serotonin reuptake, with additional antagonism at peripheral histamine and cholinergic receptors that accounts for their many side effects [140]. They are commonly used as migraine prophylaxis through a mechanism indirectly related to their antidepressant function [141] and are often used to treat chronic pain. A Cochrane review found that amitriptyline, clomipramine, and doxepin were more efficacious than placebo in reducing episodic migraine. Of these, amitriptyline is the most widely used [142] and was shown to be more likely than placebo to achieve a 50% reduction in episodic migraines [143]. Nortriptyline may occasionally be used to replace amitriptyline for less sedation; however, the increased risk of arrhythmia may necessitate regular EKGs. Additionally, at doses greater than 1 mg/kg, all TCAs may unmask a prolonged QT, and particular caution is advised in patients with epilepsy. More common side effects include sedation, orthostatic hypotension, dry mouth, dry eyes, tachycardia, blurry vision, palpitations, increased appetite, weight gain, and sexual dysfunction.

Other antidepressants, such as SSRIs and serotonin-norepinephrine reuptake inhibitors (SNRIs), have been tried for vestibular migraine prevention. Venlafaxine, an SNRI, is effective in migraine prophylaxis [124, 144] and has been shown to be equivalent to propranolol in preventing vestibular migraine, but preferred in patients with depressive symptoms [128]. Possible side effects of venlafaxine include insomnia, fatigue, somnolence, sexual dysfunction, nervousness, mydriasis, and seizures [144]. SSRIs, such as sertraline, paroxetine, and fluoxetine, have poor evidence supporting their use in migraine prevention [144], and their use in vestibular migraine prophylaxis is primarily based on expert opinion. Though SSRIs are unlikely to provide satisfactory monotherapy, they may provide additional benefit as adjunctive therapy in patients with a psychiatric comorbidity. In a study of 81 patients with migraine-associated dizziness, Reploeg et al. [109] noted that 6 patients required SSRIs in addition to other therapy for control of their symptoms. Similarly, Bisdorff [145] recommended SSRIs for migraine-anxiety-related dizziness in patients where anxiety symptoms predominate.

Acetazolamide works by inhibiting carbonic anhydrase, an enzyme distributed throughout tissue in the body and glial cells of the brain [146]. The resulting effect on carbon dioxide concentration and membrane transport has led to its use in promoting diuresis, reducing intraocular pressure, and limiting seizures. Early studies using acetazolamide to treat familial vestibulocerebellar syndromes demonstrated significant success [147, 148]. However, its use in migraine disorders is more controversial. A case series reported a response to acetazolamide in an isolated familial syndrome of migraine and essential tremor. However, a study by Shirai et al. noted that it may, in fact, trigger migraines [50, 149], and a Cochrane review found insufficient evidence to recommend its use in migraine, noting a high rate of discontinuation due to side effects [143], such as renal calculi, rash, or paresthesias. A subsequent retrospective survey of patients with vestibular migraine found significant improvement in both the severity and frequency of headaches and vertigo after treatment with at least 3 months of acetazolamide [146].

Several antiepileptic medications studied primarily in relation to migraine have also been tested against vestibular migraine, in particular topiramate, lamotrigine, valproate, and gabapentin. Topiramate inhibits carbonic anhydrase as well as voltage-sensitive sodium channels and has proven efficacy in migraine prevention [144]. Its data on vestibular migraine, though weak, is mostly promising. A study of ten patients with migraine, vertigo, and accompanying auditory symptoms reported that all patients were stabilized after 6–16 months of treatment [150], and six patients on topiramate were included in a larger study of probable or definite vestibular migraine that found patients on prophylaxis improved significantly [151]. Gode et al. reported that all 30 migrainous vertigo patients treated with 50 or 100 mg of topiramate had significantly decreased symptoms and recommended the lower dose to avoid additional adverse effects without any loss of efficacy [152]. Most recently, a retrospective study including 47 patients on topiramate concluded that it resulted in a statistically significant reduction in vestibular symptoms and headache [127]. Many side effects have been reported with topiramate, such as paresthesias, fatigue, dizziness, somnolence, memory and concentration problems, decreased appetite, and weight loss [152].

Lamotrigine also inhibits voltage-sensitive sodium channels as well as the release of glutamate to stabilize neuronal membranes; however, its usefulness in vestibular migraine is unclear. A case series of 3 patients with basilar-type migraine reported long-lasting remission after treatment with lamotrigine [153], and a study by Bisdorff noted that 19 patients with migraine-related vertigo benefited from a significant reduction in vertigo frequency, as well as a nonsignificant reduction in headache frequency after therapy with lamotrigine [154]. Two other studies have included patients on lamotrigine for vestibular migraine, but were unable to draw any significant conclusions about its efficacy due to small numbers [138, 151]. Patients on lamotrigine must always be monitored for signs of rare but serious reactions, including Stevens-Johnson syndrome, toxic epidermal necrolysis, hypersensitivity, multi-organ failure, and blood dyscrasias. Valproate increases the availability of GABA both pre- and postsynaptically and is used for migraine prophylaxis, but there is little data to support its use in vestibular migraine. A small study from 1993 reported an improvement in migraine symptoms with no relief of vestibular symptoms on valproate [155], and a recent study including three patients on valproate noted a nonsignificant clinical improvement in those patients [127]. Careful monitoring is required when prescribing valproate, as side effects include weight gain, hair loss, pancreatitis, and hepatotoxicity, and it is absolutely contraindicated in pregnancy. It is unclear if gabapentin, a GABA analog, is beneficial in migraine or vestibular migraine, but it is referenced occasionally in the literature, with one author noting anecdotally that he found it effective and well-tolerated in vestibular migraine patients [126].

Butterbur root, which acts as an anti-inflammatory, antispasmodic, and calcium channel blocker, and feverfew, an anti-inflammatory agent, are two phytoceuticals that have been effective in the prophylactic treatment of migraine in adults [142], but have only anecdotal evidence to support their use in vestibular migraine. In a randomized controlled trial, the optimal dose of feverfew extract, MIG-99, in migraine prevention was 6.25 mg TID, with good tolerability and safety but unknown long-term effects [156]. Butterbur root doses range from 50 to 150 mg daily [151]; however, it is considered a carcinogenic substance, and long-term effects are uncertain [142].

While the field awaits a conclusive randomized controlled trial of treatment, the current assortment of interventions is often able to effectively manage vestibular migraine. Whether through monotherapy, a combination of medications, or a multidisciplinary approach, patients should feel hopeful that a regimen can be optimized to successfully reduce their symptoms.

References

1. Neuhauser HK, Radtke A, von Brevern M, Feldmann M, Lezius F, Ziese T, et al. Migrainous vertigo: prevalence and impact on quality of life. Neurology. 2006;67(6):1028–33.
2. Lee JD, Kim CH, Hong SM, Kim SH, Suh MW, Kim MB, et al. Prevalence of vestibular and balance disorders in children and adolescents according to age: a multi-center study. Int J Pediatr Otorhinolaryngol. 2017;94:36–9.
3. Huppert D, Brandt T. Descriptions of vestibular migraine and Meniere's disease in Greek and Chinese antiquity. Cephalalgia. 2017;37(4):385–90.
4. Escat H. De la migraine otique. In: VII Congrés International d'Otologie. Bordeaux: Gounouillhon; 1904. p. 1176.
5. Liveing E. On megrim, sick-headache, and some allied disorders: a contribution to the pathology of nerve-storms. London: Churchill; 1873.
6. Boenheim F. Über familiäre Hemicrania vestibularis. Neurol Centralbl. 1917;36:226–9.
7. Slater R. Benign recurrent vertigo. J Neurol Neurosurg Psychiatry. 1979;42(4):363–7.
8. Kayan A, Hood JD. Neuro-otological manifestations of migraine. Brain. 1984;107(Pt 4):1123–42.
9. Dieterich M, Brandt T. Episodic vertigo related to migraine (90 cases): vestibular migraine? J Neurol. 1999;246(10):883–92.
10. Lempert T, Olesen J, Furman J, Waterston J, Seemungal B, Carey J, et al. Vestibular migraine: diagnostic criteria. J Vestib Res. 2012;22(4):167–72.
11. Neuhauser H, Leopold M, von Brevern M, Arnold G, Lempert T. The interrelations of migraine, vertigo, and migrainous vertigo. Neurology. 2001;56(4):436–41.
12. Vukovic V, Plavec D, Galinovic I, Lovrencic-Huzjan A, Budisic M, Demarin V. Prevalence of vertigo, dizziness, and migrainous vertigo in patients with migraine. Headache. 2007;47(10):1427–35.
13. Yollu U, Uluduz DU, Yilmaz M, Yener HM, Akil F, Kuzu B, et al. Vestibular migraine screening in a migraine-diagnosed patient population, and assessment of vestibulocochlear function. Clin Otolaryngol. 2017;42(2):225–33.
14. Batu ED, Anlar B, Topcu M, Turanli G, Aysun S. Vertigo in childhood: a retrospective series of 100 children. Eur J Paediatr Neurol. 2015;19(2):226–32.
15. Jahn K, Langhagen T, Heinen F. Vertigo and dizziness in children. Curr Opin Neurol. 2015;28(1):78–82.
16. Geser R, Straumann D. Referral and final diagnoses of patients assessed in an academic vertigo center. Front Neurol. 2012;3:169.
17. Zamergrad MV, Parfenov VA, Yakhno NN, Melnikov OA, Antonenko LM, Nefedovskaya LV, et al. Common causes of vertigo and dizziness in different age groups of patients. BioNanoScience. 2017;7(2):259–62.
18. Colombo B, Teggi R. Vestibular migraine: who is the patient? Neurol Sci. 2017;38:107–10.
19. Van Ombergen A, Van Rompaey V, Van de Heyning P, Wuyts F. Vestibular migraine in an otolaryngology clinic: prevalence, associated symptoms, and prophylactic medication effectiveness. Otol Neurotol. 2015;36(1):133–8.
20. Park JH, Viirre E. Vestibular migraine may be an important cause of dizziness/vertigo in perimenopausal period. Med Hypotheses. 2010;75(5):409–14.

21. Abu-Arafeh I, Russell G. Paroxysmal vertigo as a migraine equivalent in children: a population-based study. Cephalalgia. 1995;15(1):22–5; discussion 4.
22. Johnson GD. Medical management of migraine-related dizziness and vertigo. Laryngoscope. 1998;108(1 Pt 2):1–28.
23. Zhang Y, Kong Q, Chen J, Li L, Wang D, Zhou J. International Classification of Headache Disorders 3rd edition beta-based field testing of vestibular migraine in China: demographic, clinical characteristics, audiometric findings and diagnosis statues. Cephalalgia. 2016;36(3):240–8.
24. Lipton RB, Bigal ME, Diamond M, Freitag F, Reed ML, Stewart WF, et al. Migraine prevalence, disease burden, and the need for preventive therapy. Neurology. 2007;68(5):343–9.
25. Nakashima K, Yokoyama Y, Shimoyama R, Saito H, Kuno N, Sano K, et al. Prevalence of neurological disorders in a Japanese town. Neuroepidemiology. 1996;15(4):208–13.
26. Sloane PD. Dizziness in primary care. Results from the National Ambulatory Medical Care Survey. J Fam Pract. 1989;29(1):33–8.
27. Neuhauser HK, von Brevern M, Radtke A, Lezius F, Feldmann M, Ziese T, et al. Epidemiology of vestibular vertigo: a neurotologic survey of the general population. Neurology. 2005;65(6):898–904.
28. Murdin L, Schilder AGM. Epidemiology of balance symptoms and disorders in the community: a systematic review. Otol Neurotol. 2015;36(3):387–92.
29. Kroenke K, Lucas CA, Rosenberg ML, Scherokman BJ. Psychiatric disorders and functional impairment in patients with persistent dizziness. J Gen Intern Med. 1993;8(10):530–5.
30. Aragones JM, Fortes-Rego J, Fuste J, Cardozo A. Migraine: an alternative in the diagnosis of unclassified vertigo. Headache. 1993;33(3):125–8.
31. Savundra PA, Carroll JD, Davies RA, Luxon LM. Migraine-associated vertigo. Cephalalgia. 1997;17(4):505–10; discussion 487.
32. Furman JM, Marcus DA, Balaban CD. Vestibular migraine: clinical aspects and pathophysiology. Lancet Neurol. 2013;12(7):706–15.
33. Eggers SDZ, Neff BA, Shepard NT, Staab JP. Comorbidities in vestibular migraine. J Vestib Res. 2014;24(5–6):387–95.
34. Muelleman T, Shew M, Subbarayan R, Shum A, Sykes K, Staecker H, et al. Epidemiology of dizzy patient population in a neurotology clinic and predictors of peripheral etiology. Otol Neurotol. 2017;38(6):870–5.
35. Tungvachirakul V, Lisnichuk H, O'Leary SJ. Epidemiology of vestibular vertigo in a neurootology clinic population in Thailand. J Laryngol Otol. 2014;128(Suppl 2):S31–8.
36. Eggers SD, Staab JP, Neff BA, Goulson AM, Carlson ML, Shepard NT. Investigation of the coherence of definite and probable vestibular migraine as distinct clinical entities. Otol Neurotol. 2011;32(7):1144–51.
37. Gurkov R, Kantner C, Strupp M, Flatz W, Krause E, Ertl-Wagner B. Endolymphatic hydrops in patients with vestibular migraine and auditory symptoms. Eur Arch Otorrinolaringol. 2014;271(10):2661–7.
38. Neff BA, Staab JP, Eggers SD, Carlson ML, Schmitt WR, Van Abel KM, et al. Auditory and vestibular symptoms and chronic subjective dizziness in patients with Meniere's disease, vestibular migraine, and Meniere's disease with concomitant vestibular migraine. Otol Neurotol. 2012;33(7):1235–44.
39. Dieterich M, Staab JP. Functional dizziness: from phobic postural vertigo and chronic subjective dizziness to persistent postural-perceptual dizziness. Curr Opin Neurol. 2017;30(1):107–13.
40. von Brevern M, Zeise D, Neuhauser H, Clarke AH, Lempert T. Acute migrainous vertigo: clinical and oculographic findings. Brain. 2005;128(Pt 2):365–74.
41. Polensek SH, Tusa RJ. Nystagmus during attacks of vestibular migraine: an aid in diagnosis. Audiol Neurootol. 2010;15(4):241–6.
42. Espinosa-Sanchez JM, Lopez-Escamez JA. New insights into pathophysiology of vestibular migraine. Front Neurol. 2015;6:6.

43. Goadsby P, Charbit A, Andreou A, Akerman S, Holland P. Neurobiology of migraine. Neuroscience. 2009;161(2):327–41.
44. Pietrobon D, Moskowitz MA. Pathophysiology of migraine. Annu Rev Physiol. 2013;75:365–91.
45. Karatas H, Erdener SE, Gursoy-Ozdemir Y, Lule S, Eren-Koçak E, Sen ZD, et al. Spreading depression triggers headache by activating neuronal Panx1 channels. Science. 2013;339(6123):1092–5.
46. Baloh RW. Neurotology of migraine. Headache. 1997;37(10):615–21.
47. Kruit MC, Van Buchem MA, Launer LJ, Terwindt GM, Ferrari MD. Migraine is associated with an increased risk of deep white matter lesions, subclinical posterior circulation infarcts and brain iron accumulation: the population-based MRI CAMERA study. Cephalalgia. 2010;30(2):129–36.
48. Guidetti D, Rota E, Morelli N, Immovilli P. Migraine and stroke: "vascular" comorbidity. Front Neurol. 2014;5:193.
49. Baloh RW, Jacobson K, Fife T. Familial vestibulopathy: a new dominantly inherited syndrome. Neurology. 1994;44(1):20–5.
50. Baloh RW, Foster CA, Yue Q, Nelson SF. Familial migraine with vertigo and essential tremor. Neurology. 1996;46(2):458–60.
51. Oh AK, Lee H, Jen JC, Corona S, Jacobson KM, Baloh RW. Familial benign recurrent vertigo. Am J Med Genet. 2001;100(4):287–91.
52. Lee H, Jen JC, Wang H, Chen Z, Mamsa H, Sabatti C, et al. A genome-wide linkage scan of familial benign recurrent vertigo: linkage to 22q12 with evidence of heterogeneity. Hum Mol Genet. 2006;15(2):251–8.
53. Jen JC, Wang H, Lee H, Sabatti C, Trent R, Hannigan I, et al. Suggestive linkage to chromosome 6q in families with bilateral vestibulopathy. Neurology. 2004;63(12):2376–9.
54. Lee H, Jen JC, Cha YH, Nelson SF, Baloh RW. Phenotypic and genetic analysis of a large family with migraine-associated vertigo. Headache. 2008;48(10):1460–7.
55. Bahmad F Jr, DePalma SR, Merchant SN, Bezerra RL, Oliveira CA, Seidman CE, et al. Locus for familial migrainous vertigo disease maps to chromosome 5q35. Ann Otol Rhinol Laryngol. 2009;118(9):670–6.
56. De Fusco M, Marconi R, Silvestri L, Atorino L, Rampoldi L, Morgante L, et al. Haploinsufficiency of ATP1A2 encoding the Na+/K+ pump alpha2 subunit associated with familial hemiplegic migraine type 2. Nat Genet. 2003;33(2):192–6.
57. Requena T, Espinosa-Sanchez JM, Lopez-Escamez JA. Genetics of dizziness: cerebellar and vestibular disorders. Curr Opin Neurol. 2014;27(1):98–104.
58. Pietrobon D. Calcium channels and migraine. Biochim Biophys Acta. 2013;1828(7):1655–65.
59. Dichgans M, Freilinger T, Eckstein G, Babini E, Lorenz-Depiereux B, Biskup S, et al. Mutation in the neuronal voltage-gated sodium channel SCN1A in familial hemiplegic migraine. Lancet. 2005;366(9483):371–7.
60. Ophoff RA, Terwindt GM, Vergouwe MN, van Eijk R, Oefner PJ, Hoffman SM, et al. Familial hemiplegic migraine and episodic ataxia type-2 are caused by mutations in the Ca2+ channel gene CACNL1A4. Cell. 1996;87(3):543–52.
61. Gormley P, Anttila V, Winsvold BS, Palta P, Esko T, Pers TH, et al. Corrigendum: meta-analysis of 375,000 individuals identifies 38 susceptibility loci for migraine. Nat Genet. 2016;48(10):1296.
62. Gormley P, Anttila V, Winsvold BS, Palta P, Esko T, Pers TH, et al. Meta-analysis of 375,000 individuals identifies 38 susceptibility loci for migraine. Nat Genet. 2016;48(8):856–66.
63. Lopez C, Blanke O. The thalamocortical vestibular system in animals and humans. Brain Res Rev. 2011;67(1):119–46.
64. Russo A, Marcelli V, Esposito F, Corvino V, Marcuccio L, Giannone A, et al. Abnormal thalamic function in patients with vestibular migraine. Neurology. 2014;82(23):2120–6.
65. Shin JH, Kim YK, Kim HJ, Kim JS. Altered brain metabolism in vestibular migraine: comparison of interictal and ictal findings. Cephalalgia. 2014;34(1):58–67.

66. Baier B, Eulenburg PZ, Best C, Geber C, Müller-Forell W, Birklein F, et al. Posterior insular cortex–a site of vestibular–somatosensory interaction? Brain Behav. 2013;3(5):519–24.
67. Garcia-Larrea L. The posterior insular-opercular region and the search of a primary cortex for pain. Neurophysiol Clin. 2012;42(5):299–313.
68. Zu Eulenburg P, Baumgärtner U, Treede R-D, Dieterich M. Interoceptive and multimodal functions of the operculo-insular cortex: tactile, nociceptive and vestibular representations. NeuroImage. 2013;83:75–86.
69. Brandt T, Bartenstein P, Janek A, Dieterich M. Reciprocal inhibitory visual-vestibular interaction. Visual motion stimulation deactivates the parieto-insular vestibular cortex. Brain J Neurol. 1998;121(9):1749–58.
70. Russo A, Marcuccio L, Conte F, Caiazzo G, Giordano A, Conforti R, et al. No evidence of microstructural changes in patients with vestibular migraine: a diffusion tensor tract based spatial statistic (TBSS) study. J Headache Pain. 2015;16:2.
71. Obermann M, Wurthmann S, Steinberg BS, Theysohn N, Diener HC, Naegel S. Central vestibular system modulation in vestibular migraine. Cephalalgia. 2014;34(13):1053–61.
72. Messina R, Rocca MA, Colombo B, Teggi R, Falini A, Comi G, et al. Structural brain abnormalities in patients with vestibular migraine. J Neurol. 2017;264(2):295–303.
73. Lempert T, Olesen J, Furman J, Waterston J, Seemungal B, Carey J, Bisdorff A, Versino M, Evers S, Kheradmand A, Newman-Toker D. Vestibular migraine: Diagnostic criteria1. J Vestib Res. 2022;32(1):1–6. https://doi.org/10.3233/VES-201644. PMID: 34719447; PMCID: PMC9249276.
74. Moretti G, Manzoni GC, Caffarra P, Parma M. "Benign recurrent vertigo" and its connection with migraine. Headache. 1980;20(6):344–6.
75. Stolte B, Holle D, Naegel S, Diener HC, Obermann M. Vestibular migraine. Cephalalgia. 2015;35(3):262–70.
76. von Brevern M, Lempert T. Vestibular migraine. Hand. 2016;137:301–16.
77. Kuritzky A, Ziegler DK, Hassanein R. Vertigo, motion sickness and migraine. Headache. 1981;21(5):227–31.
78. Cass SP, Furman JM, Ankerstjerne K, Balaban C, Yetiser S, Aydogan B. Migraine-related vestibulopathy. Ann Otol Rhinol Laryngol. 1997;106(3):182–9.
79. Waterston J. Chronic migrainous vertigo. J Clin Neurosci. 2004;11(4):384–8.
80. Radtke A, von Brevern M, Neuhauser H, Hottenrott T, Lempert T. Vestibular migraine: long-term follow-up of clinical symptoms and vestibulo-cochlear findings. Neurology. 2012;79(15):1607–14.
81. Cutrer FM, Baloh RW. Migraine-associated dizziness. Headache. 1992;32(6):300–4.
82. Headache Classification Subcommittee of the International Headache Society. The International Classification of Headache Disorders: 2nd edition. Cephalalgia. 2004;24(Suppl 1):9–160.
83. Behan PO, Carlin J. Benign recurrent vertigo. In: Advances in migraine research and therapy. New York: Raven; 1982. p. 49–55.
84. Neuhauser H, Lempert T. Vertigo and dizziness related to migraine: a diagnostic challenge. Cephalalgia. 2004;24(2):83–91.
85. Parker W. Migraine and the vestibular system in adults. Am J Otol. 1991;12(1):25–34.
86. Olsson JE. Neurotologic findings in basilar migraine. Laryngoscope. 1991;101(1):1–41.
87. Best C, Eckhardt-Henn A, Tschan R, Dieterich M. Psychiatric morbidity and comorbidity in different vestibular vertigo syndromes. Results of a prospective longitudinal study over one year. J Neurol. 2009;256(1):58–65.
88. Best C, Tschan R, Eckhardt-Henn A, Dieterich M. Who is at risk for ongoing dizziness and psychological strain after a vestibular disorder? Neuroscience. 2009;164(4):1579–87.
89. Staab JP. Behavioural neuro-otology. In: Oxford textbook of vertigo and imbalance. Oxford: Oxford University Press; 2013. p. 333.

90. Kroenke K, Lucas CA, Rosenberg ML, Scherokman B, Herbers JE Jr, Wehrle PA, et al. Causes of persistent dizziness. A prospective study of 100 patients in ambulatory care. Ann Intern Med. 1992;117(11):898–904.
91. Post RE, Dickerson LM. Dizziness: a diagnostic approach. Am Fam Physician. 2010;82(4):361–8, 9.
92. Burch RC, Loder S, Loder E, Smitherman TA. The prevalence and burden of migraine and severe headache in the United States: updated statistics from government health surveillance studies. Headache. 2015;55(1):21–34.
93. Ricci F, De Caterina R, Fedorowski A. Orthostatic hypotension: epidemiology, prognosis, and treatment. J Am Coll Cardiol. 2015;66(7):848–60.
94. Fick DM, Cooper JW, Wade WE, Waller JL, Maclean JR, Beers MH. Updating the Beers criteria for potentially inappropriate medication use in older adults: results of a US consensus panel of experts. Arch Intern Med. 2003;163(22):2716–24.
95. Harris JP, Alexander TH. Current-day prevalence of Meniere's syndrome. Audiol Neurootol. 2010;15(5):318–22.
96. von Brevern M, Radtke A, Lezius F, Feldmann M, Ziese T, Lempert T, et al. Epidemiology of benign paroxysmal positional vertigo: a population based study. J Neurol Neurosurg Psychiatry. 2007;78(7):710–5.
97. Gannon RP, Willson GN, Roberts ME, Pearse HJ. Auditory and vestibular damage in head injuries at work. Arch Otolaryngol. 1978;104(7):404–8.
98. Kolev OI, Sergeeva M. Vestibular disorders following different types of head and neck trauma. Funct Neurol. 2016;31(2):75–80.
99. Lucas S. Posttraumatic headache: clinical characterization and management. Curr Pain Headache Rep. 2015;19(10):48.
100. Lucas S. Characterization and management of headache after mild traumatic brain injury. In: Kobeissy FH, editor. Brain neurotrauma: molecular, neuropsychological, and rehabilitation aspects, Frontiers in neuroengineering. Boca Raton: CRC Press; 2015.
101. Kim SK, Lee KJ, Hahm JR, Lee SM, Jung TS, Jung JH, et al. Clinical significance of the presence of autonomic and vestibular dysfunction in diabetic patients with peripheral neuropathy. Diabetes Metab J. 2012;36(1):64–9.
102. Alpini D, Caputo D, Pugnetti L, Giuliano DA, Cesarani A. Vertigo and multiple sclerosis: aspects of differential diagnosis. Neurol Sci. 2001;22(Suppl 2):S84–7.
103. Strupp M, Brandt T. Vestibular neuritis. Semin Neurol. 2009;29(5):509–19.
104. Kattah JC, Talkad AV, Wang DZ, Hsieh YH, Newman-Toker DE. HINTS to diagnose stroke in the acute vestibular syndrome: three-step bedside oculomotor examination more sensitive than early MRI diffusion-weighted imaging. Stroke. 2009;40(11):3504–10.
105. Foley RW, Shirazi S, Maweni RM, Walsh K, McConn Walsh R, Javadpour M, et al. Signs and symptoms of acoustic neuroma at initial presentation: an exploratory analysis. Cureus. 2017;9(11):e1846.
106. Tarnutzer AA, Lee SH, Robinson KA, Kaplan PW, Newman-Toker DE. Clinical and electrographic findings in epileptic vertigo and dizziness: a systematic review. Neurology. 2015;84(15):1595–604.
107. Maldonado FM, Birdi JS, Irving GJ, Murdin L, Kivekäs I, Strupp M. Pharmacological agents for the prevention of vestibular migraine. Cochrane Database Syst Rev. 2015;(6):CD010600. Available from: http://onlinelibrary.wiley.com/doi/10.1002/14651858.CD010600.pub2/abstract, http://onlinelibrary.wiley.com/store/10.1002/14651858.CD010600.pub2/asset/CD010600.pdf?v=1&t=j8umolu7&s=1d8aa1ff72cb0e4cb10902e7c6727f8850d99717.
108. Neuhauser H, Lempert T. Vestibular migraine. Neurol Clin. 2009;27(2):379–91.
109. Reploeg MD, Goebel JA. Migraine-associated dizziness: patient characteristics and management options. Otol Neurotol. 2002;23(3):364–71.
110. Mikulec AA, Faraji F, Kinsella LJ. Evaluation of the efficacy of caffeine cessation, nortriptyline, and topiramate therapy in vestibular migraine and complex dizziness of unknown etiology. Am J Otolaryngol. 2012;33(1):121–7.

111. Whitney SL, Wrisley DM, Brown KE, Furman JM. Physical therapy for migraine-related vestibulopathy and vestibular dysfunction with history of migraine. Laryngoscope. 2000;110(9):1528–34.
112. Wrisley DM, Whitney SL, Furman JM. Vestibular rehabilitation outcomes in patients with a history of migraine. Otol Neurotol. 2002;23(4):483–7.
113. Vitkovic J, Winoto A, Rance G, Dowell R, Paine M. Vestibular rehabilitation outcomes in patients with and without vestibular migraine. J Neurol. 2013;260(12):3039–48.
114. Whitney SL, Sparto PJ. Principles of vestibular physical therapy rehabilitation. NeuroRehabilitation. 2011;29(2):157–66.
115. Staab JP. Chronic dizziness: the interface between psychiatry and neuro-otology. Curr Opin Neurol. 2006;19(1):41–8.
116. Neuhauser H, Radtke A, von Brevern M, Lempert T. Zolmitriptan for treatment of migrainous vertigo: a pilot randomized placebo-controlled trial. Neurology. 2003;60(5):882–3.
117. Bikhazi P, Jackson C, Ruckenstein MJ. Efficacy of antimigrainous therapy in the treatment of migraine-associated dizziness. Am J Otol. 1997;18(3):350–4.
118. Cassano D, Pizza V, Busillo V. Almotriptan in the acute treatment of vestibular migraine: a retrospective study. J Headache Pain. 2015;16:2.
119. Prakash S, Chavda BV, Mandalia H, Dhawan R, Padmanabhan D. Headaches related to triptans therapy in patients of migrainous vertigo. J Headache Pain. 2008;9(3):185–8.
120. Marcus DA, Furman JM. Prevention of motion sickness with rizatriptan: a double-blind, placebo-controlled pilot study. Med Sci Monit. 2006;12(1):PI1–7.
121. Prakash S, Shah ND. Migrainous vertigo responsive to intravenous methylprednisolone: case reports. Headache. 2009;49(8):1235–9.
122. Strupp M, Dieterich M, Brandt T. The treatment and natural course of peripheral and central vertigo. Dtsch Arztebl Int. 2013;110(29–30):505–15; quiz 15–6.
123. Seemungal B, Kaski D, Lopez-Escamez JA. Early diagnosis and management of acute vertigo from vestibular migraine and Meniere's disease. Neurol Clin. 2015;33(3):619–28, ix.
124. Jackson JL, Cogbill E, Santana-Davila R, Eldredge C, Collier W, Gradall A, et al. A comparative effectiveness meta-analysis of drugs for the prophylaxis of migraine headache. PLoS One. 2015;10(7):e0130733.
125. Sanchez-Del-Rio M, Reuter U, Moskowitz MA. New insights into migraine pathophysiology. Curr Opin Neurol. 2006;19(3):294–8.
126. Eggers SD. Migraine-related vertigo: diagnosis and treatment. Curr Pain Headache Rep. 2007;11(3):217–26.
127. Salmito MC, Duarte JA, Morganti LOG, Brandao PVC, Nakao BH, Villa TR, et al. Prophylactic treatment of vestibular migraine. Braz J Otorhinolaryngol. 2017;83(4):404–10.
128. Salviz M, Yuce T, Acar H, Karatas A, Acikalin RM. Propranolol and venlafaxine for vestibular migraine prophylaxis: a randomized controlled trial. Laryngoscope. 2016;126(1):169–74.
129. Maione A. Migraine-related vertigo: diagnostic criteria and prophylactic treatment. Laryngoscope. 2006;116(10):1782–6.
130. Silberstein SD. Preventive treatment of migraine: an overview. Cephalalgia. 1997;17(2):67–72.
131. Lepcha A, Amalanathan S, Augustine AM, Tyagi AK, Balraj A. Flunarizine in the prophylaxis of migrainous vertigo: a randomized controlled trial. Eur Arch Otorrinolaringol. 2014;271(11):2931–6.
132. Visvanathan N, Kannaian S, Nimmakayala R. Flunarizine for the prophylaxis of vestibular migraine. Neurology. 2017;88(16 Supplement 1):P2.172.
133. Peer Mohamed B, Goadsby PJ, Prabhakar P. Safety and efficacy of flunarizine in childhood migraine: 11 years' experience, with emphasis on its effect in hemiplegic migraine. Dev Med Child Neurol. 2012;54(3):274–7.
134. Sanvito WL, Oliveira BC. Prophylactic treatment of migraine: a prospective open study on 100 patients. Arq Neuropsiquiatr. 1993;51(1):31–5.
135. Gordon CR, Shupak A. Prevention and treatment of motion sickness in children. CNS Drugs. 1999;12(5):369–81.

136. Taghdiri F, Togha M, Jahromi SR, Refaeian F. Cinnarizine for the prophylaxis of migraine associated vertigo: a retrospective study. Springerplus. 2014;3:5.
137. Teggi R, Colombo B, Gatti O, Comi G, Bussi M. Fixed combination of cinnarizine and dimenhydrinate in the prophylactic therapy of vestibular migraine: an observational study. Neurol Sci. 2015;36(10):1869–73.
138. Brodsky JR, Cusick BA, Zhou G. Evaluation and management of vestibular migraine in children: experience from a pediatric vestibular clinic. Eur J Paediatr Neurol. 2016;20(1):85–92.
139. Staab JP, Eggers SD, Neff BA, Shepard NT. Vestibular migraine and persistent postural-perceptual dizziness: results of a double blind, parallel group, pharmacologic dissection trial using verapamil and sertraline. Cephalalgia. 2015;35:65.
140. Frommer DA, Kulig KW, Marx JA, Rumack B. Tricyclic antidepressant overdose. A review. JAMA. 1987;257(4):521–6.
141. Walker Z, Walker RW, Robertson MM, Stansfeld S. Antidepressant treatment of chronic tension-type headache: a comparison between fluoxetine and desipramine. Headache. 1998;38(7):523–8.
142. Kacperski J, Kabbouche MA, O'Brien HL, Weberding JL. The optimal management of headaches in children and adolescents. Ther Adv Neurol Disord. 2016;9(1):53–68.
143. Linde M, Mulleners WM, Chronicle EP, McCrory DC. Antiepileptics other than gabapentin, pregabalin, topiramate, and valproate for the prophylaxis of episodic migraine in adults. Cochrane Database Syst Rev. 2013;2013:CD010608.
144. Silberstein SD. Preventive migraine treatment. Continuum. 2015;21(4 Headache):973–89.
145. Bisdorff AR. Management of vestibular migraine. Ther Adv Neurol Disord. 2011;4(3):183–91.
146. Celebisoy N, Gokcay F, Karahan C, Bilgen C, Kirazli T, Karapolat H, et al. Acetazolamide in vestibular migraine prophylaxis: a retrospective study. Eur Arch Otorhinolaryngol. 2016;273(10):2947–51. Available from: http://onlinelibrary.wiley.com/o/cochrane/clcentral/articles/193/CN-01208193/frame.html, https://link.springer.com/content/pdf/10.1007%2Fs00405-015-3874-4.pdf.
147. Baloh RW, Winder A. Acetazolamide-responsive vestibulocerebellar syndrome: clinical and oculographic features. Neurology. 1991;41(3):429–33.
148. Griggs RC, Moxley RT, Lafrance RA, McQuillen J. Hereditary paroxysmal ataxia response to acetazolamide. Neurology. 1978;28(12):1259.
149. Shirai T, Meyer J, Akiyama H, Mortel K, Wills P. Acetazolamide testing of cerebral vasodilator capacity provokes "vascular" but not tension headaches. Headache. 1996;36(10):589–94.
150. Carmona S, Settecase N. Use of topiramate (topamax) in a subgroup of migraine-vertigo patients with auditory symptoms. Ann N Y Acad Sci. 2005;1039:517–20.
151. Baier B, Winkenwerder E, Dieterich M. "Vestibular migraine": effects of prophylactic therapy with various drugs. A retrospective study. J Neurol. 2009;256(3):436–42.
152. Gode S, Celebisoy N, Kirazli T, Akyuz A, Bilgen C, Karapolat H, et al. Clinical assessment of topiramate therapy in patients with migrainous vertigo. Headache. 2010;50(1):77–84.
153. Cologno D, d'Onofrio F, Castriota O, Petretta V, Casucci G, Russo A, et al. Basilar-type migraine patients responsive to lamotrigine: a 5-year follow-up. Neurol Sci. 2013;34(Suppl 1):S165–6.
154. Bisdorff AR. Treatment of migraine related vertigo with lamotrigine an observational study. Bull Soc Sci Med Grand Duche Luxemb. 2004;2:103–8.
155. Gordon C, Kuritzky A, Doweck I, Spitzer O, Shupak A, Hering R. Vestibulo-ocular reflex in migraine patients: the effect of sodium valproate. Headache. 1993;33(3):129–32. Available from: http://onlinelibrary.wiley.com/o/cochrane/clcentral/articles/935/CN-00092935/frame.html.
156. Diener H, Pfaffenrath V, Schnitker J, Friede M, Henneicke-von ZH. Efficacy and safety of 6.25 mg t.i.d. feverfew CO2-extract (MIG-99) in migraine prevention—a randomized, double-blind, multicentre, placebo-controlled study. Cephalalgia. 2005;25(11):1031–41. Available from: http://onlinelibrary.wiley.com/o/cochrane/clcentral/articles/242/CN-00531242/frame.html.

Chapter 22
Non-Fluctuating Unilateral Vestibular Loss

Beth N. McNulty and Matthew L. Bush

Introduction

Vestibular dysfunction is a common problem, with over 35% of adults over 40 reporting some degree of balance dysfunction [1], and can lead to a significant negative impact on daily activities and quality of life [2]. Millions of doctor visits per year are attributed to the complaint of dizziness [3]. Insults to the peripheral vestibular system (either the sensory organs and/or the vestibular nerves) result in a change of the peripheral vestibular neural input to the brain. In the acute setting, isolated unilateral insults to the vestibular system can be excitatory or inhibitory from a physiological standpoint but present similarly with vertigo, motion-exacerbating disequilibrium, and visual disturbance. The loss of unilateral vestibular input results in dysfunction of the vestibular ocular reflex (VOR), which compromises image stability on the retina and presents as visual disturbance that is exacerbated by movement. Regardless of the severity and of the vestibular loss, this physiological change in sensory input results in the activation of central vestibular compensatory mechanisms to rectify the relative inequity in neural input. The process of central compensation leads to a decrease in clinical symptoms; however, the efficiency and effectiveness of compensation may vary widely and may be affected by many factors such as age, medications, and the nature of the vestibular insult.

Conditions that ablate the vestibular system may present either as an isolated insult or as a progressive process ending in destruction of remaining ipsilateral vestibular function. These conditions can be grouped into a category of physiological disorders referred to as a non-fluctuating unilateral vestibular loss. Patients may be symptomatic during the acute phase of the disease process, but central

B. N. McNulty (✉) · M. L. Bush
Division of Otology, Neurotology, & Cranial Base Surgery, Department of Otolaryngology-Head and Neck Surgery, University of Kentucky, Lexington, KY, USA
e-mail: beth.mcnulty@uky.edu; matthew.bush@uky.edu

J. C. Lucas et al. (eds.), *Diagnosis and Treatment of Vestibular Disorders*,
https://doi.org/10.1007/978-3-032-11740-3_22

compensation helps to mitigate these symptoms. As long as there is no recurrence of vestibular insult or physiological change within the ipsilateral sensory input, central compensation progresses and vertigo dissipates. During compensation, the hallmark symptom for these patients is motion-induced disequilibrium, which is typically elicited from sudden, rapid head movements. When central compensation is complete, patients with non-fluctuating unilateral vestibular loss often become asymptomatic at rest with varying degrees of motion-induced disequilibrium. Since the damage to the vestibular organ is stable in non-fluctuating unilateral vestibular loss, the status and degree of central compensation becomes the most critical factor in the prognosis and management of these patients. Impaired or delayed compensation will result in a chronic vestibulopathy with concomitant symptoms. Crucial aspects of the management of patients with these disorders include assessing the etiology of the vestibular loss, identifying impediments to compensatory mechanisms, and maximizing the central compensation process. This chapter assesses a variety of conditions, ranging from infectious to iatrogenic, that cause a non-fluctuating unilateral vestibular loss, with attention given to the underlying pathophysiology, clinical assessment, and treatment options for common conditions within this category.

Vestibular Neuritis

Vestibular neuritis is the second most common peripheral vestibular disorder, after benign paroxysmal positional vertigo (BPPV) [4]. A Japanese study from the 1990s estimated the frequency of occurrence to be 3.5 per 100,000 population [5]. A group in Germany recently published on the inpatient treatment of patients admitted for dizziness, noting acute vestibular neuritis to be the most common admission diagnosis, seen in 30.1% of their patients [6]. Acute vestibular neuritis and neuronitis are terms used interchangeably and must be differentiated from vestibular labyrinthitis, which involves associated hearing loss. The most common age at presentation is between 30 and 50. In contrast to other vestibular disorders, it is seen more commonly in males until the age of 40 [5]. The term epidemic vertigo was also used in the past, as the vertigo is often preceded by a viral illness or upper respiratory infection. As with all vestibular disorders, the history of the clinical presentation and symptoms is the most critical component in the diagnosis of vestibular neuritis. These patients present with the acute onset of intense vertigo and nausea without concurrent hearing loss. The severity may vary widely, but the intensity of the vertigo and rapid onset of the symptoms frequently lead patients to an emergency department evaluation, and they may require hospitalization for management of intractable vomiting and dehydration. Patients may experience continuous vertigo for multiple days that slowly regresses, leaving them with disequilibrium that can last from days to months. The rate of recovery depends on central compensation, which is related to factors such as the degree of vestibular insult, age of the patient, and use of vestibular suppressants.

Pathophysiology

The exact etiology is unknown, but it is thought to be due to a virus or vascular insult leading to ischemic nerve injury. The most likely viral cause is reactivation of Herpes Simplex Type 1. A resultant inflammatory cell infiltrate leads to neural degeneration and atrophy. Autopsy studies have confirmed inflammatory degeneration of the vestibular nerves and herpes simplex virus 1 (HSV-1) DNA, as well as latency-associated transcript (LAT) in the vestibular ganglia [7–10]. The superior vestibular nerve is preferentially affected, while the inferior vestibular nerve is often partially or totally spared. According to a recent review of the literature, 40–48% of all reported cases affected only the superior vestibular nerve [11, 12], while 34–56% affected both the SVN and IVN [11–13], and 1.3–18% of cases affected only the inferior vestibular nerve [11–14]. The vulnerability of the superior vestibular nerve has been attributed to its longer and narrower bony canal [15], and the resistance of the inferior vestibular nerve due to the fact that it travels in two separate bony canals [7]. The superior vestibular nerve supplies innervation to the superior and horizontal semicircular canals, utricle, and parts of the saccule, while the inferior vestibular nerve innervates the posterior semicircular canal ampulla and saccule. Anastomoses between the superior vestibular nerve and facial and cochlear nerves are also common [16]. Degeneration may extend along the innervation of the superior vestibular nerve; thus, utricular degeneration may lead to displacement of otoconia, resulting in BPPV.

Diagnosis

The diagnosis is most often made clinically, excluding other causes of a unilateral vestibular insult. Physical exam findings in the acute phase may include spontaneous nystagmus and abnormal posture, and gait findings. Spontaneous nystagmus may be observed in the acute phase, but is not often seen after central compensation has occurred. The direction of the fast phase is opposite to the involved side. During the compensation process, some posture tests, such as the Romberg, may normalize, but until compensation is complete, patients may continue to exhibit abnormal Sharpened Romberg and/or Fukuda step test findings. Diagnostic studies that augment the evaluation of these patients include an audiogram, computed tomography (CT) scan to rule out a cerebral vascular accident (CVA) in the emergency room setting, and magnetic resonance imaging (MRI) of the brain and internal auditory canal with gadolinium contrast in the outpatient setting to exclude retrocochlear pathology. This disease causes permanent peripheral vestibular injury, typically isolated to the superior vestibular nerve; thus, vestibular physiological evaluation with either electronystagmography (ENG) or videonystagmography (VNG) frequently reveals a unilateral caloric weakness. Ocular VEMP thresholds are absent or found to have a decreased amplitude on the affected side, while the cervical VEMP thresholds are within normal limits. In cases of inferior vestibular neuritis, the caloric testing (horizontal semicircular canal function) will be normal, and the cervical VEMP threshold will be absent or reduced, while the Ocular VEMP threshold will be preserved.

Treatment

Supportive treatment with vestibular suppressants and antiemetics may be very helpful in the acute phase. Vestibular suppressants should not be continued for more than a few days as they may impair central compensation. An active lifestyle with physical activity and vestibular rehabilitation with physical therapy may hasten central compensation and, thus, recovery. Patients with prolonged symptoms lasting for months are candidates for vestibular rehabilitation, which can promote central compensation.

Although there has been insufficient evidence to support the use of steroids in acute vestibular neuritis [17], a high-dose oral steroid taper may provide symptomatic relief. It is thought that the anti-inflammatory effect of steroids may stabilize damage to the vestibular nerve and promote neuronal recovery. Oral steroids should be used with caution in diabetic patients. Possible side effects and risks of steroid use must be explained to the patient.

Antivirals have also been used to treat this condition, assuming the etiology is reactivation of the Herpes Simplex Virus, Type 1. However, these medications have not been proven to be effective, and their use has fallen out of favor. Strupp et al. published a randomized study comparing methylprednisolone, valacyclovir, or a combination for the treatment of vestibular neuritis and reported that methylprednisolone significantly improved the recovery in peripheral vestibular function, while valacyclovir did not [18].

Labyrinthitis

Labyrinthitis is similar to vestibular neuritis in presentation but includes sensorineural hearing loss. The incidence of these conditions is often reported together; therefore, the true incidence of labyrinthitis is unknown. There is evidence that sudden sensorineural hearing loss occurs in 1 per 10,000 people, with about 0.4 per 10,000 people experiencing concurrent vertigo and sensorineural hearing loss [19]. Patients with labyrinthitis present with a sudden hearing loss, tinnitus, and vestibular dysfunction, similar to acute vestibular neuritis. Labyrinthitis may be bacterial or viral in etiology. Bacterial labyrinthitis may occur as a result of otitis media, cholesteatoma, or meningitis, and patients typically experience systemic toxicity signs and may become quite ill rapidly. It is important to assess for intracranial complications of otitis media when signs and symptoms of labyrinthitis are present.

These include brain abscess, meningitis, epidural abscess, and sigmoid sinus thrombosis. The most common organisms are *Streptococcus pneumoniae*, *Haemophilus influenzae*, and *Neisseria meningitidis*. Although uncommon in the current age, syphilis must always be considered as well. Viral insult to the labyrinth may be congenital (cytomegalovirus and rubella) or postnatal (mumps and measles).

Pathophysiology

In cases of otogenic labyrinthitis, spread may occur hematogenously or directly through the round window or oval window membranes, labyrinthine fistula, or a congenital temporal bone anomaly. Meningitic labyrinthitis is due to extension through the internal auditory canal, cochlear aqueduct, or through hematogenous spread. Osteoblastic bony changes within the labyrinth may occur in response to the inflammatory reaction, resulting in labyrinthitis ossificans and obliteration of the labyrinthine lumen (Fig. 22.1a, b).

Diagnosis

The diagnosis is made based on the history and physical exam, but also involves audiometric testing to demonstrate associated sensorineural hearing loss. Spontaneous nystagmus and/or gaze-directed nystagmus may be observed in the

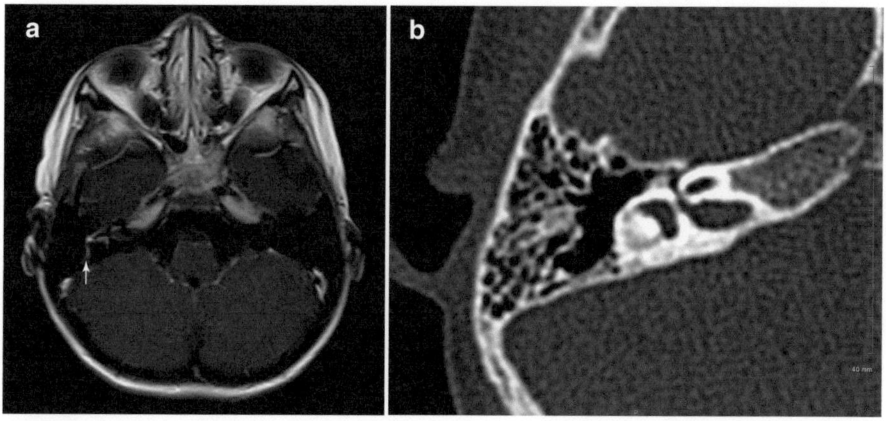

Fig. 22.1 (**a**) T1-weighted, post-gadolinium contrast axial MRI image of a two-year-old with bacterial meningitis and right-sided labyrinthitis. The white arrow points to enhancement of the right cochlea and vestibule with limited contrast seen within the right horizontal semicircular canal (SCC). (**b**) Axial CT of the temporal bone of the same child showing labyrinthitis ossificans with obliteration of the right horizontal SSC (white arrow)

direction opposite to the involved ear. Head impulse testing should also be assessed, similarly noting post-headshake nystagmus away from the affected side. Formal vestibular testing may be utilized (VNG with calorics and VEMP testing) similar to other vestibular conditions discussed in this chapter. Rotary chair testing is particularly useful to assess for residual physiological function in the event of bilateral involvement. Systemic workup involving hemogram, blood cultures, and lumbar puncture should be obtained in cases of suspected meningitis. Radiographic imaging should be obtained and may include a CT of the temporal bone to assess for bony changes of the labyrinth and an MRI of the brain with and without contrast to assess for intracranial complications.

Treatment

The underlying etiology must be addressed. Acute otitis media is typically treated with antibiotics and myringotomy with a pressure equalization tube. Coalescent otomastoiditis and cholesteatoma are typically treated surgically with tympanomastoidectomy. Meningitis is treated with culture-directed intravenous antibiotics that cross the blood-brain barrier. Supportive treatment, as described for vestibular neuritis, is also indicated as needed for nausea and vertigo.

Trauma

Mechanisms of injury to the ear and temporal bone range from blunt force head trauma, penetrating trauma, or barotrauma [20]. Temporal bone fractures have been reported to comprise 14–22% of all skull fractures, and are seen in 4% of patients with a closed head injury [21–23]. A variety of inner ear traumatic conditions can result from such temporal bone trauma, and these include complete labyrinthine deficit, labyrinthine concussion, perilymph fistula, benign paroxysmal positional vertigo, or post-traumatic endolymphatic hydrops. Direct injury to the labyrinth or labyrinthine concussion may cause a fixed vestibular deficit, while the others tend to be fluctuating.

Pathophysiology

A fracture of the temporal bone with otic capsule violation may result in immediate and profound sensorineural hearing loss with vertigo. In a landmark study, Brodie reported otic capsule violation in only 21 (2.5%) of 820 temporal bone fractures [24]. Facial nerve injury was noted in 48% of these patients, and this cohort was twice as likely to develop a cerebrospinal fluid leak. Severe to profound SNHL is usually associated with a fracture of the labyrinth, labyrinthine concussion, or perilymphatic fistula. [24].

Diagnosis

The history is most suggestive in these cases. A CT scan of the temporal bone should be obtained to assess for a temporal bone fracture (Fig. 22.2). Audiometric testing is also performed to assess for associated sensorineural hearing loss. Documentation of facial nerve function and the timing of facial nerve symptoms in relation to the trauma is an important aspect of the management of temporal bone trauma patients. The presence of a cerebrospinal fluid leak should also be assessed.

Treatment

Supportive treatment with vestibular rehabilitation is the mainstay of treatment for traumatic labyrinthine injury. Eliminating prolonged use of vestibular suppressants to allow for central compensation is of utmost importance. One may also consider addressing associated hearing loss as indicated.

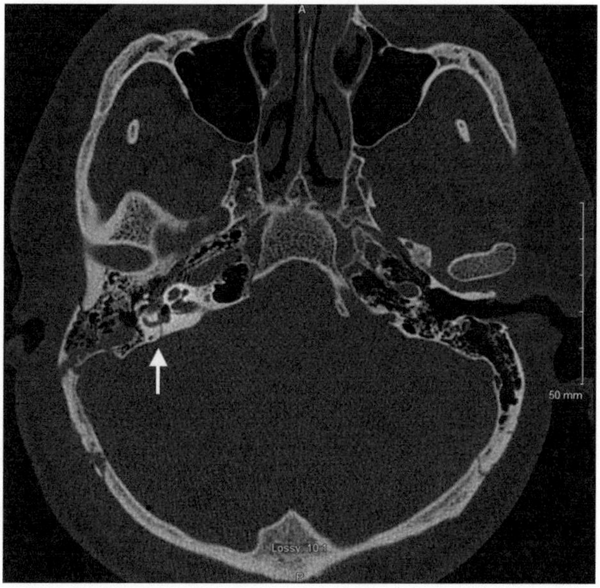

Fig. 22.2 Axial CT scan of a comminuted right-sided otic capsule violating temporal bone fracture. The white arrow points to the fracture line, which crosses the vestibule. Pneumolabyrinth is also appreciated

Advanced Meniere's Disease

Meniere's disease (MD) classically presents with fluctuating vestibular symptoms and will be described in greater detail in Chaps. 13, 14, and 15. Inactive or end-stage Meniere's disease, however, presents as a non-fluctuating unilateral vestibular disorder and is managed differently than active Meniere's disease. The following paragraphs will provide a brief description of the natural progression of the disease, resulting in a fixed vestibular deficit.

While the true incidence of MD is unknown, reports range from 4.3 to 15.3 cases per 100,000 per year [25–28]. Affected individuals are usually between the fourth and sixth decades of life, with a female/male ratio of 1.3:1. The symptoms experienced by these patients are often unilateral and characterized by fluctuating low-frequency sensorineural hearing loss (SNHL), episodic vertigo (lasting minutes to hours), tinnitus, and aural fullness [29].

Pathophysiology

Endolymphatic hydrops with periodic disruption of Reissner's membrane is thought to be the underlying etiology of symptoms related to MD and can only be confirmed on post-mortem histopathologic examination. The disturbance in the regulation of endolymphatic fluid homeostasis may be related to a variety of factors; particularly, genetic, autoimmune, allergic, viral, and post-traumatic influences have all been postulated.

Diagnosis

In the early stages of Meniere's, unilateral low-frequency sensorineural hearing loss is noted on audiometric testing. Unfortunately, as the disease progresses, all frequencies are affected, and this may even result in profound hearing loss in about 1–2% of patients. As the disease progresses, the labyrinthine dysfunction stabilizes in most patients with vertigo symptoms, resolving in 2 years in 57% of cases and 8 years in 71% of cases [30]. As the vertigo episodes resolve, a chronic disequilibrium may emerge. This is referred to as "Burned-out Meniere's," and these patients will have a stable, flat sensorineural hearing loss with a non-fluctuating unilateral vestibular hypofunction. Caloric testing may be considered in these cases to assess for degree of vestibular hypofunction and to rule out contralateral involvement. Abnormal findings on electrocochleography and VEMP testing may also support the diagnosis of Meniere's, but must not be solely relied upon [29].

Treatment

Medical management consisting of a low sodium diet, caffeine avoidance, and diuretic therapy is the first-line treatment for newly diagnosed Meniere's. Some patients may be refractory to medical management, and a progressive course is seen in one out of four patients. These patients may be more appropriate for intratympanic steroid treatments, endolymphatic sac decompression surgery, or ablative therapies as discussed in Chap. 15. Balance exercises with vestibular rehabilitation should be considered for the advanced Meniere's patient with chronic imbalance.

Vestibular Schwannoma

A vestibular schwannoma (VS) is a benign tumor of Schwann cell origin involving the eighth cranial nerve. It is the most common tumor of the cerebellopontine angle, making up 80–90% of these tumors. It is also referred to as an acoustic neuroma, although it more commonly originates from the vestibular division of the vestibulocochlear nerve, involving the superior and inferior vestibular nerves in equal incidence. A recent Danish database study estimates the overall incidence of VS to be 20 per one million population [31].

Pathophysiology

These tumors likely arise from Schwann cells within Scarpa's ganglion. A growth rate of 1–2 mm per year for these tumors has been described, and these tumors typically displace the adjacent nerves without direct invasion. There are two histopathological growth patterns, Antoni A (more densely packed with a whorled appearance) and Antoni B (more loosely organized and often seen in larger tumors). These tumors are often classified based on anatomic location and growth progression, and these categories include: intracanalicular (isolated within the internal auditory canal (IAC)), cisternal (extension into the cerebellopontine cistern), and brainstem compressive. The tumors with an intracanalicular component have compression of the acoustic, vestibular, and facial nerves with potential neuropathy. In addition to the intracanalicular symptoms, cisternal tumors may compress trigeminal nerve and/or the lower cranial nerves. Tumors that compress the brainstem can cause hydrocephalus, cerebellar tonsillar herniation, and death.

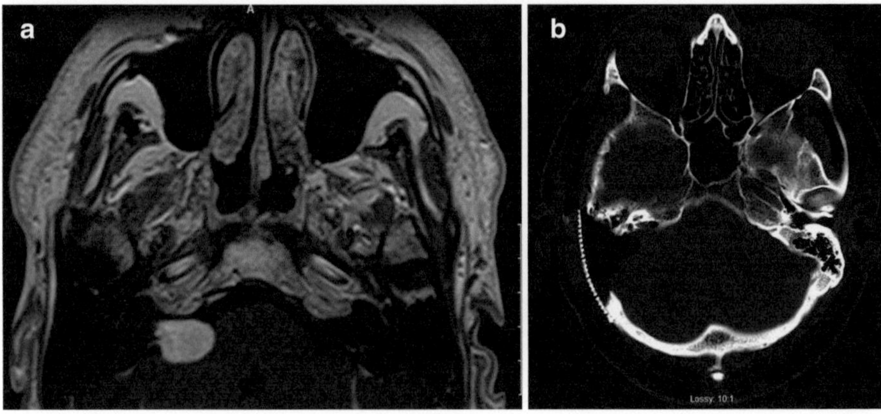

Fig. 22.3 (**a**) T1-weighted, post-gadolinium contrast axial MRI image of a right-sided, medium-sized, cisternal vestibular schwannoma. (**b**) Axial CT scan after a translabyrinthine approach for resection of the same right-sided vestibular schwannoma, with fat obliterating the posterior fossa defect and titanium mesh reconstructing the bony defect

Diagnosis

A typical presentation includes unilateral hearing loss (39–95%), tinnitus (45–75%), and dizziness (49–66%) [32, 33]. While vertigo is not typically the chief complaint, the presence of mild vertigo or disequilibrium symptoms is not uncommon, with 10 to 19% of VS patients presenting with vertigo as a primary symptom. Vertigo is more common in smaller tumors, and disequilibrium or imbalance is more common with increasing tumor size. While the majority of these tumors are non-growing or slow growing, growing tumors can cause vestibular symptoms from compression and dysfunction of the eighth cranial nerve, cerebellum, and/or pons [34]. Trigeminal nerve compression may lead to facial hypesthesia. Large tumors with brainstem compression can present with ataxia and other cerebellar symptoms. The diagnosis of these tumors is primarily through MRI of the head with and without contrast, as these tumors are avidly enhancing on T1 sequences (Fig. 22.3a). Audiological and vestibular physiological tests are also valuable in assessing the functional status of the ipsilateral vestibulocochlear nerve and may inform treatment decisions.

Treatment

Observation may be considered for small or non-growing tumors. Larger tumors or growing tumors are treated with either microsurgical resection or stereotactic radiation. There are three surgical approaches for tumor resection, and the approach chosen is most often based on the patient's pre-operative hearing status and the tumor size and location. Surgeon preference also plays a role in the surgical management of these tumors. In cases with non-serviceable hearing or tumor size greater than 1.5 cm, the translabyrinthine approach may provide the best exposure and facial nerve outcome (Fig. 22.3b). For small tumors limited to the internal auditory canal with aidable hearing and word recognition (ideally greater than 70% but no less than 50%), a middle cranial fossa approach can be utilized to resect the tumor while preserving hearing. A retrosigmoid approach may be used to remove cisternal tumors and has the potential to preserve hearing in tumors that do not involve the root entry zone of the eighth cranial nerve and do not extend beyond the lateral third of the internal auditory canal. Stereotactic radiotherapy is a nonsurgical treatment option for these tumors, and the primary objective is to halt tumor growth. The delivery of this radiation, which may be either unfractionated or fractionated, may damage actively growing tumor cells, destroy supporting cells, and impair the vascular support to VS. Often tumors lie dormant following radiation therapy, but regression of the tumor may occur. Hearing may be preserved in the acute setting and rarely long-term, as progressive hearing loss is typical in the months and years following radiation. All treatment modalities, including observation, place facial nerve function, hearing, and balance at risk. Patients with VS with chronic disequilibrium (regardless of management strategy) can be treated conservatively with vestibular rehabilitation. Patients with disabling disequilibrium due to labile vestibulopathy or brainstem compression are often treated with surgical tumor resection.

Postsurgical Vestibular Hypofunction

A unilateral vestibular hypofunction is the unfortunate consequence of most ablative treatment strategies for vestibular diseases. The translabyrinthine approach leads to a complete loss of vestibular function (Fig. 22.3b), while the other approaches may result in varying degrees of vestibular weakness based on the integrity and residual function of the labyrinth and the vestibular nerves. Similarly, a surgical labyrinthectomy, intratympanic aminoglycoside injection, or vestibular nerve section performed to treat refractory episodic vertigo in cases of Meniere's disease will result in non-fluctuating unilateral vestibular loss. Following these ablative treatments, patients have symptoms that accompany acute vestibulopathy. Most patients will become asymptomatic over the course of days to months, as a result of central compensation. Chronic disequilibrium may persist, but this is most typically more tolerable for patients than symptoms that accompany fluctuating vestibular deficits.

Treatment

Similar to other causes of a fixed vestibular deficit, treatment is aimed at optimizing central compensation. Key components of treatment include encouraging physical activity, withholding vestibular suppressants, and instituting vestibular rehabilitation.

Vestibular Rehabilitation

Management of chronic unilateral vestibular dysfunction is often best treated with vestibular rehabilitation therapy (VRT). This exercise-based treatment focuses on reducing vestibular symptoms and improving daily functioning through exercises that promote central compensation and reinforce postural stability. These exercises capitalize on the compensatory responses of the brain in response to vestibular hypofunction. Through repetitive motions, there is a habituation to symptom-inducing movements, which further supports central vestibular neural activity to lessen symptoms [35]. This rehabilitation also promotes restoration of the VOR through repetitive head movements while attempting visual fixation [36]. Additionally, these exercises promote the increased use of visual and somatosensory inputs to augment balance while improving postural control.

VRT is evidence-based, and a recent Cochrane meta-analysis found that VRT is effective in decreasing subjective dizziness symptoms, improving daily functional activities, and can lead to long-term functional recovery [37]. Additionally, the American Academy of Otolaryngology-Head and Neck Surgery has recognized VRT as "valid for the treatment of persistent dizziness due to incomplete compensation of the vestibular system, dizziness resulting from medical or surgical treatment, and acute peripheral vestibular dizziness" [38]. Furthermore, VRT was stated to be of benefit in reducing the fall risk in the elderly population suffering multiple sensory and motor deficits. The utility of VRT is expanding and can be used to treat a variety of vestibular disorders such as BPPV, unilateral and bilateral vestibulopathy, as well as patients with chronic disequilibrium without vestibular deficits.

References

1. Agrawal Y, Carey JP, Della Santina CC, Schubert MC, Minor LB. Disorders of balance and vestibular function in US adults: data from the National Health and Nutrition Examination Survey, 2001–2004. Arch Intern Med. 2009;169(10):938–44.
2. Perez N, Garmendia I, Garcia-Granero M, Martin E, Garcia-Tapia R. Factor analysis and correlation between Dizziness Handicap Inventory and dizziness characteristics and impact on quality of life scales. Acta Otolaryngol. 2001;545:145–54.
3. Gans RE. Vestibular rehabilitation: critical decision analysis. Semin Hear. 2002;23:149–59.

4. Neuhauser HK. Epidemiology of vertigo. Curr Opin Neurol. 2007;20:40–6.
5. Sekitani T, Imate Y, Noguchi T, Inokuma T. Vestibular neuronitis: epidemiological survey by questionnaire in Japan. Acta Otolaryngol. 1993;503:9–12.
6. Renner V, Geißler K, Boeger D, Buentzel J, Esser D, Hoffmann K, Jecker P, Mueller A, Radtke G, Axer H, Guntinas-Lichius O. Inpatient treatment of patients admitted for dizziness: a population-based healthcare research study on epidemiology, diagnosis, treatment, and outcome. Otol Neurotol. 2017;38(10):e460–9.
7. Arbusow V, Schulz P, Strupp M, Dieterich M, von Reinhardstoettner A, Rauch E, Brandt T. Distribution of herpes simplex virus type 1 in human geniculate and vestibular ganglia: implications for vestibular neuritis. Ann Neurol. 1999;46:416–9.
8. Arbusow V, Strupp M, Wasicky R, Horn AK, Schulz P, Brandt T. Detection of herpes simplex virus type 1 in human vestibular nuclei. Neurology. 2000;55:880–2.
9. Theil D, Arbusow V, Derfuss T, Strupp M, Pfeiffer M, Mascolo A, Brandt T. Prevalence of HSV-1 LAT in human trigeminal, geniculate, and vestibular ganglia and its implication for cranial nerve syndromes. Brain Pathol. 2001;11:408–13.
10. Theil D, Derfuss T, Paripovic I, Herberger S, Meinl E, Schueler O, Strupp M, Arbusow V, Brandt T. Latent herpesvirus infection in human trigeminal ganglia causes chronic immune response. Am J Pathol. 2003;163:2179–84.
11. Taylor RL, McGarvie LA, Reid N, Young AS, Halmagyi GM, Welgampola MS. Vestibular neuritis affects both superior and inferior vestibular nerves. Neurology. 2016;87:1704–12.
12. Magliulo G, Gagliardi S, Ciniglio Appiani M, Iannella G, Re M. Vestibular neurolabyrinthitis: a follow-up study with cervical and ocular vestibular evoked myogenic potentials and the video head impulse test. Ann Otol Rhinol Laryngol. 2014;123:162–73.
13. Chihara Y, Iwasaki S, Murofushi T, Yagi M, Inoue A, Fujimoto C, Egami N, Ushio M, Karino S, Sugasawa K, Yamasoba T. Clinical characteristics of inferior vestibular neuritis. Acta Otolaryngol. 2012;132:1288–94.
14. Kim JS, Kim HJ. Inferior vestibular neuritis. J Neurol. 2012;259:1553–60.
15. Gianoli G, Goebel J, Mowry S, Poomipannit P. Anatomic differences in the lateral vestibular nerve channels and their implications in vestibular neuritis. Otol Neurotol. 2005;26:489–94.
16. Himmelein S, Lindemann A, Sinicina I, Horn AKE, Brandt T, Strupp M, Hüfner K. Differential involvement during latent herpes simplex virus 1 infection of the superior and inferior divisions of the vestibular ganglia: implications for vestibular neuritis. J Virol. 2017;91(14):e00331-17. Print 2017 Jul 15.
17. Fishman JM, Burgess C, Waddell A. Corticosteroids for the treatment of idiopathic acute vestibular dysfunction (vestibular neuritis). Cochrane Database Syst Rev. 2011;(5):CD008607.
18. Strupp M, Zingler VC, Arbusow V, Niklas D, Maag KP, Dieterich M, Bense S, Theil D, Jahn K, Brandt T. Methylprednisolone, valacyclovir, or the combination for vestibular neuritis. N Engl J Med. 2004;351(4):354–61.
19. Byl FM. Seventy-six cases of presumed sudden hearing loss occurring in 1973: prognosis and incidence. Laryngoscope. 1977;87(5 Pt 1):817–25.
20. Yetiser S, Hıdır Y, Birket H, Satar B, Durmaz A. Traumatic ossicular dislocation: etiology and management. Am J Otolaryngol Head Neck Med Surg. 2008;29:31–6.
21. Dahiya R, Keller JD, Litofsky NS, Bankey PE, Lawrence J, Megerian CA. Temporal bone fractures: otic capsule sparing versus otic capsule violating clinical and radiographic considerations. J Trauma Inj Infect Crit Care. 1999;47(6):1079.
22. Nageris B, et al. Temporal bone fractures. Am J Emerg Med. 1995;12:211–4.
23. Virapongse C, Bhimani S, Sawar M. Radiology of the abnormal ear. In: Taveras JM, Ferrucci JT, editors. Radiology: diagnosis, imaging, intervention. Philadelphia: Lippincott; 1997.
24. Brodie HA, Thompson TC. Management of complications from 820 temporal bone fractures. Am J Otol. 1997;18:188.
25. Stahle J, Stahle C, Anerberg IK. Incidence of Ménière's disease. Arch Otolaryngol. 1978;104:99–102.

26. Nakee K, Komatuzaki K. Epidemiological study of Ménière's disease. Pract Otol (Kyoto). 1984;69:1783–8.
27. Tokumaau K, Tashiro N, Goto K, et al. Incidence and prevalence of Ménière's disease in Aagamihara City, Kanagawa-ken. Pract Otol (Kyoto). 1983;1:1165–75.
28. Kotimaki J, Sorri M, Aantaa E, Nuutinen J. Prevalence of Ménière's disease in Finland. Laryngoscope. 1999;109:748–53.
29. Semaan MT, Megerian CA. Ménière's disease: a challenging and relentless disorder. Otolaryngol Clin N Am. 2011;44(2):383–403, ix.
30. Silverstein H, Smouha E, Jones R. Natural history vs. surgery for Meniere's disease. Otolaryngol Head Neck Surg. 1989;100:6.
31. Stepanidis K, Kessel M, Caye-Thomasen P, Stangerup SE. Socio-demographic distribution of vestibular schwannomas in Denmark. Acta Otolaryngol. 2014;134(6):551–6. Epub 2014 Mar 21.
32. Arthurs BJ, Fairbanks RK, Demakas JJ, et al. A review of treatment modalities for vestibular schwannoma. Neurosurg Rev. 2011;34:265–77.
33. Humphriss RL, Baguley DM, Axon PR, Moffat DA. Preoperative audiovestibular handicap in patients with vestibular schwannoma. Skull Base. 2006;16:193–9.
34. Karatas M. Central vertigo and dizziness: epidemiology, differential diagnosis, and common causes. Neurologist. 2008;14:355–64.
35. Hain T. Neurophysiology of vestibular rehabilitation. Neuro. Rehabilitation. 2011;29:127–41.
36. Balaban C, Hoffer M, Gottshall K. Top-down approach to vestibular compensation: translational lessons from vestibular rehabilitation. Brain Res. 2012;1482:101–11.
37. McDonnell MN, Hillier SL. Vestibular rehabilitation for unilateral peripheral vestibular dysfunction. Cochrane Database Syst Rev. 2015;1:CD005397.
38. Guidelines and Policies Policy Statement: Vestibular Rehabilitation. American Academy of Otolaryngology – Head and Neck Surgery. 2007. http://www.entnet.org/Practice/policyVestibularRehab.cfm. Accessed 12 Jan 2018.

Chapter 23
Bilateral Vestibular Hypofunction

Zachary G. Schwam, Seilesh Babu, and Christopher A. Schutt

Etiology

Bilateral vestibular hypofunction was first described by Dandy in 1941 [1], accounts for 1–2% of patients undergoing electronystagmography studies [2–5], and is estimated to have a nationwide prevalence of 28 per 100,000 adults in the United States [6]. It has a profound impact on those affected by it, with the majority of those diagnosed reporting reduced participation in social activities, altered driving habits, and difficulties with activities of daily living. Those affected are also predisposed to falling, with many sustaining fall-related injuries [6]. By and large, bilateral vestibular hypofunction is attributable to ototoxicity caused by systemic drugs, most notably aminoglycoside antibiotics (gentamicin, streptomycin, tobramycin). However, it may also be found secondary to a number of systemic diseases involving the labyrinth.

Of the aminoglycoside antibiotics, gentamicin is the most frequently encountered in clinical practice. The pharmacokinetics of aminoglycosides are thought to be held responsible, with quick uptake, early saturation, and a half-life of up to 6 months in the inner ear [7, 8]. Though each aminoglycoside has cochleotoxic and vestibulotoxic capabilities streptomycin, and gentamicin are predominantly vestibulotoxic, while the remainder are predominantly cochleotoxic [9]. The exact mechanism of damage to the outer hair cells of the sensory epithelium as well as spiral ganglion cells is unknown; however, a relationship between gentamicin-induced production of free radicals in the presence of iron is thought to exist [10]. The

Z. G. Schwam
Department of Otolaryngology, Icahn School of Medicine at Mount Sinai, New York, NY, USA

S. Babu · C. A. Schutt (✉)
Department of Otology and Neurotology, Michigan Ear Institute, Farmington Hills, MI, USA

J. C. Lucas et al. (eds.), *Diagnosis and Treatment of Vestibular Disorders*,
https://doi.org/10.1007/978-3-032-11740-3_23

finding has been bolstered as diminished ototoxicity has been seen with the concurrent administration of iron chelators and radical scavengers in animal models [11–13]. Several authors have focused their efforts on preventing the cochleo- and vestibulotoxic effects of aminoglycosides with some success; Ylikoski and colleagues used CEP-1347 (an inhibitor of the c-JNK apoptotic pathway) concurrently with gentamicin and noted reduced ABR threshold shifts, less in the way of inner hair cell damage, and reduced damage to the ampullary crista hair cells [14]. Interestingly, aminoglycoside-induced oto- and nephrotoxicity are thought to be independent of each other, with reports indicating no significant relationship between the two [15, 16].

Also on the clinician's differential diagnosis of bilateral vestibular hypofunction should be autoimmune inner ear disease, history of meningitis, sequential vestibular neuritis, neurofibromatosis type 2 with bilateral vestibular schwannomas, bilateral Meniere's disease, neurosyphilis, congenital malformations, Cogan's syndrome, post-binaural cochlear implantation, and trauma causing temporal bone fractures [5, 17].

In one series of 53 patients treated at a neurological hospital in the United Kingdom, 39% had associated neurological disorders and had originally been referred for ataxia and eye movement assessment [5]. According to the authors, bilateral vestibular hypofunction was not the original concern and was unexpected. Seven of those patients were subsequently found to have cerebellar degeneration involving the vestibulocerebellum, and five were found to have various neuropathies. The authors recommend that vestibular hypofunction be considered in patients with "jerky eye movements" upon fixation and with slow head movements. In the same series, autoimmune inner ear disease was diagnosed in 9% of their population, and typically presented in one of two ways: either relapsing and episodic with progressive disequilibrium and asymmetric hearing loss, or acute, severe, and rapid bilateral vestibular failure with concomitant hearing loss. In the first group, systemic organ involvement was also evident in the way of ocular, skin, joint, and mucosal symptoms. Twenty-one percent of cases in their series had no identifiable cause and were labeled idiopathic.

Symptomatology

The hallmark symptom of bilateral vestibular hypofunction is oscillopsia, or the sensation that the environment oscillates with abrupt head movements. This is secondary to loss of the normal vestibulo-ocular reflex, which works to stabilize a given image of interest on the retina by interconnecting the vestibular pathways with the oculomotor and abducens nuclei in addition to the medial longitudinal fasciculus to synchronize movement of the globes with the head. Patients may report that their disequilibrium is worse in the dark or on uneven ground, which may reflect the loss of vestibulospinal function [5]. In 1 report of 49 patients with bilateral vestibular paresis, 39 reported unsteadiness as their chief complaint, while 11 of those patients reported additional motion-provoked vertigo, and 3 reported additional spontaneous vertigo. Three were asymptomatic. In the same analysis, there was no association between degree of paresis and prevalence of vertigo versus disequilibrium. However, oscillopsia had a strong association with a more severe paresis [18].

Diagnosis

Several tests are available that can assist in the diagnosis of bilateral vestibular hypofunction. Dynamic visual acuity testing works on the basis that head movements degrade visual acuity, and that patients with bilateral vestibular deficits have impaired visual acuity with physiologic head movements due to an inadequate vestibulo-ocular reflex. Patients view a Snellen eye chart while being subjected to passive head motions at varying frequencies (approximately 2 Hz) and displacements. A decline in visual acuity is measured. A positive test is one in which the visual acuity declines by more than two lines during rotation of the head, although much greater drops are routinely seen in patients with bilateral vestibular hypofunction [19, 20]. Another flavor of dynamic visual acuity testing is the "Dynamic illegible 'E' test," where a modified Snellen chart is again used and the head is rotated in an arc approximately 60° at a frequency of 1 Hz. One hertz frequency was chosen as it goes beyond the capabilities of the smooth pursuit system but is correctable by the vestibulo-ocular reflex in normal subjects. Decline in visual acuity is then noted in a similar fashion [21].

The Head Impulse Test (HIT) relies on the detection of overt catch-up saccades upon rapid, small-amplitude, high acceleration head thrusts in unpredictable directions. It requires no equipment and should be part of a standard physical exam for vertiginous patients. In normal patients, the vestibulo-ocular reflex maintains fixation on the point, but in patients with vestibular loss, a catch-up saccade is necessary. Overt catch-up saccades can be detected by the clinician at bedside, but covert ones that occur during head movement remain undetected. Interestingly, in one study, patients with gentamicin-induced bilateral vestibular loss only produced half the number of covert saccades during head rotation [22, 23].

A quantitative form of impulse testing, vHIT, involves high impulse head movements combined with video software that measures pupil velocity. Further information about the procedure may be found in Chap. 5. Though its use provocative tests that evaluate the VOR and, by extension, the function of any of the three paired semicircular canals may be achieved (Fig. 23.1). Benefits when compared to rotary chair testing include the ability to test at physiologic frequencies greater than 1 Hz, lower equipment cost, and isolation testing of all three canals.

Chair rotational testing is yet another way of testing the vestibulo-ocular reflex and is the most quantitative representing a clear indication for its use (Figs. 23.2 and 23.3). Sinusoidal harmonic acceleration and velocity step testing are administered to the patient in the chair while eye movements are recorded. Gain, or the ratio of

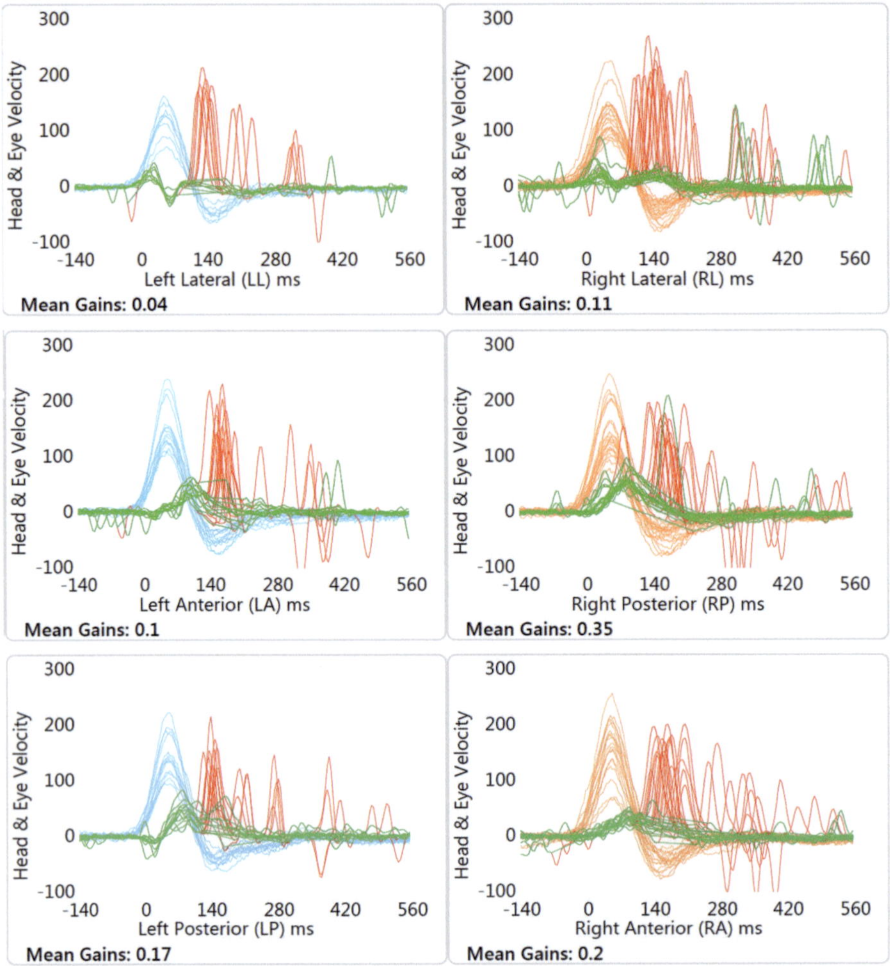

Fig. 23.1 vHIT in bilateral vestibular loss. Blue represents head thrust to the left; orange represents head thrust to the right. The green tracing is calculated vestibulo-ocular reflex activity during head thrust. Red represents compensatory saccades. Head thrust in either direction in the planes of all semicircular canals shows decreased VOR activity compared to head thrust with catch-up saccades noted. Note that for testing of the anterior and posterior canals, the contralateral thrust is to the appropriate LARP or RALP pairing. Top panel: lateral canal testing, middle panel: LARP testing, bottom panel: RALP testing. (Adapted from chapter 5, Walsh et al., figure 5.3)

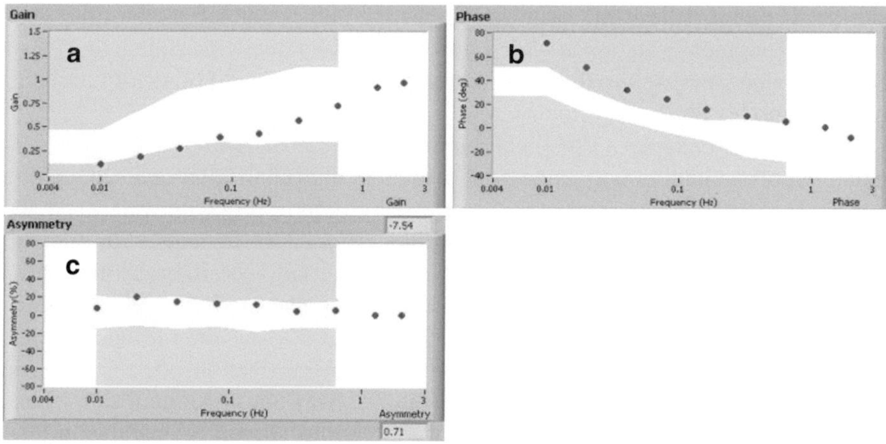

Fig. 23.2 Common Sinusoidal Harmonic Acceleration (SHA) results for bilateral labyrinthine hypofunction. Results for VOR gain (**a**), VOR phase (**b**), and VOR symmetry (**c**) from 0.01 through 2.0 Hz. Abnormal response regions are indicated by the gray regions for each results graph. (Adapted from chapter 6, Zalewski et al., figure 6.9)

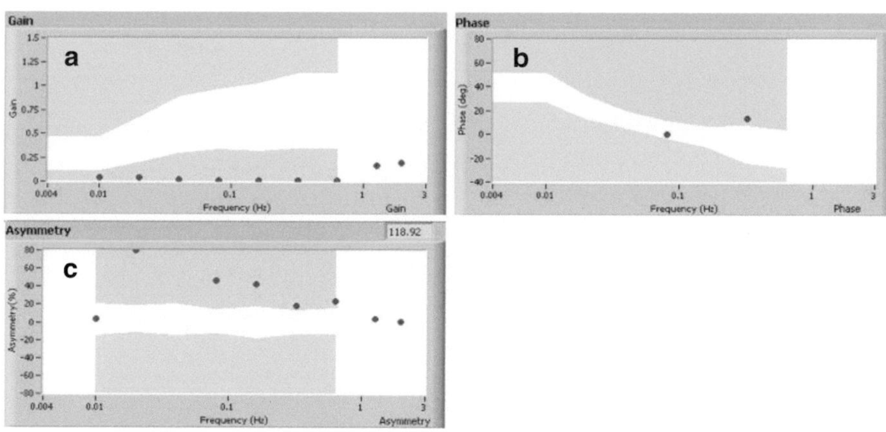

Fig. 23.3 Common Sinusoidal Harmonic Acceleration (SHA) results for bilateral labyrinthine areflexia. Results for VOR gain (**a**), VOR phase (**b**), and VOR symmetry (**c**) from 0.01 through 2.0 Hz. Since VOR phase and symmetry are calculated form VOR, these parameters should be interpreted with caution under such conditions. (Adapted from chapter 6, Zalewski et al., figure 6.10)

eye velocity to head velocity, and phase shift, or the lag timing for eye movement relative to head movement, are recorded during harmonic acceleration. A gain of 1.0 and phase shift of 180° are indicative of an optimized vestibulo-ocular reflex, while a bilateral gain of <0.4 is considered positive for bilateral vestibular hypofunction at low frequency oscillations. High frequency oscillations must be interpreted carefully and may often be misleading (Figs. 23.1 and 23.2) [20, 23, 24]. The time constant is measured during velocity step testing and is defined as the time after onset of 60 degrees/s rotation at which slow-phase eye velocity has fallen to 37% of its initial value. A value less than 10 s is considered indicative of bilateral vestibular hypofunction [5, 20].

Videonystagmography (VNG) can be helpful in the diagnosis of bilateral vestibular hypofunction but is considered less reliable than chair rotational testing due to lack of standardized normal ranges and variability in testing with water- and air-based as well as open- and closed-loop stimuli (Fig. 23.4). Patients with bilateral vestibular hypofunction undergoing traditional bithermal open-loop caloric irrigations at 30 °C and 44 °C typically display absence or a severe reduction of nystagmus (slow phase eye velocity <5–8 degrees/s), and even a diminished response (slow phase eye velocity <10 degrees/s) with ice water irrigations [5, 18, 20]. One can measure caloric response magnitudes in the way of maximum slow-phase velocities (MSPVs) and summate them for the various stimuli to calculate a total

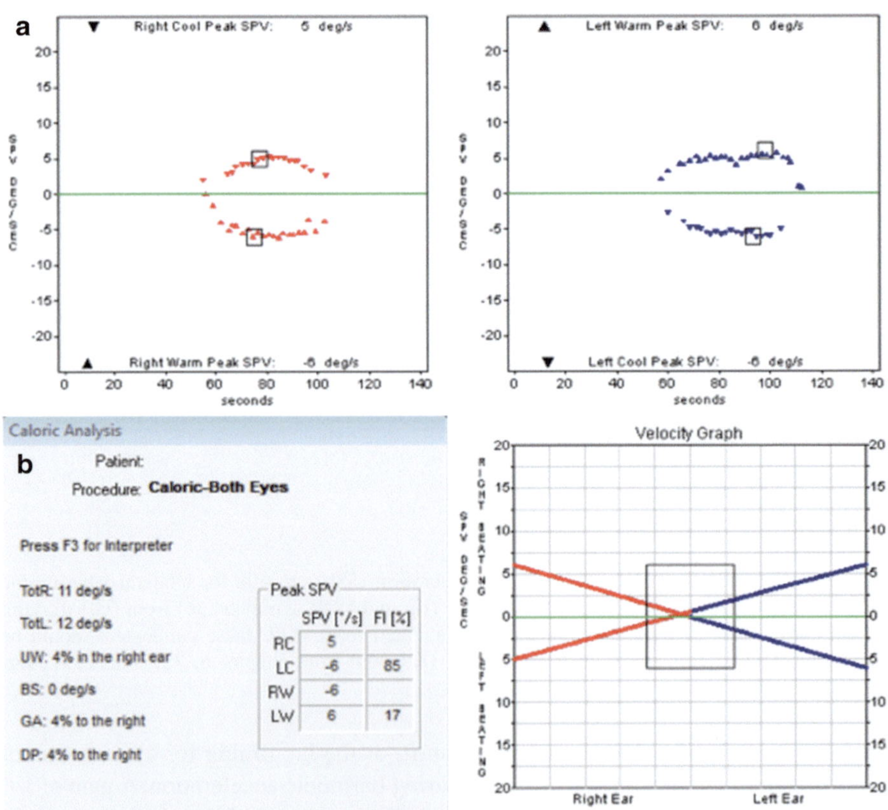

Fig. 23.4 Example of bilateral caloric weakness. Caloric responses of both ears fall at or below 12 degrees/s per side which is consistent with bilateral CW. (Adapted from chapter 4, Bojrb et al., figure 4.6b)

eye speed (TES). Bilateral vestibular hypofunction is generally diagnosed with a TES <20 degrees/s [17]. Other authors note virtually never encountering a TES <25 degrees/s in their normal groups [25].

Current Treatment

The mainstay of treatment for bilateral vestibular hypofunction is vestibular rehabilitation therapy, although it has demonstrated varied efficacy in multiple reports. A typical rehabilitation program will include exercises to optimize postural as well as gaze stability by augmenting the vestibulo-ocular and cervico-ocular reflexes. Subjects are asked to focus on an object while rotating their heads, make saccadic movements followed by head rotation, and walk while rotating their heads. These exercises are performed several times per day [20].

Krebs et al. demonstrated an 8% improvement in gait speed and a 17% decrease in time needing double support during ambulation with 16 weeks of vestibular rehabilitation [26], and Herdman et al. showed a significant improvement in dynamic visual acuity testing regardless of age with vestibular rehabilitation therapy [27]. Gillespie et al. showed normalization of dynamic visual acuity scores, improved balance with Romberg evaluation, return of gait velocity to >48 m/min, subjective feelings of improvement, and increased levels of physical activity. Improvement was seen in 51%, while 34% had no improvement, and the remainder was lost to follow-up [20]. Ototoxicity was the etiology of the vestibular hypofunction in 66% of their population and was a positive predictive factor in improvement with vestibular rehabilitation therapy (78% improved versus 50% with other etiologies). A predictive factor of no improvement was having a slowly progressive, sequential vestibular loss (found in 42% without improvement compared to 0% in those with improvement). Vertigo was also considered a negative predictive factor for improvement, as was having multiple unrelated medical comorbidities, severe hypofunction as measured by gain <0.2. Of the 18 patients that demonstrated improvement with vestibular rehabilitation therapy, only 5 returned to their subjective baseline state.

In another report of 49 patients with bilateral vestibular hypofunction [18], 22 underwent a comprehensive vestibular rehabilitation therapy program, 15 of which complete questionnaires after undergoing treatment. In combining questionnaire results with the notes of the therapist, only 3 of the 22 patients achieved a significant improvement in ambulation or equilibrium, and 50% of patients reported no improvement. None of the respondents demonstrated a significant improvement on the standardized disability scale. Additionally, the authors note that initial severity of paresis was not a predictor of degree of improvement.

Future Directions

Currently under development and with the hope to change the nature and course of bilateral vestibular hypofunction is the Johns Hopkins Multichannel Vestibular Prosthesis (MVP) project. Its goal is to selectively stimulate vestibular nerve branches using implantable sensors that detect acceleration in all directions to restore the vestibulo-ocular reflex in affected patients (Figs. 23.3 and 23.4). Using an animal model of chinchillas treated with bilateral intratympanic gentamicin to ablate their vestibular systems, prosthetic stimulation was able to partially restore the vestibulo-ocular reflex in treated animals and restore gain to that of normal animals [28]. The first-generation device was one in which the processor and three orthogonally directed sensors were fixed to the skull and connected to the electrodes percutaneously. A subsequent model was made smaller and more power efficient, with 12 electrodes, multipolar stimulation, a tri-axis linear accelerometer, and wireless control. In their earlier work in chinchillas, there was a significant risk of hearing loss, with four of six animals experiencing severe postoperative hearing loss when compared to the contralateral ear. Using an 8-electrode system in four chinchillas with surgically plugged semicircular canals and disrupted otolith end-organs, the authors noted issues of current spread to multiple canals as a result of the far more condensed rodent temporal bone anatomy [29].

In their next phase using a single adult rhesus macaque monkey, the authors implanted electrodes into the ampullae of the three semicircular canals, using fascia and dental cement to secure them [30]. Intratympanic gentmicin was then used to ablate the native vestibular organs. With use of a unilateral prosthesis, the angular vestibulo-ocular reflex was improved significantly in all axes examined, and nystagmus quick phases were observed. The authors did note, however, "prominent excitation-inhibition asymmetry," likely secondary to the inability of the device to depress afferent nerve firing rates. Of note, the authors did not attempt to stimulate the macular nerves innervating the utricle and saccule due to "the tight spacing of axons with different direction sensitivity." In a subsequent paper detailing the implantation of 5 rhesus monkeys in a similar fashion, the authors report gains that were approximately half of normal across a frequency range of 0.05–5 Hz, with an asymmetry that was amplified at higher accelerations [31]. This was in accordance with prior other studies evaluating humans and animals with one normal labyrinth. In addition, it was found that performance was improved with multisensory congruent inputs, or when a combination of total body rotation and stimulation from the prosthesis worked in tandem. The test subjects did suffer some degree of hearing loss in the implanted ears, with auditory brainstem response thresholds increased by 5–10 dB without stimulation, and 10–15 dB when the implant was activated. Distortion product otoacoustic emissions amplitudes also decreased by 2–14 dB in implanted ears [32].

There are multiple avenues for improving the prosthesis, namely in fine-tuning surgical technique, improving and miniaturizing circuit and electrode design, and optimizing stimulus parameters [30]. Human trials are the ultimate goal, and the

Multichannel Vestibular Implant Early Feasibility Study is currently underway (clinical trial #NCT02725463). While the data are unpublished, results from three implant participants showed preservation of hearing within 10 dB in one subject, and new 40–70 dB hearing loss in the 4–8 kHz range with preserved hearing in the 125–2000 Hz range. The test subjects also reported improved postural and visual stability with the prosthesis on, with modest improvements in gains.

Conclusion

Bilateral vestibular hypofunction is a debilitating disease with a reliable battery of tests to diagnose it and a variably effective method of treating it with vestibular rehabilitation therapy. A new vestibular implant is under development and is currently recruiting for a clinical trial.

References

1. Dandy WE. The surgical treatment of Meniere's disease. Surg Gynecol Obstet. 1941;72:421–5.
2. Brown KE, Whitney SL, Wrisley DM, Furman JM. Physical therapy outcomes for persons with bilateral vestibular loss. Laryngoscope. 2001;111:1812–7.
3. McGath JH, Barber HO, Stoyanoff S. Bilateral vestibular loss and oscillopsia. J Otolaryngol. 1989;18:218–21.
4. Vibert D, Liard P, Hausler R. Bilateral idiopathic loss of peripheral vestibular function with normal hearing. Acta Otolaryngol. 1995;115:611–5.
5. Rinne T, Bronstein AM, Rudge P, Gresty MA, Luxon LM. Bilateral loss of vestibular function: clinical findings in 53 patients. J Neurol. 1998;245:314–21.
6. Ward BK, Agrawal Y, Hoffman HJ, Carey JP, Della Santina CC. Prevalence and impact of bilateral vestibular hypofunction: results from the 2008 US National Health Interview Survey. JAMA Otolaryngol Head Neck Surg. 2013;139:803–10.
7. Minor LB. Gentamicin-induced bilateral vestibular hypofunction. JAMA. 1998;279:541–4.
8. Dulon D, Hiel HA, Aurousseau C, Erre JP, Aran JM. Pharmacokinetics of gentamicin in the sensory hair cells of the organ of Corti: rapid uptake and long term persistence. C R Acad Sci. 1993;III(316):682–7.
9. Matz GJ. Aminoglycoside cochlear ototoxicity. Otolaryngol Clin N Am. 1993;26:705–12.
10. Priuska EM, Schacht J. Formation of free radicals by gentamicin and iron and evidence for an iron/gentamicin complex. Biochem Pharmacol. 1995;50:1749–52.
11. Garetz SL, Altschuler RA, Schacht J. Attenuation of gentamicin ototoxiciy by glutathione in the guinea pig in vivo. Hear Res. 1994;77:81–7.
12. Song B, Schacht J. Protective effects of iron chelators on gentamicin ototoxicity. Inner Ear Biol Abst. 1995;32:O-8.
13. Conlon BJ, Smith DW. Supplemental iron exacerbated aminoglycoside ototoxicity. Hear Res. 1998;115:1–5.
14. Ylikoski J, Xing-Qun J, Virkkala U, Pirvola U. Blockage of c-jun N-terminal kinase pathway attenuates gentamicin-induced cochlear and vestibular hair cell death. Hear Res. 2002;166:33–43.
15. De Jager P, van Altena R. Hearing loss and nephrotoxicity in long-term aminoglycoside treatment in patients with tuberculosis. Int J Tuberc Lung Dis. 2002;6:622–7.

16. Smith C, Lipsky JJ, Lietman PS. Relationship between aminoglycoside-induced nephrotoxicity and auditory toxicity. Antimicrob Agents Chemother. 1979;15:780–2.
17. Hain TC, Cherchi M, Yacovino DA. Bilateral vestibular loss. Semin Neurol. 2013;33:195–203.
18. Telian SA, Shephard NT, Smith-Wheelock M, Hoberg M. Bilateral vestibular paresis: diagnosis and treatment. Otolaryngol Head Neck Surg. 1991;104:67–71.
19. Demer JL, Honrubia V, Baloh RW. Dynamic visual acuity: a test for oscillopsia and vestibulo-ocular reflex function. Am J Otol. 1994;15:340–7.
20. Gillespie MB, Minor LB. Prognosis in bilateral vestibular hypofunction. Laryngoscope. 1999;109:35–41.
21. Longridge NS, Mallinson AI. A discussion of the dynamic illegible "E" test: a new method of screening for aminoglycoside vestibulotoxicity. Otolaryngol Head Neck Surg. 1984;92:671–7.
22. Weber KP, Aw ST, Todd MJ, McGarvie LA, Curthoys IS, Halmagyi GM. Horizontal head impulse test detects gentamicin vestibulotoxicity. Neurology. 2009;72:1417–24.
23. Schubert MC, Minor LB. Vestibulo-ocular physiology underlying vestibular hypofunction. Phys Ther. 2004;84:373–85.
24. Fife TF, Tusa RJ, Furman JM, et al. Assessment: vestibular testing techniques in adults and children: report of the Therapeutic Technology Assessment Subcommittee of the American Academy of Neurology. Neurology. 2000;55:1431–41.
25. Zapala DA, Olsholt KF, Lundy LB. A comparison of water and air caloric responses and their ability to distinguish between patients with normal and impaired ears. Ear Hear. 2008;29:585–600.
26. Krebs DE, Gill-Body KM, Riley PO, Parker SW. Double-blind, placebo controlled trial of rehabilitation for bilateral vestibular hypofunction: a preliminary report. Otolaryngol Head Neck Surg. 1993;109:735–41.
27. Herdman SJ, Hall CD, Schubert MC, Das VE, Tusa RJ. Recovery of dynamic visual acuity in bilateral vestibular hypofunction. Arch Otolaryngol Head Neck Surg. 2007;133:383–9.
28. Della Santina CC, Migliaccio AA, Hayden R, et al. Current and future management of bilateral loss of vestibular sensation-an update on the Johns Hopkins Multichannel Vestibular Prosthesis Project. Cochlear Implants Int. 2010;11:2–11.
29. Della Santina C, Migliaccio A, Patel A. Electrical stimulation to restore vestibular function development of a 3-d vestibular prosthesis. Conf Proc IEEE Eng Med Biol Soc. 2005;7:7380–5.
30. Chiang B, Fridman GY, Dai C, Rahman MA, Della Santina CC. Design and performance of a multichannel vestibular prosthesis that restores semicircular canal sensation in rhesus monkey. IEEE Trans Neural Syst Rehabil Eng. 2011;19:588–98.
31. Dai C, Fridman GY, Davidovics NS, Chiang B, Ahn JH, Della Santina CC. Restoration of 3D vestibular sensation in rhesus monkeys using a multichannel vestibular prosthesis. Hear Res. 2011;281:74–83.
32. Dai C, Fridman GY, Della Santina CC. Effects of vestibular prosthesis electrode implantation and stimulation on hearing in rhesus monkeys. Hear Res. 2011;277:204–10.

Chapter 24
Post-traumatic Dizziness

Daniel Lan and Michael E. Hoffer

Introduction

Traumatic brain injury (TBI) is an increasingly common public health issue [1–10]. TBI affects an estimated incidence of 2.8 million people annually, accounting for more than 30% of the deaths and substantial number of cases of permanent disability in trauma patients [1]. TBI is defined as a head impact or blast exposure, followed by a period of alteration or loss of consciousness, and then associated with sequelae that are usually neurosensory in type. Trauma can occur through several mechanisms: motor vehicle accidents, sports injuries, assaults, falls, and work accidents. The situation is particularly serious in the military, where 25% of all individuals who have been deployed to Southwest Asia suffer at least one head injury [2]. Head trauma can be divided into several different classes, including mild, moderate, and severe TBI. Moderate and severe TBI typically involve significant brain injury and often a lengthy hospitalization. These complex neurological disorders include dizziness as one of many multi-factorial disorders, making diagnosis and treatment more difficult by the host of co-morbid conditions. Increasingly, more cases of mild TBI are diagnosed each year, while hospitalizations have stayed constant and deaths

D. Lan
Department of Otolaryngology, University of Miami, Miller School of Medicine, Miami, FL, USA
e-mail: daniel.lan@miami.edu

M. E. Hoffer (✉)
Department of Otolaryngology, University of Miami, Miller School of Medicine, Miami, FL, USA

Department of Neurological Surgery, University of Miami, Miller School of Medicine, Miami, FL, USA
e-mail: Michael.hoffer@miami.edu

J. C. Lucas et al. (eds.), *Diagnosis and Treatment of Vestibular Disorders*,
https://doi.org/10.1007/978-3-032-11740-3_24

have decreased. This chapter will focus primarily on mild TBI (herein referred to as mTBI) and the dizziness associated with this disorder.

Symptoms of Post-traumatic Dizziness

The symptoms of mTBI are primarily neurosensory [11–13], including dizziness, hearing problems, headaches, cognitive difficulties, and sleep disturbances. Symptoms of post-traumatic dizziness can be broken down to include vertigo (illusory sensation of the surrounding environment or the individual moving/rotating), head-motion induced vertigo, dizziness (sensation of disturbed or impaired spatial orientation without a false or distorted sense of motion), head-motion induced dizziness, unsteadiness (sensation of being off balance or feeling clumsy without directional preference), and visual lag (sensation of the surrounding environment following behind head movement with a delay) [14–20]. These symptoms vary depending on a number of factors, including the history of previous head trauma, undefined genetic factors, and the number, types, and forces of the primary and possible secondary impacts [21–23]. In some instances, the secondary force is obviously relevant to the head injury. For example, after a blast exposure (initial force), which itself can cause head injury, a person is thrown and hits their head on a blunt object (secondary force). In other cases, these secondary forces are less obvious, such as neck trauma (i.e., neck movement after a head impact or "whiplash") or other injuries occurring at the time of a head injury [24–26]. These forces are highly complex and unique to each individual situation.

Etiologies

Post-traumatic Dizziness After mTBI

Post-traumatic dizziness can result from several different etiologies. The acute and subacute dizziness complexes seen after head trauma are presented in Table 24.1.

A common etiology of dizziness following head trauma is benign paroxysmal positional vertigo (BPPV), in which individuals experience brief sensations of vertigo on assuming various head positions. In contrast to idiopathic BPPV, traumatic BPPV is more often persistent or recurrent despite treatment. Traumatic BPPV also presents with a higher percentage of lateral, anterior, or multi-canal damage than the idiopathic variant [27]. Nevertheless, in both cases, the posterior semicircular canal is the most common canal to be affected. The pathophysiology, diagnosis, and treatment remain the same as in idiopathic BPPV and are discussed in Chap. 11.

Exertional dizziness is dizziness (usually unsteadiness but occasionally vertigo) that occurs at the conclusion or near the very end of a period of exercise or exertion.

Table 24.1 Dizziness disorders seen after mild traumatic brain injury (mTBI)

Entity	History	Physical exam
Post-traumatic BPV	Positional vertigo	Nystagmus on Dix-Hallpike or other provocative maneuver
Post-traumatic exertion-induced dizziness	Dizziness at conclusion of exercise Dizziness when beginning exercise	Abnormalities in challenged gait with/after exertion
Post-traumatic vestibular migraine (PTVM)	Episodic vertigo with periods of unsteadiness Constant low-grade headache	Abnormalities in challenged gait Normal static posture +/− Head impulse abnormalities Satisfy ICHD-3 criteria
Post-traumatic spatial disorientation (PTSpD)	Constant feeling of unsteadiness worsened by standing and by challenged gait Drifting to one side while walking Shifting weight when standing still +/− Vertigo and headache	Abnormalities in challenged gait Abnormalities in static posture +/− Head impulse abnormalities

Vestibular migraine (otherwise known as migraine-associated vertigo) involves at least five episodes of moderate to severe vestibular symptoms with corresponding migrainous symptoms (unilateral pulsating headache, photophobia, phonophobia, or visual aura) at least 50% of the time [28, 29]. Diagnosis can be difficult if migraine symptoms are not specifically screened for. The pathophysiology is controversial, but management would seem to be the same as in other patients with vestibular migraine, including vestibular physiotherapy and anti-migraine drugs [29].

The most difficult and likely most common balance disorder seen after head injury is spatial disorientation, in which an individual feels continuously unsteady [30]. The sensation of unsteadiness is worsened by standing still or moving quickly. Slow movements tend to lessen the severity of this disorder. We, and others, have postulated that this may be due to a post-traumatic loss of the body's ability to sense the gravitoinertial vector used by the body to determine true upright. Therefore, during slow motion, the added inputs from moving help rectify this vector, whereas the fewer inputs when standing still or inputs that change quickly (fast motion) are less useful [31].

Other Causes of Vertigo

As opposed to the above discussion, there are specific, identifiable etiologies of dizziness secondary to head trauma, such as perilymphatic fistula (PLF), superior semicircular canal dehiscence (SSCD), temporal bone fracture, and Meniere's disease. While mTBI may sometimes lead to decompensation of a previously asymptomatic inner ear deformity, these disorders are not restricted to head trauma and generally behave in a similar fashion in the non-traumatic as well as the traumatic case.

PLF is a disorder caused by an abnormal defect or rupture of the fluid-filled membranous labyrinth, typically at the round or oval window [32, 33]. The injury can occur from direct head trauma, as well as an explosive blast wave or rapid scuba diving depressurization. The resulting communication allows fluid to travel between the inner ear, and middle ear cavities. Symptoms classically include vertigo, high-frequency sensorineural hearing loss, and tinnitus occurring immediately following the injury. When there is a severe sensorineural hearing loss and a very clear and a significant concussive event than treatment in the form of patching the fistula, site should be undertaken urgently. However, in the absence of significant hearing loss, because most diagnostic signs (Tullio's sign, instability or nystagmus triggered on tragal pressure or Valsalva maneuver) and tests (temporal CT, brain MRI, audiometry) do not have high sensitivity or specificity for PLF, it is difficult to diagnose with any certainty, and treatment is often delayed.

SCD is a condition where the bone over the superior semicircular canal is thinned or congenitally absent, which causes a protrusion of the membranous superior semicircular canal. This protrusion creates a "third mobile window" in the bone that enables aberrant communication from the inner ear, causing vestibular and/or auditory symptoms [34]. In classical presentations, these individuals have unsteadiness or vertigo that is intensified by loud noises (Tullio phenomenon) or pressure changes (Hennebert sign). Auditory symptoms may include an intensified sound of their own voice (autophony) and conductive hearing loss. Unlike PLF, SCD can develop more slowly as the defect (caused by damage to the bony covering of the canal) widens over time. "Third mobile window" syndromes may be associated with different patterns of performance on verbal memory, visual memory, and attention components of the Wide-Range Assessment of Learning and Memory test battery, with different post-operative recovery outcomes [35].

Meniere's disease may also be induced by trauma. The symptoms and histologic features have been reported to be identical to those of idiopathic Meniere's disease [36].

Severe head trauma may cause unilateral vestibular loss by the mechanism of temporal bone fracture. The majority of temporal bone fractures (80%) are longitudinal (in the axis of the petrous bone) rather than transverse [37]. Longitudinal temporal bone fractures are more likely to involve the inner ear while transverse fractures are more likely to transect the vestibulocochlear nerve or involve the otic capsule and inner ear [30, 38]. Vestibular loss may be seen after head trauma even without temporal bone fracture, referred to as labyrinthine concussion. This occurs as a result of traction or injury-induced demyelination of the vestibulocochlear nerve, trauma-related bleeding or micro-ischemic changes, or direct trauma or injury to the labyrinth [30, 38].

Cervical vertigo is a rare disorder that can be difficult to diagnose [39]. Because it is postulated that when traumatic the disorder is seen more often after whiplash injury, a thorough discussion of this entity goes beyond the scope of this chapter. It is mentioned here for the sake of completeness.

Examination and Diagnosis

The Role of Dizziness in the Diagnosis of mTBI

Despite a host of sideline and site of injury test platforms that have been introduced, mTBI remains difficult to diagnose [40–42], and patients suffer increased morbidity due to delayed diagnosis [12]. Many symptoms of mTBI prove difficult to evaluate, particularly headache and sleep disorders, which rely on self-report and are inherently inaccurate in this group of patients. Cognitive difficulties can be measured objectively, but tests are not necessarily efficient and test results can be difficult to interpret in mild disease. Hearing loss can be easily assessed via audiometry, but mTBI often presents with a central auditory processing abnormality, which is more difficult to assess, or tinnitus, which relies on self-report.

Work in our lab has demonstrated that a battery of antisaccade (increased error rate percentage), predictive saccade (decreased absolute number), and HIT tasks (increased absolute gain symmetry, decreased average gain) can sensitively and specifically (88% and 97%, respectively) identify individuals with acute mTBI [43–45]. Vestibular testing can be performed as early as immediately after the head trauma or later in the injury time course with nearly equal accuracy. In light of the varying reliability of many mTBI symptoms, we find that dizziness, which is almost universally present [13] in this population, is the most efficient, effective, and objective way to determine the presence or absence of mTBI.

Testing Abnormalities in Dizziness with mTBI

In evaluating a patient with suspected post-traumatic dizziness, the first and most important step is a thorough medical history and a standard vestibular physical exam. Examiners should pay particular attention to postural stability (Romberg and tandem Romberg tests), gait with horizontal and vertical head turning (museum gait), spontaneous nystagmus, smooth pursuit, and head impulse testing. Beyond these physical exam maneuvers, the most important measures are specialized vestibular function tests that can be conducted with infrared goggles and assorted visual stimuli [43–45]. These tests can be separated into oculomotor tasks (vertical and horizontal smooth pursuit, vertical and horizontal saccades, antisaccade, predictive saccade, optokinetic response, saccade-reaction time test) and vestibular tasks (head impulse test [HIT], subjective visual vertical and horizontal).

Audiological testing is also important for the evaluation of the dizzy patient after traumatic brain injury, especially for determining the degree and the site of the damage. This includes not only subjective audiometry but also objective audiometry, i.e., evoked potentials. It is also important to determine whether tinnitus is present. Other conditions that should be screened for include: migrainous symptoms (unilateral pulsating headache, photophobia, phonophobia, or visual aura), visuospatial symptoms (accommodation disorder, vergence, photosensitivity, etc.), and neurological symptoms (asthenia, headache, and concentration, memory, or mood disorder). Imaging can also be considered depending on the mechanism of injury and level of suspicion for greater than mild trauma.

Treatment

The treatment of dizziness associated with head injury requires the efforts of a multidisciplinary team. For the two specific posttraumatic vestibular disorders discussed above (PLF, SCD), surgery is the mainstay of treatment. Traumatically induced Meniere's disease can be treated in the same manner as non-traumatic Meniere's. The mainstay of treatment for other disorders is vestibular therapy [46–51]. Vestibular rehabilitation is the central pillar of non-surgical treatment for balance disorders, leading to improvements in cognitive function, dynamic visual acuity tasks, as well as shorter disability time, and time until return to activities of daily living and work [46–50]. Ocular therapy and cervical therapy have also been shown to be helpful in this population [50, 51]. In our experience, vestibular therapy is most effective when combined with a regimen that controls related symptoms, particularly headache. Moreover, despite the successes of vestibular therapy, individual patient factors (particularly young age) and less severe associated symptoms are independent predictors of a successful outcome [52]. Work is underway in a number of labs to evaluate countermeasures for mTBI. There has been some evidence shown with using antioxidant therapy, and a number of other medicines with anti-inflammatory and/or anti-apoptotic properties are currently being evaluated [12]. Hyperbaric oxygen therapy has been examined with unclear success [53], but newer treatment regimens utilizing this modality or combining this modality with other treatments might improve success. Novel therapies with non-traditional type medicines (Cannabidiol) have shown success [54]. Work is currently underway in our lab to examine the use of this type of countermeasure in mTBI.

Conclusion

TBI affects millions of people around the world and causes significant short- and long-term disability. Dizziness is one of the most common symptoms seen after head injury, and, as discussed in this chapter, recent advances have made dizziness easier to assess with objective outcomes. These developments have made vestibular testing one of the most effective and efficient methods for the diagnosis of mTBI. Once mTBI is diagnosed, a thorough evaluation of the etiology of the dizziness should follow, which will allow proper treatment of and prevention of long-term disability. Balance disorders from head injury can be treated, and this treatment is typically centered on vestibular rehabilitation therapy in addition to etiology-specific treatments. Vestibular rehabilitation therapy can result in improvement in the dizziness as well as other neurosensory symptoms.

References

1. Faul M, Xu L, Wald MM, et al. Traumatic brain injury in the United States: emergency department visits, hospitalizations and deaths 2002–2006. Atlanta: Centers for Disease Control and Prevention, National Center for Injury Prevention and Control; 2010. https://www.cdc.gov/traumaticbraininjury/pdf/blue_book.pdf. Accessed 5 Sept 2017.
2. DoD Worldwide Numbers for TBI. Defense and Veterans Brain Injury Center. 2017. http://dvbic.dcoe.mil/dod-worldwide-numbers-tbi. Accessed 5 Sept 2017.
3. Coronado VG, McGuire LC, Sarmiento K, et al. Trends in Traumatic Brain Injury in the U.S. and the public health response: 1995-2009. J Saf Res. 2012;43(4):299–307. https://doi.org/10.1016/j.jsr.2012.08.011.
4. Hendricks AM, Amara J, Baker E, et al. Screening for mild traumatic brain injury in OEF-OIF deployed US military: an empirical assessment of VHA's experience. Brain Inj. 2013;27(2):125–34. https://doi.org/10.3109/02699052.2012.729284.
5. Hoge CW, McGurk D, Thomas JL, et al. Mild traumatic brain injury in U.S. Soldiers returning from Iraq. N Engl J Med. 2008;358(5):453–63. https://doi.org/10.1056/NEJMoa072972.
6. Lew HL, Pogoda TK, Baker E, et al. Prevalence of dual sensory impairment and its association with traumatic brain injury and blast exposure in OEF/OIF veterans. J Head Trauma Rehabil. 2011;26(6):489–96. https://doi.org/10.1097/HTR.0b013e318204e54b.
7. Okie S. Traumatic brain injury in the war zone. N Engl J Med. 2005;352(20):2043–7. https://doi.org/10.1056/NEJMp058102.
8. Schneiderman AI, Braver ER, Kang HK, et al. Understanding sequelae of injury mechanisms and mild traumatic brain injury incurred during the conflicts in Iraq and Afghanistan: persistent postconcussive symptoms and posttraumatic stress disorder. Am J Epidemiol. 2008;167(12):1446–52. https://doi.org/10.1093/aje/kwn068.
9. Terrio H, Brenner LA, Ivins BJ, et al. Traumatic brain injury screening: preliminary findings in a US Army Brigade Combat Team. J Head Trauma Rehabil. 2009;24(1):14–23. https://doi.org/10.1097/HTR.0b013e31819581d8.
10. Warden D. Military TBI during the Iraq and Afghanistan wars. J Head Trauma Rehabil. 2006;21(5):398–402.
11. Hoffer ME, Balaban C, Gottshall K, et al. Blast exposure: vestibular consequences and associated characteristics. Otol Neurotol. 2010;31(2):232–6. https://doi.org/10.1097/MAO.0b013e3181c993c3.
12. Hoffer ME, Balaban C, Slade MD, et al. Amelioration of acute sequelae of blast induced mild traumatic brain injury by N-acetyl cysteine: a double-blind, placebo controlled study. PLoS One. 2013;8(1):e54163. https://doi.org/10.1371/journal.pone.0054163.
13. Hoffer ME, Szczupak M, Kiderman A, et al. Neurosensory symptom complexes after acute mild traumatic brain injury. PLoS One. 2016;11(1):e0146039. https://doi.org/10.1371/journal.pone.0146039.
14. Akin FW, Murnane OD. Head injury and blast exposure: vestibular consequences. Otolaryngol Clin N Am. 2011;44(2):323–34. https://doi.org/10.1016/j.otc.2011.01.005.

15. Bisdorff A, Von Brevern M, Lempert T, et al. Classification of vestibular symptoms: towards an international classification of vestibular disorders. J Vestib Res. 2009;19(1–2):1–13. https://doi.org/10.3233/VES-2009-0343.
16. Gottshall K, Drake A, Gray N, et al. Objective vestibular tests as outcome measures in head injury patients. Laryngoscope. 2003;113(10):1746–50.
17. Grubenhoff JA, Kirkwood MW, Deakyne S, et al. Detailed concussion symptom analysis in a paediatric ED population. Brain Inj. 2011;25(10):943–9. https://doi.org/10.3109/02699052.2011.597043.
18. Hoffer ME. Mild traumatic brain injury: neurosensory effects. Curr Opin Neurol. 2015;28(1):74–7. https://doi.org/10.1097/WCO.0000000000000164.
19. Scherer MR, Shelhamer MJ, Schubert MC. Characterizing high-velocity angular vestibulo-ocular reflex function in service members post-blast exposure. Exp Brain Res. 2011;208(3):399–410. https://doi.org/10.1007/s00221-010-2490-1.
20. Suarez H, Alonso R, Arocena M, et al. Clinical characteristics of positional vertigo after mild head trauma. Acta Otolaryngol. 2011;131(4):377–81. https://doi.org/10.3109/00016489.2010.534113.
21. Chavko M, Koller WA, Prusaczyk WK, et al. Measurement of blast wave by a miniature fiber optic pressure transducer in the rat brain. J Neurosci Methods. 2007;159(2):277–81. https://doi.org/10.1016/j.jneumeth.2006.07.018.
22. Moore DF, Jérusalem A, Nyein M, et al. Computational biology – modeling of primary blast effects on the central nervous system. Neuroimage. 2009;47(Suppl 2):T10–20. https://doi.org/10.1016/j.neuroimage.2009.02.019.
23. Wang C, Pahk JB, Balaban CD, et al. Computational study of human head response to primary blast waves of five levels from three directions. PLoS One. 2014;9(11):e113264. https://doi.org/10.1371/journal.pone.0113264.
24. Johnson CM, Perez CF, Hoffer ME. The implications of physical injury on otovestibular and cognitive symptomatology following blast exposure. Otolaryngol Head Neck Surg. 2014;150(3):437–40. https://doi.org/10.1177/0194599813515184.
25. Shah A, Ayala M, Capra G, et al. Otologic assessment of blast and nonblast injury in returning Middle East-deployed service members. Laryngoscope. 2014;124(1):272–7. https://doi.org/10.1002/lary.24169.
26. Stuhmiller JH, Phillips YY, Richmond DR. The physics and mechanisms of primary blast injury. In: Bellamy RF, Zajtchuk R, editors. Textbook of military medicine. Conventional warfare: blast ballistic and burn injuries. Washington, DC: Department of the Army, Office of the Surgeon General, Borden Institute; 1990. p. 241–70.
27. Akin FW, Murnane OD, Hall CD, et al. Vestibular consequences of mild traumatic brain injury and blast exposure: a review. Brain Inj. 2017;31(9):1188–94. https://doi.org/10.1080/02699052.2017.1288928.
28. Headache Classification Committee of the International Headache Society (IHS). The International Classification of Headache Disorders, 3rd edition (beta version). Cephalalgia. 2013;33(9):629–808. https://doi.org/10.1177/0333102413485658.
29. Lempert T, Olesen J, Furman J, et al. Vestibular migraine: diagnostic criteria. J Vestib Res. 2012;22(4):167–72. https://doi.org/10.3233/VES-2012-0453.
30. Hoffer ME, Gottshall KR, Moore R, et al. Characterizing and treating dizziness after mild head trauma. Otol Neurotol. 2004;25(2):135–8.
31. Hoffer ME, Schubert MC, Balaban CD. Early diagnosis and treatment of traumatic vestibulopathy and postconcussive dizziness. Neurol Clin. 2015;33(3):661–8. https://doi.org/10.1016/j.ncl.2015.04.004.
32. Glasscock ME, Hart MJ, Rosdeutscher JD, et al. Traumatic perilymphatic fistula: how long can symptoms persist? A follow-up report. Am J Otol. 1992;13(4):333–8.
33. Goodhill V. Traumatic fistulae. J Laryngol Otol. 1980;94(1):123–8.
34. Spasic M, Trang A, Chung LK, et al. Clinical characteristics of posterior and lateral semicircular canal dehiscence. J Neurol Surg B Skull Base. 2015;76(6):412–5. https://doi.org/10.1055/s-0035-1551667.

35. Wackym PA, Balaban CD, Mackay HT, et al. Longitudinal cognitive and neurobehavioral functional outcomes before and after repairing otic capsule dehiscence. Otol Neurotol. 2016;37(1):70–82. https://doi.org/10.1097/MAO.0000000000000928.
36. Fife TD, Giza C. Posttraumatic vertigo and dizziness. Semin Neurol. 2013;33(3):238–43. https://doi.org/10.1055/s-0033-1354599.
37. Cannon CR, Jahrsdoerfer RA. Temporal bone fractures. Review of 90 cases. Arch Otolaryngol. 1983;109(5):285–8.
38. Agrup C, Gleeson M, Rudge P. The inner ear and the neurologist. J Neurol Neurosurg Psychiatry. 2007;78(2):114–22. https://doi.org/10.1136/jnnp.2006.092064.
39. Hain TC. Cervicogenic causes of vertigo. Curr Opin Neurol. 2015;28(1):69–73. https://doi.org/10.1097/WCO.0000000000000161.
40. Choe MC, Giza CC. Diagnosis and management of acute concussion. Semin Neurol. 2015;35(1):29–41. https://doi.org/10.1055/s-0035-1544243.
41. Harmon KG, Drezner JA, Gammons M, et al. American Medical Society for Sports Medicine statement: concussion in sport. Br J Sports Med. 2013;47(1):15–26. https://doi.org/10.1136/bjsports-2012-091941.
42. Putukian M, Raftery M, Guskiewicz K, et al. Onfield assessment of concussion in the adult athlete. Br J Sports Med. 2013;47(5):285–8. https://doi.org/10.1136/bjsports-2013-092158.
43. Balaban CD, Kiderman A, Braverman A, et al. Optokinetic fast phase and saccade motor performance are depressed in acute concussion/mild traumatic brain injury. Presented at the 2015 Midwinter Meeting of the Association for Research in Otolaryngology, Baltimore, MD, 21–25 Feb 2015.
44. Hoffer ME, Braverman A, Crawford J, et al. Assessment of oculomotor, vestibular and reaction time response following a concussive event. Presented at the 2015 Midwinter Meeting of the Association for Research in Otolaryngology, Baltimore, MD, 21–25 Feb 2015.
45. Kiderman A, Hoffer ME, Braverman A. Comparing oculomotor and optokinetic findings to symptoms in patients with acute mTBI. Presented at the 2015 Midwinter Meeting of the Association for Research in Otolaryngology, Baltimore, MD, 21–25 Feb 2015.
46. Alsalaheen BA, Mucha A, Morris LO, et al. Vestibular rehabilitation for dizziness and balance disorders after concussion. J Neurol Phys Ther. 2010;34(2):87–93. https://doi.org/10.1097/NPT.0b013e3181dde568.
47. Alsalaheen BA, Whitney SL, Mucha A, et al. Exercise prescription patterns in patients treated with vestibular rehabilitation after concussion. Physiother Res Int. 2013;18(2):100–8. https://doi.org/10.1002/pri.1532.
48. Gottshall KR, Hoffer ME. Tracking recovery of vestibular function in individuals with blast-induced head trauma using vestibular-visual-cognitive interaction tests. J Neurol Phys Ther. 2010;34(2):94–7. https://doi.org/10.1097/NPT.0b013e3181dead12.
49. Munoz DP, Everling S. Look away: the anti-saccade task and the voluntary control of eye movement. Nat Rev Neurosci. 2004;5(3):218–28. https://doi.org/10.1038/nrn1345.
50. Schneider KJ, Meeuwisse WH, Nettel-Aguirre A, et al. Cervicovestibular rehabilitation in sport-related concussion: a randomised controlled trial. Br J Sports Med. 2014;48(17):1294–8. https://doi.org/10.1136/bjsports-2013-093267.
51. Thiagarajan P, Ciuffreda KJ. Versional eye tracking in mild traumatic brain injury (mTBI): effects of oculomotor training (OMT). Brain Inj. 2014;28(7):930–43. https://doi.org/10.3109/02699052.2014.888761.
52. Jacbos B, Beems T, Stulemeijer M, et al. Outcome prediction in mild traumatic brain injury: age and clinical variables are stronger predictors than CT abnormalities. J Neurotrauma. 2010;27(4):655–68. https://doi.org/10.1089/neu.2009.1059.
53. Cifu DX, Hoke KW, Wetzel PA, et al. Effects of hyperbaric oxygen on eye tracking abnormalities in males after mild traumatic brain injury. J Rehabil Res Dev. 2014;51(7):1047–56. https://doi.org/10.1682/JRRD.2014.01.0013.
54. Pazos MR, Mohammed N, Lafuente H, et al. Mechanisms of cannabidiol neuroprotection in hypoxic-ischemic newborn pigs: role of 5HT(1A) and CB2 receptors. Neuropharmacology. 2013;71:282–91. https://doi.org/10.1016/j.neuropharm.2013.03.027.

Chapter 25
Complex Dizziness

Varun V. Varadarajan and Patrick J. Antonelli

Introduction

The first step in evaluating dizziness is to obtain a clear history and classify a patient's complaint into a single subjective perception (e.g., vertigo, presyncope, disequilibrium) [1, 2]. This will usually lead to a clear diagnosis and path for further evaluation and management. Pre-syncope and syncope, for example, are largely cardiogenic, and less often, neurogenic [3]. Though patients with complaints of pre-syncope due to orthostatic hypotension are commonly referred for otologic evaluation, there is seldom a significant otologic component. In contrast, the illusion of motion, vertigo, has been heavily attributed to vestibular disorders. However, non-otologic disorders may also present with vertigo, and more mild or chronic vestibular dysfunction may present with dizziness without vertigo. Furthermore, careful inquiry into patient symptoms often reveals multiple types of dizziness [2, 4]. In a national survey, the presence of multiple descriptions of dizziness has been found to be the norm in adults in the United States, even in patients with otherwise typical presentations of a vestibular disorder [1].

The evaluation and management of patients with complex presentations of dizziness requires a solid understanding of the numerous systems that contribute to one's sense of balance. Maintaining balance requires adequate detection of environmental stimuli, integration of multisensory neural input, and execution of ocular, musculoskeletal, and autonomic responses [5, 6]. Central vestibular pathways are integrated

V. V. Varadarajan (✉)
Neurotology and Skull Base Surgery, Sacramento Ear, Nose & Throat, Sacramento, CA, USA
e-mail: vvaradarajan@sacent.com

P. J. Antonelli
Department of Otolaryngology-Head & Neck Surgery, University of Florida, Gainesville, FL, USA
e-mail: pa@ufl.edu

J. C. Lucas et al. (eds.), *Diagnosis and Treatment of Vestibular Disorders*, https://doi.org/10.1007/978-3-032-11740-3_25

with pathways responsible for autonomic control, as well as for the generation, perception, and regulation of emotional and affective states [7]. Thus, any pathology arising within the peripheral vestibular, ophthalmologic, cardiovascular, musculoskeletal, or central nervous systems may contribute to a complex presentation of dizziness. The psychological consequences of experiencing alarming symptoms, such as vertigo and imbalance, may exaggerate or color the reported complaints [8].

This chapter will discuss vestibular disorders with overlapping symptoms, comorbid conditions, and clinical features that may help establish the appropriate diagnoses in patients presenting with complex dizziness.

Commonly Recognized Balance Disorders with Overlapping Symptoms

While most balance disorders have classic presentations, there can be significant overlap among many of these. Recurrent, spontaneous vertigo carries a large differential diagnosis, and many conditions may present similarly, especially in their initial, *forme fruste* phase. This is particularly true if a precise, thorough history is not obtained.

Benign Paroxysmal Positional Vertigo

Patients presenting with classic symptoms and examination findings of benign paroxysmal positional vertigo (BPPV) are usually promptly diagnosed [9]. Patients with BPPV will, however, describe their vertigo duration in highly variable and inaccurate ways. First, many will describe the duration by the cumulative number of hours, days, weeks, or years that they are affected rather than by the duration of each episode of vertigo (i.e., less than a minute). Second, many patients avoid movements that provoke their vertigo or change positions quickly enough that they do not know its true duration. Third, BPPV may feel so severe, the vertigo likely feels longer than it truly is.

Questioning on the positional provocation may similarly lead to diagnostic confusion. Provocation of vertigo by *rolling over* in bed, typical for BPPV, may in fact result from *getting out* of bed, which is commonly due to orthostatic hypotension. As both BPPV and orthostatic hypotension are most commonly found in elderly individuals, both may be present. Furthermore, many conditions are associated with the development of BPPV, including diabetes, trauma (and post-surgical), osteoporosis, vascular, psychiatric, MD, migraine, vestibular neuritis, and autoimmune disorders [10, 11]. Thus, it is not uncommon to have a presentation of BPPV along with other types of dizziness.

Residual dizziness is common after the treatment or resolution of positional vertigo [12, 13]. Diverse explanations, including delayed compensation and underlying otolithic organ dysfunction, have been proposed as responsible mechanisms.

Semicircular Canal Dehiscence

Sound-induced (i.e., Tullio's phenomenon) or pressure-induced vertigo accompanied by autophony is pathognomonic for semicircular canal dehiscence (SCD); however, this may also present with spontaneous, ill-defined dizziness [14]. Tulio's phenomenon may occur in the absence of SCD with endolymphatic hydrops and perilymph fistula [15–18]. Clinicians must also be aware of more esoteric disorders with sound-induced dizziness, such as vestibular atelectasis, reflex epilepsy, and long QT syndrome [19–21].

Otosclerosis

Otosclerosis may be accompanied by complaints of dizziness. Though the diagnosis of otosclerosis is usually suggested by an air-borne gap on audiometry, labyrinthine dysfunction can occur without footplate fixation [22]. Vestibular complaints in the presence of otosclerosis can be highly variable. Eza-Nuñez and colleagues reported the most common presentations to be Menière's syndrome (30%), spontaneous recurrent vertigo without hearing fluctuation (27.5%), positional vertigo (32.5%), and chronic unrelapsing imbalance (7.5%) [23]. Stapedotomy may both lead to improvement with and onset of vestibular complaints [24]. Endolymphatic hydrops is more common in patients that have undergone stapedotomy than those with unoperated otosclerosis [25].

Vestibular Migraine and Ménière's Disease

As these two conditions often have similar presenting symptoms and patients are commonly without objective findings between episodes, they can be rather difficult to distinguish. Ménière's disease (MD) may present with an isolated attack of vertigo lasting less than 30 min, with minimal or no auditory complaints [26, 27]. Conversely, vestibular migraine (VM) may present with a violent attack of vertigo that lasts a few hours, is accompanied by aural fullness and/or tinnitus, and has no history of migraine headaches [26, 28]. The diagnosis of MD and VM is based on the clinical history, and there is no definitive diagnostic test to differentiate the two diseases [29–31]. Focused questioning on a history of headaches, photophobia/phonophobia, and visual stigmata (e.g., seeing lights) will often be productive, as patients will tend to neglect such events that occurred in the remote past and had no clear connection to their dizziness. Similarly, a family history of vertigo and seeing lights, as well as migraine headaches, should be solicited.

Adding to the potential confusion on the distinction between MD and VM is the lack of a clear consensus on the diagnostic criteria. Numerous authors and expert panels have promulgated diagnostic criteria. Whereas the criteria for MD are rather uniform (Table 25.1) [28], those for VM are not. Neuhauser et al. published the first diagnostic criteria for VM in 2001 and updated these in 2009 [31, 32]. However, in 2012, the International Headache Society (IHS) and Bárány Society proposed and validated slightly different criteria for the diagnosis of VM (Table 25.2) [26, 30]. The IHS/Bárány Society criteria have been found to be more specific but less sensitive for the diagnosis of VM than Neuhauser's criteria due to the type, duration, and intensity of vertigo specified in the IHS criteria [33].

Radtke et al. evaluated the validity of Neuhauser et al.'s criteria for definitive vestibular migraine (dVM) and probable vestibular migraine (pVM) and demonstrated high reliability, with a positive predictive value of 85% [34]. Patients meeting criteria for MD were excluded from the study, but 13% of patients diagnosed with dVM and 7% of patients diagnosed with pVM developed bilateral sensorineural hearing loss and met AAO-HNS criteria for bilateral MD. These patients had symptomatology atypical for MD, including symmetric and mild hearing loss, vertigo attacks of long duration (≥3 days), imbalance with head motion, or recurrent brief attacks of spontaneous or positional vertigo. The authors thus attributed these symptoms to VM with cochlear involvement. Cochlear dysfunction and hearing loss should be rare in VM and relatively mild [35, 36]. The degree of hearing loss that should be attributed to VM alone versus comorbid MD has not been established. The rate of overlapping VM and MD is likely underestimated as patients diagnosed with MD are typically excluded from studies investigating VM [27, 37].

Neff et al. compared the presentations of patients diagnosed with MD, VM, and both MD and VM (MDVM) [27]. Neuhauser's criteria were used for VM diagnosis

Table 25.1 Diagnostic criteria for Ménière's disease

Definite Ménière's disease
Two or more spontaneous episodes of vertigo, each lasting 20 min to 12 h
Audiometrically documented low- to mid-frequency sensorineural hearing loss in one ear, defining the ear on one occasion before, during, or after one episode of vertigo
Fluctuating aural symptoms (hearing, tinnitus, or fullness) in the affected ear
Not better accounted for by another vestibular diagnosis
Probable Ménière's disease
Two or more episodes of vertigo or dizziness, each lasting 20 min to 24 h
Fluctuating aural symptoms (hearing, tinnitus, or fullness) in the affected ear
Not better accounted for by another vestibular diagnosis

Adapted from Lopez-Escamez et al. [28]

Diagnostic criteria for Menière's disease jointly formulated by the Classification Committee of the Bárány Society, The Japan Society for Equilibrium Research, the European Academy of Otology and Neurotology, the Equilibrium Committee of the American Academy of Otolaryngology-Head and Neck Surgery, and the Korean Balance Society

Table 25.2 Diagnostic criteria for vestibular migraine proposed by the International Headache Society and the Bárány Society (2012)

Definite vestibular migraine
At least five episodes with vestibular symptoms of moderate or severe intensity, lasting 5 min to 72 h
Current or previous history of migraine with or without aura according to the ICHD
One or more migraine features with at least 50% of the vestibular episodes:
(a) Headache with at least two of the following characteristics: one-sided location, pulsating quality, moderate or severe pain intensity, aggravation of routine physical activity
(b) Photophobia and phonophobia
(c) Visual aura
Not better accounted for by another vestibular or ICHD diagnosis
Probable vestibular migraine
At least five episodes with vestibular symptoms of moderate or severe intensity, lasting 5 min to 72 h
Only one of the criteria B and C for vestibular migraine is fulfilled (migraine history or migraine features during the episode)
Not better accounted for by another vestibular or ICHD diagnosis

Adapted from Lempert et al. [26]
Diagnostic criteria for vestibular migraine jointly formulated by the Committee for Classification of Vestibular Disorders of the Bárány Society and the Migraine Classification Subcommittee of the International Headache Society
Abbreviations: *ICHD* International Classification of Headache Disorders

[32]. Symptom overlap between groups was significant, and there was no single clinical feature or vestibular test that reliably differentiated between groups. Increased age, male gender, vertigo lasting hours, and SNHL were more significantly associated with the MD group; a younger age, female gender, and recurrent moderate to severe headaches were more significantly associated with the VM group. Chronic Subjective Dizziness (CSD) was more commonly associated with VM than MD. Aural symptoms, decreased performance on audiometry, and evidence of peripheral vestibular deficit were more prevalent in the MD and MDVM group than the VM alone group. The presence of a peripheral vestibular deficit (e.g., positive head thrust) was unable to separate MDVM and VM patients. Patients with MDVM had a significantly higher prevalence of family history of vertigo and a greater rate of perceived hearing loss than both MD and VM alone.

Lopez-Escamez et al. investigated accompanying symptoms of vestibular attacks in 268 patients with VM (84 patients), pVM (65 patients), and MD (119 patients) using the IHC criteria for VM [38]. This study also demonstrated significant symptom overlap but identified no specific clinical feature unique to VM, pVM, or MD. Aural symptoms (tinnitus, aural fullness, hearing loss) and vomiting were more frequently seen in patients with MD than with VM during vestibular attacks. Female gender, photophobia, phonophobia, visual auras, palpitations, and anxiety were more frequently seen in patients with VM. The frequency of headaches (all types) and a migraine risk score (calculated based on headache features) was higher in patients with VM than in patients with pVM and MD. A recent systematic review of the literature comparing the clinical presentations of MD and VM showed findings consistent with the studies discussed above [30]. MD patients tend to have a greater age of onset, increased prevalence of hearing loss, tinnitus, aural fullness, abnormal nystagmus, abnormal caloric testing and VEMP testing results, and endolymphatic hydrops. VM patients demonstrated a higher frequency of headaches, photophobia, and auras.

Magnetic resonance imaging (MRI) has demonstrated gray matter volume reduction in patients with VM compared to controls; however, there is a paucity of literature describing distinguishing MRI findings between VM and MD. The structural and functional MRI changes in VM are similar to findings previously described for migraine headache; however, these changes extend to areas involved in multisensory vestibular control and central vestibular compensation [39]. Endolymphatic hydrops is more commonly identified in patients with MD; however, hydrops has been identified on MRI in patients with symptoms meeting criteria for VM but not for MD [40, 41]. Gurkov et al. reported that several patients meeting criteria for both definite VM and definite MD failed to show hydrops on MRI [41]. It is unclear if these patients truly had both disorders, if the patients were misdiagnosed with VM, if hydrops was incidentally associated with VM, or if hydrops was independently associated with VM-related labyrinthine injury.

Vestibular testing has been used to differentiate VM and MD, although the impact of these tests on management and outcomes is controversial [27]. Caloric weakness and VEMP abnormalities have not been consistently found to be more common in MD versus VM [27, 30, 42–48] Cervical-VEMP (cVEMP) asymmetry ratios for 500 Hz:1000 Hz tone bursts and cVEMP amplitudes were found to be lower in patients with MD compared to VM and control patients [45, 49]; however, other studies failed to show a difference in amplitudes or latency [47, 48]. Ocular-VEMP (oVEMP) testing has demonstrated more abnormalities, including longer latencies, lower amplitudes, and larger asymmetry ratios in patients with MD [45, 47, 50]. The rotary chair has been unable to reliably differentiate VM from MD [27, 45]. Video head impulse testing has also been recently described to demonstrate differences in vestibulo-ocular reflex gain; however, formal investigations of its utility are warranted [44, 51].

Less Established Balance Disorders

Vestibular Paroxysmia

Neurovascular compression of the vestibular nerve as a cause of episodic vertigo was first described by Janetta in 1975 [34, 52]. In 1994, Brandt introduced the term “vestibular paroxysmia” (VP), but its use has largely been limited to the European literature [53]. In 2016, an international consensus definition and criteria for VP were published (Table 25.3) [54]. VP is thought to be a rare condition in which ephaptic discharges are produced secondary to segmental, pressure-induced

Table 25.3 Diagnostic criteria for vestibular paroxysmia

Vestibular paroxysmia
At least ten attacks of spontaneous spinning or non-spinning vertigo
Duration less than 1 min
Stereotyped phenomenology in a patient
Response to a treatment with carbamazepine/oxcarbazepine
Not better accounted for by another diagnosis
Probable vestibular paroxysmia
At least five attacks of spinning or non-spinning vertigo
Duration less than 5 min
Spontaneous occurrence or provoked by certain head movements
Stereotyped phenomenology in a patient
Not better accounted for by another diagnosis

Adapted from Strupp et al. [54]

compression by blood vessels in the cerebellopontine angle, most commonly a loop of the anterior inferior cerebellar artery [34]. Episodes of rotational or non-rotational vertigo last seconds to a few minutes and can be accompanied by hearing loss, tinnitus, and hypo- or hyperacusis. Vertigo may be triggered by a change in head position or hyperventilation; however, most attacks are spontaneous. High-resolution constructive interference in steady-state magnetic resonance imaging (MRI) may support the diagnosis by demonstrating neurovascular compression; however, neurovascular compression may be identified on MRI in up to 30% of asymptomatic patients [55]. Both microvascular decompression and medical therapy (e.g., carbamazepine) have been reported to improve the severity and reduce the duration of symptoms; however, clinical trials are lacking [34].

Persistent Postural-Perceptual Dizziness

Patients with episodic vestibular symptoms or vestibular insults may experience chronic non-vertiginous disequilibrium after or in between vertiginous attacks. This phenomenon was traditionally attributed to either uncompensated peripheral vestibular deficits or a non-organic, psychogenic etiology. The term "persistent postural-perceptual dizziness" (PPPD) and its diagnostic criteria were introduced in 2015, using common features of several previously described conditions: space motion discomfort (SMD), visual vertigo (VV), and phobic postural vertigo (PPV), which was later refined as chronic subjective dizziness (CSD) syndrome [56]. It has been promoted as a unique disorder and has been described to affect patients between vertiginous episodes of MD or VM (Table 25.2) [27, 56, 57]. PPPD manifests as non-vertiginous dizziness or non-spinning vertigo that is present on most days for at least 3 months and is exacerbated by movement, upright posture, visual motion, and other complex visual stimuli [56, 58]. PPPD may also be precipitated by disorders that cause vertigo or other non-vertiginous dizziness, such as vestibular neuritis, BPPV, VM, syncope, traumatic brain injury, and panic attacks [59].

Table 25.4 Diagnostic criteria for persistent postural-perceptual dizziness

A. One or more symptoms of dizziness, unsteadiness, or non-spinning vertigo are present on most days for 3 months or more.
Symptoms last for prolonged (hours-long) periods of time, but may wax and wane in severity.
Symptoms need not be present continuously throughout the entire day.
B. Persistent symptoms occur without specific provocation but are exacerbated by three factors:
Upright posture
Active or passive motion without regard to direction or position
Exposure to moving visual stimuli or complex visual patterns
C. The disorder is precipitated by conditions that cause vertigo, unsteadiness, dizziness, or problems with balance, including acute, episodic, or chronic vestibular syndromes, other neurologic or medical illnesses, or psychological distress.
When the precipitant is an acute or episodic condition, symptoms settle into the pattern of criterion A as the precipitant resolves, but they may occur intermittently at first, and then consolidate into a persistent course.
When the precipitant is a chronic syndrome, symptoms may develop slowly at first and worsen gradually.
D. Symptoms cause significant distress or functional impairment.
E. Symptoms are not better accounted for by another disease or disorder.

Adapted from Staab et al. [56]

Differentiating VM and PPPD may be challenging as the 2012 International Headache Society (IHS) criteria for VM and PPPD overlap [8, 26, 60–62]. Comorbid conditions may include anxiety, depression, VM, or neurotologic disorders with a compensated vestibular deficit. Selective serotonin reuptake inhibitors and serotonin norepinephrine reuptake inhibitors have been reported to reduce the symptoms of PPPD in open-label studies [57]. The habituation form of vestibular and balance rehabilitation therapy has been shown to be beneficial in reducing symptoms in preliminary studies [59] (Table 25.4).

Interplay with Non-Vestibular Disorders

Psychiatric Disorders

Psychiatric comorbidity and somatization are more often seen in both adult and pediatric patients experiencing dizziness and vertigo [63–65]. Anxiety and palpitations may accompany episodic vertigo with vestibular disorders. These symptoms have been found to be more common in VM than in MD [38]. Patients with MD or VM have been shown to have higher rates of psychiatric comorbidity than patients with BPPV or vestibular neuritis. Neuroticism and panic in patients with vestibular disorders and comorbid anxiety may exacerbate the symptoms experience [8]. Anxiety associated with vertical height intolerance has been shown to adversely affect gaze control and reduce gaze stability on visual targets, potentially contributing to vestibular symptoms [66]. Psychiatric consultation is recommended for patients presenting with bothersome dizziness and comorbid psychiatric conditions.

Central Nervous System Disorders

Central nervous system (CNS) disorders affecting the pathways involving brainstem or cerebellum may be comorbid or difficult to differentiate from peripheral vestibular lesions [67]. Vertigo, imbalance, nausea, vomiting, ataxia, and multidirectional nystagmus that is not suppressed by visual fixation may be present in isolation or with other focal neurologic signs, suggesting a central vestibular disorder. The combination of head impulse, nystagmus type, and test of skew (HINTS) is likely the most accurate means of distinguishing stroke from an acute peripheral event [68, 69]. Central vestibular disorders, such as cerebrovascular disease and multiple sclerosis, are discussed in detail elsewhere in this text.

Susac's Syndrome

Susac's syndrome is thought to be an autoimmune disease of the small arteries of the brain, inner ear, and retina [70]. The classic triad includes encephalopathy with or without focal neurological signs, retinal artery branch occlusions, and hearing loss. The latter is typically bilateral, low-frequency sensorineural hearing loss, and it may be accompanied by vestibulopathy. MRI of the brain is key to making the diagnosis, particularly in the absence of retinal manifestations.

Cervicogenic Vertigo

Vertigo and dizziness have been associated with cervical pathology. Several terms have been used to describe this phenomenon, including "cervical" or "cervicogenic" dizziness or vertigo. This entity lacks a validated diagnostic test and is controversial among balance specialists [71]. Several etiologies have been described, including vertigo associated with vertebral artery impingement as well as cervical injuries, such as whiplash [72]. Rotational vertebral artery syndrome (RVAS), or "Bow-Hunter syndrome," has been described as a rare etiology in which vascular compression occurs at the atlantoaxial level, most commonly by a cervical osteophyte [71, 73]. Treatment addresses the vascular compression, as physical therapy may exacerbate symptoms and decrease blood flow.

Cervical vertigo associated with degenerative cervical spine disease and injury is more commonly described, and its etiology is based on the somatosensory input hypothesis [72]. Cervical proprioceptive pathways integrate in the vestibular nuclei and modulate peripheral vestibular discharges and posture. Somatosensory signals alone may generate vertigo or nystagmus [72]. Dysfunction of the joints, muscles, and ligaments may cause pain, limited range of motion, dizziness, imbalance, motion sickness, aural fullness, phono- and photosensitivity, and nausea [74]. Symptoms are associated with cervical movement and may be episodic, lasting minutes to hours, mimicking other episodic vestibular disorders. One may mistake cervical motion-triggered dizziness with dizziness triggered only by head and body position, such as BPPV or orthostatic hypotension. Dizziness is often comorbid with cervical disorders in the elderly population, as this population also suffers from vascular, osteoarticular, and degenerative cervical disease [72]. Proprioceptive and vestibular function deteriorates in older adults, and sensory input from cervical pain stimuli is altered; the sense of head position may thus be impaired, resulting in dizziness [75, 76]. Cervical vertigo is considered by many to be a diagnosis of exclusion, and the differential diagnosis must include presbystasis and multisensory imbalance in patients with peripheral neuropathy or visual deficits.

Trauma may also affect cervical proprioception and create a mismatch in sensory input with proprioceptive, visual, and vestibular inputs [71]. Patients with whiplash-associated disorder after cervical trauma infrequently report true vertigo; however, light- or heavy-headedness and imbalance are commonly encountered. Although vestibular therapy may be helpful, the beneficial role of physical therapy to improve neck mobility and relieve pain and spasm must not be underestimated [77]. Cervical disc decompression may be an option for patients with associated radiculopathy or severe degenerative disease [78, 79].

Ophthalmologic Conditions

Ophthalmologic conditions are not commonly the dominant etiology for dizziness; however, conditions affecting visual input and integration can produce several symptoms that mimic a vestibulopathy [80]. Ocular disorders have been reported to be responsible for instability, disequilibrium, or vertigo in both adult and pediatric populations [81]. Patients with binocular visual dysfunction in conditions such as vertical heterophoria, vergence insufficiency, or latent strabismus may report dizziness, lightheadedness, nausea, anxiety, vertigo, headache, and motion sickness [80, 81]. These conditions warrant ophthalmologic referral.

An intact visual system is necessary for central nervous system compensation to vestibular pathology. Advanced cataracts, macular degeneration, and poorly corrected refraction can prevent central compensation to simple vestibulopathies [82–84].

Oscillopsia, or the illusion of motion of the visual surroundings, may be mistaken by clinicians for vertigo. Patients may describe oscillopsia as their visual field jumping, wobbling, or becoming difficult to focus, particularly while walking [85]. In addition to bilateral vestibular hypofunction, oscillipsia may be secondary to brainstem and cerebellar lesions, head tremor (pseudonystagmus), voluntary nystagmus, ocular flutter, or superior oblique myokymia [86]. Oscillopsia must not be confused with the development of vertigo or unsteadiness associated with complex or moving visual stimuli, as seen in PPPD and other vestibular disorders [56, 86].

Cardiovascular Disease

Cardiovascular disorders are a common cause of dizziness; however, isolated vertigo is an uncommon manifestation of cardiac disease. Orthostatic hypotension is typically associated with presyncope and "light-headedness," but patients may report vertigo or the illusion of motion during tilt-table testing [87]. Vertigo has also been reported to be a primary manifestation of a cardiac arrhythmia [88]. Sound has been reported as a trigger of Long-QT syndrome, mimicking Tullio's phenomenon. Culić et al. reported that 8% of patients with acute myocardial infarction reported vertigo as one of their presenting symptoms [89]. These forms of "cardiogenic" vertigo are hypothesized to be secondary to asymmetric perfusion of the right and left-sided vestibular structures in the inner ear and cerebellum during an episode of global hypoperfusion caused by cardiovascular disease [88]. The vertebral arteries may demonstrate underlying asymmetry or atherosclerosis that may predispose patients to focal ischemia of vestibular structures. Vertigo may thus be more commonly attributed to cardiovascular disease than would be expected. Given the episodic nature of cardiac arrhythmias, these attacks of cardiogenic vertigo can mimic more common vestibular disorders.

Endocrine Disorders

A range of endocrine disorders can present with atypical forms of dizziness. Diabetes mellitus (DM) is associated with a high rate of dizziness [90]. Even in the absence of symptomatic dizziness, DM often causes vestibular dysfunction, especially utricular hypofunction [91]. In addition to the otologic impact, DM insidiously leads to multisystem organ dysfunction in the cardiovascular system, brain, peripheral nerves, and eyes. As organ involvement differs by individual, the nature of the underlying vestibular complaints can vary tremendously. As indicated above, DM may both contribute to the pathogenesis and the clinical course of common vestibular disorders, such as BPPV and MD [92–94]. There is evidence that the effects of DM on the vestibular system are mediated by hypertension [93]. Hypothyroidism is similarly associated with vestibular pathology, including MD [95–99].

Obesity and Obstructive Sleep Apnea

Obesity has long been linked to benign intracranial hypertension (BIH; aka, pseudotumor cerebri) [100]. BIH commonly presents with dizziness and pulse-synchronous tinnitus, as well headaches [101]. The presentation of headaches and dizziness can mimic migraine [102]. BIH has also been associated with the development of MD [103]. Obesity has been linked to superior semicircular canal dehiscence [104]. Though related to obesity, obstructive sleep apnea has been independently associated with hearing loss, tinnitus, increased intracranial pressures, idiopathic dizziness and vertigo, and possibly MD [105–110]. Recognition of the role of obesity and OSA is important, as treatment with weight loss and CPAP may improve functional outcomes [111].

Medications and Medication Withdrawal

Dizziness is commonly reported with a wide range of medication therapy [112]. This is particularly true in elderly patients that are taking numerous medications with overlapping effects (i.e., polypharmacy) [113]. Many have direct, central nervous system effects or side effects. Many affect the balance system secondarily, particularly in the presence of underlying pathology, such as cardiac ischemia or dysrhythmias and VM. Abrupt discontinuation of selective serotonin reuptake inhibitors is known to cause dizziness, which may be positionally provoked [114].

Aging

Advancing age brings progressive degeneration of all organ systems, making dizziness and falls common in the elderly [115–117]. This often leads to a vicious cycle that includes a more sedentary lifestyle and generalized deconditioning and further compounds the symptoms resulting from vestibular dysfunction, CNS pathology, and vision loss [118]. Treatment of numerous vestibular and non-vestibular conditions may be needed to effect clinical improvement [119, 120]. Since many conditions afflicting the elderly cannot be treated, some authors have advocated forgoing exhaustive diagnostic evaluations in favor of focusing on establishing a prognosis and managing treatable issues (e.g., BPPV and polypharmacy) [121, 122].

Conclusions

Patients with complex dizziness and vestibular symptoms overlapping multiple disorders are challenging to diagnose. Episodic vertigo carries a broad differential diagnosis. A careful history including type, duration, and triggers of dizziness, association with headaches, medical comorbidities, family history, and neurotologic examination is recommended. There is no single clinical feature or test to reliably differentiate the underlying conditions in patients with overlapping symptoms. Comorbid PPPD may complicate the diagnosis and may generate an additional sensation of dizziness between episodes of vertigo. Non-vestibular pathologies such as central nervous system, cardiac, ophthalmologic, and musculoskeletal disorders can generate vertigo and non-vertiginous dizziness by affecting multisensory input, central integration, or vestibular motor output. Clinicians must be cognizant of atypical presentations of vestibular disorders and understand the impact of comorbid psychiatric and medical disorders on the clinical manifestations of balance disorders.

References

1. Kerber KA, Callaghan BC, Telian SA, Meurer WJ, Skolarus LE, Carender W, et al. Dizziness symptom type prevalence and overlap: a US nationally representative survey. Am J Med. Elsevier Inc. 2017;130(12):1465.e1–9.
2. Neuhauser H, Lempert T. Vertigo and dizziness related to migraine: a diagnostic challenge. Cephalalgia. 2004;24:83–91.
3. Thiruganasambandamoorthy V, Stiell IG, Wells GA, Vaidyanathan A, Mukarram M, Taljaard M. Outcomes in presyncope patients: a prospective cohort study. Ann Emerg Med. 2015;65:268–276.e6. Available from: http://www.ncbi.nlm.nih.gov/pubmed/25182542.
4. Newman-Toker DE, Cannon LM, Stofferahn ME, Rothman RE, Hsieh Y-H, Zee DS. Imprecision in patient reports of dizziness symptom quality: a cross-sectional study conducted in an acute care setting. Mayo Clin Proc. 2007;82:1329–40.
5. Voelker CC, Goebel JA. Clinical evaluation of the patient with vertigo. In: Johnson JT, Rosen CA, editors. Bailey's head and neck surgery—otolaryngology. 5th ed. Philadelphia: Lippincott Williams & Wilkins; 2014. p. 2673–700.
6. Hammam E, Macefield VG. Vestibular modulation of sympathetic nerve activity to muscle and skin in humans. Front Neurol. 2017;8:1–14.
7. Balaban CCD, Jacob RG, Furman JM. Neurologic bases for comorbidity of balance disorders, anxiety disorders and migraine: neurotherapeutic implications. Expert Rev Neurother. 2011;11:379–94.
8. Eggers SDZ, Neff BA, Shepard NT, Staab JP. Comorbidities in vestibular migraine. J Vestib Res. 2014;24:387–95.
9. Parnes LS, Agrawal SK, Atlas J. Diagnosis and management of benign paroxysmal positional vertigo (BPPV). CMAJ. 2003;169:681–93.
10. Picciotti PM, Lucidi D, De Corso E, Meucci D, Sergi B, Paludetti G. Comorbidities and recurrence of benign paroxysmal positional vertigo: personal experience. Int J Audiol. 2016;2027:1–6.
11. Riga M, Bibas A, Xenellis J, Korres S. Inner ear disease and benign paroxysmal positional vertigo: a critical review of incidence, clinical characteristics, and management. Int J Otolaryngol. 2011;2011:1–7.
12. Faralli M, Lapenna R, Giommetti G, Pellegrino C, Ricci G. Residual dizziness after the first BPPV episode: role of otolithic function and of a delayed diagnosis. Eur Arch Otorhinolaryngol. 2016;273:3157–65. Available from: http://www.ncbi.nlm.nih.gov/pubmed/26926693.
13. Teggi R, Quaglieri S, Gatti O, Benazzo M, Bussi M. Residual dizziness after successful repositioning maneuvers for idiopathic benign paroxysmal positional vertigo. ORL J Otorhinolaryngol Relat Spec. 2013;75:74–81. Available from: http://www.ncbi.nlm.nih.gov/pubmed/23774304.

14. Naert L, Van de Berg R, Van de Heyning P, Bisdorff A, Sharon JD, Ward BK, et al. Aggregating the symptoms of superior semicircular canal dehiscence syndrome. Laryngoscope. 2018;128(8):1932–8. Available from: http://www.ncbi.nlm.nih.gov/pubmed/29280497.
15. Suzuki M, Kitajima N, Ushio M, Shintani M, Ishibashi T. Changes in the Tullio phenomenon and the fistula sign in the course of endolymphatic hydrops. ORL J Otorhinolaryngol Relat Spec. 2003;65:125–8. Available from: http://www.ncbi.nlm.nih.gov/pubmed/12824736.
16. Pyykkö I, Manchaiah V, Zou J, Levo H, Kentala E. Vestibular syncope: a disorder associated with drop attack in Ménière's disease. Auris Nasus Larynx. Elsevier Ireland Ltd. 2018;45(2):234–41.
17. Ildiz F, Dündar A. A case of Tullio phenomenon in a subject with oval window fistula due to barotrauma. Aviat Space Environ Med. 1994;65:67–9. Available from: http://www.ncbi.nlm.nih.gov/pubmed/8117230.
18. Fox EJ, Balkany TJ, Arenberg IK. The Tullio phenomenon and perilymph fistula. Otolaryngol Head Neck Surg. 1988;98:88–9. Available from: http://www.ncbi.nlm.nih.gov/pubmed/3124057.
19. Finn S, Dietzek M, Karvouniari P, Klingner CM, Neumann R, Guntinas-Lichius O, et al. Bilateral vestibulopathy with positive Tullio phenomenon. Laryngoscope. 2018;128(5):1223–5. Available from: http://www.ncbi.nlm.nih.gov/pubmed/28561344.
20. Wenzel A, Ward BK, Schubert MC, Kheradmand A, Zee DS, Mantokoudis G, et al. Patients with vestibular loss, tullio phenomenon, and pressure-induced nystagmus: vestibular atelectasis? Otol Neurotol. 2014;35:866–72.
21. Newman-Toker DE. Symptoms and signs of neuro-otologic disorders. Continuum. 2012;18:1016–40.
22. Balle V, Linthicum FH. Histologically proven cochlear otosclerosis with pure sensorineural hearing loss. Ann Otol Rhinol Laryngol. 1984;93:105–11. Available from: http://www.ncbi.nlm.nih.gov/pubmed/6712083.
23. Eza-Nuñez P, Manrique-Rodriguez M, Perez-Fernandez N. Otosclerosis among patients with dizziness. Rev Laryngol Otol Rhinol (Bord). 2010;131:199–206. Available from: http://www.ncbi.nlm.nih.gov/pubmed/21488576.
24. de Vilhena D, Gambôa I, Duarte D, Lopes G. Vestibular disorders after stapedial surgery in patients with otosclerosis. Int J Otolaryngol. 2016;2016:6830648. Available from: http://www.ncbi.nlm.nih.gov/pubmed/26904127.
25. Ishai R, Halpin CF, McKenna MJ, Quesnel AM. How often does stapedectomy for otosclerosis result in endolymphatic hydrops? Otol Neurotol. 2016;37:984–90. Available from: http://www.ncbi.nlm.nih.gov/pubmed/27380537.
26. Lempert T, Olesen J, Furman J, Waterston J, Seemungal B, Carey J, et al. Vestibular migraine: diagnostic criteria. J Vestib Res. 2012;22:167–72.
27. Neff BA, Staab JP, Eggers SD, Carlson ML, Schmitt WR, Van Abel KM, et al. Auditory and vestibular symptoms and chronic subjective dizziness in patients with Ménière's disease, vestibular migraine, and Ménière's disease with concomitant vestibular migraine. Otol Neurotol. 2012;33:1235–44.
28. Lopez-Escamez JA, Carey J, Chung WH, Goebel JA, Magnusson M, Mandalà M, et al. Diagnostic criteria for Menière's disease. J Vestib Res. 2015;25:1–7.
29. Neuhauser HK. Epidemiology of vertigo. Curr Opin Neurol. 2007;20:40–6.
30. Tabet P, Saliba I. Meniere's disease and vestibular migraine: updates and review of the literature. J Clin Med Res. 2017;9:733–44.
31. Neuhauser H, Leopold M, von Brevern M, Arnold G, Lempert T. The interrelations of migraine, vertigo, and migrainous vertigo. Neurology. 2001;56:436–41.
32. Neuhauser H, Lempert T. Vestibular migraine. Neurol Clin. 2009;27:379–91.
33. Salmito MC, Morganti LOG, Nakao BH, Simões JC, Duarte JA, Ganança FF. Vestibular migraine: comparative analysis between diagnostic criteria. Braz J Otorhinolaryngol. 2015;81:485–90.

34. Brandt T, Strupp M, Dieterich M. Vestibular paroxysmia: a treatable neurovascular cross-compression syndrome. J Neurol. Springer Berlin Heidelberg. 2016;263:90–6.
35. Kayan A, Hood JD. Neuro-otological manifestations of migraine. Brain. 1984;107(Pt 4):1123–42.
36. Battista RA. Audiometric findings of patients with migraine-associated dizziness. Otol Neurotol. 2004;25:987–92.
37. Radtke A, Neuhauser H, von Brevern M, Hottenrott T, Lempert T. Vestibular migraine—validity of clinical diagnostic criteria. Cephalalgia. 2011;31:906–13.
38. Lopez-Escamez JA, Dlugaiczyk J, Jacobs J, Lempert T, Teggi R, von Brevern M, et al. Accompanying symptoms overlap during attacks in Meniere's disease and vestibular migraine. Front Neurol. 2014;5:1–5.
39. Obermann M, Wurthmann S, Steinberg BS, Theysohn N, Diener H-C, Naegel S. Central vestibular system modulation in vestibular migraine. Cephalalgia. 2014;34:1053–61. Available from: http://www.ncbi.nlm.nih.gov/pubmed/24662323.
40. Nakada T, Yoshida T, Suga K, Kato M, Otake H, Kato K, et al. Endolymphatic space size in patients with vestibular migraine and Ménière's disease. J Neurol. 2014;261:2079–84.
41. Gürkov R, Kantner C, Strupp M, Flatz W, Krause E, Ertl-Wagner B. Endolymphatic hydrops in patients with vestibular migraine and auditory symptoms. Eur Arch Otorhinolaryngol. 2014;271:2661–7.
42. Sharon JD, Hullar TE. Motion sensitivity and caloric responsiveness in vestibular migraine and Meniere's disease. Laryngoscope. 2014;124:969–73.
43. Hong HR, Shim DB, Kim TS, Shim BS, Ahn JH, Chung JW, et al. Results of caloric and sensory organization testing of dynamic posturography in migrainous vertigo: comparison with Meniere's disease and vestibular neuritis. Acta Otolaryngol. 2013;133:1236–41.
44. Blödow A, Heinze M, Bloching MB, von Brevern M, Radtke A, Lempert T. Caloric stimulation and video-head impulse testing in Ménière's disease and vestibular migraine. Acta Otolaryngol. 2014;134:1239–44.
45. Taylor RL, Zagami AS, Gibson WP, Black DA, Watson SR, Halmagyi MG, et al. Vestibular evoked myogenic potentials to sound and vibration: characteristics in vestibular migraine that enable separation from Menière's disease. Cephalalgia. 2012;32:213–25.
46. Martin-Sanz E, Vargas Salamanca E, Marqués Cabrero A, Esteban J, Muerte I, Sanz-Fernández R. Value of clinical data and vestibular testing in a population of 101 patients with recurrent vestibulopathy. Clin Otolaryngol. 2014;39:311–5.
47. Zuniga MG, Janky KL, Schubert MC, Carey JP. Can vestibular-evoked myogenic potentials help differentiate Ménière disease from vestibular migraine? Otolaryngol Head Neck Surg. 2012;146:788–96.
48. Baier B, Dieterich M. Vestibular-evoked myogenic potentials in "vestibular migraine" and Meniere's disease: a sign of an electrophysiological link? Ann NY Acad Sci. 2009;1164:324–7.
49. Murofushi T, Ozeki H, Inoue A, Sakata A. Does migraine-associated vertigo share a common pathophysiology with Meniere's disease? Study with vestibular-evoked myogenic potential. Cephalalgia. 2009;29:1259–66.
50. Inoue A, Egami N, Fujimoto C, Kinoshita M, Yamasoba T, Iwasaki S. Vestibular evoked myogenic potentials in vestibular migraine: do they help differentiating from Menière's disease? Ann Otol Rhinol Laryngol. 2016;125:931–7.
51. Heuberger M, Sağlam M, Todd NS, Jahn K, Schneider E, Lehnen N. Covert anti-compensatory quick eye movements during head impulses. PLoS One. 2014;9:4–7.
52. Jannetta PJ. Neurovascular cross-compression in patients with hyperactive dysfunction symptoms of the eighth cranial nerve. Surg Forum. 1975;26:467–9.
53. Brandt T, Dieterich M. Vestibular paroxysmia: vascular compression of the eighth nerve? Lancet (London, England). 1994;343:798–9. Available from: http://www.ncbi.nlm.nih.gov/pubmed/7907760.

54. Strupp M, Lopez-Escamez JA, Kim JS, Straumann D, Jen JC, Carey J, et al. Vestibular paroxysmia: diagnostic criteria. J Vestib Res. 2017;26:409–15.
55. Best C, Gawehn J, Krämer HH, Thömke F, Ibis T, Müller-Forell W, et al. MRI and neurophysiology in vestibular paroxysmia: contradiction and correlation. J Neurol Neurosurg Psychiatry. 2013;84:1349–56. Available from: http://jnnp.bmj.com/lookup/doi/10.1136/jnnp-2013-305513.
56. Staab JP, Eckhardt-Henn A, Horii A, Jacob R, Strupp M, Brandt T, et al. Diagnostic criteria for persistent postural-perceptual dizziness (PPPD): consensus document of the committee for the Classification of Vestibular Disorders of the Barany Society. J Vestib Res. 2017;27:191–208.
57. Staab JP. Chronic subjective dizziness. Continuum. 2012;18:1118–41.
58. Ruckenstein MJ, Staab JP. Chronic subjective dizziness. Otolaryngol Clin N Am. 2009;42:71–7, ix.
59. Thompson KJ, Goetting JC, Staab JP, Shepard NT. Retrospective review and telephone follow-up to evaluate a physical therapy protocol for treating persistent postural-perceptual dizziness: a pilot study. J Vestib Res. 2015;25:97–104.
60. Cuomo-Granston A, Drummond PD. Migraine and motion sickness: what is the link? Prog Neurobiol. Elsevier Ltd. 2010;91:300–12.
61. Murdin L, Chamberlain F, Cheema S, Arshad Q, Gresty MA, Golding JF, et al. Motion sickness in migraine and vestibular disorders. J Neurol Neurosurg Psychiatry. 2015;86:585–7.
62. Golding JF, Patel M. Meniere's, migraine, and motion sickness. Acta Otolaryngol. 2017;137:495–502.
63. Neuhauser HK. The epidemiology of dizziness and vertigo. Handb Clin Neurol. 2016;137:67–82.
64. Lahmann C, Henningsen P, Brandt T, Strupp M, Jahn K, Dieterich M, et al. Psychiatric comorbidity and psychosocial impairment among patients with vertigo and dizziness. J Neurol Neurosurg Psychiatry. 2015;86:302–8.
65. Langhagen T, Schroeder AS, Rettinger N, Borggraefe I, Jahn K. Migraine-related vertigo and somatoform vertigo frequently occur in children and are often associated. Neuropediatrics. 2013;44:55–8.
66. Staab JP. The influence of anxiety on ocular motor control and gaze. Curr Opin Neurol. 2014;27:118–24. Available from: http://content.wkhealth.com/linkback/openurl?sid=WKPTLP:landingpage&an=00019052-201402000-00019.
67. Perloff MD, Patel NS, Kase CS, Oza AU, Voetsch B, Romero JR. Cerebellar stroke presenting with isolated dizziness: brain MRI in 136 patients. Am J Emerg Med. 2017;35:1724–9. Available from: http://www.ncbi.nlm.nih.gov/pubmed/28687453.
68. Newman-Toker DE, Kerber KA, Hsieh Y-H, Pula JH, Omron R, Saber Tehrani AS, et al. HINTS outperforms ABCD2 to screen for stroke in acute continuous vertigo and dizziness. Acad Emerg Med. 2013;20:986–96. Available from: http://www.ncbi.nlm.nih.gov/pubmed/24127701.
69. Saber Tehrani AS, Kattah JC, Mantokoudis G, Pula JH, Nair D, Blitz A, et al. Small strokes causing severe vertigo: frequency of false-negative MRIs and nonlacunar mechanisms. Neurology. 2014;83:169–73. Available from: http://www.ncbi.nlm.nih.gov/pubmed/24920847.
70. Kleffner I, Dörr J, Ringelstein M, Gross CC, Böckenfeld Y, Schwindt W, et al. Diagnostic criteria for Susac syndrome. J Neurol Neurosurg Psychiatry. 2016;87:1287–95. Available from: http://www.ncbi.nlm.nih.gov/pubmed/28103199.
71. Hain TC. Cervicogenic causes of vertigo. Curr Opin Neurol. 2015;28:69–73.
72. Yacovino DA, Hain TC. Clinical characteristics of cervicogenic-related dizziness and vertigo. Semin Neurol. 2013;33:244–55.
73. Lu DC, Zador Z, Mummaneni PV, Lawton MT. Rotational vertebral artery occlusion-series of 9 cases. Neurosurgery. 2010;67:1066–72; discussion 1072.

74. Borg-Stein J, Rauch S, Krabak B. Evaluation and management of cervicogenic dizziness. Crit Rev Phys Rehabil Med. 2001;13:255–64.
75. Strupp M, Arbusow V, Borges Pereira C, Dieterich M, Brandt T. Subjective straight-ahead during neck muscle vibration: effects of ageing. Neuroreport. 1999;10:3191–4.
76. Schweigart G, Chien RD, Mergner T. Neck proprioception compensates for age-related deterioration of vestibular self-motion perception. Exp Brain Res. 2002;147:89–97.
77. Racicki S, Gerwin S, DiClaudio S, Reinmann S, Donaldson M. Conservative physical therapy management for the treatment of cervicogenic headache: a systematic review. J Man Manip Ther. 2013;21:113–24.
78. Ren L, Guo B, Zhang J, Han Z, Zhang T, Bai Q, et al. Mid-term efficacy of percutaneous laser disc decompression for treatment of cervical vertigo. Eur J Orthop Surg Traumatol. 2014;24:153–8.
79. Li J, Gu T, Yang H, Liang L, Jiang D-J, Wang Z-C, et al. Sympathetic nerve innervation in cervical posterior longitudinal ligament as a potential causative factor in cervical spondylosis with sympathetic symptoms and preliminary evidence. Med Hypotheses. Elsevier Ltd. 2014;82:631–5.
80. Rosner MS, Feinberg DL, Doble JE, Rosner AJ. Treatment of vertical heterophoria ameliorates persistent post-concussive symptoms: a retrospective analysis utilizing a multi-faceted assessment battery. Brain Inj. Informa Healthcare. 2016;30:311–7.
81. Anoh-Tanon MJ, Bremond-Gignac D, Wiener-Vacher SR. Vertigo is an underestimated symptom of ocular disorders: dizzy children do not always need MRI. Pediatr Neurol. 2000;23:49–53.
82. Barin K, Dodson EE. Dizziness in the elderly. Otolaryngol Clin N Am. 2011;44:437–54.
83. Singh R, Maurya OP, Yadav VS, Samant HC. Audiometric and vestibular abnormalities in macular degeneration. Indian J Ophthalmol. 1991;39:127–8. Available from: http://www.ncbi.nlm.nih.gov/pubmed/1841887.
84. Althomali MM, Leat SJ. Binocular vision disorders and visual attention: associations with balance and mobility in older adults. J Aging Phys Act. 2017;26(2):235–47. Available from: http://www.ncbi.nlm.nih.gov/pubmed/28714802.
85. Bender M. Oscillopsia. Arch Neurol. 1965;13:204–13.
86. Bronstein AM. Vision and vertigo: some visual aspects of vestibular disorders. J Neurol. 2004;251:381–7.
87. Low PA, Opfer-Gehrking TL, McPhee BR, Fealey RD, Benarroch EE, Willner CL, et al. Prospective evaluation of clinical characteristics of orthostatic hypotension. Mayo Clin Proc. 1995;70:617–22.
88. Newman-Toker DE, Camargo CA. "Cardiogenic vertigo"—true vertigo as the presenting manifestation of primary cardiac disease. Nat Clin Pract Neurol. 2006;2:167–72; quiz 173.
89. Culić V, Mirić D, Eterović D. Correlation between symptomatology and site of acute myocardial infarction. Int J Cardiol. 2001;77:163–8.
90. Agrawal Y, Carey JP, Della Santina CC, Schubert MC, Minor LB. Disorders of balance and vestibular function in US adults: data from the National Health and Nutrition Examination Survey, 2001-2004. Arch Intern Med. 2009;169:938–44. Available from: http://archinte.jamanetwork.com/article.aspx?doi=10.1001/archinternmed.2009.66.
91. Jáuregui-Renaud K, Aranda-Moreno C, Herrera-Rangel A. Utricular hypofunction in patients with type 2 diabetes mellitus. Acta Otorhinolaryngol Ital. 2017;37:430–5. Available from: http://www.ncbi.nlm.nih.gov/pubmed/28530263.
92. Warninghoff JC, Bayer O, Ferrari U, Straube A. Co-morbidities of vertiginous diseases. BMC Neurol. 2009;9:29. Available from: http://www.ncbi.nlm.nih.gov/pubmed/19583869.
93. D'Silva LJ, Staecker H, Lin J, Sykes KJ, Phadnis MA, McMahon TM, et al. Retrospective data suggests that the higher prevalence of benign paroxysmal positional vertigo in individuals with type 2 diabetes is mediated by hypertension. J Vestib Res. 2016;25:233–9. Available from: http://www.ncbi.nlm.nih.gov/pubmed/26890424.

94. Pieskä T, Kotimäki J, Männikkö M, Sorri M, Hietikko E. Concomitant diseases and their effect on disease prognosis in Meniere's disease: diabetes mellitus identified as a negative prognostic factor. Acta Otolaryngol. 2018;138:36–40. Available from: http://www.ncbi.nlm.nih.gov/pubmed/28914106.
95. Wojtczak R, Narożny W, Kuczkowski J, Siebert J. Epidemiology of dizziness in northern Poland – the first Polish neurootologic survey of the general population. Ann Agric Environ Med. 2017;24:502–6. Available from: http://www.ncbi.nlm.nih.gov/pubmed/28954498.
96. Rybak LP. Metabolic disorders of the vestibular system. Otolaryngol Head Neck Surg. 1995;112:128–32. Available from: http://www.ncbi.nlm.nih.gov/pubmed/7816447.
97. Bhatia PL, Gupta OP, Agrawal MK, Mishr SK. Audiological and vestibular function tests in hypothyroidism. Laryngoscope. 1977;87:2082–9. Available from: http://www.ncbi.nlm.nih.gov/pubmed/926972.
98. Brenner M, Hoistad DL, Hain TC. Prevalence of thyroid dysfunction in patients with Ménière's disease. Arch Otolaryngol Head Neck Surg. 2004;130:226–8. Available from: http://www.ncbi.nlm.nih.gov/pubmed/14967756.
99. Santosh UP, Rao MSS. Incidence of hypothyroidism in Meniere's disease. J Clin Diagn Res. 2016;10:MC01–3. Available from: http://www.ncbi.nlm.nih.gov/pubmed/27437251.
100. Hannerz J, Greitz D, Ericson K. Is there a relationship between obesity and intracranial hypertension? Int J Obes Relat Metab Disord. 1995;19:240–4. Available from: http://www.ncbi.nlm.nih.gov/pubmed/7627247.
101. Wall M, Kupersmith MJ, Kieburtz KD, Corbett JJ, Feldon SE, Friedman DI, et al. The idiopathic intracranial hypertension treatment trial: clinical profile at baseline. JAMA Neurol. 2014;71:693–701. Available from: http://www.ncbi.nlm.nih.gov/pubmed/24756302.
102. Lee EB, Edelman FS, Stafstrom CE. Evidence of diplopia in children's headache drawings helps to differentiate pseudotumor cerebri from migraine. Pediatr Neurol. 2018;79:40–4. Available from: http://www.ncbi.nlm.nih.gov/pubmed/29413638.
103. Ranieri A, Cavaliere M, Sicignano S, Falco P, Cautiero F, De Simone R. Endolymphatic hydrops in idiopathic intracranial hypertension: prevalence and clinical outcome after lumbar puncture. Preliminary data. Neurol Sci. 2017;38:193–6. Available from: http://www.ncbi.nlm.nih.gov/pubmed/28527079.
104. Rizk HG, Hatch JL, Stevens SM, Lambert PR, Meyer TA. Lateral skull base attenuation in superior semicircular canal dehiscence and spontaneous cerebrospinal fluid otorrhea. Otolaryngol Head Neck Surg. 2016;155:641–8. Available from: http://www.ncbi.nlm.nih.gov/pubmed/27221578.
105. Chopra A, Jung M, Kaplan RC, Appel DW, Dinces EA, Dhar S, et al. Sleep apnea is associated with hearing impairment: the Hispanic Community Health Study/Study of Latinos. J Clin Sleep Med. 2016;12:719–26. Available from: http://www.ncbi.nlm.nih.gov/pubmed/26951413.
106. Koo M, Hwang J-H. Risk of tinnitus in patients with sleep apnea: a nationwide, population-based, case-control study. Laryngoscope. 2017;127:2171–5. Available from: http://www.ncbi.nlm.nih.gov/pubmed/27666578.
107. Jennum P, Børgesen SE. Intracranial pressure and obstructive sleep apnea. Chest. 1989;95:279–83. Available from: http://www.ncbi.nlm.nih.gov/pubmed/2914475.
108. Sowerby LJ, Rotenberg B, Brine M, George CFP, Parnes LS. Sleep apnea, daytime somnolence, and idiopathic dizziness—a novel association. Laryngoscope. 2010;120:1274–8. Available from: http://www.ncbi.nlm.nih.gov/pubmed/20513051.
109. Tsai M-S, Lee L-A, Tsai Y-T, Yang Y-H, Liu C-Y, Lin M-H, et al. Sleep apnea and risk of vertigo: a nationwide population-based cohort study. Laryngoscope. 2018;128:763–8. Available from: http://www.ncbi.nlm.nih.gov/pubmed/28771753.
110. Nakayama M, Kabaya K. Obstructive sleep apnea syndrome as a novel cause for Ménière's disease. Curr Opin Otolaryngol Head Neck Surg. 2013;21:503–8. Available from: http://www.ncbi.nlm.nih.gov/pubmed/23989598.

111. Thurtell MJ, Wall M. Idiopathic intracranial hypertension (pseudotumor cerebri): recognition, treatment, and ongoing management. Curr Treat Options Neurol. 2013;15:1–12. Available from: http://www.ncbi.nlm.nih.gov/pubmed/23136035.
112. Chimirri S, Aiello R, Mazzitello C, Mumoli L, Palleria C, Altomonte M, et al. Vertigo/dizziness as a drugs' adverse reaction. J Pharmacol Pharmacother. 2013;4:S104–9. Available from: http://www.ncbi.nlm.nih.gov/pubmed/24347974.
113. Shoair OA, Nyandege AN, Slattum PW. Medication-related dizziness in the older adult. Otolaryngol Clin North Am. 2011;44:455–71, x. Available from: http://www.ncbi.nlm.nih.gov/pubmed/21474017.
114. Smith PF, Darlington CL. A possible explanation for dizziness following SSRI discontinuation. Acta Otolaryngol. 2010;130:981–3. Available from: http://www.ncbi.nlm.nih.gov/pubmed/20144124.
115. Fernández L, Breinbauer HA, Delano PH. Vertigo and dizziness in the elderly. Front Neurol. 2015;6:144. Available from: http://www.ncbi.nlm.nih.gov/pubmed/26167157.
116. Ciorba A, Bianchini C, Scanelli G, Pala M, Zurlo A, Aimoni C. The impact of dizziness on quality-of-life in the elderly. Eur Arch Otorhinolaryngol. 2017;274:1245–50. Available from: http://www.ncbi.nlm.nih.gov/pubmed/27450383.
117. Iwasaki S, Yamasoba T. Dizziness and imbalance in the elderly: age-related decline in the vestibular system. Aging Dis. 2015;6:38–47. Available from: http://www.ncbi.nlm.nih.gov/pubmed/25657851.
118. Mueller M, Strobl R, Jahn K, Linkohr B, Peters A, Grill E. Burden of disability attributable to vertigo and dizziness in the aged: results from the KORA-Age study. Eur J Public Health. 2014;24:802–7. Available from: http://www.ncbi.nlm.nih.gov/pubmed/24213583.
119. Jahn K, Kressig RW, Bridenbaugh SA, Brandt T, Schniepp R. Dizziness and unstable gait in old age: etiology, diagnosis and treatment. Dtsch Arztebl Int. 2015;112:387–93. Available from: http://www.ncbi.nlm.nih.gov/pubmed/26157011.
120. Ahearn DJ, Umapathy D. Vestibular impairment in older people frequently contributes to dizziness as part of a geriatric syndrome. Clin Med. 2015;15:25–30. Available from: http://www.ncbi.nlm.nih.gov/pubmed/25650194.
121. Maarsingh OR, Stam H, van der Horst HE. A different approach of dizziness in older patients: away from the diagnostic dance between patient and physician. Front Med. 2014;1:50. Available from: http://www.ncbi.nlm.nih.gov/pubmed/25593923.
122. Dros J, Maarsingh OR, Beem L, van der Horst HE, ter Riet G, Schellevis FG, et al. Functional prognosis of dizziness in older adults in primary care: a prospective cohort study. J Am Geriatr Soc. 2012;60:2263–9. Available from: http://www.ncbi.nlm.nih.gov/pubmed/23231549.

Chapter 26
Multisensory Imbalance and Presbystasis

Bradley W. Kesser and A. Tucker Gleason

Aging and Population Health Statistics: Prevalence of Dizziness

The United States population aged 65 and over ("older adults" according to the US Census Bureau and the term used in this chapter) is projected to jump from 43.1 million in 2012 (13.7% of the population) to 72.8 million (20.3% of the population) in 2030 [10]. In one analysis of over 131,000 consecutive visits to an otolaryngology practice, geriatric patients showed a statistically significant increase from 14.3% to 17.9% between 2004 and 2010; predictive analysis estimates that by 2030, 30% of all patients presenting to an otolaryngology clinic will be over 65, and that 74% of their diagnoses will be otologic in nature [11]. Practitioners—otolaryngologists, neurologists, family medicine doctors, internists, audiologists, physical therapists, and others—will increasingly see and evaluate more and more older "dizzy" patients.

While not all elderly patients complain of dizziness, the prevalence of dizziness clearly increases with increasing age. These increased prevalence rates with age span population-based studies, community-based studies, and primary and specialty care clinic population studies. Population-based studies estimate the prevalence of dizziness among the older population (65 and older) to be 20–30% [12–14] and as high as 50% in the over 85 age group [15]. Women seem to be affected more

B. W. Kesser (✉) · A. T. Gleason
University of Virginia, Department of Otolaryngology-Head and Neck Surgery, Charlottesville, VA, USA
e-mail: Bwk2n@uvahealth.org

J. C. Lucas et al. (eds.), *Diagnosis and Treatment of Vestibular Disorders*,
https://doi.org/10.1007/978-3-032-11740-3_26

commonly than men [14, 15], with 36% of women age 70 and 29% of men age 70 complaining of dizziness in one survey study [15]. Among the 2751 Blue Mountain patient cohort in Australia, participants reporting dizziness/vertigo had lower quality of life scores [12]. The 2001–2004 National Health and Nutrition Examination Survey assessed vestibular function objectively with the modified Romberg test, and vestibular impairment was inferred from an inability to stand with eyes closed on a foam pad. With this criterion, 35% of the US population over 40 had balance dysfunction; the odds of vestibular dysfunction increased significantly with age, and 85% of people over 80 surveyed had balance impairment [16].

With regard to healthcare utilization, the 2008 National Health Interview Survey reported that 50% of older individuals with dizziness and balance complaints saw one medical provider—86% saw a general practitioner, 24% saw a neurologist, and 17% saw an otolaryngologist; 35% of these patients saw three or more providers, and approximately 57% had an imaging study. Interestingly, according to the report, despite these resources, >40% of older individuals still did not have a clear diagnosis for their symptoms [17]. Hence, the term "presbystasis," age-related decline in balance function, a term patients can carry with them as their diagnosis.

Fall Injury Statistics

Perhaps the greatest concern regarding dizziness in the elderly is the risk of falling. One in three to one in four older adults falls each year, and 50% of those falling once will fall again [18, 19]. Dizziness and vestibular disorders have been shown to be independent risk factors for falling [18, 20–22] and have been estimated to increase the risk of falling by two to three-fold [23–25]. In a meta-analysis of 12 large studies, Rubinstein and Josephson estimated that balance disorders and dizziness are the second and third leading causes of falls in older persons [21, 26–28]. Symptoms of dizziness, imbalance, and lightheadedness also lead to a fear of falling [26–28], and fear of falling is another risk factor for falling [26].

Falls carry a tremendous risk of morbidity and cost and are the leading cause of fatal and non-fatal injuries among adults over 65. The Centers for Disease Control and Prevention (CDC) analyzed data from the 2014 Behavioral Risk Factor Surveillance System (BRFSS) survey and found that 28.7% of older adults reported falling in the previous year. The CDC further documents 29 million falls among 46 million older adults in the United States with 7 million fall-related injuries in 2014 and estimates 12 million fall injuries among 49 million falls in 2030 (74 million older adults) [19, 29]. Falls are the leading cause of accidental death among the elderly and are the main reason for hospital admission in this age group [4]. According to the CDC in 2014:

- 27,000 older adults died because of falls
- 2.8 million patients were treated in emergency departments for fall-related injuries
- 800,000 of these patients were subsequently hospitalized

- Women were more likely to fall than men
- Fall risk increases with increasing age to as high as 36.5% among persons 85 and over [29, 30]

The cost of falls is exorbitant—in 2012, there were 24,190 fatal and 3.2 million medically treated non-fatal fall-related injuries. Direct medical costs totaled $616.5 million for fatal and $30.3 billion for non-fatal injuries and rose to $637.5 million and $31.3 billion, respectively, in 2015. Fall incidence and total cost increased with age and were higher among women [31]. Clearly, falls, and those conditions leading to falls, create a substantial direct and indirect physical, emotional, and financial cost to patients, families, and society.

Physiological Considerations of Aging

Balance and postural control are complex processes maintained and mediated by central neurological control of three primary peripheral sensory systems: vestibular, visual, and proprioceptive. Dysfunction in any peripheral sensory system can lead to imbalance or dizziness as can dysregulation of central control of these processes. Aging has multiple effects on all of these processes, and the next section discusses each sensory system and factors that can lead to loss of central neurologic control, including efferent pathways and the musculoskeletal system, cardiovascular abnormalities, including the baroreceptor reflex, medication and polypharmacy, cognitive decline, and other specific central neurologic and neurovascular disease states.

Vestibular

The primary purpose of the vestibular system is to maintain or stabilize gaze despite head or body motion (vestibulo-ocular reflex [VOR]) and to maintain upright posture and stabilize the trunk and limbs despite head motion (postural control; vestibulo-spinal reflex [VSR]).

Age-related loss of vestibular function ("presbyvestibulopathy") has been documented both histologically and functionally. Hair cell loss or degeneration has been implicated in presbycusis [32]; so too, vestibular hair cells in the cristae of the semicircular canals and maculae of the otolith organs [33] as well as vestibular ganglion cells [34], primary afferents [35], and brainstem vestibular nucleus cell populations [36] are all subject to age related decline and degeneration [32, 37–39].

With such anatomic decline and change in morphology of vestibular cell populations comes potential concomitant functional decline. Functional decline in the vestibulo-ocular reflex manifests as "dizziness" (abnormal sensation of motion), and functional decline in the vestibulo-spinal reflex manifests as imbalance or postural instability [40]. Interestingly, one series of studies did not show a significant age-related decline in rotary chair testing, caloric testing, or postural control in subjects ranging from 7 to 81 [41, 42].

Other tests, however, have shown functional decline in the vestibular system with age when looking at the VOR, especially at higher frequencies [43, 44], ocular counter-roll, and postural sway [45]. One study reported only subtle age changes in rotary chair and caloric testing, with more pronounced age-related changes in vestibular evoked myogenic potential (VEMP) testing with decreasing amplitudes, increasing thresholds, and decreasing N1 latencies [46]. When seeking normative data for the head impulse test (HIT), Mossman et al. showed very little decline in age-related VOR and stated, "Normative data with respect to HVOR velocity gain decreases slightly with age, but with careful attention to methodology, the 2 standard deviation lower limit of normal is relatively robust across a wide age range and into the eighth decade, without requirement for adjustment with age" [47].

Taken together, age-related changes in the vestibular system seem to show relative preservation or small declines in peripheral (at least horizontal) semicircular canal function (VOR), with greater deterioration in otolith function. One study suggests that age-related changes in the otolith-ocular reflex and semicircular canal-otolith interaction are a result primarily of degradation in central vestibular processing of otolith signals rather than a decline of peripheral vestibular function [48]. Despite changes in the VOR over time in a cohort of older subjects followed longitudinally, patients did not show signs or symptoms of disequilibrium. Clinically, the implications are for poorer postural control and a higher risk of falling for elderly patients (females more so than males [45]), but older patients' ability to turn the head and maintain gaze remains intact.

Visual

Changes in visual acuity, contrast sensitivity, depth perception, and low-light vision all show age-related decline and contribute to presbystasis. Older patients have difficulty judging distance—steps, curbs—and can thus be at risk for falls. When standing on a firm surface, visual acuity and contrast sensitivity were not associated with body sway, but on a compliant surface, body sway was associated with poor visual acuity and contrast sensitivity [49]. These authors also found a difference in contrast sensitivity between those who had fallen and those who had not, and concluded that reduced vision, particularly impaired depth perception, slow reaction time, and increased body sway on a compliant surface, were the strongest predisposing risk factors for postural imbalance and falls [49, 50]. Patients reporting multiple falls had decreased vision on all tests of vision, with impaired depth perception, contrast sensitivity, and low-contrast visual acuity being the strongest risk factors [50]. Reduced contrast sensitivity and impaired low contrast visual acuity and depth perception seem to be the greatest visual risk factors for falls [51]. One author has suggested that multifocal lenses increase the risk for falls by impairing distance contrast sensitivity and depth perception in the lower visual field (where the hazards are); further, cataract surgery may help prevent falls [51].

The complex interactions between an aging visual system and an aging vestibular system, especially the otolith organs involved in postural control, further place elderly patients at fall risk. In addition, when exposed to a moving visual scene, older subjects exhibited greater postural sway than younger subjects [52].

Referral to ophthalmology for vision assessment can greatly improve balance, as can ensuring good lighting. As humans age, we rely more on vision to assist in balance function (even in subjects age 44–60) [53], especially when proprioceptive information may be compromised by comorbid diseases, such as the peripheral neuropathy of diabetes and renal disease, rheumatoid arthritis, and other autoimmune disorders, as well as degenerative changes in the spine (see also section "Proprioception" below).

Proprioception

Comorbidities that often accompany aging, such as rheumatoid arthritis and osteoarthritis, contribute to presbystasis through alterations in joint proprioception, joint stiffness and decreased mobility, and structural changes in the vertebral spine and its associated ligaments. Spinal stenosis, herniated nucleus pulposus, foraminal stenosis, kyphosis, lordosis, scoliosis, etc. can lead to aberrations of the sensory input to the brain and vestibular centers leading to postural instability and increased risk of falling. Motor changes as a result of the above spinal diseases also predispose to falling.

Peripheral neuropathy can be caused by numerous disease states, including diabetes and chronic renal disease; medications, including cancer chemotherapeutic agents, can also cause derangements in proprioceptive sense (not to mention vestibular toxicity). In patients with vestibulopathy, peripheral neuropathy is an independent risk factor for falls [54]. Reduction of vibration and tactile sensation at the ankle and knee joints has also been associated with an increased risk of falls in the elderly [49, 55]. In this study of elderly residents of an assisted living facility, proprioception in the lower limbs, visual contrast sensitivity, ankle dorsiflexion strength, reaction time, and sway with the eyes closed significantly discriminated between subjects who did not fall or fell only once during the 1 year study period and those who fell multiple times; interestingly, there was little difference in the mean scores of tests of vestibular function among the non-fallers, once-only fallers, and multiple fallers [55].

Finally, peripheral sensory receptors and the axons that propagate their signals are subject to age-related change. These sensors in the foot and ankle are critical for postural control and assessing the contact of the foot with the ground or pavement, and thus, the orientation and movement of the body. Vibration and touch thresholds decline in older individuals adversely affecting tactile information arising from the feet at their contact point with the ground [56]. In addition, the ability to detect the position and direction of joint movements declines with age [57].

Sensors in the neck are also important for head stability and detecting head orientation, providing a stable platform for visual and vestibular input [58]. Sensitivity of proprioceptive neck receptors also declines with age [59], an important consideration given the age-related decline in otolith organ function noted above.

Other Physiological Contributors to Presbystasis (Table 26.1)

Table 26.1 Other body systems and health disorders contributing to presbystasis

Body System	Cause or Condition	Comments
Cerebrovascular—particularly with involvement of posterior circulation (i.e., vertebrobasilar vascular system)	Vertebrobasilar insufficiency or ischemia Cerebral artery atherosclerotic disease or stenosis Transient ischemic attack (TIA) Global cerebral hypoperfusion	Cardiovascular comorbidities are common; stroke risk factors include hypertension, smoking, hyperlipidemia, diabetes, obesity, and alcohol abuse
Cardiovascular	Hypertension Hypotension Arrhythmia Coronary artery atherosclerotic disease or stenosis Autonomic dysregulation	Symptoms of impairment include presyncope, syncope, orthostatic hypotension
Musculoskeletal	Age-related muscle changes	30–50% loss of skeletal muscle mass between ages of 40–80
	Arthritis	Significant implications for living independently—ADL impacts particularly on ability to bathe, dress, and transfer from bed to chair
	Osteoporosis, osteopenia, and fractures	High risk of serious injury from falls
	Joint replacement surgery	Disruption of proprioceptive cues importance for balance and postural stability
Metabolic/endocrine	Diabetes	Secondary sequelae include effects on vision and proprioception (e.g., retinopathy, peripheral neuropathy)
	Vitamin deficiency	B complex and D +/− calcium
Neurologic	Parkinson's disease	Loss of postural reflexes is a cardinal sign
	Cognitive impairment/ Alzheimer's disease	Cognitive decline and medication side effects increase fall risk
	Cerebellar degeneration	Gait disturbance with/without nystagmus; failure of fixation suppression is common
Psychiatric	Anxiety Depression Fear of falling	Associated with increased fall risk; adverse effects of medications used to treat these conditions are also associated with increased fall risk

As discussed above, age-related changes in the "vestibular triad" of sensory systems are well-known contributors to the development of *dizziness* in older patients; however, changes in other body systems, as well as specific disorders that are more prevalent in the elderly, have been shown to be dominant factors in the development of *presbystasis* and require particular consideration by managing healthcare providers [42, 57, 58, 60, 61]. These conditions alone can be associated with disequilibrium and, when combined with age-related decline or pathology in the vestibular triad, can produce devastating effects on social participation, personal safety, and quality of life.

In addition to body systems and health conditions contributing to presbystasis summarized in Table 26.1, adverse drug effects from medications used to treat common conditions in older patients further complicate the ability to maintain and control balance and postural stability. Adverse drug effects associated with imbalance in the elderly are grossly under-reported and inherently difficult to study, and while this is a significant consideration, detailed discussion is beyond the scope of this chapter. In a recent review, Min et al. reported that the most common classes of medications prescribed to patients over age 65 are antihypertensives, benzodiazepines and related drugs, sedative/hypnotics, anxiolytic drugs, and antiepileptic drugs [62].

Cerebrovascular disease, particularly involving the posterior circulation, can result in symptoms of true vertigo as well as imbalance and ataxia, whereas involvement of the anterior circulation system is more likely to produce lightheadedness and orthostatic symptoms. The vertebrobasilar, or posterior circulatory system, provides blood supply to the brainstem, cerebellum, and labyrinth. Elderly patients with health issues that are more prevalent with advancing age (e.g., hypertension, hyperlipidemia, diabetes mellitus, coronary artery disease, peripheral vascular disease, past strokes, or TIAs) should be evaluated carefully for evidence of vertebral or basilar artery stenosis and atherosclerotic disease. Typically, vertebrobasilar insufficiency is associated with atherosclerotic disease, and in a large study of patients who had TIA and/or stroke, Marquardt et al. found that more than 25% of patients had significant stenosis in the posterior circulatory system [63]. Elderly patients with imbalance and ataxia related to cerebrovascular disease may present with cerebellar signs that can run the gamut from subtle to pronounced depending on the site and extent of the lesion(s).

Cardiovascular health is vital for the health of all body tissues. Alterations in cardiovascular system functions associated with aging are well-known, and in general include left ventricular hypertrophy, left ventricular diastolic and systolic dysfunction, increased arterial stiffness, atrial fibrillation, cardiac valvular dysfunction, and impaired endothelial function [64–66]. Abnormalities may manifest as hypertension, hypotension, or arrhythmia, producing alterations in cerebral blood flow. Any of these impairments can result in patient complaints of lightheadedness and imbalance or falls when standing or walking. The baroreflex appears to be particularly vulnerable to aging effects resulting from stiffening of large vessels, and this in turn reduces the sensitivity of vascular stretch receptors typically activated upon standing [67]. In addition, age-related changes have been shown to adversely affect sympathetic nervous system signals that provide critical cardiovascular responses to changes in posture [68]. Interestingly, autoregulation of cerebral blood flow appears to be resistant to aging effects [69]. Of note, emerging evidence suggests that vestibular signals may provide rapid and important cues to cardiovascular control centers of the brain regarding changes in posture [70–73]. This, of course, has crucial implications for elderly patients with known vestibular deficits.

Musculoskeletal anatomy and physiology are characterized by relentless change throughout life. Beginning around age 40, decrease in bone and muscle mass and increase in adipose tissue occur, resulting in significant deterioration in physical performance [74, 75]. Even in conditioned athletes, muscle atrophy, bone fragility, and decline in physical performance occur with aging in both men and women [75]. These physical changes are even more pronounced in individuals who adopt a sedentary lifestyle, leading to increased risk of obesity, diabetes, and falls [76]. Furthermore, the prevalence of arthritis, most commonly osteoarthritis, increases dramatically with age and is linked to significant disability in activities of daily living [77, 78]. Osteoporosis, another well-known condition associated with aging, is mainly determined by genetics, although modifiable lifestyle factors such as weight-bearing exercise, nutrition (including calcium and vitamin D intake), as well as reducing alcohol consumption and nicotine use, are additional factors in altering its development [79]. The combination of osteoporosis and increased risk of falls can produce disastrous and potentially fatal injury. Sterling et al. indicate that 20% of all falls in the elderly result in serious injury [80], and direct costs of treating falls in older adults in the United States are estimated at $31 billion annually [31]. Joint replacement surgery, necessitated by either disease or injury, increases the likelihood of imbalance and gait disturbance in the elderly. This is due in part to alteration or elimination of joint proprioception signals considered by most to be essential sensory inputs for balance competence. By all measures, musculoskeletal changes associated with aging have important implications for presbystasis.

Type II diabetes represents the most common and serious metabolic/endocrine disorder associated with presbystasis. Studies estimate that nearly 20% of the population develops type 2 diabetes by age 75 [81]. In addition to the high risk of compromise to two sensory systems of the vestibular triad (i.e., vision: diabetic retinopathy; proprioception: peripheral neuropathy), diabetes is associated with increased incidence of atherosclerosis and abnormal insulin-mediated vasodilation in older adults [82]. This in turn increases the likelihood of comorbid cardiovascular and cerebrovascular disease, frequently with early warning signs of lightheadedness, dizziness, and unsteadiness. Patients who develop diabetes over the age of 65 have poorer quality of life and shorter life expectancy than age-matched controls and demonstrate more rapid functional decline (i.e., loss of independence) in longitudinal studies [83–85].

Elderly patients experiencing dizziness or unsteadiness are likely to be referred to an otolaryngologist or neurologist at some point in the diagnostic process. Evaluation and management of several peripheral vestibular disorders are covered in other chapters of this book. A few neurological disorders that are common in the elderly and associated with imbalance and falling may mimic peripheral vestibular disorders in their early stages. For example, although peripheral vestibular function typically is preserved in patients with Parkinson's disease, impaired kinesthesia and bradykinetic anticipatory postural adjustments have been demonstrated early in disease progression and may manifest as imbalance or frequent falls prior to the development of tremor, joint rigidity, or other classic features of Parkinson's disease [86, 87]. Interestingly, cervical VEMPs are frequently abnormal in patients in early stages of Parkinson's disease [88], which can mislead management decisions.

Patients will use the term "dizzy" to describe the spatial disorientation found to accompany degeneration of the hippocampus that occurs very early in the course of Alzheimer's disease [89, 90], and this symptom description may result in referral and diagnostic evaluation through the otolaryngology clinic. The situation becomes more perilous for patients with Parkinson's disease and Alzheimer's disease as cognitive decline occurs and the risk and frequency of falls increase. Cerebellar ataxia encompasses a wide range of etiologies, some of which are reversible (e.g., vitamin B12 deficiency) and some are irreversible degenerative processes (hereditary and non-hereditary). Patients may present with symptoms of imbalance, unsteadiness and falls [91]. Occasionally, these patients are diagnosed with BPPV as a result of the presence of nystagmus during Dix-Hallpike testing. Careful ocular motor examination reveals nystagmus with central (i.e., non-vestibular) characteristics, including spontaneous or immediate onset, persistence, non-fatigability, and little or no dizziness.

Finally, normal pressure hydrocephalus (NPH) carries the classic triad of memory loss/dementia, urinary incontinence, and ataxia. The gait associated with NPH is characterized as bradykinetic, broad-based, magnetic, and shuffling [92]. Computed tomography (CT) or magnetic resonance (MR) imaging is diagnostic showing dilation of the ventricles, and large volume lumbar puncture can be both diagnostic and therapeutic. Referral to neurology or neurosurgery is indicated.

Complex interactions exist among anxiety, depression, fear of falling, and postural instability in the elderly. It is estimated that 20% of community-dwelling older adults experience anxiety and/or depression, although this may be greatly underestimated, as patients may be reluctant to report symptoms of these disorders to their healthcare provider. With the growth in the aging baby-boomer population, these common psychological disorders have become significant societal concerns. Several studies have evaluated the association between anxiety/depression and dizziness [93, 94]; however, the relationship of psychiatric disorders to presbystasis is quite a bit murkier. Despite this, there is clear evidence that fear of falling is itself a risk factor for imbalance and actual falls [95, 96].

History and Physical Exam of the Elderly Patient

History

Taking a thorough history is the cornerstone in the evaluation of any dizzy patient. Onset of dizziness, episodic vs continuous nature of the dizziness, character of the dizziness, exacerbating and relieving factors, and associated symptoms, including hearing loss and tinnitus, are the key elements of a good history. In elderly patients who come to the office for evaluation of "dizziness," onset is important because it gives the examiner a time frame of reference for the dizziness—acute or chronic. Patients with presbystasis most typically have subacute or chronic, often progressive dizziness, described more as an off-balance feeling or disequilibrium, maybe a rocking or swaying sensation, and not true vertigo. The symptoms may have been present at a low level or infrequently for years with a more recent (weeks or months or even "in the last year") worsening. Otologic symptoms such as hearing loss/asymmetric hearing loss, otorrhea, otalgia, and tinnitus should be elicited. Lightheadedness/presyncope, especially on arising, may also be a complaint and should direct the examiner to a cardiovascular source of dizziness. "Cardiovascular dizziness" tends to be chronic but wax and wane, better in the morning and worsening over the day or with fatigue. Patients may have hearing loss and tinnitus, but the hearing does not fluctuate. Patients do not complain of nausea or vomiting but often have associated fatigue. Headache, if present, may or may not be related.

An important line of questioning relates to falls and fall prevention. The Centers for Disease Control and Prevention has launched the STEADI campaign—Stopping Elderly Accidents, Deaths, and Injuries (https://www.cdc.gov/steadi/), and urges physicians to ask three simple questions:

1. Have you fallen in the past year?
2. Do you feel unsteady when standing or walking?
3. Do you worry about falling?

A "yes" answer to any one of these questions puts the patient at increased risk of falling. As mentioned above, approximately 30% of adults older than 65 years will fall at least once, and about 50% of those will fall again [97, 98]. Fear of falling is a strong predictor of an actual fall [21]. Hip weakness, poor balance, and number of prescribed medications (see below) were the factors most strongly associated with falls among institutionalized subjects [99].

Past medical history, including a history of a single episode of room-spinning vertigo with nausea and vomiting lasting 24 h or longer, followed by motion-induced disequilibrium that eventually resolved (i.e., vestibular neuritis), may steer the examiner to diagnose an uncompensated, previously undiagnosed unilateral vestibular loss (see Chaps. 2 and 19). Otologic history, including history of ear surgery, Meniere's disease, vestibular schwannoma, and cholesteatoma, may clue the practitioner in to the etiology of dizziness. History of atherosclerotic heart disease, heart valvular disease, or heart failure indicates a cardiovascular source of dizziness.

History of peripheral vascular disease, cerebrovascular disease, or atherosclerotic heart disease points to vertebrobasilar insufficiency as a potential diagnosis. A prior neurologic diagnosis (e.g., Parkinson's disease, Alzheimer's disease, myasthenia gravis, multiple sclerosis, FamilNPH) would be a likely etiology as well.

Review of medications is important in elderly patients as several classes of medications, including antihypertensive medications (all classes), gastrointestinal agents, antihistamines, anxiolytics (benzodiazepines), cancer chemotherapeutic agents, sedative-hypnotics, and anti-epileptics can all cause dizziness through various mechanisms. Among elderly patients, altered pharmacokinetics (how much drug reaches the systemic circulation and is subsequently eliminated—absorption, distribution, metabolism, and excretion) and altered pharmacodynamics (the effect of the drug on the person) can cause adverse drug events such as dizziness [100].

Polypharmacy, the concurrent use of multiple medications by a patient, is a major contributor to dizziness in the elderly, as is the prescribing cascade—using one medication to treat the side effects of another medication. Medication reconciliation and review of current medications with an eye toward reducing the number of medications and the dosages of each medication (especially considering possible altered renal and hepatic metabolism in the elderly) will go a long way toward helping the elderly dizzy patient.

History of smoking predisposes to peripheral vascular disease (claudication, peripheral neuropathy), heart disease (valvular and atherosclerotic coronary artery disease), and cerebrovascular disease (vertebrobasilar insufficiency), all contributing to presbystasis. History of alcohol or drug abuse also contributes to postural instability; Wernicke's encephalopathy, caused by depletion and insufficiency of B vitamins (thiamine in particular), is characterized by ophthalmoplegia, ataxia, and confusion. Tabes dorsalis, from tertiary syphilis, is a rare but potential cause of ataxia due to neuropathic degeneration (demyelination) of the posterior (dorsal) columns of the spinal tract. Family history of disequiibrium or falls may point toward an inherited spinocerebellar degeneration.

A focused review of systems should be directed at the sensory (proprioceptive, visual, and vestibular) and motor components of balance and postural stability—e.g., numbness, tingling, or hypoesthesia of the toes, feet, hands, which could be caused by diabetes, renal disease, neurologic disease, medication; visual loss, double vision, or change in vision; and dizziness, vertigo, or hearing loss. Cardiovascular (lightheadedness/presyncope, especially when standing, syncopal episodes, rapid heartbeat/palpitations) and neurological (weakness, slurring of speech, dysphagia, dysphonia, dysarthria, numbness, unilateral loss of pain and temperature sensation) systems review may also reveal the source of dizziness and/or contributing factors.

Physical Exam

The physical exam, much like the review of systems, is directed at the sensory systems contributing to balance along with central neurologic control and cardiovascular perfusion.

Simply watching a patient walk into (or out of) the office can often lead the examiner to the source and degree of presbystasis. Does the patient use a walking stick? Walker? Wheelchair? Assistance from a family member? Touch the wall (or hold a family member's hand or arm) walking down the hall? Listing to one side when walking down the hall? Vital signs are necessity and should include evaluation for orthostatic hypotension, defined as a decrease in systolic blood pressure of 20 mm Hg or a decrease in diastolic blood pressure of 10 mm Hg within 3 min of standing when compared with blood pressure from the sitting or supine position. This change in position can also be accompanied by an increase in pulse. Patients may also complain of presyncopal symptoms, (i.e., lightheadedness). Asking if the dizziness experienced when standing for the orthostatic test mirrors the dizziness complaint may make the diagnosis.

The visual system is a critical component of balance, and investigation into visual acuity can be simple and straightforward with a Snellen eye chart. Alternatively, simply querying the patient about a change in vision may be enough to discuss visual loss or a change in vision as a contributor to presbystasis. Cataracts in the elderly are quite common, and a thorough visual exam and evaluation by an ophthalmologist may address visual change or visual loss as a source of presbystasis.

Ears should be examined for evidence of middle ear disease. Even serous otitis media can cause subtle labyrinthine dysfunction and imbalance. Cholesteatoma can erode bone over the horizontal semicircular canal and contribute to imbalance. Tuning fork testing or pneumatic otoscopy can elicit symptoms of dizziness in superior semicircular canal dehiscence, although this condition seems to be rare in the elderly.

Vestibulo-ocular reflex testing can diagnose a unilateral vestibular deficit. Tests of static and especially dynamic visual acuity can reveal a vestibular deficit. Have the patient hold the Snellen card (or cellphone or tablet app) at a comfortable distance. Move the card and have the patient read the lowest line possible. Then, move the patient's head back and forth and have the patient read the lowest line. An increase by two lines is significant.

Head impulse testing can diagnose unilateral and bilateral vestibular loss. The patient's head is rotated slowly to one side, about 30 degrees off midline. The patient is asked to keep the eyes trained on the examiner's eyes as the head is rapidly thrust to the midline. The patient should be able to track the examiner's eyes fluidly through the movement. In the setting of vestibular loss, the eyes will overshoot, and the patient will bring the eyes back to the examiner's eyes after a quick delay—a "refixation saccade." If the refixation saccade occurs when the patient's head is thrust to the right, the vestibular loss maps to the right vestibular system. Chapter 3 describes the physical examination of the vestibular system.

Central testing includes cerebellar testing to elicit dysdiadochokinesia with rapidly alternating hand movements and dysmetria with finger-to-nose/finger-to-finger testing. Strength and motor testing give the examiner an overall sense of the frailty of the patient. Romberg and tandem Romberg tests may reveal unilateral vestibular loss (falling to the side of the loss), and Fukuda step testing can also uncover unilateral vestibular loss (marching to the side of the loss). Specific tests of balance function are addressed in the next section.

Audiometry should be performed, mostly assessing for asymmetric sensorineural hearing loss and the possibility of an occult vestibular schwannoma. Several studies have suggested audiometric parameters predictive of vestibular schwannoma including the presence of rollover (greater than 20% decrease in word recognition score [WRS] when the stimulus intensity is increased 30–40 dB above the initial presenting stimulus level); difference of greater than 20% in the WRS between ears; greater than 15 dB difference in pure tone average at 3000 Hz between ears, and others.

The decision to pursue magnetic resonance imaging is based on history, physical exam, audiometry, and a frank discussion between doctor and patient acknowledging the relative rarity of finding a causative lesion and the possibility that if a vestibular schwannoma were found, it may simply be observed given its slow growth over time. Imaging simply for presbystasis in the absence of localizing findings on physical exam or audiometry is of low diagnostic yield although it may reveal global parenchymal volume loss or signs of cerebrovascular disease that may help explain symptoms.

Tests of Balance, Equilibrium, and Fall Risk

Vestibular laboratory testing is highlighted in other chapters of this book, and the reader is encouraged to review these sections. There are additional tools that can be very useful for evaluating gait, balance, and fall risk in the older adult. These measures include self-report and provider-administered questionnaires, as well as physical tests of static and dynamic balance capability. Whether considered adjuncts to results from vestibular laboratory tests or as screening instruments, information from these tests can provide a multidimensional assay of a patient's self-perceived and functional gait, balance, and mobility competence, and fall risk. Any of these measures can be easily incorporated into an office examination of an older adult reporting unsteadiness or imbalance. Several of the most widely used tests require little or no equipment and take little time to complete. An excellent collection of materials is available online for clinicians and patients at the STEADI website: https://www.cdc.gov/steadi/materials.html. These materials include downloadable screening tools for balance and fall risk assessment, brochures, and fact sheets regarding safety tips and fall prevention.

Questionnaires for balance and fall risk range from simple, few-item screening forms to elaborate surveys querying multiple domains. The three-item screening in the STEADI toolkit mentioned earlier suggests additional assessment if the patient answers "yes" to falling in the past 12 months, feeling unsteady when standing or walking, or worrying about falling. The Morse Fall Scale [101], widely used on inpatient units, examines six categories: history of fall(s) in the past 3 months, secondary diagnosis, use of ambulatory aid (i.e., crutches, cane, etc.), IV/heparin lock, gait characteristics (e.g., stooped posture, difficulty rising from chair), and mental status. Scores >24 indicate the need to implement fall precautions.

The Johns Hopkins Fall Risk Assessment Tool (JHFRAT) judges seven areas linked to fall risk: age, history of falls in the past 6 months, bladder/bowel elimination, medication review, the number of patient care equipment in use (e.g., IV infusion, indwelling catheter, etc.), mobility/transfer assistance needs, and cognition [102]. The JHFRAT has been shown to be reliable with high specificity as well as high negative predictive value [103]. The Activities-Specific Balance Confidence (ABC) Scale is a self-report instrument that asks patients to evaluate their confidence in their ability to perform 16 common activities (e.g., walk around the house, get out of a car, step onto or off an escalator) without becoming unsteady [104]. Scores below 50% indicate a moderate or low level of functioning, and scores below 67% are predictive of future falls [105].

Static and dynamic tests of balance typically involve components to assess balance, gait speed or gait characteristics, mobility, and endurance. In the modified Clinical Test of Sensory Interaction and Balance (mCTSIB), the examiner tests whether a patient can stand for 30 s in each of four test conditions: firm surface with eyes open; firm surface with eyes closed; foam surface with eyes open; and foam surface with eyes closed. This inexpensive test has demonstrated utility in examining static standing balance, and results compare favorably with platform posturography [106]. The Berg Balance Scale (BBS) is a 14-item performance test that examines the patient's ability to perform progressively more complex standing and walking tasks, such as standing with eyes open and closed, picking up an object from the floor, and standing on 1 foot, to name a few [107]. The BBS has high sensitivity and specificity for predicting falls, and norms have been established at different age groups, as have confidence intervals for minimal detectable change [108]; however, a ceiling effect has been noted for high-functioning individuals.

Gait speed is a well-known proxy for general health status as well as fall risk. Age-appropriate gait speed requires body support, physical power, coordination, and balance. In addition, decrease in gate speed over time has been associated with worsening condition [109, 110]. The Timed Up and Go (TUG) test is a widely used gait speed test in which the patient is asked to stand up from a chair, walk 10 feet, turn around, and return to their starting position [111]. Variations of the TUG include performing a cognitive task (e.g., counting by intervals) while walking or adding a dual attention task (e.g., carrying a cup of water). Patients who take more than 13.5 s to complete the TUG have a high likelihood of falling and will have limited ability to walk independently in the community [112]. The 30-Second Chair Stand Test assesses balance and endurance by having the patient stand from a seated position, with arms crossed, and sit back down as many times as possible within 30 s [113]. Norms have been established by age and gender, and patients aged 65–80 should be able to come to a full stand at least 10 times within 30 s.

The Performance-Oriented Mobility Assessment (POMA) scores the patient's balance and gait characteristics as they attempt to perform 16 sitting, standing, and walking tasks of varying complexity. Scores are based on the level of independence with which the patient is able to complete each component, and higher scores indicate more independent function, whereas lower scores indicate fall risk. Likewise, higher scores on the Dynamic Gait Index (DGI) indicate greater independence and lower fall risk [114]. The 8-item DGI judges gait impairment while walking on a level surface, changing gait speed, adding horizontal and vertical head movements, turning, stepping over and around obstacles, and walking up steps. The 4-item DGI (walking on a level surface, changing gait speed, walking with horizontal head turns, and walking with vertical head turns) is often used as a screening tool, with recommendations for additional testing in patients whose score is less than 10 points [115].

Management of the Patient with Presbystasis

While there is no "cure" for presbystasis, many measures can help patients and improve confidence, mobility, and independence. Perhaps the most important management strategy in counseling and rehabilitating the older dizzy patient is fall prevention. As referenced in several areas of this chapter, the CDC has resources for doctors and patients to address fall prevention (https://www.cdc.gov/steadi/index.html). Simple suggestions such as removing area rugs, securing railings and bannisters in the house, installing grab bars and non-skid mats in bathrooms, and having a night light on at night go a long way to giving the patient confidence and instituting measures to prevent falls.

We find it helpful to counsel patients on the physiology of the balance system and how it is composed of the sensory systems—visual, vestibular, and proprioceptive—all sending information to the brain. The brain, then, coordinates this information and maintains balance. Derangement in any of these systems and structures can lead to imbalance and falls. This simple explanation gives patients and their families a framework to consider the dizziness and identify for themselves specific factors that predispose to presbystasis. Changes in vision, comorbid conditions such as diabetes mellitus, polypharmacy/medication, trauma, central neurologic disease, spine and joint problems, and others all predispose to presbystasis. Families and patients are thus empowered to "be the doctor" and identify and address risk factors.

Use of a walking stick, walker, or rollator reinforces the proprioceptive sensory system by allowing the patient to "touch" the ground through the walking stick, four-pronged walker, or balance with the more stable walker. Many patients are resistant to using a walking stick, but acknowledge they feel safer and more secure using one. Walking sticks or trekking poles can also be decorative and fun (golf putter, ski pole, or colorful wooden "staff"). Doctors should not be reticent to write a prescription for a medical device such as cane or walker as these will be covered by insurance with a prescription.

Referral to ophthalmology for an assessment of vision may go a long way to helping the patient with imbalance. Cataract surgery has been shown to help prevent falls. Other corrective eyewear may also help.

Addressing medications and polypharmacy by eliminating unnecessary medications, especially vestibular suppressants, such as meclizine and benzodiazepines often given for "dizziness," allows the brain to compensate for the factors predisposing to imbalance and stops the pharmacological "dumbing down" of the brain. Antihypertensive medications can be particularly tricky to manage in the patient with presyncopal symptoms or orthostatic hypotension. Patients should have a frank discussion with their cardiologist or primary care provider about "balancing" the goal of normotension with the symptoms of dizziness that these medications may be exacerbating. Interestingly, recent guidelines on blood pressure control by the American Heart Association and American College of Cardiology have recommended stricter control—defining elevated blood pressure as 120–129 systolic and less than 80 diastolic (with Stage 1 Hypertension as 130–139 systolic and 80–89 diastolic) [116]. These new guidelines will likely increase the number of patients on antihypertensives and the subsequent sequelae, including dizziness and postural dizziness clinicians will encounter [62]. Finding the right medication at the right dosage may be challenging. Very high blood pressures also cause dizziness; thus, the need for a sometimes delicate balance with adjustments in dose and antihypertensive medication itself.

Vestibular rehabilitation exercises or other exercise programs that may include strength training, fitness training, or other planned exercises, specifically with attention to postural control and balance, have been shown to help the older "at risk" dizzy patient and reduce the risk of falling (Table 26.2) [58, 117, 118]. Novel interventions to help elderly patients with balance and postural stability include the use of virtual reality (a "virtual reality supermarket"), Tai Chi, the Nintendo Wii®, vibrotactile feedback devices, habituation exercises with optokinetic stimulation, and balance-enhancing insoles (for an excellent review of these newer technologies, see Alrwaily and Whitney [119]).

Rest is an important adjunct to balance. When people are tired or fatigued, they are more off balance, and having a balance disorder makes people more tired because they are expending much more "cognitive energy" simply to avoid falling or veering off course. Stressing the importance of a bedtime routine and a good night's sleep (7–9 h) can be helpful. In addition, a nap in the afternoon "recharges the brain's battery," is refreshing, and improves balance late in the day and evening.

Table 26.2 Older adults should be referred to rehabilitation if they have one or more of the following signs

Positive Dix-Hallpike test
Positive Romberg test
Dizziness with movement of the head
Dizziness associated with neck pain
Slow gait
History of falling two or more times within the past 6 months
Inability to rise from a chair without using arm support
Fear of falling that prohibits the person from participating in activities of interest
Arrhythmic gait

Adapted from [119]

Conclusions

Presbystasis, age-related change in balance function, can (and usually does) have multiple causes in each patient. An understanding of the basic physiology of balance and inquiry into the sensory systems and central neurologic processes that control balance will point the clinician (and patient and family) to the specific etiologic factor(s) that contribute(s) to imbalance. A clear discussion with patient and family is a critical part of this diagnostic and rehabilitative process.

Addressing comorbidities, polypharmacy (eliminating meclizine and other vestibular suppressants), and predisposing factors helps. A formal program of therapist-directed vestibular rehabilitation directed at balance, postural control, and fall prevention will also help. Making simple changes in the home and environment and use of a walking stick can go a long way to prevent the devastating sequela of presbystasis and falls.

References

1. Popp P, Wulff M, Finke K, Ruhl M, Brandt T, Dieterich M. Cognitive deficits in patients with a chronic vestibular failure. J Neurol. 2017;264(3):554–63.
2. Mueller M, Strobl R, Jahn K, Linkohr B, Ladwig KH, Mielck A, et al. Impact of vertigo and dizziness on self-perceived participation and autonomy in older adults: results from the KORA-Age study. Qual Life Res. 2014;23(8):2301–8.
3. Mueller M, Strobl R, Jahn K, Linkohr B, Peters A, Grill E. Burden of disability attributable to vertigo and dizziness in the aged: results from the KORA-Age study. Eur J Pub Health. 2014;24(5):802–7.
4. Kannus P, Parkkari J, Koskinen S, Niemi S, Palvanen M, Jarvinen M, et al. Fall-induced injuries and deaths among older adults. JAMA. 1999;281(20):1895–9.
5. Ciorba A, Bianchini C, Scanelli G, Pala M, Zurlo A, Aimoni C. The impact of dizziness on quality-of-life in the elderly. Eur Arch Otorrinolaringol. 2017;274(3):1245–50.
6. Inouye SK, Studenski S, Tinetti ME, Kuchel GA. Geriatric syndromes: clinical, research, and policy implications of a core geriatric concept. J Am Geriatr Soc. 2007;55(5):780–91.
7. Tinetti ME, Inouye SK, Gill TM, Doucette JT. Shared risk factors for falls, incontinence, and functional dependence. Unifying the approach to geriatric syndromes. JAMA. 1995;273(17):1348–53.
8. Tinetti ME, Williams CS, Gill TM. Dizziness among older adults: a possible geriatric syndrome. Ann Intern Med. 2000;132(5):337–44.
9. Kao AC, Nanda A, Williams CS, Tinetti ME. Validation of dizziness as a possible geriatric syndrome. J Am Geriatr Soc. 2001;49(1):72–5.
10. Ortman JM, Velkoff VA, Hogan H. An aging nation: the older population in the United States. Washington, DC: U.S. Census Bureau; 2014. p. 25–1140.
11. Creighton FXJ, Poliashenko SM, Statham MM, Abramson P, Johns MM3. The growing geriatric otolaryngology patient population: a study of 131,700 new patient encounters. Laryngoscope. 2013;123(1):97–102.
12. Gopinath B, McMahon CM, Rochtchina E, Mitchell P. Dizziness and vertigo in an older population: the Blue Mountains prospective cross-sectional study. Clin Otolaryngol. 2009;34(6):552–6.

13. Stevens KN, Lang IA, Guralnik JM, Melzer D. Epidemiology of balance and dizziness in a national population: findings from the English Longitudinal Study of Ageing. Age Ageing. 2008;37(3):300–5.
14. Lin HW, Bhattacharyya N. Balance disorders in the elderly: epidemiology and functional impact. Laryngoscope. 2012;122(8):1858–61.
15. Jonsson R, Sixt E, Landahl S, Rosenhall U. Prevalence of dizziness and vertigo in an urban elderly population. J Vestib Res. 2004;14(1):47–52.
16. Agrawal Y, Carey JP, Della Santina CC, Schubert MC, Minor LB. Disorders of balance and vestibular function in US adults: data from the National Health and Nutrition Examination Survey, 2001–2004. Arch Intern Med. 2009;169(10):938–44.
17. Roberts DS, Lin HW, Bhattacharyya N. Health care practice patterns for balance disorders in the elderly. Laryngoscope. 2013;123(10):2539–43.
18. Graafmans WC, Ooms ME, Hofstee HM, Bezemer PD, Bouter LM, Lips P. Falls in the elderly: a prospective study of risk factors and risk profiles. Am J Epidemiol. 1996;143(11):1129–36.
19. Centers for Disease Control and Prevention. Stopping elderly accidents, deaths, and injuries (STEADI). 2017. Available at: https://www.cdc.gov/steadi/. Accessed 16 Jan 2018.
20. O'Loughlin JL, Boivin JF, Robitaille Y, Suissa S. Falls among the elderly: distinguishing indoor and outdoor risk factors in Canada. J Epidemiol Community Health. 1994;48(5):488–9.
21. Rubenstein LZ, Josephson KR. Falls and their prevention in elderly people: what does the evidence show? Med Clin North Am. 2006;90(5):807–24.
22. Whitney SL, Marchetti GF, Schade AI. The relationship between falls history and computerized dynamic posturography in persons with balance and vestibular disorders. Arch Phys Med Rehabil. 2006;87(3):402–7.
23. Agrawal Y, Ward BK, Minor LB. Vestibular dysfunction: prevalence, impact and need for targeted treatment. J Vestib Res. 2013;23(3):113–7.
24. Agrawal Y, Davalos-Bichara M, Zuniga MG, Carey JP. Head impulse test abnormalities and influence on gait speed and falls in older individuals. Otol Neurotol. 2013;34(9):1729–35.
25. Ekvall Hansson E, Magnusson M. Vestibular asymmetry predicts falls among elderly patients with multi-sensory dizziness. BMC Geriatr. 2013;13:77.
26. Burker EJ, Wong H, Sloane PD, Mattingly D, Preisser J, Mitchell CM. Predictors of fear of falling in dizzy and nondizzy elderly. Psychol Aging. 1995;10(1):104–10.
27. Perez-Jara J, Enguix A, Fernandez-Quintas JM, Gomez-Salvador B, Baz R, Olmos P, et al. Fear of falling among elderly patients with dizziness and syncope in a tilt setting. Can J Aging. 2009;28(2):157–63.
28. Holmberg J, Karlberg M, Harlacher U, Magnusson M. Experience of handicap and anxiety in phobic postural vertigo. Acta Otolaryngol (Stockh). 2005;125(3):270–5.
29. Bergen G, Stevens MR, Burns ER. Falls and fall injuries among adults aged ≥ 65 years – United States, 2014. MMWR Morb Mortal Wkly Rep. 2016;65:993–8.
30. Centers for Disease Control and Prevention. Home and Recreational Safety > Older Adult Falls. 2017. Available at: https://www.cdc.gov/homeandrecreationalsafety/falls/index.html. Accessed 16 Jan 2018.
31. Burns ER, Stevens JA, Lee R. The direct costs of fatal and non-fatal falls among older adults – United States. J Saf Res. 2016;58:99–103.
32. Merchant SN. Degeneration of auditory and vestibular end organs. In: Merchant SN, Nadol JB, editors. Schuknecht's pathology of the ear. 3rd ed. Shelton: People's Medical Publishing House; 2010. p. 632–63.
33. Rosenhall U, Rubin W. Degenerative changes in the human vestibular sensory epithelia. Acta Otolaryngol (Stockh). 1975;79(1–2):67–80.
34. Richter E. Quantitative study of human Scarpa's ganglion and vestibular sensory epithelia. Acta Otolaryngol (Stockh). 1980;90(3–4):199–208.
35. Ishiyama A, Lopez I, Ishiyama G, Tang Y. Unbiased quantification of the microdissected human Scarpa's ganglion neurons. Laryngoscope. 2004;114(8):1496–9.

36. Tang Y, Lopez I, Baloh RW. Age-related change of the neuronal number in the human medial vestibular nucleus: a stereological investigation. J Vestib Res. 2001;11(6):357–63.
37. Merchant SN, Velazquez-Villasenor L, Tsuji K, Glynn RJ, Wall C, Rauch SD. Temporal bone studies of the human peripheral vestibular system. Normative vestibular hair cell data. Ann Otol Rhinol Laryngol Suppl. 2000;181:3–13.
38. Rauch SD, Velazquez-Villasenor L, Dimitri PS, Merchant SN. Decreasing hair cell counts in aging humans. Ann N Y Acad Sci. 2001;942:220–7.
39. Walther LE, Westhofen M. Presbyvertigo-aging of otoconia and vestibular sensory cells. J Vestib Res. 2007;17(2–3):89–92.
40. Agrawal Y. Dizziness demographics and population health. In: Gleason AT, Kesser BW, editors. Dizziness and vertigo across the lifespan. 1st ed. Philadelphia: Elsevier; 2018. p. 1–7.
41. Peterka RJ, Black FO, Schoenhoff MB. Age-related changes in human vestibulo-ocular reflexes: sinusoidal rotation and caloric tests. J Vestib Res. 1990;1(1):49–59.
42. Peterka RJ, Black FO. Age-related changes in human posture control: sensory organization tests. J Vestib Res. 1990;1(1):73–85.
43. Paige GD. The aging vestibulo-ocular reflex (VOR) and adaptive plasticity. Acta Otolaryngol Suppl (Stockh). 1991;481:297–300.
44. Paige GD. Senescence of human visual-vestibular interactions. 1. Vestibulo-ocular reflex and adaptive plasticity with aging. J Vestib Res. 1992;2(2):133–51.
45. Serrador JM, Lipsitz LA, Gopalakrishnan GS, Black FO, Wood SJ. Loss of otolith function with age is associated with increased postural sway measures. Neurosci Lett. 2009;465(1):10–5.
46. Maes L, Dhooge I, D'haenens W, Bockstael A, Keppler H, Philips B, et al. The effect of age on the sinusoidal harmonic acceleration test, pseudorandom rotation test, velocity step test, caloric test, and vestibular-evoked myogenic potential test. Ear Hear. 2010;31(1):84–94.
47. Mossman B, Mossman S, Purdie G, Schneider E. Age dependent normal horizontal VOR gain of head impulse test as measured with video-oculography. J Otolaryngol Head Neck Surg. 2015;44:29.
48. Furman JM, Redfern MS. Effect of aging on the otolith-ocular reflex. J Vestib Res. 2001;11(2):91–103.
49. Lord SR, Clark RD, Webster IW. Visual acuity and contrast sensitivity in relation to falls in an elderly population. Age Ageing. 1991;20(3):175–81.
50. Lord SR, Dayhew J. Visual risk factors for falls in older people. J Am Geriatr Soc. 2001;49(5):508–15.
51. Lord SR. Visual risk factors for falls in older people. Age Ageing. 2006;35(Suppl 2):42–5.
52. Borger LL, Whitney SL, Redfern MS, Furman JM. The influence of dynamic visual environments on postural sway in the elderly. J Vestib Res. 1999;9(3):197–205.
53. Poulain I, Giraudet G. Age-related changes of visual contribution in posture control. Gait Posture. 2008;27(1):1–7.
54. Schniepp R, Schlick C, Schenkel F, Pradhan C, Jahn K, Brandt T, et al. Clinical and neurophysiological risk factors for falls in patients with bilateral vestibulopathy. J Neurol. 2017;264(2):277–83.
55. Lord SR, Clark RD, Webster IW. Physiological factors associated with falls in an elderly population. J Am Geriatr Soc. 1991;39(12):1194–200.
56. Wiles PG, Pearce SM, Rice PJ, Mitchell JM. Vibration perception threshold: influence of age, height, sex, and smoking, and calculation of accurate centile values. Diabet Med. 1991;8(2):157–61.
57. Sturnieks DL, St George R, Lord SR. Balance disorders in the elderly. Neurophysiol Clin. 2008;38(6):467–78.
58. Barin K, Dodson EE. Dizziness in the elderly. Otolaryngol Clin N Am. 2011;44(2):437–54.
59. Deshpande N, Patla AE. Postural responses and spatial orientation to neck proprioceptive and vestibular inputs during locomotion in young and older adults. Exp Brain Res. 2005;167(3):468–74.

60. Belal AJ, Glorig A. Dysequilibrium of ageing (presbyastasis). J Laryngol Otol. 1986;100(9):1037–41.
61. Peterka RJ, Black FO. Age-related changes in human posture control: motor coordination tests. J Vestib Res. 1990;1(1):87–96.
62. Min Y, Shoair OA, Slattum PW. Medication-related dizziness in the older adult. In: Gleason AT, Kesser BW, editors. Dizziness and vertigo across the lifespan. Philadelphia: Elsevier; 2018.
63. Marquardt L, Kuker W, Chandratheva A, Geraghty O, Rothwell PM. Incidence and prognosis of > or = 50% symptomatic vertebral or basilar artery stenosis: prospective population-based study. Brain. 2009;132(Pt 4):982–8.
64. Lakatta EG, Levy D. Arterial and cardiac aging: major shareholders in cardiovascular disease enterprises: part I: aging arteries: a "set up" for vascular disease. Circulation. 2003;107(1):139–46.
65. Lakatta EG, Levy D. Arterial and cardiac aging: major shareholders in cardiovascular disease enterprises: part II: the aging heart in health: links to heart disease. Circulation. 2003;107(2):346–54.
66. Antelmi I, de Paula RS, Shinzato AR, Peres CA, Mansur AJ, Grupi CJ. Influence of age, gender, body mass index, and functional capacity on heart rate variability in a cohort of subjects without heart disease. Am J Cardiol. 2004;93(3):381–5.
67. Monahan KD. Effect of aging on baroreflex function in humans. Am J Physiol Regul Integr Comp Physiol. 2007;293(1):R3–R12.
68. Joyner MJ, Charkoudian N, Wallin BG. Sympathetic nervous system and blood pressure in humans: individualized patterns of regulation and their implications. Hypertension. 2010;56(1):10–6.
69. Deegan BM, Sorond FA, Galica A, Lipsitz LA, O'Laighin G, Serrador JM. Elderly women regulate brain blood flow better than men do. Stroke. 2011;42(7):1988–93.
70. Tiecks FP, Planck J, Haberl RL, Brandt T. Reduction in posterior cerebral artery blood flow velocity during caloric vestibular stimulation. J Cereb Blood Flow Metab. 1996;16(6):1379–82.
71. Yates BJ, Miller AD. Physiological evidence that the vestibular system participates in autonomic and respiratory control. J Vestib Res. 1998;8(1):17–25.
72. Heckmann JG, Leis S, Muck-Weymann M, Hilz MJ, Neundorfer B. Vestibular evoked blood flow response in the basilar artery. Acta Neurol Scand. 1999;100(1):12–7.
73. Wilson TD, Serrador JM, Shoemaker JK. Head position modifies cerebrovascular response to orthostatic stress. Brain Res. 2003;961(2):261–8.
74. Taaffe DR, Marcus R. Musculoskeletal health and the older adult. J Rehabil Res Dev. 2000;37(2):245–54.
75. Akima H, Kano Y, Enomoto Y, Ishizu M, Okada M, Oishi Y, et al. Muscle function in 164 men and women aged 20–84 yr. Med Sci Sports Exerc. 2001;33(2):220–6.
76. Burr DB. Muscle strength, bone mass, and age-related bone loss. J Bone Miner Res. 1997;12(10):1547–51.
77. Song J, Chang RW, Dunlop DD. Population impact of arthritis on disability in older adults. Arthritis Rheum. 2006;55(2):248–55.
78. Covinsky K. Aging, arthritis, and disability. Arthritis Rheum. 2006;55(2):175–6.
79. Pietschmann P, Rauner M, Sipos W, Kerschan-Schindl K. Osteoporosis: an age-related and gender-specific disease—a mini-review. Gerontology. 2009;55(1):3–12.
80. Sterling DA, O'Connor JA, Bonadies J. Geriatric falls: injury severity is high and disproportionate to mechanism. J Trauma. 2001;50(1):116–9.
81. Harris MI, Flegal KM, Cowie CC, Eberhardt MS, Goldstein DE, Little RR, et al. Prevalence of diabetes, impaired fasting glucose, and impaired glucose tolerance in U.S. adults. The Third National Health and Nutrition Examination Survey, 1988–1994. Diabetes Care. 1998;21(4):518–24.
82. Meneilly GS, Elliott T. Metabolic alterations in middle-aged and elderly obese patients with type 2 diabetes. Diabetes Care. 1999;22(1):112–8.

83. Gu K, Cowie CC, Harris MI. Mortality in adults with and without diabetes in a national cohort of the U.S. population, 1971–1993. Diabetes Care. 1998;21(7):1138–45.
84. Fillenbaum GG, Pieper CF, Cohen HJ, Cornoni-Huntley JC, Guralnik JM. Comorbidity of five chronic health conditions in elderly community residents: determinants and impact on mortality. J Gerontol A Biol Sci Med Sci. 2000;55(2):M84–9.
85. Miller DK, Lui LY, Perry HM, Kaiser FE, Morley JE. Reported and measured physical functioning in older inner-city diabetic African Americans. J Gerontol A Biol Sci Med Sci. 1999;54(5):M230–6.
86. Wright WG, Gurfinkel VS, King LA, Nutt JG, Cordo PJ, Horak FB. Axial kinesthesia is impaired in Parkinson's disease: effects of levodopa. Exp Neurol. 2010;225(1):202–9.
87. Rocchi L, Chiari L, Mancini M, Carlson-Kuhta P, Gross A, Horak FB. Step initiation in Parkinson's disease: influence of initial stance conditions. Neurosci Lett. 2006;406(1–2):128–32.
88. Venhovens J, Meulstee J, Bloem BR, Verhagen WIM. Neurovestibular analysis and falls in Parkinson's disease and atypical Parkinsonism. Eur J Neurosci. 2016;43(12):1636–46.
89. Alzheimer's Association. Alzheimer's disease facts and figures. Alzheimer Dement. 2016;12(4):459–509.
90. Braak H, Braak E. Neuropathological stageing of Alzheimer-related changes. Acta Neuropathol (Berl). 1991;82(4):239–59.
91. Cherchi MO. Uncommon causes of dizziness in the adult. In: Gleason AT, Kesser BW, editors. Dizziness and vertigo across the lifespan. Philadelphia: Elsevier; 2018.
92. Schnek MJ. Normal pressure hydrocephalus clinical presentation. 2017. Available at: https://emedicine.medscape.com/article/1150924-clinical. Accessed 30 Jan 2018.
93. Sloane PD, Hartman M, Mitchell CM. Psychological factors associated with chronic dizziness in patients aged 60 and older. J Am Geriatr Soc. 1994;42(8):847–52.
94. Eckhardt-Henn A, Breuer P, Thomalske C, Hoffmann SO, Hopf HC. Anxiety disorders and other psychiatric subgroups in patients complaining of dizziness. J Anxiety Disord. 2003;17(4):369–88.
95. Delbaere K, Crombez G, Vanderstraeten G, Willems T, Cambier D. Fear-related avoidance of activities, falls and physical frailty. A prospective community-based cohort study. Age Ageing. 2004;33(4):368–73.
96. Li F, Fisher KJ, Harmer P, McAuley E, Wilson NL. Fear of falling in elderly persons: association with falls, functional ability, and quality of life. J Gerontol B Psychol Sci Soc Sci. 2003;58(5):P283–90.
97. Vivrette RL, Rubenstein LZ, Martin JL, Josephson KR, Kramer BJ. Development of a fall-risk self-assessment for community-dwelling seniors. J Aging Phys Act. 2011;19(1):16–29.
98. Rubenstein LZ, Josephson KR. The epidemiology of falls and syncope. Clin Geriatr Med. 2002;18(2):141–58.
99. Robbins AS, Rubenstein LZ, Josephson KR, Schulman BL, Osterweil D, Fine G. Predictors of falls among elderly people. Results of two population-based studies. Arch Intern Med. 1989;149(7):1628–33.
100. Shoair OA, Nyandege AN, Slattum PW. Medication-related dizziness in the older adult. Otolaryngol Clin N Am. 2011;44(2):455–71.
101. Morse JM, Black C, Oberle K, Donahue P. A prospective study to identify the fall-prone patient. Soc Sci Med. 1989;28(1):81–6.
102. Poe SS, Cvach MM, Gartrelu DG, Radzik BR, Joy TL. An evidence-based approach to fall risk assessment, prevention, and management: lessons learned. J Nurs Care Qual. 2005;20(2):107–16; quiz 117–8.
103. Klinkenberg WD, Potter P. Validity of the Johns Hopkins fall risk assessment tool for predicting falls on inpatient medicine services. J Nurs Care Qual. 2017;32(2):108–13.
104. Powell LE, Myers AM. The Activities-specific Balance Confidence (ABC) scale. J Gerontol A Biol Sci Med Sci. 1995;50A(1):M28–34.

105. Lajoie Y, Gallagher SP. Predicting falls within the elderly community: comparison of postural sway, reaction time, the Berg balance scale and the Activities-specific Balance Confidence (ABC) scale for comparing fallers and non-fallers. Arch Gerontol Geriatr. 2004;38(1):11–26.
106. Cohen H, Blatchly CA, Gombash LL. A study of the clinical test of sensory interaction and balance. Phys Ther. 1993;73(6):346–51; discussion 351–4.
107. Berg KO, Wood-Dauphinee SL, Williams JI, Maki B. Measuring balance in the elderly: validation of an instrument. Can J Public Health. 1992;83(Suppl 2):S7–11.
108. Donoghue D, Stokes EK, Physiotherapy Research and Older People (PROP) Group. How much change is true change? The minimum detectable change of the Berg Balance Scale in elderly people. J Rehabil Med. 2009;41(5):343–6.
109. Guralnik JM, Ferrucci L, Pieper CF, Leveille SG, Markides KS, Ostir GV, et al. Lower extremity function and subsequent disability: consistency across studies, predictive models, and value of gait speed alone compared with the short physical performance battery. J Gerontol A Biol Sci Med Sci. 2000;55(4):M221–31.
110. Studenski S. Bradypedia: is gait speed ready for clinical use? J Nutr Health Aging. 2009;13(10):878–80.
111. Shumway-Cook A, Brauer S, Woollacott M. Predicting the probability for falls in community-dwelling older adults using the Timed Up & Go Test. Phys Ther. 2000;80(9):896–903.
112. Studenski S, Perera S, Patel K, Rosano C, Faulkner K, Inzitari M, et al. Gait speed and survival in older adults. JAMA. 2011;305(1):50–8.
113. Jones CJ, Rikli RE, Beam WC. A 30-s chair-stand test as a measure of lower body strength in community-residing older adults. Res Q Exerc Sport. 1999;70(2):113–9.
114. Shumway-Cook A. Motor control: theory and practical applications. Philadelphia: Lippincott, Williams & Wilkins; 1995.
115. Marchetti GF, Whitney SL. Construction and validation of the 4-item dynamic gait index. Phys Ther. 2006;86(12):1651–60.
116. American Heart Association, American College of Cardiology. High blood pressure redefined for first time in 14 years: 130 is the new high. 2017. Available at: https://newsroom.heart.org/news/high-blood-pressure-redefined-for-first-time-in-14-years-130-is-the-new-high. Accessed 28 Jan 2018.
117. Rossi-Izquierdo M, Gayoso-Diz P, Santos-Perez S, Del-Rio-Valeiras M, Faraldo-Garcia A, Vaamonde-Sanchez-Andrade I, et al. Short-term effectiveness of vestibular rehabilitation in elderly patients with postural instability: a randomized clinical trial. Eur Arch Otorrinolaringol. 2017;274(6):2395–403.
118. Alrwaily M, Whitney SL. Vestibular rehabilitation of older adults with dizziness. Otolaryngol Clin N Am. 2011;44(2):473–96.
119. Alrwaily M, Whitney SL. Older adults with dizziness: rehabilitation strategies and novel interventions. In: Gleason AT, Kesser BW, editors. Dizziness and vertigo across the lifespan. Philadelphia: Elsevier; 2018.

Chapter 27
Pediatric Vestibular Disorders

Zachary G. Schwam and George Wanna

As in the adult population, evaluating the vertiginous child must take into consideration potential malfunction of the vestibular, proprioceptive, and visual systems. In one large series analyzing over 2000 children seen in a vestibular clinic, the most common causes of pediatric vertigo included migrainous equivalent, benign paroxysmal positional vertigo, trauma, ocular disorders, and congenital malformations [1]. The workup of pediatric vertigo should be based on the particular patient; with that provision, we recommend obtaining an audiogram and vestibular testing as needed, a CT scan of the temporal bones if labyrinthine malformations or trauma are suspected, an MRI if there is suspicion for tumor or intracranial lesion, and a neurologic/ophthalmologic evaluation should the workup otherwise be negative.

Z. G. Schwam (✉)
Department of Otolaryngology, Icahn School of Medicine at Mount Sinai,
New York, NY, USA

G. Wanna
Department of Otolaryngology at New York Eye and Ear Infirmary of Mount Sinai and
Mount Sinai Beth Israel, New York, NY, USA

Division of Otology-Neurotology at the Mount Sinai Health System, New York, NY, USA

Audiology, Hearing and Balance Center at the Mount Sinai Health System,
New York, NY, USA

Ear Institute at the Mount Sinai Health System, New York, NY, USA
e-mail: gwanna@nyee.edu

J. C. Lucas et al. (eds.), *Diagnosis and Treatment of Vestibular Disorders*,
https://doi.org/10.1007/978-3-032-11740-3_27

Migraine Equivalent

Migraine and benign paroxysmal vertigo of childhood (BPVC) were found in one publication to account for 50–75% of vertiginous children with normal tympanic membranes [2, 3]. BPVC is similar to adult benign paroxysmal positional vertigo (BPPV) (discussed in Chaps. 14 and 15) and requires ≥5 episodes of severe vertigo that are self-limited and occur over minutes to hours, normal audiometric and vestibular exams between attacks, and a normal electroencephalogram (EEG) [4]. It is of particular significance in children 2–3 years of age [1]. Nausea, vomiting, diaphoresis, and pallor may occur [5], but headache is uncommon [1].

Basilar artery migraine is another migrainous equivalent that frequently presents with vertigo and may be secondary to vasospasm or abnormal central processing [6, 7]. Other presenting symptoms include tinnitus, hearing loss, diplopia, ataxia, or loss of consciousness [8]. According to guidelines put forth by the International Headache Society and the Bárány society, criteria for diagnosis of vestibular migraine include ≥5 episodes of moderate-to-severe vestibular symptoms lasting 5 min to 72 h, current or previous migraine +/− aura, ≥1 migraine features with ≥50% of vestibular episodes, and symptomatology not better accounted for by another diagnosis [9].

Trauma

Recent head trauma should not be overlooked in trying to ascertain the etiology of a child's vertigo. For a more in-depth discussion on trauma-induced vertigo, please refer to Chap. 21. Temporal bone fracture involving the labyrinth may cause vertigo in addition to facial nerve palsy and hearing loss. A comprehensive neurologic and trauma exam should be performed, looking for cranial neuropathies as well as stigmata of temporal bone fracture, including external auditory canal lacerations, hemotympanum, and battle sign (ecchymosis over the mastoid process). The tuning fork exam may demonstrate a Weber that lateralizes to the ipsilateral ear if there is hemotympanum secondary to a conductive loss. Fracture through the otic capsule would be most consistent with a sensorineural loss. Once imaging is complete and the patient is stable, then prompt audiometric evaluation should be performed.

Perilymphatic fistula is defined as an abnormal communication between the middle ear space and the fluid of the membranous labyrinth and may be found in the context of (baro)trauma, significant exertion, congenital anomalies, or after recent stapes surgery [10, 11]. Unfortunately, there is no non-invasive test to confirm the diagnosis; middle ear exploration with direct visualization is the only definitive option. The clinical presentation is nonspecific and may include tinnitus, high-frequency hearing loss, vertigo, or aural fullness. Tullio phenomenon (sound-induced vertigo) as well as Hennebert sign (vertigo and nystagmus with pneumatic otoscopy) were only present in 4% and 24% of a series of 91 patients from the

University of Iowa [11], which is in concordance with the established literature [12, 13]. In one series of 71 cases, the presence of Hennebert sign did not correlate with the diagnosis [14]. Surgical repair of the fistula is the most definitive therapy, and in the same series of patients from the University of Iowa, 94% had improvement in vertigo, and approximately half had an improvement in hearing loss. However, only 23% had serviceable hearing. While there are undoubtedly microleaks that spontaneously heal [13], surgical intervention is recommended for significant, persistent leaks not only because of the debilitating symptom profile, but because of the risk of meningitis [10]. A trial of conservative therapy, including vestibular suppressants, bedrest, and avoidance of straining, is a reasonable first step for many [13].

Labyrinthine contusion, hemorrhage, and concussion may all cause labyrinthine failure, which is characterized by nausea and vomiting, gait instability, rotatory vertigo, and horizontal rotatory nystagmus to the contralateral side in the absence of temporal bone fracture [15]. Concussion typically presents with high-frequency sensorineural hearing loss with or without vestibulopathies, and symptom resolution typically occurs within days to weeks [16].

Ocular Disorders

While a comprehensive discussion on ophthalmologic disorders is beyond the scope of this chapter, it is prudent for the otolaryngologist to know that ocular disorders such as vergence insufficiency, ametropia, anisometropia, strabismus, and amblyopia are often-overlooked causes of pediatric vertigo and should be on the differential diagnosis in the context of a normal neurologic and vestibular exam [1]. In one study, approximately 5% of the 523 children in their sample were found to have various ocular disorders, and two-thirds of cases were resolved after ophthalmologic intervention [17]. The authors found that children over 6 years of age were most often affected, and that symptoms worsened after prolonged concentration or after focusing on a screen. Referral to an ophthalmologist should be performed for evaluation in which another cause cannot better explain the symptomatology.

Congenital Malformations and Syndromes

Large vestibular aqueduct syndrome (LVAS) refers to an aqueduct with diameter >1.5 mm and classically presents with congenital sensorineural hearing loss but may also have vestibular symptoms in as many as 71% of patients [18]. LVAS is frequently found in conjunction with other congenital anomalies, including cochlear aplasia, hypoplasia, and incomplete partition [19, 20]. In children, vertigo may manifest as incoordination and imbalance for minutes to hours, notably after minor head trauma or strenuous physical activity [19, 21]. LVAS is also a component of Pendred syndrome, which includes SNHL, cochlear aplasia, and defects in thyroid hormone organification [21]. While the etiology of auditory and vestibular symptoms is unknown, it has been postulated that pressure gradients are transmitted across the enlarged duct and somehow alter the labyrinthine epithelium. Treatment of LVAS largely focuses on restoration of audition in the way of hearing amplification and cochlear implantation. Endolymphatic sac surgery is avoided, as there is a significant risk of worsened hearing postoperatively [22].

Cogan syndrome is classically described as the coupling of episodic acute interstitial keratitis with vestibuloauditory dysfunction. Most cases were found to occur in patients aged 15–30 years, and a significant percentage thereof reported a recent upper respiratory tract infection. Meniere-like attacks were common and included symptoms of nausea, vertigo, vomiting, tinnitus, and profound unilateral to bilateral hearing loss. Aortitis was found in 10% of patients with the typical form of the disease, while patients with atypical forms, or other ocular inflammatory disorders, were found to have other rheumatologic diseases and had a less favorable prognosis. Otologic symptoms were occasionally controlled with systemic steroids or cytotoxic drugs, but irreversible deafness was found in the majority of patients [23, 24]. Cochlear implantation was reported to be successful for these patients [25].

Superior Semicircular Canal Dehiscence

Superior semicircular canal dehiscence is a rare cause of vertigo in children and typically presents in middle age. It is confirmed with computed tomography (CT) of the temporal bones using 0.5 mm cuts in the plane of the superior semicircular canal. Vertigo may be elicited by sound or pressure (via pneumatic otoscopy or Valsalva maneuver). The characteristic nystagmus is one that is intorsional and upward in the affected side from ampullofugal deflection of the superior canal cupula with a "third window" from a dehiscence. The direction of eye movement is in the plane of the dehiscent semicircular canal. The Weber tuning fork exam is typically ipsilateral to the lesion, and bone conduction sensitivity may be elevated. This may also explain some of the other characteristic symptomatology of affected patients hearing their own pulse or extraocular movements. While in one series of 65 patients with canal dehiscence, a cause could not be identified in nearly half of patients, trauma or straining was found to precede the development of symptoms in the remainder. A minority of patients had solely auditory symptoms; their audiograms displayed the largest air-bone gaps in lower frequencies. In patients in whom surgical repair was performed utilizing a middle cranial fossa approach to plug the canal with fascia, bone pate, and cortical bone, nearly 90% had a significant improvement in their symptoms, while 10% experienced some degree of significant hearing loss. Therefore, it is critical to gauge the severity of symptoms and to consider everything from conservative management to surgical repair [26, 27].

Vestibular Neuritis

Vestibular neuritis is a clinical syndrome that is characterized by an acute attack consisting of vertigo without associated auditory symptoms. The vertigo typically resolves over days to weeks and is associated with an impaired caloric response in the affected ear. An upper respiratory tract infection is usually antecedent to the episode and is thought to cause inflammation of the vestibular nerve [28]. Several viral entities are associated with the disorder, notably herpes simplex virus, cytomegalovirus, measles, mumps, rubella, influenza, parainfluenza, varicella-zoster, coxsackie, retroviruses, and enterovirus. While there is an association with viral disease, a complete serologic workup is often not necessary and of limited utility. Treatment is primarily symptomatic and may consist of anti-histamines, anti-cholinergics, anti-dopaminergics, and gamma-aminobutyric acid agonists. A vestibular exercise regimen may be added as an adjunct [29]. In one randomized control trial, the addition of systemic methylprednisolone was found to significantly improve symptoms, while adding valacyclovir to the regimen did not change the course of the disease [30].

Chronic Otitis Media and Cholesteatoma

The prevalence of chronic otitis media (COM) has been decreasing with the use of antibiotics in the last several years, and with it, many of the feared intra- and extra-cranial complications. In one series of over 3200 patients in Taiwan, labyrinthitis was diagnosed in 1.43%, secondary endolymphatic hydrops in 1.00%, and labyrinthine fistula of the horizontal SCC in three patients [31]. Vertigo has been thought to be secondary to labyrinthine inflammation, exotoxins produced by bacterial pathogens, changes in pressure gradients across the oval and round windows, and labyrinthine fistula. In the setting of cholesteatomatous otitis media, the incidence of labyrinthine fistula is significantly higher, likely due to collagenase-induced bone erosion as well as the local pressure from the cholesteatoma matrix [32]; in one series of over 1200 patients who underwent surgery for cholesteatoma, 92 were found to have labyrinthine fistulas (7.7%). Of those patients with fistulas, 84% of them involved the lateral SCC [33]. The diagnosis of fistula is primarily one made intraoperatively, although extensive fistulas may be reliably diagnosed based on imaging alone [34]. Surgical treatment of labyrinthine fistulas varies; some authors prefer to excise all cholesteatoma matrix overlying the fistula and seal it with various materials, while other authors will leave residual matrix over the fistula to minimize the risk of sensorineural deafness.

Psychiatric Disorders

By some reports, psychiatric disorders exert much influence on the course of disease in the dizzy patient, with those who experience a psychiatric component remaining more symptomatic and disabled than their purely organic counterparts [35]. In several studies of pediatric vertigo, psychogenic causes were in the top three most common etiologies [3, 36–39]. In one report of 100 children with vertigo, psychogenic causes were found in 21% and were more prevalent in those >5 years of age and female [39]. Of those patients, three had a known psychiatric disorder, and nine had associations between stressful situations and vertigo. Anxiety, depression, panic disorder, and various somatoform disorders have all been associated with vertigo and should prompt referral to a mental health practitioner should the suspicion arise that comorbid psychiatric illness is at play.

Central Nervous System Disorders

Differentiating central and peripheral causes of vertigo is a crucial initial step in diagnosing the dizzy child, with central lesions usually causing more severe imbalance, slower compensation, and other neurologic symptoms. Auditory symptoms are rare in central causes of vertigo, and nystagmus may be purely vertical, horizontal, or torsional, as opposed to the horizontal and torsional nystagmus often found in peripheral lesions. Nystagmus secondary to a central cause is not often suppressed with visual fixation and may change direction [40].

While uncommon, epileptic vertigo has been reported in the literature. Electroencephalogram (EEG) recordings show the posterior middle frontal gyrus to receive vestibular input and may be implicated in the symptomatology of seizures affecting this area [41]. In one series of 42 children with central vertigo, patients often reported headaches, nausea, vomiting, loss of postural control, and loss of consciousness. Symptoms consistent with focal seizures were rare [42]. In cases where epilepsy is thought to be at play, referral to a pediatric neurologist for EEG and anti-epileptic medications is warranted.

Despite multiple sclerosis (MS) being an uncommon disorder in children with an incidence of 0.51 per 100,000 person-years [43], up to 10% of adult patients report that their symptoms began before the age of 18 [44]. Vertigo is a common presenting symptom and indicates demyelination along the vestibular tract. Diagnostic criteria include MRI findings of T2-intense lesions in characteristic locations, oligoclonal IgG bands in the CSF, as well as clinical evidence of the lesions [45]. Prompt referral to a pediatric neurologist is recommended.

Episodic ataxia type 2, of which there are six subtypes, is the most common and presents with vertigo, imbalance, and ataxia. The episodes have been known to last between hours and days, with triggers that include ingestion of alcohol, stress, and physical exertion [46, 47]. The vast majority of patients have central ocular disturbances, including downbeat nystagmus, internuclear ophthalmoplegia, and impaired visual suppression of the vestibulo-ocular reflex [48]. History and physical exam alone are insufficient to differentiate the disorder from vestibular migraine. Atrophy of the anterior cerebellar vermis is a common finding on MRI [49], and genetic testing often, but does not always, reveals mutations of the CACNA1A calcium channel gene on chromosome 19 [50]. Treatment options include acetazolamide, which is thought to alter the pH and therefore the conductance of neuronal membranes, and 4-aminopyridine, which may increase the release of gamma-aminobutyric acid in Purkinje cells [51].

Posterior Fossa Lesions

Among lesions of the posterior fossa, those of the cerebellopontine angle (CPA) dominate. Vestibular schwannoma (VS) is the most common CPA lesion and comprises more than 90% of lesions in this area. Meningiomas compose 3% of lesions, and the remaining include epidermoid lesions, arachnoid cysts hemangiomas, metastatic tumors, lipomas, dermoids, teratomas, chordomas, chondrosarcomas, and giant cell tumors. Lesions of the petrous apex and intraaxial tumors should also be considered in the differential diagnosis, but will not be discussed here.

While unilateral, sporadically formed vestibular schwannomas are typically diagnosed between 40 and 60 years of age, those associated with neurofibromatosis type 2 (NF2) typically are diagnosed before the age of 21 years [52], are often bilateral, and are frequently associated with concomitant Schwannomas, ependymomas, and meningiomas [53]. Symptoms may be related to compression of adjacent cranial nerves and vascular structures as well as the fourth ventricle, leading to hydrocephalus and increased intracranial pressure. While true vertigo is uncommon, dysequilibrium is often a presenting symptom in addition to hearing loss, tinnitus, and facial hypoesthesia. Audiometry may demonstrate asymmetric sensorineural hearing loss or speech discrimination out of proportion to the hearing loss. Auditory brainstem response testing and gadolinium-enhanced MRI are the most sensitive and specific tests for diagnosing vestibular schwannomas. While not useful in diagnosing a vestibular schwannoma, vestibular testing may be useful in localizing the lesion to the superior or inferior vestibular nerve [52, 54]. Treatment may include observation with serial imaging, radiotherapy, or surgical resection based on age, symptomatology, growth rate, and family/surgeon preference.

References

1. Wiener-Vacher SR. Vestibular disorders in children. Int J Audiol. 2008;47:578–83.
2. Choung YH, Park K, Moon SK, Kim CH, Ryu SJ. Various causes and clinical characteristics in vertigo in children with normal eardrums. Int J Pediatr Otorhinolaryngol. 2003;67:889–94.
3. Erbek SH, Erbek SS, Yilmaz I, et al. Vertigo in childhood: a clinical experience. Int J Pediatr Otorhinolaryngol. 2006;70:1547–54.
4. International Headache Society. Benign paroxysmal vertigo of childhood. http://www.ihs-klassifikation.de/en/02_klassifikation/02_teil1/01.03.03_migraine.html. Accessed 24 Sept 2017.
5. Baloh RW. Neurotology of migraine. Headache. 1997;37:615–21.
6. Koenigsberger MR, Chutorian AM, Gold AP, Schvey MS. Benign paroxysmal vertigo of childhood. Neurology. 1970;20:1108–11.
7. Baloh RW, Honrubia V. Clinical neurophysiology of the vestibular system. 3rd ed. New York: Oxford University Press; 2001. p. 161.
8. Kirchmann M, Thomsen LL, Olesen J. Basilar-type migraine: clinical, epidemiologic, and genetic features. Neurology. 2006;28:880–6.
9. O'Connell Ferster AP, Priesol AJ, Isildak H. The clinical manifestations of vestibular migraine: a review. Auris Nasus Larynx. 2017;44:249–52.
10. Althaus SR. Perilymph fistulas. Laryngoscope. 1981;91:538–62.
11. Seltzer S, McCabe BF. Perilymph fistula: the Iowa experience. Laryngoscope. 1986;94:37–49.
12. Fox EJ, Balkany TJ, Arenberg IK. The Tullio phenomenon and perilymph fistula. Otolaryngol Head Neck Surg. 1988;98:88–9.
13. Hughes GB, Sismanis A, House JW. Is there consensus in perilymph fistula management? Otolaryngol Head Neck Surg. 1990;102:111–7.
14. Alzahrani M, Fadous R, Dufour JJ, Saliba I. Perilymphatic fistulas: can we predict the diagnosis? Eur Arch Otorrinolaringol. 2015;272:1885–91.
15. Brandt T, Dieterich M, Strupp M. Traumatic forms of vertigo. In: Vertigo and dizziness. London: Springer; 2013.
16. Elzière M, Devèze A, Bartoli C, Levy G. Post-traumatic balance disorder. Eur Ann Otorhinolaryngol Head Neck Dis. 2017;134:171–5.
17. Anoh-Tanon MJ, Bremond Gignac D, Wiener-Vacher SR. Vertigo is an underestimated symptom of ocular disorders: dizzy children do not always need an MRI. Pediatr Neurol. 2000;23:49–53.
18. Grimmer JF, Hedlund G. Vestibular symptoms in children with enlarged vestibular aqueduct anomaly. Int J Pediatr Otorhinolaryngol. 2007;71:275–82.
19. Jackler RK, De La Cruz A. The large vestibular aqueduct syndrome. Laryngoscope. 1989;99:1238–43.
20. Jackler RK, Luxfor WM, House WF. Congenital malformations of the inner ear: a classification based on embryogenesis. Laryngoscope. 1987;97:2–14.
21. Oh AK, Ishiyama A, Baloh RW. Vertigo and the enlarged vestibular aqueduct syndrome. J Neurol. 2001;248:971–4.
22. Wilson DF, Hodgson RS, Talbot JM. Endolymphatic sac obliteration for large vestibular aqueduct syndrome. Am J Otol. 1997;18:101–7.
23. Haynes BF, Kaiser-kupfer MI, Mason P, Fauci AS. Cogan syndrome: studies in thirteen patients, long-term follow-up, and a review of the literature. Medicine. 1980;59:426–41.
24. Mcdonald TJ, Vollertsen RS, Younge BR. Cogan's syndrome: audiovestibular involvement and prognosis in 18 patients. Laryngoscope. 1985;95:650–4.
25. Pasanisi E, Vincenti V, Bacciu A, Guida M, Berghenti T, Barbot A, Orsoni JG, Bacciu S. Cochlear implantation and Cogan syndrome. Otol Neurotol. 2003;24:601–4.
26. Minor LB, Solomon D, Zinreich JS, Zee DS. Sound-and/or pressure-induced vertigo due to bone dehiscence of the superior semicircular canal. Arch Otolaryngol Head Neck Surg. 1998;124:249–58.

27. Minor LB. Clinical manifestations of superior semicircular canal dehiscence. Laryngoscope. 2005;115:1717–27.
28. Schuknecht HF, Kitamura K. Vestibular neuritis. Ann Otol Rhinol Laryngol Suppl. 1981;90:1–9.
29. Baloh RW. Vestibular neuritis. N Engl J Med. 2003;348:1027–32.
30. Strupp M, Zingler VC, Arbusow V, et al. Methylprednisolone, valacyclovir, or the combination for vestibular neuritis. N Engl J Med. 2004;351:354–61.
31. Lin YS, Lin LC, Lee FP, Lee KJ. The prevalence of chronic otitis media and its complication rates in teenagers and adult patients. Otolaryngol Head Neck Surg. 2009;140:165–70.
32. Soda-Merhy A, Betancourt-Suarez MA. Surgical treatment of labyrinthine fistula caused by cholesteatoma. Otolaryngol Head Neck Surg. 2000;122:739–42.
33. Magliulo G, Terranova G, Varacalli S, Sepe C. Labyrinthine fistula as a complication of cholesteatoma. Otol Neurotol. 1997;18:697–701.
34. Gersdorff MC, Nouwen J, Decat M, et al. Labyrinthine fistula after cholesteatomatous chronic otitis media. Am J Otol. 2000;21:32–5.
35. Eckhardt-Henn A, Breuer P, Thomalske C, Hoffmann SO, Hopf HC. Anxiety disorders and other psychiatric subgroups in patients complaining of dizziness. J Anxiety Disord. 2003;17:369–88.
36. Szirmai A. Vestibular disorders in childhood and adolescents. Eur Arch Otorrinolaringol. 2010;267:1801–4.
37. Jahn K, Langhagen T, Schroeder AS, Heinen F. Vertigo and dizziness in childhood-update on diagnosis and treatment. Neuropediatrics. 2011;42:129–34.
38. Langhagen T, Schroeder AS, Rettinger N, Borggraefe I, Jahn K. Migraine-related vertigo and somatoform vertigo frequently occur in children and are often associated. Neuropediatrics. 2013;44:55–8.
39. Batu ED, Anlar B, Topçu M, Turanlı G, Aysun S. Vertigo in childhood: a retrospective series of 100 children. Eur J Pediatr Neurol. 2015;19:226–32.
40. Baloh RW. Differentiating between peripheral and central causes of vertigo. Otolaryngol Head Neck Surg. 1998;119:55–9.
41. Altay EE, Serdaroglu A, Gucuyener K, Bilir E, Karabacak NI, Thio LL. Rotational vestibular epilepsy from the temporo-parieto-occipital junction. Neurology. 2005;65:1675–6.
42. Eviatar L, Eviatar A. Vertigo in children: differential diagnosis and treatment. Pediatrics. 1977;59:833–8.
43. Langer-Gould A, Zhang JL, Chung J, et al. Incidence of acquired CNS demyelinating syndromes in a multiethnic cohort of children. Neurology. 2011;77:1143–8.
44. Ferreira ML, Machado MI, Dantas MJ, Moreira AJ, Souza AM. Pediatric multiple scleoris: analysis of clinical and epidemiological aspects according to National MS Society Consensus 2007. Arq Neuropsiquiatr. 2008;66:665–70.
45. Polman CH, Reingold SC, Banwell B, et al. Diagnostic criteria for multiple sclerosis: 2010 revisions to the McDonald criteria. Ann Neurol. 2011;69:292–302.
46. Strupp M, Zwergal A, Brandt T. Episodic ataxia type 2. Neurotherapeutics. 2007;30:267–73.
47. Griggs RC, Nutt JG. Episodic ataxia as channelopathies. Ann Neurol. 1995;37:285–7.
48. Sasaki O, Jen JC, Baloh RW, Kim GW, Isawa M, Usami S. Neurotological findings in a family with episodic ataxia. J Neurol. 2003;250(3):373–5.
49. Vighetto A, Froment JC, Trillet M, Aimard G. Magnetic resonance imaging in familial paroxysmal ataxia. Arch Neurol. 1988;45:547–9.
50. Ophoff RA, Terwindt GM, Vergouwe MN, et al. Familial hemiplegic migraine and episodic ataxia type-2 are caused by mutations in the Ca2+ channel gene CACNL1A4. Cell. 1996;87:543–52.
51. Kalla R, Teufel J, Fail K, Muth C, Strupp M. Update on the pharmacotherapy of cerebellar and central vestibular disorders. J Neurol. 2016;263:S24–9.
52. Flint PW, Haughey BW, Lund VJ, et al. Cummings otolaryngology: head & neck surgery. 6th ed. Philadelphia: Elsevier/Saunders; 2015.

53. Martuza RL, Eldridge R. Neurofibromatosis 2 (bilateral acoustic neurofibromatosis). N Engl J Med. 1988;318:684.
54. Linthicum FH, Waldorf R, Luxford WM, et al. Infrared/video ENG recording of eye movements to evaluate the inferior vestibular nerve using the minimal caloric test. Otolaryngol Head Neck Surg. 1988;98:207–10.

Chapter 28
Central Vestibular Disorders and Emergent Vertigo

Omolara Lawal and Dhasakumar Navaratnam

Introduction

Central vertigo is vertigo that arises due to an abnormality in the central nervous system (CNS). Traditionally, the vestibular system, and by implication the causes of vertigo, have been divided into the central and peripheral subcategories. Peripheral causes of vertigo involve the semicircular canal and saccule/utricle. Central causes of vertigo are primarily located in the brainstem and the 8th nerve. This is not surprising given the centrality of connections from the peripheral system that relay in the brainstem, including postural control, eye movements, spinal reflexes, and the adjacent cerebellum with which it connects intimately.

A plethora of disease entities implicate the brainstem. Included in this exhaustive list are common and uncommon diseases including vascular disorders (strokes, aneurysm, basilar ectasia), inflammatory disorders (multiple sclerosis, Miller Fisher variant of Guillain-Barre acute demyelinating polyneuropathy, Whipple's disease), degenerative disorders (Parkinson's disease, progressive supranuclear palsy, multi-system atrophy, spinocerebellar atrophy, Friedreich's ataxia), tumors (8th nerve tumors, meningiomas of the CP angle, gliomas of the brainstem and astrocytomas of the cerebellum), nutritional deficiencies (thiamine), and toxic/metabolic anomalies (Metronidazole overdose). We have chosen to concentrate on the evidence for a number of selective disorders.

O. Lawal · D. Navaratnam (✉)
Yale School of Medicine, Department of Neurology, New Haven, CT, USA
e-mail: omolara.lawal@yale.edu; dhasakumar.navaratnam@yale.edu

J. C. Lucas et al. (eds.), *Diagnosis and Treatment of Vestibular Disorders*,
https://doi.org/10.1007/978-3-032-11740-3_28

Vascular Causes of Central Vertigo

Introduction

Dizziness/vertigo is a common presentation of a cerebrovascular accident (CVA), particularly in the posterior circulation. Thirty-seven percent of posterior strokes can be initially misdiagnosed compared with 16% of anterior strokes ($P < 0.001$) [1]. Furthermore, atypical symptoms associated with posterior circulation strokes lead to misdiagnoses with two- and fourfolds' higher risk of misdiagnosis [1, 2].

Twenty percent of all ischemic strokes involve regions of the brain supplied by the vertebrobasilar (posterior) circulation [3]. Vertigo has been described as the most common symptom of vertebrobasilar insufficiency [3]. In a recent study, it was found that the patients who visited the emergency department with dizziness/vertigo had a twofold (95% CI, 1.35–2.96; $P < 0.001$) higher risk of stroke than those without dizziness/vertigo during a follow-up of 3 years [4]. It was also demonstrated that the patients hospitalized with isolated vertigo have a 3.01-times (95% CI, 2.20–4.11; $P < 0.001$) higher risk for stroke than the general population during the 4-year follow-up [4]. Patients with vertigo who had 3 or more risk factors were found to have a 5.51-fold higher risk for stroke (95% CI, 3.10–9.79; $P < 0.001$) than those without risk factors [4].

Another study in California showed that the incidence rate for cerebrovascular events in ED patients discharged after vertigo was highest in the first month (30.2 [24.4–37.0] per 10,000 person-months) and then decreased during the study period to 6.5 (5.3–8.0) events per 10,000 person-months thereafter [5].

Vertebrobasilar Insufficiency

The brainstem, cerebellum, and peripheral labyrinths are all supplied by the vertebrobasilar arterial system.

The vertebrobasilar arterial system originates with the union of the two vertebral arteries to form the basilar artery. The cerebellum is supplied by the posterior inferior cerebellar artery (PICA), which arises from the vertebral artery, and the anterior inferior cerebellar artery (AICA) and the superior cerebellar artery (SCA), which arise from the basilar artery (Fig. 28.1).

Brainstem Infarct (Associated with Hearing Loss)

The AICA usually arises from the caudal third of the basilar artery and supplies the inner ear, lateral pons, middle cerebellar peduncle, and anterior inferior cerebellum, including the flocculus [6]. It is an important artery for the blood supply to the peripheral and central vestibular structures; thus, its occlusion commonly results in

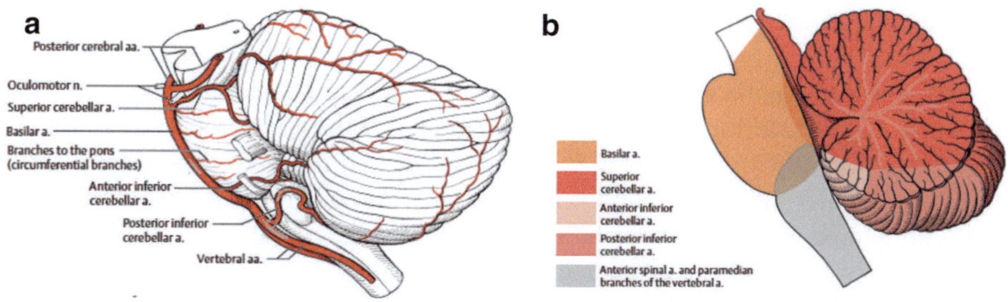

Fig. 28.1 (**a**) Blood supply of the cerebellum. (**b**) Territories of the cerebellum and brainstem arteries in midline sagittal section. (Picture credit: Baehr [60])

vertigo of either peripheral or central etiology [7]. AICA infarction is characterized by acute audiovestibular loss with or without other neurological symptoms and signs of brainstem or cerebellar involvement [7].

One study demonstrated that nearly all (98%) patients with AICA territory infarction presented with an acute onset of prolonged (>24 h) vertigo and had a vestibular dysfunction of peripheral, central, or combined origin, with ocular, motor, or vestibular signs, seen in a third of the study population [7]. This was attributed to the fact that AICA supplies the peripheral vestibular structures, such as the inner ear and CN VIII, as well as the central vestibular structures. In lieu of this, complete AICA infarction usually results in combined peripheral and central vestibular damage in addition to symptoms of hearing loss, facial weakness, sensory loss, gait ataxia, and cerebellar dysmetria [7]. However, it is difficult to determine the exact mechanism responsible for prolonged vertigo in patients with AICA infarction, as ischemia of any of the structures supplied by AICA can lead to vertigo [7]. In another study, 65% of the subjects with AICA infarction had a unilateral weakness to caloric stimulation, which suggests that the vertigo resulted from a peripheral vestibular structure dysfunction, while in 33% of the subjects, a normal caloric response was elicited, which points to vertigo resulting from ischemia to the central vestibular structures [7].

Patients with cerebellar infarcts often report dizziness, occasionally in conjunction with frank vertigo, blurred vision, difficulty walking, and vomiting. Other commonly reported symptoms include gait instability, ataxia, hypotonia ipsilateral to the side of the lesion, and notably, nystagmus [3]. Patients with pure cerebellar infarcts do not typically have hemiparesis or hemisensory loss [3]. In a study [8] of patients with vertigo due to vertebrobasilar insufficiency, 62% had a history of at least one isolated episode of vertigo, and 19% developed vertigo as the initial symptom. Patients with infarction in the territory of anterior inferior cerebellar artery (AICA) may have isolated recurrent vertigo, fluctuating hearing loss, and/or tinnitus (similar to Meniere's disease) as the initial symptoms 1–10 days prior to the permanent infarction [8].

Labyrinthine Infarction

The blood supply to the inner ear originates from the internal auditory artery (IAA), a branch of the anterior inferior cerebellar artery. Thus vertebrobasilar ischemic stroke can present with vertigo and hearing loss due to infarction of the inner ear [9]. The IAA supplies the cochlea and vestibular labyrinth, resulting in loss of auditory and vestibular function when occluded [10], and being an end artery, the labyrinth is particularly susceptible to ischemia due to limited collateral circulation from the otic capsule [9, 11]. Internal auditory artery infarction mostly occurs due to thrombotic narrowing of the AICA itself, or in the basilar artery at the orifice of the AICA [9].

Sudden onset of unilateral deafness and vertigo should prompt a suspicion of labyrinthine infarction, particularly in the elderly [12]. A definite diagnosis is not possible as an MRI cannot visualize the inner ear [12]. However, the apical region of the cochlea is more vulnerable to ischemia, and this may be clinically detected with the presence of low-frequency hearing loss [12].

Brainstem Infarct (No Hearing Loss)

Posterior Inferior Cerebellar Artery

Infarction in the dorsolateral medulla (Wallenberg's syndrome) commonly involves the inferior and medial vestibular nuclei and usually manifests with nausea/vomiting, vertigo, and imbalance [9]. Vertigo in the lateral medullary infarction is usually associated with other neurologic symptoms or signs, but a tiny infarct in the lateral medulla can present with vertigo without other localizing symptoms [9, 13].

One study reported that about 11% (25/240) of patients with isolated cerebellar infarction presented as isolated vertigo only, and most (24/25, 96%) patients with isolated vertigo had an infarct in the territory of the medial branch of the PICA, including the nodulus [14]. It has also been reported that the caudal cerebellum in the medial branch of the PICA is the most common site responsible for central isolated vertigo of vascular cause [3].

Acute Vestibular Syndrome (AVS)

Acute vestibular syndrome can be described as a sudden onset of dizziness accompanied by nausea or vomiting, unsteady gait, nystagmus, and intolerance to head motion that persists for a day or more [15]. Isolated acute vestibular syndrome (with or without hearing loss) may be defined as vertigo/dizziness occurring in the absence of focal neurologic signs such as hemiparesis, hemisensory loss, or gaze palsy [16].

Most lesions that result in AVS from a stroke etiology occur within the territory of the PICA [15]. A systematic review assessed the central causes of AVS as follows: cerebrovascular event in posterior fossa (83%), ischemic stroke (cerebellum or brainstem) (79%), hemorrhage (cerebellum or brainstem) (4%), multiple sclerosis (11%), and other central/equivocal causes (6%) [16].

An infarction in the brainstem localized to the vestibular nuclei may mimic an acute peripheral vestibulopathy. These must be differentiated from AVS due to other causes (vestibular neuronitis, Meniere's) with careful clinical examination, including HINTS (Head Impulse Nystagmus and Test of Skew) testing and caloric testing [17, 18]. A normal head impulse and normal calorics point to a central cause of AVS [17, 18]. These criteria initially proposed by Newman-Toker's group have been subsequently validated by other groups. In their initial report, the authors demonstrated that among patients with AVS, the presence of any one of these bedside findings—normal horizontal HIT, skew deviation, impaired vertical smooth pursuit, or central-appearing nystagmus—identified stroke with 100% sensitivity and 96% specificity [15, 16, 19–22].

Non-vascular Causes of Central Vertigo

There are several non-vascular causes of central vertigo. Some are well established in their pathophysiology; others are still not well understood with little data available on them. A literature review study reported that none of its included studies were large enough to identify rare causes such as post-CNS infections [16].

Tumors

Tumors of the cerebellopontine angle often cause vertigo. Vestibular schwannoma (VS) is the most frequent benign lesion that occurs at the cerebellopontine angle, representing about 90% of tumors at this site [23, 24]. A bilateral occurrence of VS is usually associated with neurofibromatosis Type II. NF2 is an autosomal dominant tumor-suppressor syndrome characterized by schwannomas, meningiomas, and ependymomas that develop throughout the central and peripheral nervous systems [23]. However, the mechanism differs for different tumor types [25]. Vertigo may result from a lesion of the labyrinth, compression or invasion of the endolymphatic sac, compression of the vestibular nerve, cerebellar compression, or compression of the key blood supply to the vestibular organs [25].

A study [26] to characterize the clinical picture obtained with vestibular schwannomas in 122 subjects showed that only half of them reported vertigo attacks, the predominant features being hearing loss (94%) and tinnitus (83%). The vertigo associated with VS differed, however, from that of other causes by the absence or low intensity of nausea [26]. The duration of vertigo attacks ranged from 5 min to 4 h, with the intensity varying from mild to moderate. The occurrence of vertigo was not associated with the duration of disease or the size of tumor [26].

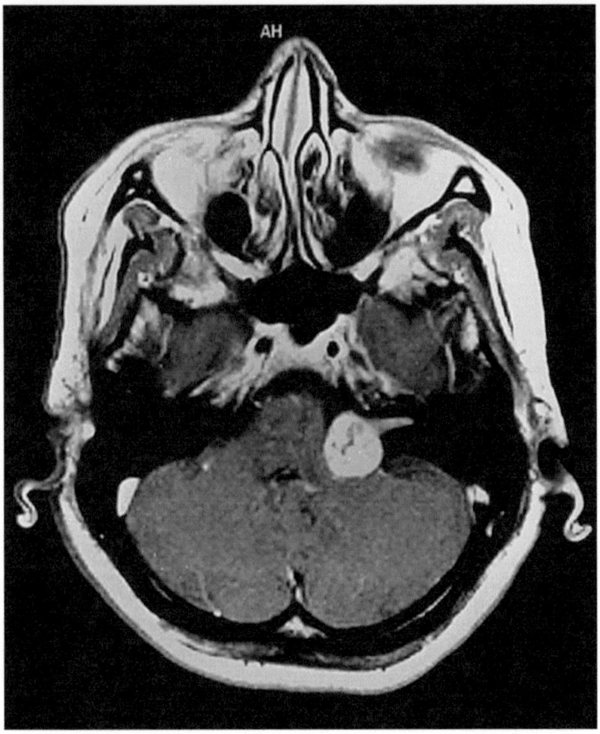

Fig. 28.2 Acoustic neuroma, seen in an axial, T1-weighted MR image at the level of the internal acoustic meatus, obtained after intravenous administration of contrast material. (Picture credit: Baehr [60])

Microvascular compression of the vestibulocochlear nerve is also known to cause disabling vertigo usually at the cerebellopontine angle. Comorbid symptoms include tinnitus, hearing loss, and imbalance. Successful treatment may be accomplished through microvascular decompression [27]. Compressional symptoms have been attributed largely to the wide variability in the anatomy of the neurovascular complex of the cerebellopontine angle [27]. Attempts to link the symptomatic presentation to the anatomical location of the vestibulocochlear nerve compression site have yet to produce conclusive data [27, 28] (Fig. 28.2).

Vestibular Migraine

There is a definite association between vertigo and migraine; however, the pathophysiologic mechanism remains largely unclear [29]. Using the Classification and Diagnostic criteria [30] for the diagnosis of migraine, vertigo was redefined as being a form of migraine aura, and the duration of aura was extended [30]. A diagnosis of migraine with aura is often made when vertigo occurs within 60 min before or after the onset of headache [29].

Recent collaboration between the Bárány Society and the International Headache Society has led to establishing the newest diagnostic criteria for VM with subsequent creation of the classification systems of VM [31, 32].

Savundra et al. [29] retrospectively analyzed 363 patients who presented to a neurotology clinic with vertigo and found 116 patients (32%) possessed migraines. Eighty-five percent of these had no other explanation for their vertigo in contrast to only 51% of nonmigraineurs with idiopathic vertigo, suggesting that in a large proportion of patients with vertigo, VM is underdiagnosed. This underdiagnosis may be due to several factors, including the wide variability in presentation of patients with VM, lack of a widely accepted pathophysiologic model linking migraine and vertigo, and significant overlap with depression or anxiety [29, 31].

The study also noted significantly higher prevalence of a central vestibular disturbance and of a combined central and peripheral vestibular disturbance in migraineurs with vertigo [29]. Migraineurs with vertigo may also experience transient vestibular dysfunction occurring at any site between the end organ and the cerebral cortex [29]. Likely causes include ischemia of the labyrinth, vestibular nerve, vestibular nuclei, reticular activating system, or cerebellar modulating pathways [29, 33]. Other possibilities include ischemia at the cortical level at the temporoparietal junction, anterior cingulate gyrus, and primary sensory cortex [29, 33].

Demyelinating Disorder

Demyelinating disorders like multiple sclerosis (MS), although uncommon, have been estimated to be the cause of central vertigo in 10–15% of cases [16, 34]. These are largely attributed to demyelinating plaques within and around the 8th nerve fascicle or vestibular nuclei [35, 36]. MS patients have been reported to develop vertigo either as an initial symptom or during the course of the disease, with several reporting chronicity [37].

Acute symptoms of vertigo in MS may be classified into two groups: acute vestibular syndrome and positional vertigo [38]. It is widely accepted that the major cause of AVS in MS is due to damage to the vestibular nucleus or fascicular portion of the 8th CN by a lesion in the lower pons or upper medulla [39].

In a study [38] of patients presenting with AVS, 4% of the study population were identified with demyelinating disease as the cause of vertigo, with AVS occurring in demyelinating attacks in all the subjects. The most prominent clinical features were ocular motility limitation and vertical nystagmus. This, along with a normal h-HIT, suggested the presence of central localization in the subjects. MRI revealed lesions throughout the brainstem and in each cerebellar peduncle, with more than half showing gadolinium enhancement. All the lesions were noted to occur in anatomic structures involved in vestibular signaling (Fig. 28.3).

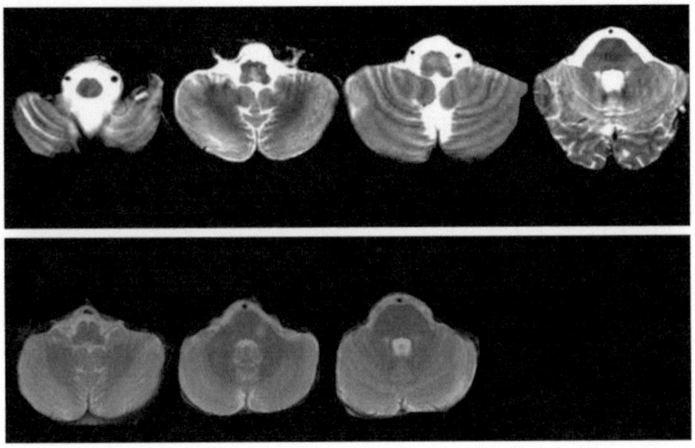

Fig. 28.3 Representative axial T2-weighted brain MRIs in subjects with MS presenting with acute vestibular syndrome. Axial MRI images include cuts caudal and cranial to the purported responsible lesion in order to present the extent of visible demyelination [38]. (Picture credit: Springer link)

Metronidazole-Induced Central Vertigo

Metronidazole is relatively safe when used at appropriate doses, but prolonged use may result in peripheral neuropathies and cerebellar dysfunction. Patients with the condition often present with dizziness, vertigo, and headache [40]. MRI shows the unique characteristic of increased T2/FLAIR signal in the dentate and red nucleus [41–43]. This finding is only alternatively seen in Wernicke's encephalopathy. Although the pathophysiology of metronidazole neurotoxicity remains unclear, most lesions secondary to metronidazole neurotoxicity are completely reversible.

Prior studies done in rats have shown axonal degeneration after treatment with Metronidazole, with symmetric lesions in the cerebellar and cochlear nuclei [44, 45]. It was postulated that Metronidazole, and its metabolites bind to neuronal RNA and inhibit protein synthesis, resulting in reversible axonal swelling [45]. Metronidazole also crosses the blood-brain barrier and can result in imaging and histological findings similar to Wernicke's encephalopathy [44] (Fig. 28.4).

Central Vestibulopathy After Heat Exposure

Heat exposure is a potentially fatal condition with the CNS being reported to be particularly susceptible to heat injury [46]. Jung et al. reported a case study of patients post exposure to extreme heat, in which subjects were noted to develop vertigo and imbalance about a week after heat exposure, with positive HITs bilaterally alongside signs of cerebellar dysfunction [46]. All patients showed abnormal downward corrective saccades during horizontal head impulses along with rare head-shaking nystagmus [46].

A post-mortem study found a loss of cerebellar Purkinje cells in certain patients with heat stroke [47, 48]. Additionally, an increased expression of heat shock protein 72 (HSP 72) was present near residual Purkinje cells, indicating a selective vulnerability [47, 48]. CT and MRIs have shown atrophy in the cerebellar

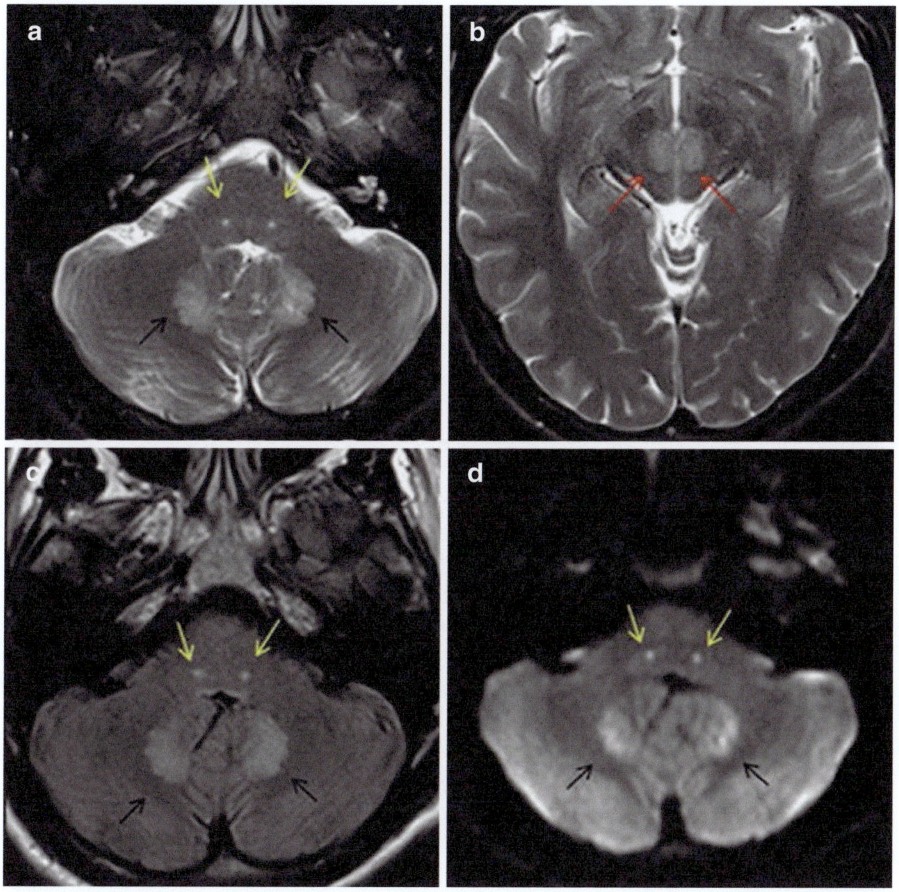

Fig. 28.4 Multiple axial magnetic resonance imaging of the brain in a 22-year-old male on metronidazole presenting with cerebellar symptoms. Axial T2 images (**a**, **b**) reveal symmetric areas of increased signal in the dentate (black arrows), the facial (yellow arrows), and the red nuclei (red arrows), bilaterally. Axial fluid attenuated inversion recovery images (**c**) showing similar changes with restricted diffusion noted on the diffusion-weighted image (**d**) [44]

hemisphere and vermis in patients with heat stroke [49]. Nystagmus is thought to be attributed to damage to the vestibulocerebellum [49].

Wernicke's Encephalopathy

While oculomotor findings and memory dysfunction are the well-known correlates of thiamine deficiency, dizziness has also been described. Differential susceptibility of the vestibular systems to thiamine deficiency can be demonstrated using the head impulse test. [50]

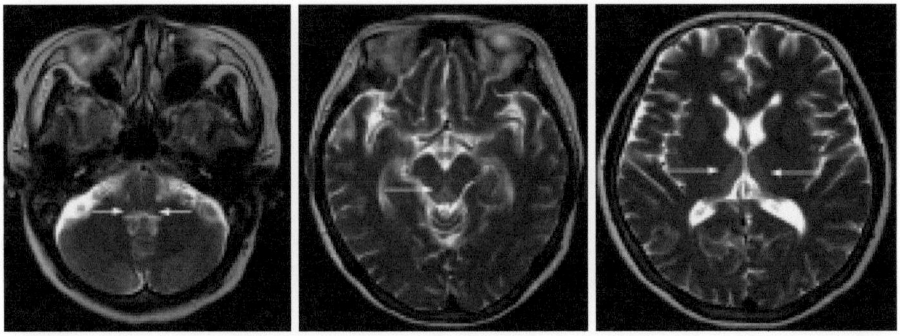

Fig. 28.5 T2-weighted MRIs of a patient with Wernicke's showing symmetrical hyperintense lesions are shown at dorsal portions of both the medulla, periaqueductal gray matter, and medial portions of both thalami [51] . (Picture credit: Journal of Neurology, Neurosurgery & Psychiatry)

Kwang et al. [50] studied two patients with thiamine deficiency: one with anoxia and the other with excessive alcohol consumption. They both presented with vertigo, ataxia, and psychomotor slowing, among other symptoms. Vestibular function, assessed using the bithermal caloric testing, in the anorexic patient showed minimal responses in both ears initially, which markedly improved 6 months after thiamine replacement [50].

Neuropathological examinations of patients with WE have revealed lesions in the VN, especially in the medial VN (MVN), nucleus prepositus hypoglossi, nodulus, and uvula [50], with MVN being most vulnerable to thiamine deprivation [51]. Previous studies have attributed vestibular paresis in WE to be due to lesions in the vestibular nucleus [52] (Fig. 28.5).

Epileptiform Activity

Vestibular symptoms may be associated with seizures, with those resulting directly from focal, intermittent epileptic discharges collectively known as epileptic vertigo [53]. They may present as an aura symptom preceding a seizure, be the result of a side effect of anti-epileptic medications, or may constitute the seizure itself [53, 54]. Vertigo and dizziness are also known to manifest in non-convulsive status epilepticus (NCSE) [53], a picture consistent with transient neurological attack (TNA) [55].

Penfield et al. reported that electrical stimulation of the posterior half of the superior temporal gyrus and the parieto-temporal junction produced vertiginous experiences similar to those of spontaneous seizures [54, 56].

In a recent study by Kim et al. [57] in which the importance of vertigo was assessed in epileptic patients using video-EEG monitoring, it was reported that cortical stimulation studies of patients with epilepsy identified both the temporal and parietal lobes as vestibular cortical areas [58]; however, epileptic discharges in patients with epileptic vertigo were observed in more expansive areas, including the frontal and temporo-parieto-occipital junctional areas, suggesting either processing of vestibular-related input across large cortical regions or spread of excitation to or from nearby areas [59]. This study also revealed that vertigo or dizziness was the most frequently encountered first aura [57]. Patients with epileptic vertigo respond well to anti-epileptics, as depicted by Tarnutzer et al. [53] in which response rates to anti-epileptic treatment were as high as 90%.

References

1. Arch AE, et al. Missed ischemic stroke diagnosis in the emergency department by emergency medicine and neurology services. Stroke. 2016;47(3):668–73.
2. Lever NM, et al. Missed opportunities for recognition of ischemic stroke in the emergency department. J Emerg Nurs. 2013;39(5):434–9.
3. Savitz SI, Caplan LR. Vertebrobasilar disease. N Engl J Med. 2005;352(25):2618–26.
4. Lee CC, et al. Risk of stroke in patients hospitalized for isolated vertigo: a four-year follow-up study. Stroke. 2011;42(1):48–52.
5. Kim AS, Fullerton HJ, Johnston SC. Risk of vascular events in emergency department patients discharged home with diagnosis of dizziness or vertigo. Ann Emerg Med. 2011;57(1):34–41.
6. Amarenco P, et al. Anterior inferior cerebellar artery territory infarcts. Mechanisms and clinical features. Arch Neurol. 1993;50(2):154–61.
7. Lee H, et al. Infarction in the territory of anterior inferior cerebellar artery: spectrum of audiovestibular loss. Stroke. 2009;40(12):3745–51.
8. Grad A, Baloh RW. Vertigo of vascular origin. Clinical and electronystagmographic features in 84 cases. Arch Neurol. 1989;46(3):281–4.
9. Kim JS, Lee H. Vertigo due to posterior circulation stroke. Semin Neurol. 2013;33(3):179–84.
10. Navi BB, et al. Application of the ABCD2 score to identify cerebrovascular causes of dizziness in the emergency department. Stroke. 2012;43(6):1484–9.
11. Oas JG, Baloh RW. Vertigo and the anterior inferior cerebellar artery syndrome. Neurology. 1992;42(12):2274–9.
12. Lee H, Yi HA, Baloh RW. Sudden bilateral simultaneous deafness with vertigo as a sole manifestation of vertebrobasilar insufficiency. J Neurol Neurosurg Psychiatry. 2003;74(4):539–41.
13. Kim JS. Vertigo and gait ataxia without usual signs of lateral medullary infarction: a clinical variant related to rostral-dorsolateral lesions. Cerebrovasc Dis. 2000;10(6):471–4.
14. Lee H, et al. Cerebellar infarction presenting isolated vertigo: frequency and vascular topographical patterns. Neurology. 2006;67(7):1178–83.
15. Kattah JC, et al. HINTS to diagnose stroke in the acute vestibular syndrome: three-step bedside oculomotor examination more sensitive than early MRI diffusion-weighted imaging. Stroke. 2009;40(11):3504–10.
16. Tarnutzer AA, et al. Does my dizzy patient have a stroke? A systematic review of bedside diagnosis in acute vestibular syndrome. CMAJ. 2011;183(9):E571–92.
17. Kim HA, Lee H. Isolated vestibular nucleus infarction mimicking acute peripheral vestibulopathy. Stroke. 2010;41(7):1558–60.
18. Chang TP, Wu YC. A tiny infarct on the dorsolateral pons mimicking vestibular neuritis. Laryngoscope. 2010;120(11):2336–8.
19. Chen L, et al. Diagnostic accuracy of acute vestibular syndrome at the bedside in a stroke unit. J Neurol. 2011;258(5):855–61.
20. Saber Tehrani AS, et al. Small strokes causing severe vertigo: frequency of false-negative MRIs and nonlacunar mechanisms. Neurology. 2014;83(2):169–73.

21. Edlow JA, Newman-Toker D. Using the physical examination to diagnose patients with acute dizziness and vertigo. J Emerg Med. 2016;50(4):617–28.
22. Nouh A, Remke J, Ruland S. Ischemic posterior circulation stroke: a review of anatomy, clinical presentations, diagnosis, and current management. Front Neurol. 2014;5:30.
23. Teggi R, et al. Vestibular assessment in patients with vestibular schwannomas: what really matters? Acta Otorhinolaryngol Ital. 2014;34(2):123–8.
24. Barbara M, et al. Double localization of a unilateral sporadic vestibular schwannoma. Acta Otorhinolaryngol Ital. 2008;28(1):34–7.
25. Franco-Vidal V, Negrevergne M, Darrouzet V. Vertigo and pathology of the cerebello-pontine angle. Rev Laryngol Otol Rhinol (Bord). 2005;126(4):223–6.
26. Kentala E, Pyykko I. Clinical picture of vestibular schwannoma. Auris Nasus Larynx. 2001;28(1):15–22.
27. Wuertenberger CJ, Rosahl SK. Vertigo and tinnitus caused by vascular compression of the vestibulocochlear nerve, not intracanalicular vestibular schwannoma: review and case presentation. Skull Base. 2009;19(6):417–24.
28. Ryu H, et al. Neurovascular compression syndrome of the eighth cranial nerve. Can the site of compression explain the symptoms? Acta Neurochir. 1999;141(5):495–501.
29. Savundra PA, et al. Migraine-associated vertigo. Cephalalgia. 1997;17(4):505–10; discussion 487.
30. Classification and diagnostic criteria for headache disorders, cranial neuralgias and facial pain. Headache Classification Committee of the International Headache Society. Cephalalgia. 1988;8 Suppl 7:1–96.
31. Headache Classification Committee of the International Headache, S. The international classification of headache disorders, 3rd edition (beta version). Cephalalgia. 2013;33(9):629–808.
32. O'Connell Ferster AP, Priesol AJ, Isildak H. The clinical manifestations of vestibular migraine: a review. Auris Nasus Larynx. 2017;44(3):249–52.
33. Bottini G, et al. Identification of the central vestibular projections in man: a positron emission tomography activation study. Exp Brain Res. 1994;99(1):164–9.
34. Zaffaroni M, Baldini SM, Ghezzi A. Cranial nerve, brainstem and cerebellar syndromes in the differential diagnosis of multiple sclerosis. Neurol Sci. 2001;22(Suppl 2):S74–8.
35. Commins DJ, Chen JM. Multiple sclerosis: a consideration in acute cranial nerve palsies. Am J Otol. 1997;18(5):590–5.
36. Frohman EM, et al. Vertigo in MS: utility of positional and particle repositioning maneuvers. Neurology. 2000;55(10):1566–9.
37. Rae-Grant AD, et al. Sensory symptoms of multiple sclerosis: a hidden reservoir of morbidity. Mult Scler. 1999;5(3):179–83.
38. Pula JH, Newman-Toker DE, Kattah JC. Multiple sclerosis as a cause of the acute vestibular syndrome. J Neurol. 2013;260(6):1649–54.
39. Schumacher GA. Demyelinating diseases as a cause for vertigo. Arch Otolaryngol. 1967;85(5):537–8.
40. Patel K, et al. Cerebellar ataxia following prolonged use of metronidazole: case report and literature review. Int J Infect Dis. 2008;12(6):e111–4.
41. Woodruff BK, Wijdicks EF, Marshall WF. Reversible metronidazole-induced lesions of the cerebellar dentate nuclei. N Engl J Med. 2002;346(1):68–9.
42. Bottenberg MM, et al. Metronidazole-induced encephalopathy: a case report and review of the literature. J Clin Pharmacol. 2011;51(1):112–6.
43. Ralph ED. Clinical pharmacokinetics of metronidazole. Clin Pharmacokinet. 1983;8(1):43–62.
44. Agarwal A, et al. Metronidazole-induced cerebellar toxicity. Neurol Int. 2016;8(1):6365.
45. Bradley WG, Karlsson IJ, Rassol CG. Metronidazole neuropathy. Br Med J. 1977;2(6087):610–1.
46. Jung I, et al. Delayed vestibulopathy after heat exposure. J Neurol. 2017;264(1):49–53.
47. Bouchama A, Knochel JP. Heat stroke. N Engl J Med. 2002;346(25):1978–88.
48. Bazille C, et al. Brain damage after heat stroke. J Neuropathol Exp Neurol. 2005;64(11):970–5.

49. Albukrek D, et al. Heat-stroke-induced cerebellar atrophy: clinical course, CT and MRI findings. Neuroradiology. 1997;39(3):195–7.
50. Choi KD, et al. The vestibulo-ocular reflexes during head impulse in Wernicke's encephalopathy. J Neurol Neurosurg Psychiatry. 2007;78(10):1161–2.
51. Witt ED, Goldman-Rakic PS. Intermittent thiamine deficiency in the rhesus monkey. I. Progression of neurological signs and neuroanatomical lesions. Ann Neurol. 1983;13(4):376–95.
52. Furman JM, Becker JT. Vestibular responses in Wernicke's encephalopathy. Ann Neurol. 1989;26(5):669–74.
53. Tarnutzer AA, et al. Clinical and electrographic findings in epileptic vertigo and dizziness: a systematic review. Neurology. 2015;84(15):1595–604.
54. Alpers BJ. Vertiginous epilepsy. Laryngoscope. 1960;70:631–7.
55. Nagayama M, et al. Novel clinical features of nonconvulsive status epilepticus. F1000Res. 2017;6:1690.
56. Penfield W, Kristiansen K. Seizure onset and the localization of epileptic discharge. Trans Am Neurol Assoc. 1948;73(73 Annual Meet):73–80.
57. Kim DW, Sunwoo JS, Lee SK. Incidence and localizing value of vertigo and dizziness in patients with epilepsy: video-EEG monitoring study. Epilepsy Res. 2016;126:102–5.
58. Guldin WO, Grusser OJ. Is there a vestibular cortex? Trends Neurosci. 1998;21(6):254–9.
59. Hewett R, et al. Benign temporo-parieto-occipital junction epilepsy with vestibular disturbance: an underrecognized form of epilepsy? Epilepsy Behav. 2011;21(4):412–6.
60. Baehr M. Duus' topical diagnosis in neurology. 4th ed. New York/Stuttgart: Thieme Medical Publishers; 2005.

Index

J. C. Lucas et al. (eds.), *Diagnosis and Treatment of Vestibular Disorders*,
https://doi.org/10.1007/978-3-032-11740-3

MIX
Papier aus verantwortungsvollen Quellen
Paper from responsible sources
FSC® C105338

If you have any concerns about our products,
you can contact us on
ProductSafety@springernature.com

In case Publisher is established outside the EU,
the EU authorized representative is:
Springer Nature Customer Service Center GmbH
Europaplatz 3, 69115 Heidelberg, Germany

Printed by Libri Plureos GmbH
in Hamburg, Germany